Pruritus in Clinical Medicine

Pruritus in Clinical Medicine

Editor: Elise Walters

AMERICAN
MEDICAL PUBLISHERS
www.americanmedicalpublishers.com

AMERICAN
MEDICAL PUBLISHERS
www.americanmedicalpublishers.com

Cataloging-in-Publication Data

Pruritus in clinical medicine / edited by Elise Walters.
p. cm.
Includes bibliographical references and index.
ISBN 979-8-88740-402-8
1. Itching. 2. Skin--Diseases. 3. Dermatology. 4. Clinical medicine. I. Walters, Elise.
RL721 .P78 2023
616.5--dc23

American Medical Publishers,
41 Flatbush Avenue,
1st Floor, New York,
NY 11217, USA

ISBN 979-8-88740-402-8 (Hardback)

Contents

Preface

In my initial years as a student, I used to run to the library at every possible instance to grab a book and learn something new. Books were my primary source of knowledge and I would not have come such a long way without all that I learnt from them. Thus, when I was approached to edit this book; I became understandably nostalgic. It was an absolute honor to be considered worthy of guiding the current generation as well as those to come. I put all my knowledge and hard work into making this book most beneficial for its readers.

Pruritus (itch) is a sensation that leads to the desire or reflex to scratch. If the sensation lasts for six weeks or beyond, then it is referred to as chronic pruritus. The signs and symptoms of chronic pruritus include contagious itch and itch inhibition due to pain. There are various causes leading to this condition that include factors such as infections, allergy and environment, and skin disorders. Infections like body louse, cutaneous larva migrans, head lice, herpes, insect bites, tungiasis, etc. and skin disorders such as dandruff, xerosis, and punctate palmoplantar keratoderma are some factors that lead to chronic pruritus. It can develop in the peripheral nervous system (dermal or neuropathic) or in the central nervous system (neuropathic, neurogenic, or psychogenic). Treatment methods include anti-itch drugs and some plant products that act as effective anti-pruritic. Certain non-chemical remedies such as cooling, warming, and soft stimulation are also used. If severe itching is caused due to kidney failure, then phototherapy can also be used as a treatment. This book strives to provide a fair idea about pruritus and will help develop a better understanding of the latest advances in its diagnosis and management. It includes contributions of experts and researchers, which will provide innovative insights to all involved in the study and management of this disease.

I wish to thank my publisher for supporting me at every step. I would also like to thank all the authors who have contributed their researches in this book. I hope this book will be a valuable contribution to the progress of the field.

Editor

1

Attentional Bias Modification Training for Itch: A Proof-of-Principle Study in Healthy Individuals

Antoinette I. M. van Laarhoven[1,2*], *Jennifer M. Becker*[1,2], *Dimitri M. L. van Ryckeghem*[3,4,5], *Stefaan Van Damme*[3], *Geert Crombez*[3,6] *and Reinout W. H. J. Wiers*[7]

[1] Health, Medical, and Neuropsychology Unit, Faculty of Social and Behavioural Sciences, Leiden University, Leiden, Netherlands, [2] Leiden Institute for Brain and Cognition, Leiden University, Leiden, Netherlands, [3] Department of Experimental-Clinical and Health Psychology, Ghent University, Ghent, Belgium, [4] Research Unit Integrative Research Unit on Social and Individual Development (INSIDE), Institute of Health and Behaviour, Faculty of Humanities and Social Sciences, University of Luxembourg, Esch-sur-Alzette, Luxembourg, [5] Section Experimental Health Psychology, Clinical Psychological Science Departments, Faculty of Psychology and Neuroscience, Maastricht University, Maastricht, Netherlands, [6] Centre for Pain Research, University of Bath, Bath, United Kingdom, [7] Addiction Development and Psychopathology Laboratory, Department of Psychology, University of Amsterdam, Amsterdam, Netherlands

***Correspondence:**
Antoinette I. M. van Laarhoven
a.vanlaarhoven@fsw.leidenuniv.nl

Itch draws our attention to allow imposing action against bodily harm (e.g., remove insects). At the same time, itch is found to interfere with ongoing tasks and daily life goals. Despite the key role of attention in itch processing, interventions that train individuals to automatically disengage attention from itch cues are lacking. The present proof-of-principle attention bias modification (ABM) training study was aimed at investigating whether attention to itch as well as sensitivity to mild itch can be changed. Healthy volunteers were randomized over three ABM-training conditions. Training was done via a modified pictorial dot-probe task. In particular, participants were trained to look away from itch stimuli (n = 38), toward itch stimuli (n = 40) or not trained toward or away from itch at all (sham training, n = 38). The effects of the ABM-training were tested primarily on attention to itch pictures. Secondarily, it was investigated whether training effects generalized to alterations in attention to itch words and mechanical itch sensitivity. The ABM-training did not alter attention toward the itch pictures, and there was no moderation by baseline levels of attention bias for itch. Also, attention bias to the itch words and itch sensitivity were not affected by the ABM-training. This study was a first step toward trainings to change attention toward itch. Further research is warranted to optimize ABM-training methodology, for example increasing motivation of participants. Eventually, an optimized training could be used in patient populations who suffer most from distraction by their symptoms of itch.

Clinical Trial Registration: Identifier: NL6134 (NTR6273). The website URL is: https://www.trialregister.nl/

Keywords: itch, attention, attention bias, attention bias modification (ABM), attention training, pruritus, psychodermatology, dot-probe paradigm

INTRODUCTION

Itch, and particularly chronic itch interferes with one's behavior and psychosocial functioning (1–3). In turn, reduced psychosocial well-being can intensify itch, resulting in a vicious cycle (4, 5). Unique for itch compared to pain is that it can be further amplified or even induced audiovisually (e.g., by hearing scratch sounds or looking at pictures of scratching people); i.e., itch is contagious and this is amplified in itch patients (6). A key mechanism of contagious itch is attention (7, 8). Focusing attention on potential threat is essential to sort its nocifensive function and protect skin integrity (9, 10). Since attention may play a central role in the vicious circle of itch amplification (11) and psychological burden (12–16), interventions targeting attention to itch seem promising.

Research indicates that patients with chronic itch may have increased attention (AB; attention bias) toward words related to itch compared to neutral words (17), and compared with healthy controls (18). Similarly, healthy individuals display an AB toward itch words and pictures (12, 14), although evidence is equivocal (16). Some techniques have been investigated to reduce itch temporarily (19, 20), but no strategies exist that reduce AB to itch; hence attention strategies effectuating longer-term itch relief are lacking. Attention bias modification (ABM) training for itch may offer a solution, as such a training has been shown effective in other fields (21).

In the domain of pain, closely related to itch (9, 22), ABM-trainings have been developed to alter AB for pain. Such ABM-trainings aim to train individuals to automatically focus attention at neutral stimuli while concurrently displaying pain-stimuli (pain-related words and/or painful faces). Initial studies in patients with chronic pain indicated that single- as well as multi-session ABM-trainings could reduce pain sensitivity (23–25). In healthy individuals, ABM-trainings affected pain thresholds, pain tolerance, or experienced pain (26–29), and some studies demonstrated altered AB for pain (26, 27). In addition, a study has shown that effects of an ABM-training with words generalized to effects on AB for painful faces after the training (27). Furthermore, individual characteristics, like catastrophizing or the ability to inhibit attention to irrelevant information (as feature of executive control), may play a role in (the retraining of) AB for pain (30–32). All in all, evidence on ABM-training effectiveness in pain as well as the role of individual characteristics is equivocal (28, 29, 33–35). Overall, based on theory and promising evidence in pain, it seems worthwhile to investigate whether an ABM-training for itch would be effective to reduce itch sensitivity and/or AB toward itch. However, to our knowledge, an ABM-training for itch has not yet been developed. As a first step of intervention-development, it should be verified whether AB toward itch can be trained—in either direction (i.e., in a proof-of-principle study) (36).

In this proof-of-principle study, we aimed to investigate whether AB to itch pictures can be altered by an ABM-training away from and toward pictorial itch stimuli. Furthermore, we investigated whether these effects would generalize to altered AB to itch words and actual itch sensitivity. It was hypothesized that, when compared to sham training, an ABM-training away from itch pictures would result in AB away from itch pictures and words as well as a lowered itch sensitivity, whereas an ABM-training toward itch would effectuate the opposite. Additionally, the possible role of individual characteristics, including general attentional inhibition, neuroticism, and itch catastrophizing, in the ABM-training effects was explored. Moreover, given some recent evidence (37), we explored *post-hoc* whether the training effects were moderated by the baseline AB for itch.

MATERIALS AND METHODS

Design

This study comprises a 2 (pre-training, post-training) × 3 (ABM-training away from itch, ABM-training toward itch, sham training: equal allocation ratio) mixed research design with AB to itch pictures, AB to itch words and sensitivity to mechanically induced itch as dependent variables. This study was pre-registered in the Netherlands Trial Registry under number: NL6134 (/NTR6273). The protocol was approved by the Psychology Research Ethics Committee of Leiden University (CEP17-0228/116).

Participants

Participants were recruited through advertisements on social media, at Leiden University, and via the Leiden University Research Participation system SONA systems Ltd. (Tallinn, Estonia). Recruitment and testing took place between March and May 2017. Inclusion criteria for participation were being aged between 18 and 30 years and being proficient in the Dutch language. Exclusion criteria were current itch or pain $\geq$3 on a numeric rating scale (NRS) from 0 (no itch/pain) to 10 (worst imaginable itch/pain), diagnosis of a chronic itch or pain condition (e.g., eczema or rheumatoid arthritis), psychiatric diagnosis (e.g., major depression or ADHD), color blindness, dyslexia, and impairment in visual acuity that is not corrected with glasses or contact lenses. All participants provided written informed consent for their participation in the study.

Procedure

Potential participants were informed about the study via written information and, when interested in participation, they were asked to fill out (online) self-report questionnaires, which also included questions regarding the in- and exclusion criteria (see section Self-Report Questionnaires). When found eligible for participation, participants were instructed to refrain from intake of alcohol and drugs 24 h before the test session and of caffeinated drinks within 1 h before the session started. Adherence to this guideline was checked in the lab (n = 1 missing), resulting in 15 participants who had taken alcohol the preceding 24 h (11 of them drank $\leq$2 units), 5 participants who had taken caffeinated drinks in the preceding hour (all $\leq$2 units), and none had used drugs. During each session, two experimenters were present, one conducting the practical tasks (e.g., starting computer tasks and itch stimulus application) and the other one guiding participants through the procedures, mainly by providing instructions. Upon arrival at the Leiden University

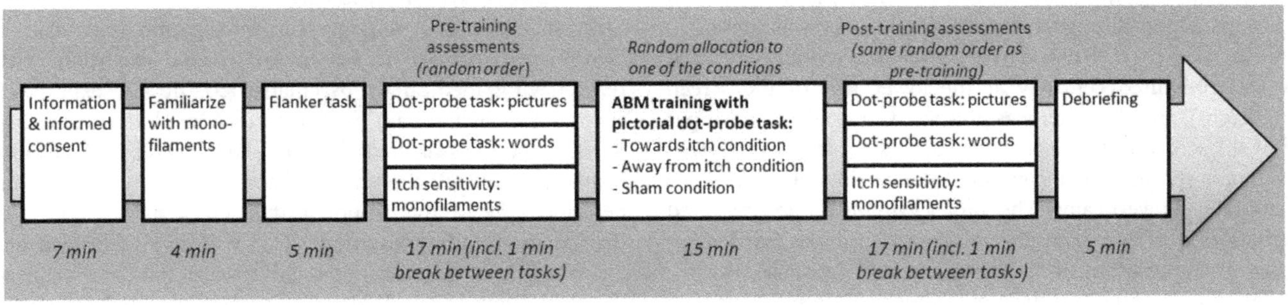

FIGURE 1 | Timeline of the experimental session (total ca. 1 h:10 min).

lab (see **Figure 1** for a timeline), participants were verbally informed about the study procedures and told that they were free to terminate the experiment at any time. Next, participants signed the informed consent and rated their current levels of spontaneous itch and pain on the NRSs. Participants were familiarized with the mechanical itch induction by applying Touch test evaluators as described in the section Mechanical Itch Sensitivity (ca. 4 min). Thereafter, the Flanker task (ca. 5 min) was conducted measuring general response inhibition (Flanker task). Consecutively, participants performed the pre-training AB assessments using the dot-probe task with pictures (ca. 5 min), the dot-probe task with words (Dot-Probe Tasks; ca. 5 min), and the mechanical itch induction (ca. 2 min). These tasks were provided in random order, i.e., an independent person had put the randomization information in opaque envelopes stratified by participant's sex and handedness. After these pre-training assessments, participants were randomized to one of the three ABM-training (ca. 15 min) conditions (participants were blind for receiving any intervention). Post-training assessments were carried out in the same order as the pre-training assessments of that specific participant. Upon completion of the tasks, participants were debriefed about the purposes of the study and reimbursed for their participation.

Measures

All computer tasks were run on a desktop computer with Microsoft Windows 7 attached to a Philips Brilliance 220B TFT screen (Resolution 1,280px × 1,024px, 60 Hz). Both the Dot-probe task and the Flanker task were programmed and run in E-prime 2.0 (Psychology Software Tools Inc., Sharpsburg, PA, USA). Randomization to one of the ABM-training conditions was also done in E-prime based on participant number (this was unknown to the experimenters), with separate lists for males and females. E-prime automatically started the correct condition the participant was randomized to, so the participant was blinded. Responses were given using finger response buttons, one for each hand [Pushbutton Switch, SPDT, Off-(On)] connected to a serial response box model 200A (Psychology Software Tools Inc. Sharpsburg, PA, USA). During the tasks, participants kept their head in a chin rest to keep the distance to the screen at 54 cm.

Dot-Probe Tasks

A dot-probe paradigm was used to measure AB toward itch pictures and words. The dot-probe paradigm assumes that being attentive to a stimulus speeds up responding to targets at the focused location (congruent trials) when compared to the opposite location (incongruent trials). There were in total 60 stimulus pairs of an itch-related and a neutral stimulus (40 picture-pairs and 20 word-pairs with Dutch words). Itch stimuli depicted a hand scratching him-/herself on e.g., the head, limb and back. Neutral stimuli depicted objects, e.g., light bulb, doorbell, and spoon. The itch stimuli had been validated earlier [see (38)] on the basis of their applicability to itch (average itch scores per task ranged from 2.7 to 2.8 for the dot-probe tasks assessing AB and the ABM-training task rated on a Likert scale from 1 (not applicable to itch) to 5 (very applicable to itch), non-applicability to pain (average pain scores ranged from 1.0 to 1.4 on a 1 to 5 Likert scale for pain) and slightly negative valence [ranging from −1.2 to −1.1 on a Likert scale ranging from −5 (very negative) to 5 (very positive)], whereas the neutral stimuli were characterized as neither itchy nor painful (average itch and pain scores were 1.1 at maximum), and were of neutral valence (average score ranging from 0.1 to 0.2) (38). Based on the validation scores, the picture-pairs were randomized in advance over three pictorial dot-probe tasks, i.e., two regular dot-probe tasks (10 stimulus-pairs each) and one training dot-probe task (20 stimulus-pairs). The word-pairs were randomized in advance, across two regular dot-probe tasks. Randomization of the stimulus-pairs occurred on basis of the previously acquired validation ratings on itch in order to make sure that the itch ratings would overall be comparable across the dot-probe tasks used. For each participant, the order of the two dot-probe tasks was randomized (i.e., one was administered pre-training and the other post-training). The regular dot-probe tasks contained 40 trials each (14). Half of the trials were congruent (itch stimulus and target at same location) and half of the trials were incongruent (itch stimulus and target at opposite location). The proportion of itch stimuli displayed in the upper and lower half of the screen was equal over all trials. Right before the experimental trials in the pre-training dot-probe tasks only, there were 16 practice trials with neutral-neutral stimulus pairs. Feedback on the accuracy of responses to the targets was included. A trial was constructed as follows:

First, a fixation point was shown in the middle of the screen for 500 ms. Upon disappearance, a stimulus pair was presented on the screen for 500 ms (27, 29, 34). One stimulus of each pair was presented centrally at the lower half of the screen (20% height), and the other was presented centrally at the upper half of the screen (80% height). The stimulus-pair was followed by a target stimulus that consisted of two dots aligned either horizontally or vertically. The target stimulus was presented at either one of the stimulus locations until the participant pressed a response button, with a maximum response window of 1,500 ms. Correct response-mapping was counterbalanced across participants, i.e., right button for horizontally oriented target stimuli and left button for vertically oriented target stimuli or vice versa (e.g., a participant responded with the right button to horizontally oriented targets in all dot-probe tasks). Reaction times and accuracy in responding to the targets were measured.

The ABM-training exclusively contained pictorial stimuli. The training task was comparable to the regular dot-probe tasks, but contained 320 trials (24) and the locations of the targets as opposed to the itch pictures was manipulated in the ABM-training conditions that were trained towards and away from itch. Specifically, in the training condition towards itch, 100% of the trials were congruent (i.e., at the itch picture location), whereas in the ABM-training away from itch condition, 100% of the trials were incongruent (i.e., at the neutral picture location). In the sham training condition, 50% of the targets were displayed congruently and 50% were shown incongruently to the itch picture location, akin the regular dot-probe tasks. One minute breaks were built-in after every 40 trials.

Mechanical Itch Sensitivity

Sensitivity to touch evoked itch (STI) was assessed, using three von Frey monofilaments (4.08 mN, 4.17 mN, and 4.31 mN; Stoelting, North Coast Medical, Gilroy, CA) as described in previous research (39). The monofilaments were applied to the non-dominant inner forearm. Each filament was applied for 1 s in triplicate after which the participants rated the evoked itch per filament on the NRS for itch.

Flanker Task

This task (40, 41) was used to measure general attentional inhibition. In each trial, 5 numbers were shown. The middle number was the target stimulus, which was flanked by non-target stimuli. The flankers could be congruent to the target stimulus, e.g., 44444 or incongruent, e.g., 44244. Half of the trials were congruent and half were incongruent and the use of 2's and 4's was balanced across the task. The task contained 120 experimental trials and 8 practice trials without feedback at the beginning of the task. The left response button was used to indicate "2" as target and the right button was used to indicate "4." A short break was included half-way the task if desired. The average reaction time to the congruent vs. the incongruent target stimuli is the outcome measure.

Self-Report Questionnaires

Questions assessing demographic information (e.g., age) and information required to screen for in- and exclusion criteria (e.g., having medical or psychiatric conditions, experiencing spontaneous itch or pain) were included. In addition, *attentional focus on bodily sensations* was measured using both the Body Vigilance Scale (BVS with Cronbach alpha 0.70) as previously described (i.e., only including the sub items of question 4 that concern bodily sensations) (11) with two additional items assessing one's attention directed toward itch and pain and the Pain Vigilance and Awareness Questionnaire adjusted for itch (PVAQ-I with Cronbach alpha 0.88). Adjustments for itch were made by substituting the word "pain" by "itch" for all concerning items. This procedure was also applied to the following questionnaires originating from the pain field. *Catastrophizing* about itch was measured using the Pain Catastrophizing Scale adjusted for itch (PCS-I with Cronbach alpha 0.91) (39). *Experience of Cognitive Intrusion of itch* was assessed using the Experience of Cognitive Intrusion of pain scale adjusted for itch and, accidentally, with scales ranging from 1 to 6 for each item instead of 0 to 6 like the original version (ECIP-I with Cronbach alpha 0.96). *Attentional disengagement from itch and pain* was assessed using two Likert scales ranging from 1 (not at all able to disengage attention) to 5 (always able to disengage attention) (12). Finally, *Neuroticism* was measured with the Eysenck Personality Questionnaire revised short scale (EPQ-RSS with Cronbach alpha = 0.72) (42). All self-report questionnaires were administered in Dutch using the online system Qualtrics (Provo, Utah, USA).

Statistical Analyses

All statistical analyses were conducted using SPSS 25.0 software (IBM SPSS Statistics for Windows, Armonk, NY, USA) if not specified otherwise. All values displayed are means ± standard deviation (SD), if not stated otherwise. Effect sizes were reported as partial eta squared (η_p^2). A $p < 0.05$ was considered statistically significant.

For the dot-probe tasks, reaction times (RT) were extracted from E-prime for trials with RT ≥ 150 ms (0.2 and 0.08% of the RT were excluded for the picture and word tasks, respectively) and trials with correct responses (7.2 and 8.5% of the RT were excluded from the picture and word tasks, respectively). Cases for which no responses were recorded due to a programming error (see section Sample) were excluded from the respective analysis. Participants' data that had accuracy levels below 70% were excluded from the respective analyses; in the case that <70% of the trials in the training were incorrect, this participant was not included in any of the analyses. For the pre- and post-training dot-probe tasks, AB-indices were calculated by subtracting the RT of the congruent trials from the RT of the incongruent trials ($RT_{incongruent}$-$RT_{congruent}$). A positive AB-index indicates an AB toward itch, whilst a negative AB-index indicates an AB away from itch. All variables to be included in the statistical analyses were checked for normality.

First, baseline between-group differences in demographics, current spontaneous itch and pain, total scores of the questionnaires, AB toward itch pictures and words, mechanically evoked itch, and general attentional inhibition (i.e., Flanker task) were assessed using Kruskal-Wallis-tests for interval variables (due to a violation of normality for most variables) and a Chi-square-test for the dichotomous variable sex. Second, the presence of ABs toward itch pictures and words at baseline was tested using one sample *t*-tests checking whether the AB-index significantly differed from 0. Additionally, effectiveness of participants' attentional inhibition (entire group) was checked by comparing the RT on the congruent and incongruent trials of the Flanker task as within-subjects factor in a repeated measures analysis of variance (RM-ANOVA).

For the primary aim to assess whether ABM-training resulted in altered attention to itch pictures, a 2 × 2 × 3 RM-ANOVA was conducted with the within-factors *itch congruency* (congruent vs. incongruent trials) and *time* (pre- vs. post-training assessments) and the between-factor *condition* (ABM-training away, ABM-training towards, sham training). Additionally, *post-hoc* moderation analyses were carried out using the Process Macro v3.3 (43) (model 1) in SPSS to investigate whether the effects of the training were different depending on the baseline level of AB toward the main outcome of itch pictures. Here, *condition* was the independent variable (X), the training effect on itch pictures ($\text{AB-index}_{\text{post-training}}\text{-AB-index}_{\text{pre-training}}$) was the dependent variable (Y; centered) and the pre-training AB towards itch pictures was the moderator variable. Another *post-hoc* RM-ANOVA tested the change in AB-index for the itch pictures before vs. after the training in the entire sample.

For the secondary aim to assess the effect of the ABM-training on itch words, a RM-ANOVA akin the one with pictures was conducted with the RT of the word dot-probe tasks. For the mechanical itch sensitivity outcome, pre- and post-training levels of evoked itch, as subjectively rated on NRS, were compared using a RM-ANOVA with the within-factor *time* (mechanically evoked itch pre- vs. post-training) and the between-factor *condition* (ABM-training away, ABM-training towards, sham training). Finally, to test associations between the main study outcomes and the individual characteristics, Spearman correlation coefficients (ρ) were calculated for each condition separately. Specifically, the ABM-training effects on the AB toward itch pictures and AB toward itch words (both AB-index post-training–AB-index pre-training) as well as itch sensitivity (pre–post assessment) were correlated with both the Flanker index ($\text{RT}_{\text{incongruent}}\text{-RT}_{\text{congruent}}$) and the total scores of the self-report questionnaires. The Sidak-Holm correction was applied for all RM-ANOVAs when performing *post-hoc* tests.

Reliability of the dot-probe tasks was assessed with split-half reliabilities. These were calculated with R (R version 4.0.3) (44) with the "splithalfr" package (45). Reliability of the AB index was calculated for all four versions of the dot-probe task (version 1 and version 2 with pictures as well as version 1 and version 2 with words) of all participants that were included in the analyses. The function used a Monte-Carlo splitting technique to estimate 5,000 split-half samples that were used to estimate Spearman-Brown correlations for all 5,000 samples. The resulting mean and median coefficients of all 5,000 samples accompanied by the minimum, maximum, and interquartile range were calculated per task.

RESULTS

Sample

We aimed to include 40 participants per condition as this would be sufficient to detect a small effect (in GPower 3.1.6, effect size f of 0.10; with an alpha of 0.05, power of 0.80 and an estimated correlation between the pre- and post- measurements between 0.75 and 0.80). On top, 5% participants extra were tested in order to be able to overcome potential data loss. Therefore, 126 participants had been included in the study. For the following reasons, data of several participants could not be used in data analyses: Seven participants responded differently to the orientation of the dots during the training task as opposed to the pre- and post-training dot-probe tasks due to incorrectly provided instructions (e.g., they were instructed to respond to horizontal oriented targets with the right button during the pre- and post-training dot-probe tasks and with the left button during training). Due to a programming error, data of the dot-probe picture and word tasks had not been recorded /could not be retrieved for two participants and for similar reasons data of another 12 participants was unavailable for the word tasks (amongst them, there was one participant of whom data of the mechanically evoked itch were missing, too). Moreover, one participant was excluded from the main analysis because of exceeding the pre-determined 30% error rate (specifically 33% errors) for the post-training dot-probe picture task. None of the participants had to be excluded based on their number of errors during the ABM-training; at maximum 18% of the trials were incorrect ($n = 1$). Finally, 116 participants could be included in the main analysis with the pictorial stimuli, 105 in the secondary analyses with the word stimuli, and 116 in the analyses for mechanically evoked itch. The sample of 116 participants was mostly female (74%), right-handed (89%) and most participants were following or had finished tertiary education (85%). Participants' baseline characteristics did not differ across training conditions (**Table 1**). Median levels of spontaneous itch and pain at baseline were 0.0.

Dot-Probe Tasks

Reliability was good for all versions of the task with a mean Spearman-Brown coefficient between 0.61 and 0.71, based on 5,000 split-half samples, see **Table 2**. For the dot-probe task with pictures and the itch sensitivity analyses, one outlier (>3 interquartile range) was excluded (final $n = 115$ for both outcomes). Variables for the dot-probe task with pictures were log-transformed to obtain normal distribution.

Pre-training AB Toward Itch Pictures and Words

The one-sample *t*-test with the pre-training AB-index differed significantly from zero [$t_{(114)} = -2.26, p = 0.026$], indicating that participants overall were focused away from the itch pictures at baseline (see **Table 3** for descriptive values). There was no pre-training AB for itch words [$t_{(104)} = 0.248, p = 0.805$] (**Table 4**). The RM-ANOVA demonstrated that ABM-training conditions did not significantly differ in their pre-training AB-index for itch pictures [$F_{(2,113)} = 0.09, p = 0.911, \eta_p{}^2 = 0.002$] or words [$F_{(2,102)} = 0.559, p = 0.574, \eta_p{}^2 = 0.011$].

TABLE 1 | Baseline individual characteristics per attention bias modification (ABM) training condition.

	Total sample	ABM-training away from itch (n = 38)	ABM-training towards itch (n = 40)	Sham training (n = 38)	Statistic for condition difference
Prior to session					
Sex (n M/F)	30/86	11/27	10/30	9/29	$\chi^2_{(2)} = 0.298$, $p = 0.861$
Age	22 (21; 23)	22 (21; 23)	22 (21; 23)	21 (21; 23)	$H_{(2)} = 0.021$, $p = 0.990$
Body vigilance (BVS)	3.1 (2.1; 4.2)	3.2 (1.6; 4.0)	2.9 (1.8; 3.8)	3.1 (1.9; 3.9)	$H_{(2)} = 0.044$, $p = 0.978$
Single item for attentional focus on itch/pain (0–10)	1.7 (0.3; 3.8)/2.5 (0.3; 4.7)	1.3 (0.2; 3.9)/2.2 (1.5; 5.0)	1.6 (0.7; 3.2)/2.9 (0.6; 5.0)	1.7 (0.1; 3.8)/1.8 (0.5; 5.0)	$H_{(2)} = 0.418$, $p = 0.811$/$H_{(2)} = 0.910$, $p = 0.635$
Itch vigilance and awareness (PVAQ-I)	25.0 (17.5; 32.5)	24.5 (17.8; 31.0)	22.5 (15.3; 32.0)	28.0 (16.8; 32.8)	$H_{(2)} = 1.067$, $p = 0.587$
Single item for attentional disengagement from itch/pain	4.0 (3.0; 5.0)/4.0 (3.0; 4.0)	4.0 (3.0; 5.0)/4.0 (3.0; 4.0)	4.0 (3.0; 5.0)/4.0 (3.0; 4.0)	5.0 (3.8; 5.0)/4.0 (3.0; 5.0)	$H_{(2)} = 3.883$, $p = 0.143$/$H_{(2)} = 2.770$, $p = 0.250$
Itch catastrophizing (PCS-I)	6.0 (1.0; 11.0)	7.5 (3.5; 12.0)	6.0 (2.0; 12.8)	5.5 (2.0; 12.3)	$H_{(2)} = 0.454$, $p = 0.797$
Cognitive intrusions of itch (ECIP-I)	13.5 (8.0; 19)	14.0 (11.0; 22.0)	15.0 (11.0; 22.3)	13.0 (11.0; 22.3)	$H_{(2)} = 0.372$, $p = 0.830$
Neuroticism (EPQ-RSS)	3.0 (2.0; 5.0)	3.0 (2.0; 5.0)	3.5 (2.0; 6.0)	3.0 (1.0; 6.0)	$H_{(2)} = 1.806$, $p = 0.405$
During session					
General response inhibition (Flanker index)	51.0 (37.3; 64.7)	52.9 (40.8; 66.0)	54.7 (39.4; 64.1)	47.2 (31.8; 60.8)	$H_{(2)} = 1.820$, $p = 0.403$

Values displayed are medians (interquartile range: IQR) and absolute numbers for the variable sex.
EPQ-RSS, Eysenck Personality Questionnaire revised short scale (theoretical range 0–12 neuroticism subscale); Single items assessing attentional focusing on itch and pain (theoretical range 0–10); BVS, Body Vigilance Scale (theoretical range 0–10); PVAQ-I, Pain Vigilance and Awareness Scale, adjusted for itch (theoretical range 0–80); PCS-I, Pain Catastrophizing Scale, adjusted for itch (theoretical range 0–52); ECIP-I, Experience of Cognitive Intrusions of Pain, adjusted for itch (theoretical range original version 0–60—in the current study 10–60); Single items about attentional disengagement (theoretical range 1–5). The flanker index was calculated by subtracting the RT for congruent trials from the RT from incongruent trials. Because most questionnaires were not-normally distributed, the conditions were compared using non-parametric Kruskal-Wallis-tests (H) on most outcomes, except for sex, which was compared in a Chi-square-test.

TABLE 2 | Reliability coefficients for the different versions of the dot-probe tasks.

		Mean (range)	Median (IQR)
Dot-probe tasks with pictures	Version 1	0.68 (0.34–0.84)	0.68 (0.64; 0.72)
	Version 2	0.71 (0.41–0.70)	0.72 (0.68; 0.75)
Dot-probe tasks with words	Version 1	0.67 (0.23–0.86)	0.68 (0.62; 0.72)
	Version 2	0.60 (0.20–0.84)	0.61 (0.55; 0.66)

Mean and the range of the Spearman-Brown coefficient of 5,000 split-half samples are reported, as well as the median and interquartile range (IQR).

Training AB Toward Itch Pictures

The 2 (time: pre- vs. post- training) × 2 (itch congruency: itch-congruent vs. itch-incongruent) × 3 (training condition) RM-ANOVA, testing the main hypothesis whether training attention away and towards pictorial itch stimuli altered attention toward itch pictures (**Figure 2** and **Tables 3A,B**) showed no significant time × itch congruency ×condition effect [$F_{(2,112)} = 0.41$, $p = 0.663$, ${\eta_p}^2 = 0.007$]. There was a significant main effect of time [$F_{(1,112)} = 199.87$, $p < 0.001$, ${\eta_p}^2 = 0.641$], showing that RT were shorter after the training than before (**Tables 3A,B**). There was neither a significant main effect of congruency [$F_{(1,112)} = 2.46$, $p = 0.120$, $\eta^2_p = 0.022$] nor of condition [$F_{(2,112)} = 0.753$, $p = 0.473$, $\eta^2_p = 0.013$].

Training AB Toward Itch Words

The 2 × 2 × 3 RM-ANOVA testing the secondary hypothesis whether ABM-training away and towards pictorial itch stimuli would generalize to changes in AB toward itch words showed no significant time x itch congruency x condition effect [$F_{(2,102)} = 0.091$, $p = 0.913$, $\eta^2_p = 0.002$]. The significant main effect of time [$F_{(1,102)} = 118.29$, $p < 0.0001$, $\eta^2_p = 0.537$] showed RT to be shorter after the training than before (**Table 4**). No significant main effect of itch congruency [$F_{(1,102)} = 0.194$, $p = 0.661$, $\eta^2_p = 0.002$], but a significant main effect of condition was found [$F_{(2,102)} = 5.842$, $p = 0.004$, $\eta^2_p = 0.103$] with contrasts showing that RT for targets was faster in both, the condition trained away and towards itch, than in the sham training condition [mean difference (MD) = −39.4, standard error (SE) = 15.2, $p = 0.032$, and $MD = -47.7$, $SE = 14.9$, $p = 0.005$, respectively].

Itch Sensitivity

On the pre-training assessment of mechanically evoked itch (log-transformed), training conditions did not significantly differ [$F_{(2,112)} = 0.458$, $p = 0.634$, $\eta^2_p = 0.008$]. The 2 × 3 RM-ANOVA testing the secondary hypothesis whether ABM-training attention away and towards pictorial itch stimuli would generalize to changes in itch sensitivity (residuals were normally distributed after excluding the outlier, so variables were not transformed) obtained no significant time × condition effect [$F_{(2,112)} = 0.259$, $p = 0.772$, $\eta^2_p = 0.005$]. There was neither a significant main effect of time [$F_{(1,112)} = 0.294$, $p = 0.588$, $\eta^2_p = 0.003$] nor of condition [$F_{(2,112)} = 0.625$, $p = 0.537$, $\eta^2_p = 0.011$]. See **Table 5** for descriptive values.

Table 3A | Mean ± standard deviation of reaction times for the trials congruent and incongruent to the itch pictures of the dot-probe tasks administered pre- and post-attention bias modification (ABM)-training, displayed for the total sample and per training condition.

		Total sample (n = 115)	ABM-training away from itch (n = 38)	ABM-training towards itch (n = 40)	Sham training (n = 37)
Pre-training	Congruent trials	545.4 ± 77.5	544.7 ± 67.8	537.1 ± 75.2	555.0 ± 89.5
	Incongruent trials	536.2 ± 77.8	532.1 ± 65.8	528.7 ± 83.8	548.5 ± 83.0
	AB-index	−9.1 ± 43.4	−12.6 ± 38.0	−8.4 ± 41.5	−6.5 ± 51.0
Post-training	Congruent trials	474.0 ± 63.3	475.1 ± 62.0	462.7 ± 50.2	485.0 ± 75.8
	Incongruent trials	475.1 ± 68.9	473.4 ± 65.4	467.8 ± 58.7	484.9 ± 82.1
	AB-index	1.2 ± 31.5	−1.7 ± 30.0	5.1 ± 31.8	−0.1 ± 33.2

Table 3B | Median (and interquartile range; IQR) of reaction times for the trials congruent and incongruent to the itch pictures of the dot-probe tasks administered pre- and post-attention bias modification (ABM)-training, displayed for the total sample, and per training condition.

	Trial type	Total sample (n = 115)	ABM-training away from itch (n = 38)	ABM-training towards itch (n = 40)	Sham training (n = 37)
Pre-training	Congruent	534.2 (488.9; 580.7)	535.0 (492.7; 579.7)	529.3 (485.5; 567.1)	537.4 (491.3; 605.4)
	Incongruent	521.3 (473.0; 579.8)	515.6 (480.2; 574.2)	511.1 (468.6; 566.5)	531.6 (476.0; 613.0)
Post-training	Congruent	464.3 (429.0; 507.5)	453.7 (430.2; 510.5)	458.8 (426.9; 501.8)	480.2 (424.5; 536.1)
	Incongruent	463.2 (426.4; 516.6)	460.6 (423.2; 513.6)	462.6 (424.4; 503.6)	480.9 (430.3; 533.6)

Table 4 | Mean ± standard deviation of reaction times for the trials congruent and incongruent to the itch words of the dot-probe tasks administered pre- and post-training, displayed for the total sample and per attention bias modification (ABM)-training condition.

		Total sample (n = 105)	ABM-training away from itch (n = 33)	ABM-training towards itch (n = 36)	Sham training (n = 36)
Pre-training	Congruent trials	557.6 ± 84.9	544.6 ± 87.9	535.9 ± 67.4	591.1 ± 89.4
	Incongruent trials	558.5 ± 85.0	550.2 ± 90.7	537.9 ± 69.5	586.8 ± 88.2
	AB-index	0.9 ± 39.2	5.5 ± 35.9	2.0 ± 32.0	−4.3 ± 48.1
Post-training	Congruent trials	497.6 ± 62.9	483.1 ± 47.6	481.6 ± 62.4	527.0 ± 66.5
	Incongruent trials	494.1 ± 61.3	487.3 ± 55.4	476.7 ± 55.3	517.8 ± 66.2
	AB-index	−3.5 ± 36.0	4.2 ± 34.9	−4.9 ± 38.1	−9.2 ± 34.7

Post-hoc Analyses

Post-hoc moderation analysis showed that the effect of the ABM-training on AB for itch pictures was not moderated by the pre-training level of AB for itch pictures (**Table 6**). Additionally, over the entire sample, AB for itch pictures increased significantly [$F_{(1,114)} = 5.16, p = 0.025, \eta_p^2 = 0.043$].

Flanker Effect

A significant Flanker effect [$F_{(1,115)} = 419.76$, $p < 0.001$, $\eta_p^2 = 0.785$], with faster RT for congruent (423.8 ± 78.7) than incongruent trials (472.2 ± 69.6) indicated attentional inhibition across the sample.

Associations With Individual Characteristics

Of all Spearman correlation coefficients between the individual characteristics and the ABM-training effect on the different outcomes, only a significant correlation was found between high levels of neuroticism and larger increases in mechanically induced itch in the ABM-training condition towards itch ($\rho_S = 0.35$, $p = 0.03$). Another significant correlation emerged in the sham training condition, which was between a better disengagement ability from itch and a larger decrease in mechanically induced itch ($\rho_S = 0.46, p = 0.004$).

DISCUSSION

We assessed the effects of attention bias modification (ABM)-training on healthy individuals' attentional bias (AB) toward itch pictures and itch words as well as on sensitivity to mild itch. This is the first proof-of-principle ABM-training study in the field of itch. Specifically, we also included a condition in which attention was trained toward itch, besides the training away from itch and a sham condition. In contrast to expectations, ABM-training did not alter attention to itch pictures. Furthermore, ABM-training using itch pictures did not affect AB toward itch words nor itch sensitivity. Additionally, of the individual characteristics, only neuroticism was associated with a larger training effect, specifically with an increase in mechanically evoked itch in the condition trained towards itch. In sum, although we expected

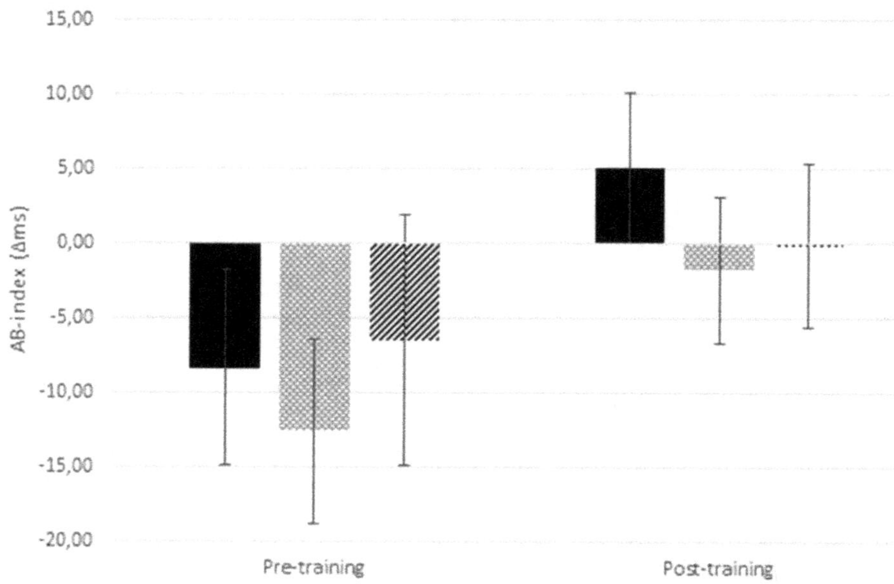

FIGURE 2 | Attentional Bias (AB)-index for the itch pictures pre- and post-ABM-training. Results are displayed for the ABM-training away from itch (black; $n = 38$), ABM-training toward itch (light gray dots; $n = 40$), and the sham training (intermediate gray stripes; $n = 37$). Positive values indicate an AB toward itch. Error bars represent standard errors of the mean.

Table 5 | Mean ± standard deviation of mechanically evoked itch measured on a numeric rating scale from 0 (no itch) to 10 (worst itch imaginable) displayed for the total sample and per attention bias modification (ABM) training condition.

	Total sample ($n = 115$)	ABM-training away from itch ($n = 37$)	ABM-training toward itch ($n = 39$)	Sham training ($n = 39$)
Pre-training itch[a]	1.8 ± 1.5	2.0 ± 1.5	1.7 ± 1.4	1.8 ± 1.5
Post-training itch	1.8 ± 1.5	2.0 ± 1.8	1.6 ± 1.4	1.9 ± 1.5

[a]*For the pre-training analysis, the variables were not-normally distributed, hence the medians and interquartile ranges are reported here. Median (IQR) was for the total sample 1.5 (0.7; 2.7), for the ABM-training away from itch 1.7 (0.9; 2.8), for the ABM-training toward itch 1.3 (0.5; 2.8), and for the sham training 1.7 (0.5; 2.7).*

Table 6 | Linear model of pre-training attention bias (AB)-index for itch pictures as predictor (moderator) of the attention bias modification (ABM) training effect [$n = 115$; 95% confidence intervals (CI) and standard errors based on 1,000 bootstrap samples].

	B (CI)	*SE B*	*t*	*p*
Constant	−10.40 (−16.21, −4.60)	2.93	−3.551	0.001
Condition	2.56 (−4.88, 10.01)	3.76	0.683	0.496
Pre-training AB-index for itch pictures (Centered)	0.85 (0.71, 0.98)	0.07	12.516	< 0.001
Pre-training AB-index for itch pictures X Condition effect	0.12 (−0.04, 0.28)	0.08	1.478	0.142

$R^2 = 0.61$. The training effect is defined by the change in AB-index before minus after the training (a positive value indicates a decreased AB after training).

ABM-training to be promising for itch, given the contagiousness and attention-capturing characteristics of itch (6, 13, 15), we can conclude that the hypotheses could not be confirmed.

Given the novelty of an ABM-training for itch, comparing current findings with findings of previous ABM-trainings for pain may provide some further insight. Largely inspired upon previous ABM research on pain (27, 29, 34), we opted for a 500-ms stimulus display time, the use of pictures, and a target discrimination instead of a localization task. Yet, we can conclude that although results are not in line with our hypotheses, current findings are also not completely unexpected when inspecting the ABM-training literature. Indeed, although initial results of ABM for pain-related information showed promising results (26, 27), more recent studies indicate that ABM-trainings for pain are ineffective in changing AB toward pain in healthy participants (28, 29, 35). For both, potential moderation of ABM-training effects by baseline levels of AB for itch and generalization to another type of AB (i.e., from pictures to words), only preliminary evidence from the pain literature is available (37). Moreover, generalization occurred only from words to pictures and not vice versa (27). That itch sensitivity was unaffected by the ABM-training is also partly in line with previous pain studies. Specifically, some studies favored effectiveness of ABM-training on experienced pain or pain thresholds (26, 27, 29), while others did not find effects on pain outcomes or only for some pain outcomes (28, 29, 35). Furthermore, in multiple studies changes in somatosensory pain outcomes were not accompanied by changes in AB for pain (27, 29). Comparable mixed results emerged in other fields, such as anxiety for which ABM-trainings were originally developed (21, 46). Overall, previous findings of the effects of ABM-training are mixed or preliminary.

Various explanations of current findings in relation to the inconsistent evidence for ABM-training studies for pain [see also (35)] can be considered. First, the present study included a sham training to inform about potential distinct effects of each training condition. Nonetheless, previous pain research often compared an ABM-training toward pain with an ABM-training away from pain, which likely obtains larger effects due to comparison of the most "extreme" conditions. Noteworthy, *post-hoc* analyses comparing our extreme conditions does not change the conclusions. Second, lack of effectiveness on AB for pictures and words may relate to the fact that after the active training conditions (including either congruent or incongruent trials), both congruent and incongruent trials were offered in the dot-probe tasks to assess AB for itch. This may have diluted potential training effects. Moreover, given the null-findings of an AB towards itch pictures, the lack of a generalization towards the itch words and sensitivity is not surprising. Third, participants did not have a baseline AB for itch stimuli, as would be expected (14, 17). This generally hampers the possibility to train attention away, although also no moderation by the baseline AB levels was found. Moreover, this does not explain the lack of training effects for those trained towards itch, particularly because at baseline average RT pointed in the opposite direction, which could be interpreted as attentional avoidance of itch pictures. Nevertheless, previous ABM-trainings away from pain have shown to be effective in reducing pain outcomes despite the absence of a baseline AB towards pain (26, 28, 29). However, the current study did not find effects on itch sensitivity either. This does not seem to be due to the levels of itch induced, which were comparably moderate in previous studies (39, 47), in which itch reduction was effectuated (by heterotopic stimulation) (39). Fourth, as elaborated on by Wiers et al. (36) a proof-of-principle study in healthy individuals entails that participants are not aware of receiving an intervention and have no motivation to change responses. Motivation to pursue certain goals, e.g., getting rid of itch, as well as having positive expectations about an intervention play an important role in the experience and treatment of various symptoms (13, 32, 48–50). Therefore, possible effects to be obtained are probably smaller in healthy individuals than in patients.

Interestingly, at baseline, participants were faster on itch incongruent than congruent trials for the itch pictures [also seen in (16); this may be related to the picture content, e.g., the itch pictures are of weak emotional valence (50) to the healthy individuals], which could be indicative of attentional avoidance of itch. This "avoidance bias" hampered the ability to train attention away, and simultaneously increased the opportunity to train attention towards itch. In fact, the "avoidance bias" was abolished, as demonstrated by the lack of a significant itch-congruency effect after the training irrespective of the condition participants were in (though seemingly mostly in the training towards itch; **Figure 2**). This unexpected finding of increased attention to itch in the entire sample is in the direction opposite to what is desirable. This may have been caused by participants becoming generally more familiar with the picture content over time. Additionally, particularly in the pre-training assessment, the stimuli were new to the participants and the neutral pictures apparently drew more attention than the itch pictures. This may be related to the more heterogeneous content of the neutral (various objects) than the itch pictures (scratching hand), making the neutral pictures more novel (51). It may be worthwhile to explore if the attention increase to the itch pictures would still occur when presenting stimuli subliminally. Noteworthy, participants' responses were significantly faster after the training than before, which can be attributed to a task learning effect.

Several limitations and directions for future research should be mentioned. First, although reliability of the dot-probe tasks in the current study was adequate, generally the use of dot-probe tasks to measure AB (not so much to train attention) has recently been questioned because attention may vary highly across trials which is not reflected by the calculated average reaction times (50, 52). However, the majority of, if not all, ABM-trainings used the dot-probe paradigm with comparable analyses, and some were successful. Nevertheless, future studies may benefit from using other tasks, e.g., the dual probe task variant (53), as well as eye-tracking methodology to fully capture the fluctuating process of attention over time (50, 54). Second, training effects could be assessed on more intense itch stimuli, e.g., cowhage (55). Third, including somatosensory itch stimuli as opposed to visual stimuli in the task would enhance ecological validity. However, because of the lack of spatial attention allocation effects toward somatosensory itch (12, 14, 16), translating the ABM-training paradigm into a somatosensory variant remains challenging. Fourth, current ABM-trainings may be improved by incorporating motivational components, e.g., by implementing reward, gamification, or creating a more representable context (32, 35). It is also worthwhile to explore how to extend and personalize cognitive bias trainings for itch in line with the innovative, promising, theory-driven ABC-training for addiction (49). Actually, the itch-scratch cycle behavior and addiction share common neurobiological mechanisms (56). Finally, when ABM-training for itch would eventually be successful, future studies should also include patients with chronic itch, who are generally motivated to diminish the itch, hence have a baseline AB toward itch that can be targeted [e.g., (50, 57, 58) for results in related fields].

ETHICS STATEMENT

The studies involving human participants were reviewed and approved by Psychology Research Ethics Committee of Leiden

University. The patients/participants provided their written informed consent to participate in this study.

AUTHOR CONTRIBUTIONS

AvL, DvR, SVD, GC, and RW designed the study and interpreted the data. AL lead the data acquisition, conducted the analyses, and wrote the initial draft. JB supported the conduction of analyses. AvL and JB revised the manuscript according to the critical feedback of DvR, SD, GC, and RW. All authors provided approval for publication of the content and agreed to be accountable for all aspects of the work in ensuring that questions related to the accuracy or integrity of any part of the work are appropriately investigated and resolved.

ACKNOWLEDGMENTS

The authors would like to thank Elisa Kovacs, Jolijn Giesbers, and Sjoerd Dobbinga for their contribution to the collection of stimuli used in both dot-probe tasks. Elisa Kovacs and Bao Fang are also acknowledged for their help with stimulus validation. Fien Akkersdijk, Bao Fang, Leandra Gentenaar, Bart de Jonge, Bas Rikers, Jolien Schurg, and Naomi Wiebing are acknowledged for their help with participant recruitment and/or testing. We are very grateful for the support of Stephen Brown and Maureen Meekel in the dot-probe task programming. Data-manager Jaap-Willem Mink is acknowledged for the randomization. We highly appreciate that Christopher Eccleston, Edmund Keogh, and Nina Attridge shared their programming of the Flanker task with us, so we could use it in this study. Lastly, we thank Ralph Rippe and Thomas Pronk for their advice concerning the dot-probe reliability analyses.

REFERENCES

1. Matterne U, Apfelbacher CJ, Loerbroks A, Schwarzer T, Buttner M, Ofenloch R, et al. Prevalence, correlates and characteristics of chronic pruritus: a population-based cross-sectional study. *Acta Derm Venereol.* (2011) 91:674–9. doi: 10.2340/00015555-1159
2. Jensen P, Zachariae C, Skov L, Zachariae R. Sleep disturbance in psoriasis: a case-controlled study. *Br J Dermatol.* (2018) 179:1376–84. doi: 10.1111/bjd.16702
3. Strom MA, Fishbein AB, Paller AS, Silverberg JI. Association between atopic dermatitis and attention deficit hyperactivity disorder in U.S. children and adults. *Br J Dermatol.* (2016) 175:920–9. doi: 10.1111/bjd.14697
4. Van Laarhoven AI, Walker AL, Wilder-Smith OH, Kroeze S, van Riel PL, van de Kerkhof PC, et al. Role of induced negative and positive emotions in sensitivity to itch and pain in women. *Br J Dermtol.* (2012) 167:262–9. doi: 10.1111/j.1365-2133.2012.10933.x
5. Mochizuki H, Lavery MJ, Nattkemper LA, Albornoz C, Valdes Rodriguez R, Stull C, et al. Impact of acute stress on itch sensation and scratching behaviour in patients with atopic dermatitis and healthy controls. *Br J Dermatol.* (2019) 180:821–7. doi: 10.1111/bjd.16921
6. Schut C, Grossman S, Gieler U, Kupfer J, Yosipovitch G. Contagious itch: what we know and what we would like to know. *Front Hum Neurosci.* (2015) 9:57. doi: 10.3389/fnhum.2015.00057
7. van Laarhoven AIM, Holle H. Optimizing audiovisual itch induction: the role of attention and expectancy. *Br J Dermtol.* (2020) 182:1088–9. doi: 10.1111/bjd.18596
8. Holle H, Warne K, Seth AK, Critchley HD, Ward J. Neural basis of contagious itch and why some people are more prone to it. *Proc Natl Acad Sci USA.* (2012) 109:19816–21. doi: 10.1073/pnas.1216160109
9. Ross SE. Pain and itch: insights into the neural circuits of aversive somatosensation in health and disease. *Curr Opin Neurobiol.* (2011) 21:880–7. doi: 10.1016/j.conb.2011.10.012
10. Paus R, Schmelz M, Biro T, Steinhoff M. Frontiers in pruritus research: scratching the brain for more effective itch therapy. *J Clin Investig.* (2006) 116:1174–86. doi: 10.1172/jci28553
11. van Laarhoven AIM, Kraaimaat FW, Wilder-Smith OH, Evers AWM. Role of attentional focus on bodily sensations in sensitivity to itch and pain. *Acta Derm Venereol.* (2010) 90:46–51. doi: 10.2340/00015555-0743
12. van Laarhoven AIM, van Damme S, Lavrijsen A, van Ryckeghem DM, Crombez G, Evers AWM. Do tonic itch and pain stimuli draw attention towards their location? *Biomed Res Int.* (2017) 2017:2031627. doi: 10.1155/2017/2031627
13. Evers AWM, Peerdeman KJ, van Laarhoven AIM. What is new in the psychology of chronic itch? *Exp Dermatol.* (2019) 28:1442–7. doi: 10.1111/exd.13992
14. van Laarhoven AIM, van Damme S, Lavrijsen APM, van Ryckeghem DM, Crombez G, Evers AWM. Attentional processing of itch. *Psychol Res.* (2018) 82:876–88. doi: 10.1007/s00426-017-0878-2
15. Van Laarhoven AIM, Peerdeman KJ, Van Ryckeghem DM, Evers AWM. Cognitive processing of itch and pain: the role of attention and expectations. In: Yosipovitch G, Arendt-Nielsen L, Andersen HH, editors. *Itch and Pain: Similarities, Interactions, and Differences*. Philadelphia, PA: Wolters-Kluwer (2020). p. 289–98.
16. Becker JM, Vreijling SR, Van Damme S, Kovacs EA, Veldhuijzen DS, Lavrijsen APM, et al. Attentional interference, but no attentional bias, by tonic pain and itch stimulation. (submitted).
17. van Laarhoven AI, Ulrich DJ, Wilder-Smith OH, van Loey NE, Nieuwenhuis M, van der Wee NJ, et al. Psychophysiological processing of itch in patients with chronic post-burn itch: an exploratory study. *Acta Derm Venereol.* (2016) 96:613–8. doi: 10.2340/00015555-2323
18. Fortune DG, Richards HL, Corrin A, Taylor RJ, Griffiths CE, Main CJ. Attentional bias for psoriasis-specific and psychosocial threat in patients with psoriasis. *J Behav Med.* (2003) 26:211–24. doi: 10.1023/a:1023408503807
19. Leibovici V, Magora F, Cohen S, Ingber A. Effects of virtual reality immersion and audiovisual distraction techniques for patients with pruritus. *Pain Res Manag.* (2009) 14:283–6. doi: 10.1155/2009/178751
20. Stumpf A, Pfleiderer B, Schneider G, Heuft G, Schmelz M, Phan NQ, et al. Distraction from itch shows brainstem activation without reduction in experimental itch sensation. *Acta Derm Venereol.* (2017) 97:1074–80. doi: 10.2340/00015555-2732
21. Jones EB, Sharpe L. Cognitive bias modification: a review of meta-analyses. *J Affect Disord.* (2017) 223:175–83. doi: 10.1016/j.jad.2017.07.034
22. Ikoma A, Steinhoff M, Stander S, Yosipovitch G, Schmelz M. The neurobiology of itch. *Nat Rev Neurosci.* (2006) 7:535–47. doi: 10.1038/nrn1950
23. Carleton RN, Richter AA, Asmundson GJ. Attention modification in persons with fibromyalgia: a double blind, randomized clinical trial. *Cogn Behav Ther.* (2011) 40:279–90. doi: 10.1080/16506073.2011.616218
24. Sharpe L, Ianiello M, Dear BF, Nicholson Perry K, Refshauge K, Nicholas MK. Is there a potential role for attention bias modification in pain patients? Results of 2 randomised, controlled trials. *Pain.* (2012) 153:722–31. doi: 10.1016/j.pain.2011.12.014

25. Schoth DE, Georgallis T, Liossi C. Attentional bias modification in people with chronic pain: a proof of concept study. *Cogn Behav Ther.* (2013) 42:233–43. doi: 10.1080/16506073.2013.777105
26. McGowan N, Sharpe L, Refshauge K, Nicholas MK. The effect of attentional re-training and threat expectancy in response to acute pain. *Pain.* (2009) 142:101–7. doi: 10.1016/j.pain.2008.12.009
27. Sharpe L, Johnson A, Dear BF. Attention bias modification and its impact on experimental pain outcomes: comparison of training with words versus faces in pain. *Eur J Pain.* (2015) 19:1248–57. doi: 10.1002/ejp.648
28. Todd J, Sharpe L, Colagiuri B. Attentional bias modification and pain: the role of sensory and affective stimuli. *Behav Res Ther.* (2016) 83:53–61. doi: 10.1016/j.brat.2016.06.002
29. Bowler JO, Bartholomew KJ, Kellar I, Mackintosh B, Hoppitt L, Bayliss AP. Attentional bias modification for acute experimental pain: a randomized controlled trial of retraining early versus later attention on pain severity, threshold and tolerance. *Eur J Pain.* (2017) 21:112–24. doi: 10.1002/ejp.908
30. Heathcote LC, Vervoort T, Eccleston C, Fox E, Jacobs K, Van Ryckeghem DM, et al. The relationship between adolescents' pain catastrophizing and attention bias to pain faces is moderated by attention control. *Pain.* (2015) 156:1334–41. doi: 10.1097/j.pain.0000000000000174
31. Goubert L, Crombez G, Van Damme S. The role of neuroticism, pain catastrophizing and pain-related fear in vigilance to pain: a structural equations approach. *Pain.* (2004) 107:234–41. doi: 10.1016/j.pain.2003.11.005
32. Van Ryckeghem DML, Noel M, Sharpe L, Pincus T, Van Damme S. Cognitive biases in pain: an integrated functional-contextual framework. *Pain.* (2019) 160:1489–93. doi: 10.1097/j.pain.0000000000001508
33. Heathcote LC, Jacobs K, Van Ryckeghem DML, Fisher E, Eccleston C, Fox E, et al. Attention bias modification training for adolescents with chronic pain: a randomized placebo-controlled trial. *Pain.* (2018) 159:239–51. doi: 10.1097/j.pain.0000000000001084
34. Crombez G, Van Ryckeghem DM, Eccleston C, Van Damme S. Attentional bias to pain-related information: a meta-analysis. *Pain.* (2013) 154:497–510. doi: 10.1016/j.pain.2012.11.013
35. Van Ryckeghem DML, Van Damme S, Vervoort T. Does attention bias modification training impact on task performance in the context of pain: an experimental study in healthy participants. *PLoS ONE.* (2018) 13:e0200629. doi: 10.1371/journal.pone.0200629
36. Wiers RWHJ, Boffo M, Field M. What's in a trial? On the importance of distinguishing between experimental lab studies and randomized controlled trials: the case of cognitive bias modification and alcohol use disorders. *J Stud Alcohol Drugs.* (2018) 79:333–43. doi: 10.15288/jsad.2018.79.333
37. Fox E, Zougkou K, Ashwin C, Cahill S. Investigating the efficacy of attention bias modification in reducing high spider fear: the role of individual differences in initial bias. *J Behav Ther Exp Psychiatry.* (2015) 49:84–93. doi: 10.1016/j.jbtep.2015.05.001
38. Becker JM, Vreijling SR, Dobbinga S, Giesbers JJJ, Evers AWM, Veldhuijzen DS, et al. Attentional bias towards visual itch and pain stimuli in itch- and pain-free individuals? *Acta Derm Venereol.* (2020) 100:adv00199. doi: 10.2340/00015555-3537
39. Andersen HH, van Laarhoven AIM, Elberling J, Arendt-Nielsen L. Modulation of itch by conditioning itch and pain stimulation in healthy humans. *J Pain.* (2017) 18:1437–50. doi: 10.1016/j.jpain.2017.07.002
40. Eriksen BA, Eriksen CW. Effects of noise letters upon the identification of a target letter in a nonsearch task. *Percept Psychophys.* (1974) 16:143–9.
41. Moore DJ, Keogh E, Eccleston C. The interruptive effect of pain on attention. *Q J Exp Psychol (Hove).* (2012) 65:565–86. doi: 10.1080/17470218.2011.626865
42. Eysenck HJ, Eysenck SBG. *Manual of the Eysenck Personality Scales (EPS Adult).* London: Hodder & Stoughton (1991).
43. Hayes AF. *An Introduction to Mediation, Moderation, and Conditional Process Analysis: A Regression-Based Approach.* 2nd ed. New York, NY: Guilford Press (2018).
44. R Foundation for Statistical Computing, Vienna, Austria. *R Core Team. R: A Language and Environment for Statistical Computing.* (2019). Available online at: https://www.r-project.org/ (accessed October 13, 2020).
45. Pronk T. *splithalfr: Extensible Bootstrapped Split-Half Reliabilities.* (2020). Available online at: https://CRAN.R-project.org/package=splithalfr (accessed October 13, 2020).
46. Mogg K, Waters AM, Bradley BP. Attention bias modification (ABM): review of effects of multisession ABM training on anxiety and threat-related attention in high-anxious individuals. *Clin Psychol Sci.* (2017) 5:698–717. doi: 10.1177/2167702617696359
47. Andersen HH, Elberling J, Lo Vecchio S, Arendt-Nielsen L. Topography of itch: evidence of distinct coding for pruriception in the trigeminal nerve. *Itch (Phila).* (2017) 2:e2. doi: 10.1097/itx.0000000000000002
48. Van Ryckeghem DM, Crombez G, Eccleston C, Legrain V, Van Damme S. Keeping pain out of your mind: the role of attentional set in pain. *Eur J Pain.* (2013) 17:402–11. doi: 10.1002/j.1532-2149.2012.00195.x
49. Wiers RWHJ, Van Dessel P, Köpetz C. ABC-training: a new theory-based form of cognitive bias modification to foster automatization of alternative choices in the treatment of addiction and related-disorders. *Curr Dir Psychol.* (2020) 29:499–505. doi: 10.1177/0963721420949500
50. Field M, Werthmann J, Franken I, Hofmann W, Hogarth L, Roefs A. The role of attentional bias in obesity and addiction. *Health Psychol.* (2016) 35:767–80. doi: 10.1037/hea0000405
51. Ernst D, Becker S, Horstmann G. Novelty competes with saliency for attention. *Vision Res.* (2020) 168:42–52. doi: 10.1016/j.visres.2020.01.004
52. Dear BF, Sharpe L, Nicholas MK, Refshauge K. The psychometric properties of the dot-probe paradigm when used in pain-related attentional bias research. *J Pain.* (2011) 12:1247–54. doi: 10.1016/j.jpain.2011.07.003
53. MacLeod C, Grafton B, Notebaert L. Anxiety-linked attentional bias: is it reliable? *Annu Rev Clin Psychol.* (2019) 15:529–54. doi: 10.1146/annurev-clinpsy-050718-095505
54. Jiang MYW, Vartanian LR. A review of existing measures of attentional biased in body image and eating disorders research. *Aust J Pychol.* (2018) 70:3–17. doi: 10.1111/ajpy.12161
55. Andersen HH, Elberling J, Arendt-Nielsen L. Human surrogate models of histaminergic and non-histaminergic itch. *Acta Derm Venereol.* (2015) 95:771–7. doi: 10.2340/00015555-2146
56. Ishiuji Y. Addiction and the itch-scratch cycle. What do they have in common? *Exp Dermatol.* (2019) 28:1448–54. doi: 10.1111/exd.14029
57. Todd J, van Ryckeghem DML, Sharpe L, Crombez G. Attentional bias to pain-related information: a meta-analysis of dot-probe studies. *Health Psychol Rev.* (2018) 12:419–36. doi: 10.1080/17437199.2018.1521729
58. Van Ryckeghem DML, Crombez G. Pain and attention: towards a motivational account. In: Karoly P, Crombez G, editors. *Motivational Perspectives on Chronic Pain: Theory, Research, and Practice.* New York, NY: Oxford University Press (2018).

2

Vulvar Pruritus: A Review of Clinical Associations, Pathophysiology and Therapeutic Management

Haya S. Raef[1,2] and Sarina B. Elmariah[1]**

[1] *Tufts University School of Medicine, Boston, MA, United States,* [2] *Massachusetts General Hospital, Boston, MA, United States*

***Correspondence:**
Haya S. Raef
haya.raef@tufts.edu
Sarina B. Elmariah
sbelmariah@mgh.harvard.edu

Vulvar pruritus is an unpleasant sensation and frequent symptom associated with many dermatologic conditions, including infectious, inflammatory and neoplastic dermatoses affecting the female genitalia. It can lead to serious impairment of quality of life, impacting sexual function, relationships, sleep and self-esteem. In this review, common conditions associated with vulvar itch are discussed including atopic and contact dermatitis, lichen sclerosus, psoriasis and infectious vulvovaginitis. We review the potential physiologic, environmental and infectious factors that contribute to the development of vulvar itch and emphasize the importance of addressing their complex interplay when managing this disruptive and challenging symptom.

Keywords: vulva, pruritus, itch, neurogenic itch, barrier function, neuropathic itch

INTRODUCTION

Vulvar pruritus is a frequently chronic and debilitating symptom associated with many vulvar disorders. The exact prevalence of vulvar pruritus is unknown as epidemiologic data are limited and most reports focus on individual conditions involving genital itch. In a study that surveyed 480 women from the general population in Boston, Massachusetts, 6.6% of women reported experiencing vulvar itch or burning (1). This is similar to rates of vulvar pruritus reported amongst the general German population, which was noted to range from 5 to 10% (2). The true prevalence of vulvar pruritus may be difficult to assess as it is likely underreported given the embarrassment many women feel when discussing genital symptoms (3). Itch was found to be the most frequent symptom, occurring in 70% of patients presenting to a clinic specializing in vulvar conditions (4). Similarly, in a survey study performed in the United Kingdom, 67.3% of general practitioners reported that they see more than five patients per month with vulvar symptoms, with vulvar pruritus being the most common (5).

Vulvar pruritus can have a profound impact on quality of life (6). In patients with genital psoriasis, itch was reported to be the most bothersome symptom with substantial impact on sexual relationships and psychosocial well-being (7). Moreover, several studies have demonstrated the negative impact of lichen sclerosus, a condition characterized by genital itch and pain, on sexual satisfaction (8–10).

PRURITIC VULVAR DERMATOSES

Vulvar pruritus arises in the setting of many inflammatory, infectious, and neoplastic processes that can affect the female genitalia (11).

Inflammatory

Common Etiologies

Common inflammatory vulvar dermatoses characterized by marked pruritus include atopic and contact dermatitis, lichen planus, lichen simplex chronicus, psoriasis and lichen sclerosus, among others. Atopic dermatitis (AD), irritant contact dermatitis (ICD) and allergic contact dermatitis (ACD) are the most common causes of vulvar itch in women (12). In one study of 144 adult women with vulvar complaints, 66% of patients had an eczematous process confirmed on pathology (13). In a separate prospective cohort study, 81.4% of patients with vulvar itch were found to have at least one positive contact allergen on patch testing (14). Similarly, AD and ICD have been reported to be the most common cause of vulvar symptoms in prepubertal girls (15).

AD is a genetic skin disease characterized by an altered skin barrier and chronic pruritus. It presents acutely as erythematous edematous or vesiculated plaques. Lichenification and dyspigmentation may be observed in chronic cases. It is important to note that due to the altered skin barrier, patients with AD may be at higher risk for the development of both irritant and allergic contact dermatoses (16–19).

Contact dermatitis consists of inflammation of the skin resulting from an external agent that acts as an irritant or as an allergen. The manifestation of both forms of dermatitis is very similar, varying from mild erythema and scaling to more severe erythema and edema (20). The area of involvement may be localized to the exposed site or be more extensive as the product spreads, with moisture or scratching (20). In addition to itch, pain and burning may also be present. Ulceration and erosions may be seen with primary irritants (21). In ACD, vesiculation in the acute phase may be observed (22). In more chronic cases, lichenification with excoriation are common features. Secondary infection can be seen in both ICD and ACD with pustules, crusting and fissuring.

Many substances can cause irritation of the vulva, including body fluids, feminine hygiene products or various topical medications (20). Physical and thermal irritants like tight fitting clothes, wash cloths, sponges and hair dryers have been implicated in ICD development (20, 22). Similarly, allergens often contribute to itch and dermatitis in patients with vulvar disease. Common allergens include fragrances and preservatives in products like soaps and detergents, cleansing wipes, antiseptics, spermicides, sanitary pads, lubricants, and even topical treatments like steroids, anesthetics, antibacterial and antifungal agents (20, 23). Rubber products, like pessaries, condoms, diaphragms, and gloves may also be sensitizers (20). Additionally, pantyhose and clothing with azo dyes may contribute to ACD (20). Patch testing may identify the allergens responsible for ACD.

Lichen simplex chronicus (LSC), or circumscribed neurodermatitis, is an eczematous disorder that commonly affects vulvar skin. It presents as scaly, thickened plaques that develop in response to persistent and vigorous scratching of intensely pruritic sites (24). LSC accounts for 35% of patient visit to vulvar specialty clinics, predominately affecting adult women but may also occur in children (25). Although often considered a primary diagnosis, LSC often arises as a secondary finding in the setting of neuropathic or other underlying primary cutaneous diseases such as AD, ACD or LP (26). It can also occur in patients with psychiatric disorders like depression and obsessive-compulsive disorder (27, 28). Pruritus in systemic diseases such as end stage renal disease, obstructive biliary disease or Hodgkin's lymphoma can also provoke LSC (29). LSC is characterized by a self-perpetuating itch-scratch cycle. In patients with primary LSC, the itch-scratch cycle is often triggered by initial skin irritation from tight-fitting clothing, irritating fabrics or personal care items which provoke scratching (11, 30). Damage to the vulvar epithelium due to scratching compromises the skin barrier, potentially provoking release of epithelial cytokines and making the skin more vulnerable to potential infection, which in turn drives itch and inflammation (26). If sufficiently pronounced, scratching results in hypertrophy and lichenification of the genital skin. Clinical examination usually reveals lichenified plaques with excoriations and variable levels of erythema and scale (25).

Psoriasis is another common inflammatory skin disease that affects genital skin and is often accompanied by pruritus (31). In most cases, genital psoriasis arises in the setting of more widespread cutaneous involvement, but isolated presentation of genital psoriasis may occur in 2–5% of psoriatic patients (32). Psoriatic lesions of the vulva are more common in children than in adults. In a study that evaluated 130 prepubertal girls with vulvar complaints, 17% had psoriasis, which was the third most common cutaneous condition after AD and LS (15). Clinical features of vulvar psoriasis consist of well-demarcated, brightly erythematous plaques with or without scale on the labia majora (33). Plaques may extend to the inguinal folds and maceration may be present (27).

Lichen sclerosus (LS) is another inflammatory dermatosis that affects the vulvar and vaginal mucosa, and not uncommonly extends to the perineum and perianal skin. While vulvar LS can occur at any age, most cases are observed in prepubertal girls or in postmenopausal women, when endogenous estrogen production is low (34). Pruritus and pain are predominant symptoms of the disease, although rarely LS may be asymptomatic. Other symptoms include dyspareunia and dysuria. In children, constipation may be a presenting symptom due to pain with defecation (35). The exact prevalence of LS is unknown, but estimates range from 1:300 to 1:1,000 of all adult patients referred to dermatology departments (36). The estimated prevalence in prepubertal girls is 1 in 900 (37). At a general gynecology practice, the rate of vulvar LS was estimated to be 1.7% (38). Again, the discrepancy in reported prevalence among gynecology and dermatology practices may reflect the hesitance of patients to discuss genital symptoms outside of a dedicated health visit focused on genitourinary care. LS typically manifests as atrophic, pale to white patches or plaques that often form a figure-of-eight pattern encompassing the vulva and anus (39). Erosions and painful fissures may be observed due to underlying inflammation as well as scratching or irritation of the inflamed, fragile tissue. Loss of normal vulvar architecture may be observed in more advanced cases, with burying of the clitoris and agglutination of the labia. Lichen sclerosus is associated with increased risk of developing genital squamous cell carcinoma (SCC). While the exact risk of malignant transformation is uncertain, estimates of the development of SCC are between 3 and 5% (40, 41). In a more recent study that used data from the Dutch Pathology Registry and included 3,038 women diagnosed with lichen sclerosus, the risk of SCC development after 10 and 20 years was 3.3 and 6.7%, respectively (42).

Lichen planus (LP) is a highy pruritic, autoimmune mucocutaneous disorder in which activated T-cells target basal keratinocytes of keratinized and non-keratinized squamous epithelium (43). The prevalence of LP is estimated to be 1% of the general population (44). Although LP most commonly affects the oral mucosa, ~25% of women with oral LP also have vulvovaginal involvement (45). LP predominately affects adult women, although isolated cases have been reported in young girls (46). Vulvovaginal LP may manifest in several ways, presenting in erosive, papulosquamous, and hypertrophic forms (47). Erosive LP, the most common presentation affecting genital skin, is characterized by well-demarcated glassy, erythematous to violaceous patches with a hyperkeratotic border and primarily affects the non-keratinized epithelium of the vestibule, labia minora and vagina (48). Several cohort studies have examined the distribution of LP subtypes arising on keratinized skin of the labia majora (48, 49). Papulosquamous LP, also referred to as classic LP, arises in 4–33% of cases and manifests with purple, brown or pink polygonal papules or small plaques which may have associated Wickham's striae (48, 49). Hypertrophic lichen planus arises in 29–46% of cases and presents with thicker, violaceous and hyperkeratotic plaques (47). One cohort study describing clinical and histologic features in 63 vulvar LP cases reported pruritus as the primary symptom affecting 79 and 81% of hypertrophic and papulosquamous LP patients, respectively, while pain was a primary manifestation in only 10 and 14%, respectively (48). Similar to LS, longstanding and untreated disease may lead to alterations in the normal architecture with narrowing of the vaginal introitus (50).

Other Etiologies

Inflammatory vulvar pruritus may also be caused by seborrheic dermatitis, plasma cell vulvitis, and Fox-Fordyce disease. Seborrheic dermatitis is an inflammatory condition that affects the sebum-rich areas of the body and should be considered in patients with vulvar pruritus. While uncommon, seborrheic dermatitis can occasionally present on the vulva, and is usually associated with simultaneous appearance of characteristic seborrhea on the scalp and face (51). It manifests on the vulva as erythematous plaques mainly on the labia, majora, perineum, and mons pubis. Scale is frequently absent in the vulva and the severity of pruritus is often more marked than would be expected based on the clinical signs (52).

Plasma cell vulvitis (PCV) is an extremely rare cause of vulvar pruritus characterized by a well-circumscribed erythematous plaque composed of predominately plasma cells (53, 54). It is typically located within the vulvar vestibule, often extending to the medial labia minora. The most common symptoms associated with PCV are pruritus, pain, burning, and dyspareunia (55).

Fox-Fordyce disease is another rare inflammatory condition which can affect vulvar skin and may provoke intense itching. The primary pathophysiologic process involves obstruction of the apocrine sweat duct and subsequent ductal rupture causing inflammation and enlargement of the glands (56). The mons pubis and labia majora are most commonly affected. Clinically, Fox-Fordyce disease manifests as intensely pruritic, numerous, flesh-colored to slightly yellow papules (57, 58).

Infectious

Common Etiologies

Vulvar pruritus may be associated with several types of infections and these vary with age. In prepubertal females, infection with *Group A beta-hemolytic streptococcus* (GABHS) commonly provokes vulvar symptoms including pruritus and pain, and manifests with sharply demarcated, edematous, red plaques (59). In contrast, adult women are less susceptible to acute GABHS-mediated vulvitis. Oropharyngeal GABHS infection often, but not always, precedes the development of vulvar symptoms (60).

In adult women, vulvovaginal candidiasis is a frequent cause of vulvar pruritus, with some studies suggesting candidiasis accounts for 35–40% of vulvar itch cases in this age group (2). Multiple epidemiologic studies have indicated that *Candida albicans* is responsible for the excess of episodes of vulvovaginal candidiasis, although reports indicate than non-*albicans Candida* species, notably *Candida glabrata,* account for 10–20% of episodes in certain regions (61–63). Increased estrogen levels, which have been implicated in reducing the inhibitory activity of epithelial cells against *Candida*, are thought to account for the rise in candidiasis in women of reproductive age (64). It is estimated that 75% of women have been affected by vulvovaginal candidiasis at some point in their lifetime (61, 65). Pregnancy, antibiotics, oral contraceptives and hormonal replacement therapies may increase estrogen levels resulting in an increased frequency of disease (66, 67). Tamoxifen, an estrogen antagonist in breast tissue, has been reported to have estrogen-like effects on vaginal epithelium in postmenopausal women, increasing risk of vulvovaginal candidiasis (68–70). In addition, compromised immune function is also associated with increased risk of yeast infections, as has been observed in patients with diabetes, HIV or who regularly use systemic or topical corticosteroids (23). Patients with recurrent candidal vulvovaginitis, defined as the occurrence of at least four episodes in 1 year, may have a predisposing genetic factor underlying their susceptibility (71). Clinical presentation of vulvar erythema, pustules or erosions and vaginal discharge may vary, but symptoms of pruritus and burning are commonly observed. Additional symptoms may include dysuria and dyspareunia. Identification of the specific *Candida* species can be considered in patients with refractory or recurrent vulvovaginal candidiasis as some species are often resistant to treatment (72).

Other Etiologies

In contrast to GABHS, which commonly affects prepubertal females, *Staphylococcus aureus*, *Haemophilus* and *Shigella* infections are less common infectious causes of vulvovaginal pruritus (23). *Enterobius vermiuclaris* (pinworm) infestation may be another source of vulvar and perineal pruritus in younger females worldwide (73).

In adults, the two most common parasitic vulvar infestations are pediculosis pubis (pubic lice) and scabies (52). Both cutaneous infections are often seen in young adults and are typically acquired during sexual contacts. Vulvar pruritus is the predominant symptom that develops following allergic sensitization (52, 74). In pediculosis pubis, adult lice and their eggs (nits) can be visible to the naked eye. Infection may spread from the genital area to other parts of the body, such as the thighs or trunk (74). Infestation with scabies causes widespread itching with nocturnal predominance. Unlike in other areas of the body, burrows on the vulva are uncommon and may be masked by excoriations or secondary infection (52).

Tinea cruris is an additional infection that can cause vulvar pruritus in women (52, 75). It can involve the inguinal creases and the labia majora. The typical lesions consist of mildly pruritic plaques with a raised erythematous scaly edge and central clearing. Viral infections, such as herpes simplex virus (HSV), human papilloma virus (HPV), and molluscum contagiosum may also trigger a sensation of vulvar itch (52). However, herpetic infections predominately manifest as pain, and HSV and molluscum are typically asymptomatic.

Neoplastic

Benign or malignant neoplasms are uncommon causes of vulvar pruritus. Rarely, pruritus may be an indication of vulvar malignancy such as SCC, melanoma, extramammary Paget's disease (EMPD) or vulvar intraepithelial neoplasia (VIN). Vulvar malignancy is uncommon and represents approximately 2–5% of all gynecologic cancers, with SCC representing the vast majority (>80%) of cases, followed by melanoma, BCC, verrucous carcinoma, EMPD, adenocarcinoma and Bartholin gland carcinoma (76). Although frequently overlooked, pruritus is the most common initial symptom of vulvar malignancy, with reports of up to 50–60% of patients endorsing moderate to severe pruritus (11, 77). In a multi-center, retrospective study describing 76 women with vulvar cancer in Tunisia, 48.7% of patients experienced chronic pruritus as the presenting symptom and the mean interval of time from symptom onset to cancer diagnosis was ~12.9 months (+/- 6.38) (77). Squamous cell carcinoma typically presents as persistent papules, plaques or ulcers with associated bleeding, itch and/or pain that is refractory to anti-inflammatory treatment (78). It is more common in postmenopausal women and is often associated with LS. Paget's disease of the vulva is an uncommon lesion that represents <1% of vulvar neoplasms (79). It predominately affects postmenopausal Caucasian women and presents as a white to red, velvety pruritic thin plaques (80). Although usually confined to the epithelium, invasive disease is observed in 15–25% of patients (81). VIN is a premalignant finding and is associated with HPV infection, particularly subtypes 16 and 18 (82). It can cause itch leading to varying degrees of excoriation and crusting (11).

Additionally, a variety of benign neoplastic processes may contribute to vulvar pruritus. For example, syringomas are rare tumors derived from eccrine sweat glands. While they typically involve the face, neck or chest, they occasionally present as multiple small, flesh-colored pruritic papules on the vulva (83). Moreover, hidradenoma papilliferum (HP), a tumor thought to originate from apocrine glands or mammary glands, can occasionally occur on the vulva and cause pruritus (84). In one series, HP represented up to 60% of vulvar adnexal tumors (85). It usually manifests as a firm, flesh to red-colored nodule that may or may not be accompanied with pruritus (86). It can be confused with adenocarcinoma due to its tendency to ulcerate (83, 87).

PATHOPHYSIOLOGY OF VULVAR ITCH

Impaired Barrier Function

Many pruritic vulvar disorders, such as atopic dermatitis and psoriasis, are associated with altered skin barrier function (88). Disruption of the skin barrier can be caused from a variety of factors including epidermal inflammation and mechanical or environmental insults, which in turn activate itch receptors (89). The barrier function of vulvar skin is substantially weaker than at other anatomical sites, and thus may be particularly prone to developing pruritus. The rate of transepidermal water loss (TEWL), a marker of barrier function, is significantly higher in vulvar skin than the skin of other cutaneous sites such as the forearm, suggesting a weaker epidermal barrier at the vulva (90, 91). Indeed, several studies have shown vulvar skin to be more reactive to irritants compared to other skin areas. In one study, two irritants, bezalkonium chloride and maleic acid, were applied the labia majora and forearm, and the intensity of skin reactions were assessed (92). Vulvar skin was found to be significantly more reactive than forearm skin to the two irritants, although this reactivity was not reproduced in studies with another irritant, sodium lauryl sulfate (93). Sweat, urine, friction by clothes and feminine hygiene products may all contribute to vulvar irritation by weakening barrier function (94). Moreover, low estrogen levels occurring with menopause, breast-feeding, postpartum and medications can also result in impaired barrier function as estrogen is important to maintain the structural integrity of the vulvovaginal space (20). Thinning of the vulvar epithelium in postmenopausal women combined with elevated skin pH and reduced corneum hydration cause barrier dysfunction (95).

Once disrupted, the skin barrier is more susceptible to exogenous and endogenous itch-triggers. In addition to the potential itch or pain associated with microbial colonization, mechanical irritation and chemical injury discussed above, epithelial damage leads to immune activation via release of skin-specific cytokines, including thymic stromal lymphopoietin (TSLP) and interleukin (IL)-33, which directly activate pruriceptive afferent nerve fibers (96, 97). Moreover, cysteine and serine proteases, such as cathepsin S and various kallikreins (KLKs), may be released by keratinocytes upon barrier disruption and are capable of directly stimulating or modulating itch via activation of Mas-related G-protein coupled receptors (MRGPRs) and protease-activated receptors (PARs) (98–100).

Neural Dysfunction

Neural dysfunction, due to neurogenic or neuropathic insults, is common but often-overlooked cause of vulvar pruritus. Neurogenic itch originates from endogenous or exogenous factors that activate the central nervous system at the level of the brain or spinal cord without evidence of nerve damage (101). Growing evidence suggests that neurogenic factors may contribute to vulvar pruritus. Epithelial and stromal tissue of the vulvar skin and vaginal mucosa express the transient receptor potential cationic channel type A1 (TRPA1), a channel known for its role in mediating and modulating non-histaminergic itch (102). Animal models of neonatal vaginal irritation suggest that hypersensitivity of the vagina is driven in part by increased hypothalamic-pituitary-adrenal (HPA) axis activation and subsequent increases in TRPA1 expression and functional activity in nerve terminals innervating the vaginal mucosa (103). Similarly, separate studies have demonstrated that expression of the transient receptor potential vanilloid 1 (TRPV1) ion channel, also well-known for its role in modulating pain and itch signals, is increased in vulvovaginal epithelia in patients with vulvodynia compared to controls (104, 105). Although vulvodynia is classically regarded as a type of neuropathic pain, itch and burning can accompany vulvodynia in 20 and 70%, respectively (106). Future studies will be needed to specifically evaluate whether the expression and function of TRP ion channels as well as primary itch-sensing receptors are altered in disorders associated with vulvar pruritus.

In contrast to neurogenic pruritus in which neural architecture is considered normal but stimulated abnormally, neuropathic pruritus results from injury or damage to nerve fibers. Small fiber polyneuropathy (SFPN), which affects the small, unmyelinated C-fibers and thinly myelinated A-delta fibers that conduct itch and pain may arise secondary to systemic diseases such as diabetes mellitus, sarcoidosis, amyloidosis, B12 deficiency, and viral infections, among others (107). While individuals with SFPN usually present with symptoms in their distal extremities or generalized symptoms, itch can also be localized entirely to the vulva. Vulvar itch may also be caused by nerve or nerve root compression at the levels of L4 through S2 vertebrae secondary to spinal injuries or lumbosacral arthritis (11, 23, 108). Another source of potential nerve irritation or injury may be caused by reactivation of varicella zoster, as 8.4% of shingles cases affect the dermatomes that innervate the vulva (109). Despite a robust immune response, long-lasting damage to the affected nerves may result in persistent pain and/or itch in affected vulvar skin (110). It is estimated that 30% of people with post-herpetic neuralgia suffer from itch (111), and thus postherpetic itch (PHI) should be considered in women presenting with genital pruritus.

Hormonal Influence

Hormonal changes play an important role in regulating vulvar epithelium by influencing vaginal pH and microflora composition. Similar to the vagina, vulvar pH is related to hormonal status and will change over a lifetime (112). In childhood, the vulvar and vaginal epithelia are neutral or alkaline, due to a lack of acid-producing vaginal microbes, lactobacilli (113). With the onset of menstruation, cyclic changes in estrogen and progesterone create a new epithelial micro-environment. Estrogen stimulation increases glycogen levels in the vulvar epithelium and lactobacilli subsequently colonize the vulvovaginal area, causing the pH to decrease (114). During parts of the menstrual cycle and following menopause, decreases in systemic estrogen result in an increase in vulvovaginal pH.

At more alkaline pH, the activity of various epithelial or immune-cell derived proteases may increase and thereby lead to greater activation of neuronal itch receptors (100, 115). Consistent with this hypothesis, abnormal expression of proteases and PAR activation has been implicated in several pruritic inflammatory skin disorders, such as AD and psoriasis (116–119). In addition to their effects on neuronal PARs, serine proteases such as KLKs and mast cell tryptase may also activate PARs expressed by keratinocytes or endothelial cells, stimulating the release of neuropeptides and cytokines which drive neurogenic inflammation and further propagation of endogenous pruritogens (120–123). Furthermore, the interactions between proteases and their endogenous inhibitors, present in the skin to ensure skin homeostasis, are influenced by the pH, with the greatest inhibitory capacity occurring in neutral pH environments (124). Thus, fluctuations in vulvovaginal pH due to hormonal status could shift the balance between protease and protease inhibitor activity, further contributing to PAR-mediated inflammation and itch.

Microbiome

The composition of the human vaginal microbiome may contribute to the pathogenesis of vulvar pruritus, particularly with respect to itch triggered by the mucocutaneous pathogens discussed previously. Interestingly, compared to the microbiota that colonize other regions of the body, such as the oropharynx and gut, the vaginal microbiome exhibits much lower diversity with Lactobacillus as the dominating species (125). Vaginal pH correlates with microbiome composition. Indeed, the composition of the vulvovaginal microbiome is dynamic and influenced by hormone-driven pH changes throughout the woman's reproductive life (126). Lactobacillus dominance increases with high estrogen levels because of proliferation and accumulation of glycogen. Ethnic differences also correlate with microbiome composition, with Blacks and Hispanics demonstrating higher levels of anaerobic bacterial species (125–127). By acidifying the vagina and producing antimicrobial substances, such as lactic acid and hydrogen peroxide, lactobacilli protect against opportunistic infections (2). Similarly, in keratinized squamous epithelia like that of the labia majora, resident microbiota such as *Cutibacterium acnes* promotes reduces skin pH via production of short-chain fatty acids (128). Other commensal microbes, such as *Staphylococcus epidermidis*, not only produce biofilms and other enzymes that enhance the function of antimicrobial peptides (AMPs) such as human b-defensins (HbDs) against dysbiosis, but also promote production of anti-inflammatory cytokines such as IL-10 from antigen presenting cells and reduce pro-inflammatory signals released by keratinocytes (129, 130).

Dysbiosis may lead to pruritus or sensory disturbance via multiple mechanisms. First, bacterial and viral pathogens directly engage keratinocytes via cell surface toll-like receptors (TLRs), triggering their release of the alarmins TSLP and IL-33 as well as AMPs such as HbDs and canthelicidins. While the alarmins directly activate itch by binding to their receptors on peripheral afferents (96, 97), they also initiate T_H2 immune cascades that contribute to barrier inflammation that fuels ongoing pruritus (131). Keratinocyte-derived AMPs trigger itch indirectly by stimulating mast cell release of histamine and IL-31 which in turn activate pruriceptors (132). Moreover, mast cells may also detect microbiota via their own TLRs or their ability to respond to a host of endogenous molecules released as part of a coordinated tissue response to infection including substance P and complements (133). Consistent with these data, derived primarily from animal models and human studies in allergic disorders, one study found that compared to healthy controls, women with LS has increased expression of AMPs including HbD-2 and psoriasin (134).

Pathogenic bacteria, such as *Staphylococcus aureus*, *Streptococcus pneumoniae*, *Pseudomonas aeruginosa* and others have also been shown to directly activate peripheral afferent nociceptive fibers (135). In animal models, bacteria-derived N-formylated peptides and the pore-forming toxin a-haemolysin stimulated calcium influx in nociceptive dorsal root ganglia by binding to neuronal formyl-peptide receptor 1 or by direct pore-formation, respectively (135). Once activated, nociceptors are capable of releasing neuropeptides that in turn modulate the inflammatory response, which may further influence the development of pain and/or itch. Similarly, in colonic epithelium, bacterial cell products have also been shown to directly activate dorsal root ganglion neurons and subsequently trigger elaboration of inflammatory cytokines (136). In addition, lipopolysaccharide (LPS) contained in the cell envelope of Gram-negative bacteria is also capable of stimulating calcium influx in trigeminal dorsal root ganglia neurons and sensitizing TRPV1 via a TLR4-mediated mechanism (137). How these processes specifically contribute to the development of itch or sensory disturbance in vulvovaginal epithelia remains to be examined.

MANAGEMENT CONSIDERATIONS

Recognizing the numerous factors that contribute to the pathogenesis of vulvar pruritus is crucial for appropriate diagnostic evaluation and management. The approach to therapy should be directed against the primary underlying mechanism suspected (e.g., inflammation due to AD or ACD, candidiasis, etc), but must also account for other exacerbating factors.

Pharmacologic Treatments

Topical corticosteroids are commonly used to alleviate itch caused by inflammatory skin disease (26). The potency used in a patient should be determined based on the age of the patient, diagnosis and severity of symptoms. Some vulvar conditions, such as LS and LP, may require more potent or prolonged corticosteroid therapy like clobetasol and halobetasol, whereas a less potent formulation may be sufficient for other diagnoses (52). The topical calcineurin inhibitors, tacrolimus or pimecrolimus, are non-steroidal anti-inflammatory agents that may also be useful in reducing vulvar inflammation or pruritus, particularly when prolonged courses are required to avoid steroid-induced side effects. Additional topical therapy targeting pruritus may be considered, for instance capsaicin or doxepin preparations (101). Doxepin should be used with caution due to high sensitizing capacity (138, 139). If capsaicin cream is being considered for use on genital skin, lower concentrations (0.012%) are advised (140). Systemic steroid preparations should be considered only after topical approaches have been exhausted or in severe dermatitis. Systemic immunomodulators, such as azathioprine, methotrexate, mycophenolate mofetil and infliximab have been evaluated for their potential use in AD, however further research is needed to specifically determine their utility in pruritic vulvar dermatoses (141–144).

Excoriated epidermis can become superinfected, and thus practitioners should have a low threshold to investigate and treat potential fungal and/or bacterial superinfections even when women have other underlying reasons for genital pruritus. For infectious causes of vulvar pruritus, treatment should depend on the inciting pathogen. Specific single bacterial infections require appropriate topical or oral antibiotics. For fungal infections like candidiasis, topical or oral azole agents are effective. There is no evidence to suggest that a specific azole results in better cure rates (72, 145). However, it is important to note that *Candida glabrata* is less responsive to azoles. Vaginal boric acid or amphotericin B can be used for refractory cases (72). Treatment of pediculosis and scabies infestations is best accomplished with permethrin or pyrethrins with piperonyl butoxide (146). Accepted therapies for pinworms include pyrantel pamoate or mebendazole, which should be administered to all household members (147). For viral causes of vulvar pruritus, acyclovir or valacyclovir are considered standard treatment for genital herpes (147). In patients with condyloma acuminatum caused by HPV infection, treatment with podophyllin, liquid nitrogen, or imiquimod are effective (147).

Although few studies address using neuromodulators for neuropathic vulvar itch, some reports suggest that oral gabapentin and topical lidocaine may be effective (148, 149). Use of tricyclic antidepressants, selective serotonin reuptake inhibitors and other antidepressants may also be considered and have shown benefit in patients with chronic itch and prurigo (5). In postmenopausal women or in the setting of a hypoestrogenic state, topical estrogen therapy may be suitable to reduce symptoms of dryness, atrophy and pruritus. As our understanding of itch pathophysiology grows, targeted anti-pruritic treatments may emerge and will need to be evaluated in randomized control trials for vulvar pruritus.

Non-pharmacologic Treatments

Because barrier dysfunction arises so frequently in conditions associated with vulvar pruritus, it is important to counsel patients to avoid all sources of irritation or potential allergic sensitization, including fragrances, lubricants and cleaning products. Patch testing should be performed for patients with physical exam or histologic findings suspicious of allergic contact dermatitis. Patch testing may also be a useful tool in patients with persistent vulvar symptoms that is unresponsive to treatment after 8 weeks, to avoid delays in diagnosis (150). Simple steps of cleansing with mild or no detergents when bathing and rinsing genital skin with water following urination when possible should be emphasized. Moreover, lipid-replenishing formulations such as petrolatum or barrier creams such as zinc oxide paste should be used to enhance barrier function of the vulvar skin and mucosa.

Behavioral modification strategies, such as skin rubbing and cooling rather than scratching can be effective when used in combination with pharmacotherapy. Patients should also be advised to keep fingernails short to minimize trauma caused by excoriation. Moreover, psychological interventions to control the urge to scratch, such as cognitive behavioral therapy, may be beneficial for some patients. A randomized controlled trial with AD patients receiving cognitive-behavioral treatment have shown significantly decreased itch intensity and scratching behavior after 1 year, as compared to those receiving only standard dermatologic care (151).

Phototherapy is another therapeutic modality that may be considered for the management of itch in various inflammatory pruritic conditions affecting the vulva, such as AD, psoriasis and LS (152). Several studies have documented the efficacy of phototherapy at various wavelengths for improving AD severity and associated pruritus, with medium-dose ultraviolet A (UVA) and narrowband UVB (NBUVB) being the preferred modalities (152–155). Similarly ultraviolet B (UVB) has been shown to reduce itch in psoriasis patients (156). Phototherapy on genital skin may best be considered in refractory cases and when handheld devices are available.

CONCLUSIONS

Vulvar pruritus is a common symptom of multifactorial etiology that may be driven by primary inflammatory disorders, barrier disruption, hormonal changes and infectious causes. Vulvar itch has a significant impact on the quality of life of affected patients and should be addressed by gynecologists, dermatologists, urologists and general practitioners when possible. Effective therapeutic strategies require that practitioners understand the multidimensional nature of vulvar pruritus and simultaneously address the many contributing factors that underly this challenging symptom.

AUTHOR CONTRIBUTIONS

HR conducted the literature review and drafted the manuscript. SE participated in reviewing and revising the manuscript. Both authors read and approved the final version of the manuscript including references.

REFERENCES

1. Harlow BL, Wise LA, Stewart EG. Prevalence and predictors of chronic lower genital tract discomfort. *Am J Obstet Gynecol.* (2001) 185:545–50. doi: 10.1067/mob.2001.116748
2. Woelber L, Prieske K, Mendling W, Schmalfeldt B, Tietz H-J, Jaeger A. Vulvar pruritus-causes, diagnosis and therapeutic approach. *Dtsch Arztebl Int.* (2020) 116:126–33. doi: 10.3238/arztebl.2020.0126
3. Gokdemir G, Baksu B, Baksu A, Davas I, Koslu A. Features of patients with vulvar dermatoses in dermatologic and gynecologic practice in Turkey: is there a need for an interdisciplinary approach? *J Obstet Gynaecol Res.* (2005) 31:427–31. doi: 10.1111/j.1447-0756.2005.00314.x
4. Sullivan AK, Straughair GJ, Marwood RP, Staughton RC, Barton SE. A multidisciplinary vulva clinic: the role of genito-urinary medicine. *J Eur Acad Dermatol Venereol.* (1999) 13:36–40. doi: 10.1111/j.1468-3083.1999.tb00841.x
5. Kandanearachchi P, Sahu B, Antonakou A, Papoutsis D. A survey of management of vulvar disorders in the primary health care setting in an urban area of England. *Arch Hell Med.* (2018) 35:405–11. Available online at: http://www.mednet.gr/archives/2018-3/pdf/405.pdf
6. Hickey S, Bell H. Quality of life in the vulvar clinic: a pilot study. *J Low Genit Tract Dis.* (2010) 14:225–9. doi: 10.1097/LGT.0b013e3181dc1e45
7. Cather JC, Ryan C, Meeuwis K, Potts Bleakman AJ, Naegeli AN, Edson-Heredia E, et al. Patients' perspectives on the impact of genital psoriasis: a qualitative study. *Dermatol Ther.* (2017) 7:447–61. doi: 10.1007/s13555-017-0204-3
8. Haefner HK, Aldrich NZ, Dalton VK, Gagné HM, Marcus SB, Patel DA, et al. The impact of vulvar lichen sclerosus on sexual dysfunction. *J Womens Health.* (2014) 23:765–70. doi: 10.1089/jwh.2014.4805
9. Felmingham C, Chan L, Doyle LW, Veysey E. The Vulval Disease Quality of Life Index in women with vulval lichen sclerosus correlates with clinician and symptom scores. *Australas J Dermatol.* (2020) 61:110–8. doi: 10.1111/ajd.13197
10. Vittrup G, Moerup L, Heilesen T, Jensen D, Laursen BS, Westmark S, et al. PO-02-015 Quality of life and sexuality in Danish women with lichen sclerosus. *J Sex Med.* (2019) 16:S80. doi: 10.1016/j.jsxm.2019.03.256
11. Savas JA, Pichardo RO. Female genital itch. *Dermatol Clin.* (2018) 36:225–43. doi: 10.1016/j.det.2018.02.006
12. Fischer GO. The commonest causes of symptomatic vulvar disease: a dermatologist's perspective. *Australas J Dermatol.* (1996) 37:12–8. doi: 10.1111/j.1440-0960.1996.tb00988.x
13. Fischer G, Spurrett B, Fischer A. The chronically symptomatic vulva: aetiology and management. *Br J Obstet Gynaecol.* (1995) 102:773–9. doi: 10.1111/j.1471-0528.1995.tb10841.x
14. Haverhoek E, Reid C, Gordon L, Marshman G, Wood J, Selva-Nayagam P. Prospective study of patch testing in patients with vulval pruritus. *Australas J Dermatol.* (2008) 49:80–5. doi: 10.1111/j.1440-0960.2008.00442.x
15. Fischer G, Rogers M. Vulvar disease in children: a clinical audit of 130 cases. *Pediatr Dermatol.* (2000) 17:1–6. doi: 10.1046/j.1525-1470.2000.01701.x
16. Milam EC, Jacob SE, Cohen DE. Contact dermatitis in the patient with atopic dermatitis. *J Allergy Clin Immunol Pract.* (2019) 7:18–26. doi: 10.1016/j.jaip.2018.11.003
17. Kohli N, Nedorost S. Inflamed skin predisposes to sensitization to less potent allergens. *J Am Acad Dermatol.* (2016) 75:312–7.e1. doi: 10.1016/j.jaad.2016.03.010
18. Shaughnessy CN, Malajian D, Belsito DV. Cutaneous delayed-type hypersensitivity in patients with atopic dermatitis: Reactivity to surfactants. *J Am Acad Dermatol.* (2014) 70:704–8. doi: 10.1016/j.jaad.2013.12.009
19. Machler BC, Sung CT, Darwin E, Jacob SE. Dupilumab use in allergic contact dermatitis. *J Am Acad Dermatol.* (2019) 80:280–1.e1. doi: 10.1016/j.jaad.2018.07.043
20. Margesson LJ. Contact dermatitis of the vulva. *Dermatol Ther.* (2004) 17:20–7. doi: 10.1111/j.1396-0296.2004.04003.x
21. Bauer A, Rodiger C, Greif C, Kaatz M, Elsner P. Vulvar dermatoses-irritant and allergic contact dermatitis of the vulva. *Dermatology.* (2005) 210:143–9. doi: 10.1159/000082570
22. Connor CJ, Eppsteiner EE. Vulvar contact dermatitis. *Proc Obstet Gynecol.* (2014) 4:1–14. doi: 10.17077/2154-4751.1255

23. Rimoin LP, Kwatra SG, Yosipovitch G. Female-specific pruritus from childhood to postmenopause: clinical features, hormonal factors, and treatment considerations. *Dermatol Ther.* (2013) 26:157–67. doi: 10.1111/dth.12034
24. Patterson JW. *Weedon's Skin Pathology.* 4th ed. Charlottesville, VA: Elsevier (2016).
25. Lynch PJ. Lichen simplex chronicus (atopic/neurodermatitis) of the anogenital region. *Dermatol Ther.* (2004) 17:8–19. doi: 10.1111/j.1396-0296.2004.04002.x
26. Thorstensen KA, Birenbaum DL. Recognition and management of vulvar dermatologic conditions: lichen sclerosus, lichen planus, and lichen simplex chronicus. *J Midwifery Womens Health.* (2012) 57:260–75. doi: 10.1111/j.1542-2011.2012.00175.x
27. Charifa A, Badri T, Harris BW. Lichen Simplex Chronicus. In: *StatPearls.* Treasure Island (FL): StatPearls Publishing. (2020).
28. Konuk N, Koca R, Atik L, Muhtar S, Atasoy N, Bostanci B. Psychopathology, depression and dissociative experiences in patients with lichen simplex chronicus. *Gen Hosp Psychiatry.* (2007) 29:232–5. doi: 10.1016/j.genhosppsych.2007.01.006
29. Bolognia JL, Schaffer JV, Cerroni L, editors. *Dermatology E-Book.* 4th ed. New Haven, CT: Elsevier (2017).
30. Corazza M, Borghi A, Minghetti S, Toni G, Virgili A. Effectiveness of silk fabric underwear as an adjuvant tool in the management of vulvar lichen simplex chronicus: results of a double-blind randomized controlled trial. *Menopause.* (2015) 22:850–6. doi: 10.1097/GME.0000000000000410
31. Zamirska A, Reich A, Berny-Moreno J, Salomon J, Szepietowski JC. Vulvar pruritus and burning sensation in women with psoriasis. *Acta Derm Venereol.* (2008) 88:132–5. doi: 10.2340/00015555-0372
32. Meeuwis KAP, de Hullu JA, Massuger LFAG, van de Kerkhof PCM, van Rossum MM. Genital psoriasis: a systematic literature review on this hidden skin disease. *Acta Derm Venereol.* (2011) 91:5–11. doi: 10.2340/00015555-0988
33. Kapila S, Bradford J, Fischer G. Vulvar psoriasis in adults and children: a clinical audit of 194 cases and review of the literature. *J Low Genit Tract Dis.* (2012) 16:364–71. doi: 10.1097/LGT.0b013e31824b9e5e
34. Powell JJ, Wojnarowska F. Lichen sclerosus. *Lancet.* (1999) 353:1777–83. doi: 10.1016/S0140-6736(98)08228-2
35. Lagerstedt M, Karvinen K, Joki-Erkkilä M, Huotari-Orava R, Snellman E, Laasanen S-L. Childhood lichen sclerosus–a challenge for clinicians. *Pediatr Dermatol.* (2013) 30:444–50. doi: 10.1111/pde.12109
36. Wallace HJ. Lichen sclerosus et atrophicus. *Trans St Johns Hosp Dermatol Soc.* (1971) 57:9–30.
37. Powell J, Wojnarowska F. Childhood vulvar lichen sclerosus: an increasingly common problem. *J Am Acad Dermatol.* (2001) 44:803–6. doi: 10.1067/mjd.2001.113474
38. Goldstein AT, Marinoff SC, Christopher K, Srodon M. Prevalence of vulvar lichen sclerosus in a general gynecology practice. *J Reprod Med.* (2005) 50:477–80.
39. Smith YR, Haefner HK. Vulvar lichen sclerosus. *Am J Clin Dermatol.* (2004) 5:105–25. doi: 10.2165/00128071-200405020-00005
40. Hart WR, Norris HJ, Helwig EB. Relation of lichen sclerosus et atrophicus of the vulva to development of carcinoma. *Obstet Gynecol.* (1975) 45:369–77.
41. Carlson JA, Ambros R, Malfetano J, Ross J, Grabowski R, Lamb P, et al. Vulvar lichen sclerosus and squamous cell carcinoma: a cohort, case control, and investigational study with historical perspective; implications for chronic inflammation and sclerosis in the development of neoplasia. *Hum Pathol.* (1998) 29:932–48. doi: 10.1016/S0046-8177(98)90198-8
42. Bleeker MCG, Visser PJ, Overbeek LIH, van Beurden M, Berkhof J. Lichen sclerosus: Incidence and risk of vulvar squamous cell carcinoma. *Cancer Epidemiol Biomarkers Prev.* (2016) 25:1224–30. doi: 10.1158/1055-9965.EPI-16-0019
43. Terlou A, Santegoets LAM, van der Meijden WI, Heijmans-Antonissen C, Swagemakers SMA, van der Spek PJ, et al. An autoimmune phenotype in vulvar lichen sclerosus and lichen planus: a Th1 response and high levels of microRNA-155. *J Invest Dermatol.* (2012) 132:658–66. doi: 10.1038/jid.2011.369
44. Eisen D. The clinical features, malignant potential, and systemic associations of oral lichen planus: a study of 723 patients. *J Am Acad Dermatol.* (2002) 46:207–14. doi: 10.1067/mjd.2002.120452
45. Eisen D. The evaluation of cutaneous, genital, scalp, nail, esophageal, and ocular involvement in patients with oral lichen planus. *Oral Surg Oral Med Oral Pathol Oral Radiol Endod.* (1999) 88:431–6. doi: 10.1016/S1079-2104(99)70057-0
46. Handa S, Sahoo B. Childhood lichen planus: a study of 87 cases. *Int J Dermatol.* (2002) 41:423–7. doi: 10.1046/j.1365-4362.2002.01522.x
47. Goldstein AT, Metz A. Vulvar lichen planus. *Clin Obstet Gynecol.* (2005) 48:818–23. doi: 10.1097/01.grf.0000179670.98939.b7
48. Day T, Weigner J, Scurry J. Classic and hypertrophic vulvar lichen planus. *J Low Genit Tract Dis.* (2018) 22:387–95. doi: 10.1097/LGT.0000000000000419
49. Chew A, Stefanato CM, Savarese I, Neill SM, Fenton DA, Lewis FM. Clinical patterns of lichen planopilaris in patients with vulval lichen planus. *Br J Dermatol.* (2014) 170:218–20. doi: 10.1111/bjd.12609
50. Fruchter R, Melnick L, Pomeranz MK. Lichenoid vulvar disease: a review. *Int J Womens Dermatol.* (2017) 3:58–64. doi: 10.1016/j.ijwd.2017.02.017
51. Stewart KMA. Clinical care of vulvar pruritus, with emphasis on one common cause, lichen simplex chronicus. *Dermatol Clin.* (2010) 28:669–80. doi: 10.1016/j.det.2010.08.004
52. Bohl TG. Overview of vulvar pruritus through the life cycle. *Clin Obstet Gynecol.* (2005) 48:786–807. doi: 10.1097/01.grf.0000179636.64663.e6
53. Mensing H, Jänner M. Vulvitis plasmacellularis Zoon (author's transl). *Z Hautkr.* (1981) 56:728–32.
54. Bharatia PR, Pradhan AM, Zawar VP. Plasma cell vulvitis. *Indian J Sex Transm Dis AIDS.* (2015) 36:185–7. doi: 10.4103/0253-7184.167172
55. Goldstein AT, Christopher K, Burrows LJ. Plasma cell vulvitis: a rare cause of intractable vulvar pruritus. *Arch Dermatol.* (2005) 141:789–90. doi: 10.1001/archderm.141.6.789
56. Yost J, Robinson M, Meehan SA. Fox-Fordyce disease. *Dermatol Online J.* (2012) 18:28.
57. Gurusamy L, Jegadeesan M, Jayakumar S. Fox-Fordyce disease of the vulva. *Indian J Sex Transm Dis AIDS.* (2016) 37:65–7. doi: 10.4103/0253-7184.180293
58. Mahajan R, Bang D, Nagar A, Bilimoria F. Rare sweat gland tumors of vulva: report of two cases. *Indian J Sex Transm Dis AIDS.* (2012) 33:124–7. doi: 10.4103/0253-7184.102128
59. Mogielnicki NP, Schwartzman JD, Elliott JA. Perineal group A streptococcal disease in a pediatric practice. *Pediatrics.* (2000) 106:276–81. doi: 10.1542/peds.106.2.276
60. Fischer GO. Vulval disease in pre-pubertal girls. *Australas J Dermatol.* (2001) 42:225–34. doi: 10.1046/j.1440-0960.2001.00526.x
61. Corsello S, Spinillo A, Osnengo G, Penna C, Guaschino S, Beltrame A, et al. An epidemiological survey of vulvovaginal candidiasis in Italy. *Eur J Obstet Gynecol Reprod Biol.* (2003) 110:66–72. doi: 10.1016/S0301-2115(03)00096-4
62. Okungbowa FI, Isikhuemhen OS, Dede APO. The distribution frequency of Candida species in the genitourinary tract among symptomatic individuals in Nigerian cities. *Rev Iberoam Micol.* (2003) 20:60–3.
63. Buscemi L, Arechavala A, Negroni R. Study of acute vulvovaginitis in sexually active adult women, with special reference to candidosis, in patients of the Francisco J. Muñiz Infectious Diseases Hospital. *Rev Iberoam Micol.* (2004) 21:177–81.
64. Fidel PL Jr, Cutright J, Steele C. Effects of reproductive hormones on experimental vaginal candidiasis. *Infect Immun.* (2000) 68:651–7. doi: 10.1128/IAI.68.2.651-657.2000
65. Lambert J. Pruritus in female patients. *Biomed Res Int.* (2014) 2014:541867. doi: 10.1155/2014/541867
66. Xu J. Response: Re: Effect of antibiotics on vulvovaginal candidiasis: a metronet study. *J Am Board Fam Med.* (2009) 22:223. doi: 10.3122/jabfm.2009.02.080258
67. Ahmad A, Khan AU. Prevalence of Candida species and potential risk factors for vulvovaginal candidiasis in Aligarh, India. *Eur J Obstet Gynecol Reprod Biol.* (2009) 144:68–71. doi: 10.1016/j.ejogrb.2008.12.020
68. Ferrazzi E, Cartei G, Mattarazzo R, Fiorentino M. Oestrogen-like effect of tamoxifen on vaginal epithelium. *Br Med J.* (1977) 1:1351–2. doi: 10.1136/bmj.1.6072.1351-e
69. Sobel JD, Chaim W, Leaman D. Recurrent vulvovaginal candidiasis associated with long-term tamoxifen treatment in postmenopausal women. *Obstet Gynecol.* (1996) 88:704–6. doi: 10.1016/0029-7844(96)00123-8
70. Lahti E, Vuopala S, Kauppila A, Blanco G, Ruokonen A, Laatikainen T. Maturation of vaginal and endometrial epithelium in postmenopausal

breast cancer patients receiving long-term tamoxifen. *Gynecol Oncol.* (1994) 55:410–4. doi: 10.1006/gyno.1994.1314
71. Smeekens SP, van de Veerdonk FL, Kullberg BJ, Netea MG. Genetic susceptibility to Candida infections. *EMBO Mol Med.* (2013) 5:805–13. doi: 10.1002/emmm.201201678
72. Sobel JD. Vulvovaginal candidosis. *Lancet.* (2007) 369:1961–71. doi: 10.1016/S0140-6736(07)60917-9
73. Siegfried EC, Frasier LD. Anogenital skin diseases of childhood. *Pediatr Ann.* (1997) 26:321–31. doi: 10.3928/0090-4481-19970501-11
74. Bignell C. Lice and scabies. *Medicine.* (2014) 42:382–4. doi: 10.1016/j.mpmed.2014.04.008
75. Ingram JT. Tinea of vulva. *BMJ.* (1955) 2:1500. doi: 10.1136/bmj.2.4954.1500
76. Rogers LJ, Cuello MA. Cancer of the vulva. *Int J Gynaecol Obstet.* (2018) 143(Suppl. 2):4–13. doi: 10.1002/ijgo.12609
77. Kehila M, Harabi S, Mhiri R, Touhami O, Abouda HS, Khlifi A, et al. Vulvar cancer in Tunisia: epidemiological and clinicopathological features multicentric study. *J Egypt Natl Canc Inst.* (2017) 29:95–8. doi: 10.1016/j.jnci.2017.02.001
78. Kingston A. Vulval disease in the postmenopausal patient: a guide to current management. *Menopause Int.* (2010) 16:117–20. doi: 10.1258/mi.2010.010031
79. Fanning J, Lambert HCL, Hale TM, Morris PC, Schuerch C. Paget's disease of the vulva: prevalence of associated vulvar adenocarcinoma, invasive Paget's disease, and recurrence after surgical excision. *Am J Obstet Gynecol.* (1999) 180:24–7. doi: 10.1016/S0002-9378(99)70143-2
80. Tebes S, Cardosi R, Hoffman M. Paget's disease of the vulva. *Am J Obstet Gynecol.* (2002) 187:281–3. doi: 10.1067/mob.2002.125700
81. Hoffmann PE. Malignancies of the vulva. *Am J Obstet Gynecol.* (1937) 33:60–7. doi: 10.1016/S0002-9378(15)32743-5
82. Ngan HY, Cheung AN, Liu SS, Yip PS, Tsao SW. Abnormal expression or mutation of TP53 and HPV in vulvar cancer. *Eur J Cancer.* (1999) 35:481–4. doi: 10.1016/S0959-8049(98)00407-9
83. Heller DS. Benign tumors and tumor-like lesions of the vulva. *Clin Obstet Gynecol.* (2015) 58:526–35. doi: 10.1097/GRF.0000000000000133
84. El-Khoury J, Renald M-H, Plantier F, Avril M-F, Moyal-Barracco M. Vulvar hidradenoma papilliferum (HP) is located on the sites of mammary-like anogenital glands (MLAGs): analysis of the photographs of 52 tumors. *J Am Acad Dermatol.* (2016) 75:380–4. doi: 10.1016/j.jaad.2016.01.034
85. Baker GM, Selim MA, Hoang MP. Vulvar adnexal lesions: a 32-year, single-institution review from Massachusetts General Hospital. *Arch Pathol Lab Med.* (2013) 137:1237–46. doi: 10.5858/arpa.2012-0434-OA
86. Kambil SM, Bhat RM, D'Souza DC. Hidradenoma papilliferum of the vulva. *Indian Dermatol Online J.* (2014) 5:523–4. doi: 10.4103/2229-5178.142541
87. Dabral R, Jetly D, Goel D. Hidradenoma papilliferum of the vulva with extensive squamous metaplasia mimicking malignancy: rare entity with diagnostic challenge. *Oncol J India.* (2019) 3:38. doi: 10.4103/oji.oji_23_19
88. Cork MJ, Danby SG, Vasilopoulos Y, Hadgraft J, Lane ME, Moustafa M, et al. Epidermal barrier dysfunction in atopic dermatitis. *J Invest Dermatol.* (2009) 129:1892–908. doi: 10.1038/jid.2009.133
89. Potenzieri C, Undem BJ. Basic mechanisms of itch. *Clin Exp Allergy.* (2012) 42:8–19. doi: 10.1111/j.1365-2222.2011.03791.x
90. Elsner P, Maibach HI. The effect of prolonged drying on transepidermal water loss, capacitance and pH of human vulvar and forearm skin. *Acta Derm Venereol.* (1990) 70:105–9.
91. Britz MB, Maibach HI. Human labia majora skin: transepidermal water loss *in vivo*. *Acta Derm Venereol Suppl.* (1979) 59:23–5.
92. Britz MB, Maibach HI. Human cutaneous vulvar reactivity to irritants. *Contact Dermat.* (1979) 5:375–7. doi: 10.1111/j.1600-0536.1979.tb04908.x
93. Elsner P, Wilhelm D, Maibach HI. Effect of low-concentration sodium lauryl sulfate on human vulvar and forearm skin. Age-related differences. *J Reprod Med.* (1991) 36:77–81.
94. Pichardo-Geisinger R. Atopic and contact dermatitis of the vulva. *Obstet Gynecol Clin North Am.* (2017) 44:371–8. doi: 10.1016/j.ogc.2017.05.003
95. Yong AA, Cao T, Tan V, Yosipovitch G, Tey HL. Skin physiology in pruritus of advanced ageing. *J Eur Acad Dermatol Venereol.* (2016) 30:549–50. doi: 10.1111/jdv.12948
96. Liu B, Tai Y, Achanta S, Kaelberer MM, Caceres AI, Shao X, et al. IL-33/ST2 signaling excites sensory neurons and mediates itch response in a mouse model of poison ivy contact allergy. *Proc Natl Acad Sci U S A.* (2016) 113:E7572–9. doi: 10.1073/pnas.1606608113
97. Wilson SR, Thé L, Batia LM, Beattie K, Katibah GE, McClain SP, et al. The epithelial cell-derived atopic dermatitis cytokine TSLP activates neurons to induce itch. *Cell.* (2013) 155:285–95. doi: 10.1016/j.cell.2013.08.057
98. Reddy VB, Sun S, Azimi E, Elmariah SB, Dong X, Lerner EA. Redefining the concept of protease-activated receptors: cathepsin S evokes itch via activation of Mrgprs. *Nat Commun.* (2015) 6:7864. doi: 10.1038/ncomms8864
99. Hägermark O. Studies on experimental itch induced by kallikrein and bradykinin. *Acta Derm Venereol.* (1974) 54:397–400.
100. Akiyama T, Lerner EA, Carstens E. Protease-activated receptors and itch. *Handb Exp Pharmacol.* (2015) 226:219–35. doi: 10.1007/978-3-662-44605-8_13
101. Yosipovitch G, Greaves MW, Schmelz M. Itch. *Lancet.* (2003) 361:690–4. doi: 10.1016/S0140-6736(03)12570-6
102. Ückert S, Sonnenberg JE, Albrecht K, Kuczyk MA, Hedlund P. Expression and distribution of the transient receptor potential cationic channel ankyrin 1 (TRPA1) in the human vagina. *Int J Impot Res.* (2015) 27:16–9. doi: 10.1038/ijir.2014.23
103. Pierce AN, Zhang Z, Fuentes IM, Wang R, Ryals JM, Christianson JA. Neonatal vaginal irritation results in long-term visceral and somatic hypersensitivity and increased hypothalamic-pituitary-adrenal axis output in female mice. *Pain.* (2015) 156:2021–31. doi: 10.1097/j.pain.0000000000000264
104. Tympanidis P, Terenghi G, Dowd P. Increased innervation of the vulval vestibule in patients with vulvodynia. *Br J Dermatol.* (2003) 148:1021–7. doi: 10.1046/j.1365-2133.2003.05308.x
105. Tympanidis P, Casula MA, Yiangou Y, Terenghi G, Dowd P, Anand P. Increased vanilloid receptor VR1 innervation in vulvodynia. *Eur J Pain.* (2004) 8:129–33. doi: 10.1016/S1090-3801(03)00085-5
106. Phillips NA, Brown C, Foster D, Bachour C, Rawlinson L, Wan J, et al. Presenting symptoms among premenopausal and postmenopausal women with vulvodynia: a case series. *Menopause.* (2015) 22:1296–300. doi: 10.1097/GME.0000000000000526
107. Stumpf A, Ständer S. Neuropathic itch: diagnosis and management. *Dermatol Ther.* (2013) 26:104–9. doi: 10.1111/dth.12028
108. Cohen AD, Vander T, Medvendovsky E, Biton A, Naimer S, Shalev R, et al. Neuropathic scrotal pruritus: anogenital pruritus is a symptom of lumbosacral radiculopathy. *J Am Acad Dermatol.* (2005) 52:61–6. doi: 10.1016/j.jaad.2004.04.039
109. Oaklander AL, Rissmiller JG. Postherpetic neuralgia after shingles: an under-recognized cause of chronic vulvar pain. *Obstet Gynecol.* (2002) 99:625–8. doi: 10.1016/S0029-7844(01)01663-5
110. Oaklander AL. The pathology of postherpetic neuralgia and postherpetic itch. In: *Herpes Zoster: Postherpetic Neuralgia and Other Complications.* Cham: Springer International Publishing. (2017). p. 141–56. doi: 10.1007/978-3-319-44348-5_12
111. Oaklander AL, Bowsher D, Galer B, Haanpää M, Jensen MP. Herpes zoster itch: preliminary epidemiologic data. *J Pain.* (2003) 4:338–43. doi: 10.1016/S1526-5900(03)00637-0
112. Farage M, Maibach H. Lifetime changes in the vulva and vagina. *Arch Gynecol Obstet.* (2006) 273:195–202. doi: 10.1007/s00404-005-0079-x
113. Hammerschlag MR, Alpert S, Rosner I, Thurston P, Semine D, McComb D, et al. Microbiology of the vagina in children: normal and potentially pathogenic organisms. *Pediatrics.* (1978) 62:57–62.
114. Brabin L, Roberts SA, Fairbrother E, Mandal D, Higgins SP, Chandiok S, et al. Factors affecting vaginal pH levels among female adolescents attending genitourinary medicine clinics. *Sex Transm Infect.* (2005) 81:483–7. doi: 10.1136/sti.2005.014621
115. Paus R, Schmelz M, Bíró T, Steinhoff M. Frontiers in pruritus research: scratching the brain for more effective itch therapy. *J Clin Invest.* (2006) 116:1174–86. doi: 10.1172/JCI28553
116. Steinhoff M, Buddenkotte J, Shpacovitch V, Rattenholl A, Moormann C, Vergnolle N, et al. Proteinase-activated receptors: transducers of proteinase-mediated signaling in inflammation and immune response. *Endocr Rev.* (2005) 26:1–43. doi: 10.1210/er.2003-0025
117. Stefansson K, Brattsand M, Roosterman D, Kempkes C, Bocheva G, Steinhoff M, et al. Activation of proteinase-activated receptor-2 by

human kallikrein-related peptidases. *J Invest Dermatol.* (2008) 128:18–25. doi: 10.1038/sj.jid.5700965

118. Komatsu N, Saijoh K, Kuk C, Liu AC, Khan S, Shirasaki F, et al. Human tissue kallikrein expression in the stratum corneum and serum of atopic dermatitis patients. *Exp Dermatol.* (2007) 16:513–9. doi: 10.1111/j.1600-0625.2007.00562.x
119. Komatsu N, Saijoh K, Kuk C, Shirasaki F, Takehara K, Diamandis EP. Aberrant human tissue kallikrein levels in the stratum corneum and serum of patients with psoriasis: dependence on phenotype, severity and therapy. *Br J Dermatol.* (2007) 156:875–83. doi: 10.1111/j.1365-2133.2006.07743.x
120. Steinhoff M, Vergnolle N, Young SH, Tognetto M, Amadesi S, Ennes HS, et al. Agonists of proteinase-activated receptor 2 induce inflammation by a neurogenic mechanism. *Nat Med.* (2000) 6:151–8. doi: 10.1038/72247
121. Brain SD. New feelings about the role of sensory nerves in inflammation. *Nat Med.* (2000) 6:134–5. doi: 10.1038/72218
122. Kempkes C, Buddenkotte J, Cevikbas F, Buhl T, Steinhoff M. 11 role of PAR-2 in neuroimmune communication and itch. In: *Itch: Mechanisms and Treatment*. Davis, CA: CRC Press (2014). p. 193.
123. Steinhoff M, Corvera CU, Thoma MS, Kong W, McAlpine BE, Caughey GH, et al. Proteinase-activated receptor-2 in human skin: tissue distribution and activation of keratinocytes by mast cell tryptase. *Exp Dermatol.* (1999) 8:282–94. doi: 10.1111/j.1600-0625.1999.tb00383.x
124. Lee SE, Jeong SK, Lee SH. Protease and protease-activated receptor-2 signaling in the pathogenesis of atopic dermatitis. *Yonsei Med J.* (2010) 51:808–22. doi: 10.3349/ymj.2010.51.6.808
125. Human Microbiome Project Consortium. Structure, function and diversity of the healthy human microbiome. *Nature.* (2012) 486:207–14. doi: 10.1038/nature11234
126. Amabebe E, Anumba DOC. The vaginal microenvironment: the physiologic role of lactobacilli. *Front Med.* (2018) 5:181. doi: 10.3389/fmed.2018.00181
127. MacIntyre DA, Chandiramani M, Lee YS, Kindinger L, Smith A, Angelopoulos N, et al. The vaginal microbiome during pregnancy and the postpartum period in a European population. *Sci Rep.* (2015) 5:8988. doi: 10.1038/srep08988
128. Grice EA, Segre JA. The skin microbiome. *Nat Rev Microbiol.* (2011) 9:244–53. doi: 10.1038/nrmicro2537
129. Iwase T, Uehara Y, Shinji H, Tajima A, Seo H, Takada K, et al. Staphylococcus epidermidis Esp inhibits Staphylococcus aureus biofilm formation and nasal colonization. *Nature.* (2010) 465:346–9. doi: 10.1038/nature09074
130. Lai Y, Di Nardo A, Nakatsuji T, Leichtle A, Yang Y, Cogen AL, et al. Commensal bacteria regulate Toll-like receptor 3-dependent inflammation after skin injury. *Nat Med.* (2009) 15:1377–82. doi: 10.1038/nm.2062
131. Roan F, Obata-Ninomiya K, Ziegler SF. Epithelial cell-derived cytokines: more than just signaling the alarm. *J Clin Invest.* (2019) 129:1441–51. doi: 10.1172/JCI124606
132. Sung Kim H, Yosipovitch G. The skin microbiota and itch: is there a link? *J Clin Aesthet Dermatol.* (2020) 13:39–46. doi: 10.3390/jcm9041190
133. Corbière A, Loste A, Gaudenzio N. MRGPRX2 sensing of cationic compounds-A bridge between nociception and skin diseases? *Exp Dermatol.* (2021) 30:193–200. doi: 10.1111/exd.14222
134. Gambichler T, Skrygan M, Tigges C, Kobus S, Gläser R, Kreuter A. Significant upregulation of antimicrobial peptides and proteins in lichen sclerosus. *Br J Dermatol.* (2009) 161:1136–42. doi: 10.1111/j.1365-2133.2009.09273.x
135. Chiu IM, Heesters BA, Ghasemlou N, Von Hehn CA, Zhao F, Tran J, et al. Bacteria activate sensory neurons that modulate pain and inflammation. *Nature.* (2013) 501:52–7. doi: 10.1038/nature12479
136. Ochoa-Cortes F, Ramos-Lomas T, Miranda-Morales M, Spreadbury I, Ibeakanma C, Barajas-Lopez C, et al. Bacterial cell products signal to mouse colonic nociceptive dorsal root ganglia neurons. *Am J Physiol Gastrointest Liver Physiol.* (2010) 299:G723–32. doi: 10.1152/ajpgi.00494.2009
137. Diogenes A, Ferraz CCR, Akopian AN, Henry MA, Hargreaves KM. LPS sensitizes TRPV1 via activation of TLR4 in trigeminal sensory neurons. *J Dent Res.* (2011) 90:759–64. doi: 10.1177/0022034511400225
138. Taylor JS. Allergic contact dermatitis from doxepin cream. *Arch Dermatol.* (1996) 132:515. doi: 10.1001/archderm.1996.03890290049006
139. Bonnel RA, La Grenade L, Karwoski CB, Beitz JG. Allergic contact dermatitis from topical doxepin: food and drug administration's postmarketing surveillance experience. *J Am Acad Dermatol.* (2003) 48:294–6. doi: 10.1067/mjd.2003.46
140. Szmulowicz UM. Pruritus Ani. In: Zutshi M, editor. *Anorectal Disease: Contemporary Management*. Cham: Springer International Publishing. (2016). p. 153–87. doi: 10.1007/978-3-319-23147-1_7
141. Berth-Jones J, Takwale A, Tan E, Barclay G, Agarwal S, Ahmed I, et al. Azathioprine in severe adult atopic dermatitis: a double-blind, placebo-controlled, crossover trial. *Br J Dermatol.* (2002) 147:324–30. doi: 10.1046/j.1365-2133.2002.04989.x
142. Goujon C, Nicolas JF, Nosbaum A. Methotrexate in atopic eczema. Comments to: Consensus-based European guidelines for treatment of atopic eczema (atopic dermatitis) in adults and children: part II. *J Eur Acad Dermatol Venereol.* (2019) 33:e154–5. doi: 10.1111/jdv.15386
143. Grundmann-Kollmann M, Podda M, Ochsendorf F, Boehncke WH, Kaufmann R, Zollner TM. Mycophenolate mofetil is effective in the treatment of atopic dermatitis. *Arch Dermatol.* (2001) 137:870–3. doi: 10-1001/pubs.Arch Dermatol.-ISSN-0003-987x-137-7-dst10044
144. Jacobi A, Antoni C, Manger B, Schuler G, Hertl M. Infliximab in the treatment of moderate to severe atopic dermatitis. *J Am Acad Dermatol.* (2005) 52:522–6. doi: 10.1016/j.jaad.2004.11.022
145. Reef SE, Levine WC, McNeil MM, Fisher-Hoch S, Holmberg SD, Duerr A, et al. Treatment options for vulvovaginal candidiasis, 1993. *Clin Infect Dis.* (1995) 20(Suppl. 1):S80–90. doi: 10.1093/clinids/20.Supplement_1.S80
146. Wendel K, Rompalo A. Scabies and pediculosis pubis: an update of treatment regimens and general review. *Clin Infect Dis.* (2002) 35:S146–51. doi: 10.1086/342102
147. Paek SC, Merritt DF, Mallory SB. Pruritus vulvae in prepubertal children. *J Am Acad Dermatol.* (2001) 44:795–802. doi: 10.1067/mjd.2001.112578
148. Fishman SM, Caneris OA, Stojanovic MP, Borsook D. Intravenous lidocaine for treatment-resistant pruritus. *Am J Med.* (1997) 102:584–5. doi: 10.1016/S0002-9343(97)00057-0
149. Bueller HA, Bernhard JD, Dubroff LM. Gabapentin treatment for brachioradial pruritus. *J Eur Acad Dermatol Venereol.* (1999) 13:227–8. doi: 10.1111/j.1468-3083.1999.tb00890.x
150. Trivedi MK, Woodruff CM, Kornik R, Botto N. Patch testing in vulvar allergic contact dermatitis. *Dermatitis.* (2018) 29:95–6. doi: 10.1097/DER.0000000000000345
151. Ehlers A, Stangier U, Gieler U. Treatment of atopic dermatitis: a comparison of psychological and dermatological approaches to relapse prevention. *J Consult Clin Psychol.* (1995) 63:624–35. doi: 10.1037/0022-006X.63.4.624
152. Zhong CS, Elmariah SB. Phototherapy for itch. *Dermatol Clin.* (2020) 38:145–55. doi: 10.1016/j.det.2019.08.008
153. Rivard J, Lim HW. Ultraviolet phototherapy for pruritus. *Dermatol Ther.* (2005) 18:344–54. doi: 10.1111/j.1529-8019.2005.00032.x
154. von Kobyletzki G, Pieck C, Hoffmann K, Freitag M, Altmeyer P. Medium-dose UVA1 cold-light phototherapy in the treatment of severe atopic dermatitis. *J Am Acad Dermatol.* (1999) 41:931–7. doi: 10.1016/S0190-9622(99)70249-5
155. Reynolds NJ, Franklin V, Gray JC, Diffey BL, Farr PM. Narrow-band ultraviolet B and broad-band ultraviolet A phototherapy in adult atopic eczema: a randomised controlled trial. *Lancet.* (2001) 357:2012–6. doi: 10.1016/S0140-6736(00)05114-X
156. Narbutt J, Olejniczak I, Sobolewska-Sztychny D, Sysa-Jedrzejowska A, Słowik-Kwiatkowska I, Hawro T, et al. Narrow band ultraviolet B irradiations cause alteration in interleukin-31 serum level in psoriatic patients. *Arch Derm Res.* (2013) 305:191–5. doi: 10.1007/s00403-012-1293-6

3

The 12-Item Pruritus Severity Scale – Determining the Severity Bands

Katarzyna Stępień[†] *and Adam Reich*[*†]

Department of Dermatology, Institute of Medical Sciences, Medical College of Rzeszow University, Rzeszów, Poland

***Correspondence:**
Adam Reich
adamandrzejreich@gmail.com

[†]*These authors have contributed equally to this work*

Introduction: Assessment of pruritus still remains a challenge due to its subjective character. Various itch questionnaires are widely used to evaluate the severity of pruritus. The aim of the current study was to define the cut off values for the 12-Item Pruritus Severity Scale (12-PSS).

Methods: A total of 240 patients (86 males and 154 females) in the age between 19 and 87 years (mean 52.9 ± 20.7 years) suffering from pruritic dermatological conditions were asked to assess their maximal pruritus with the 12-PSS, the Verbal Rating Scale (VRS) and the Numerical Rating Scale (NRS). All subjects also completed the Dermatology Life Quality Index (DLQI). VRS, NRS, and DLQI scorings were used as anchor measures to define cut-offs of 12-PSS.

Results: According to VRS, 43 (17.9%) patients suffered from mild, 96 (40%) from moderate, 65 (27.1%) from severe and 36 (15%) from very severe pruritus. Mean 12-PSS scoring for each VRS category was 7.6 ± 3.9, 10.4 ± 3.9, 13.0 ± 3.8, and 13.9 ± 3.8 points, respectively ($p < 0.001$). Each VRS category significantly differed from the others regarding the mean 12-PSS scoring, except the mean scoring of severe and very severe pruritus ($p = 0.72$). Thus, three pruritus severity categories of 12-PSS were defined with following score ranges: mild pruritus–3–6 points of 12-PSS, moderate pruritus–7–11 points of 12-PSS and severe pruritus–12–22 points of 12-PSS based on calculation of weighted κ coefficient against VRS, NRS, and DLQI as anchor measures.

Conclusions: The 12-PSS is able to differentiate between patients suffering from mild, moderate, and severe pruritus.

Keywords: itch, measurement, questionnaire, validation, pruritus

INTRODUCTION

Pruritus is a subjective sensation which causes a desire to scratch. It is a common symptom of many dermatological as well as non-dermatological conditions. However, due to its subjective nature, its objective assessment, both in clinical trials as well as in routine daily practice, still remains a challenge (1). Among various methods of pruritus assessments, unidimensional scales, and itch questionnaires are most commonly used (1). The Special Interest Group (SIG) on itch questionnaires of the International Forum on the Study of Itch (IFSI) provided recommendations on the dimensions which should be addressed in an itch questionnaire in order to properly assess pruritus (2).

Recently, our group has developed the 12-Item Pruritus Severity Scale (12-PSS), which has been shown to be a valid and reliable assessment tool for patients suffering from dermatological itch (3). This questionnaire was validated in a group of 148 Polish patients with chronic pruritic dermatoses. It has also been successfully used by other researchers in patients with post-burn pruritus and uremic pruritus, indicating that the 12-PSS may also be applied in other pruritus types (4). As mentioned by Almeida et al. (5), the 12-PSS is probably not as specific as the 5-D itch scale for itch distribution, but it has the advantage of incorporating extent and consequences of scratching along with numerous aspects of quality of life. In a recent systematic review on itch questionnaires by Dominick et al., the 12-PSS was indicated as covering several dimensions of itch characteristics: localization, frequency, intensity, scratch response, affective qualities, sleep disturbances, and quality of life (6). In order to provide more data on the 12-PSS validity and give more information on interpretability of this scale we performed a study to define the cut off values for the 12-PSS.

MATERIALS AND METHODS

Patients

Overall, 336 patients were asked to participate in this prospective study. Fifteen (4.5%) patients did not agree to participate, and further 81 (24.1%) individuals, after initial approval, were found not to have pruritus and subsequently were excluded from the study. Finally, a total of 240 subjects were included into this research projects. All active participants signed a written informed consent before any procedures related to the study.

The final analysis group consisted of 154 (64.2%) females and 86 (35.8%) males aged between 19 and 87 years (mean 50.6 ± 16.3 years). They suffered from psoriasis (n = 45, 18.7%), atopic dermatitis (AD) (n = 27, 11.2%), lichen planus (n = 61, 25.4%), cutaneous lupus erythematosus (CLE) (n = 79, 32.9%), eczema (n = 10, 4.2%), or other pruritic dermatoses (n = 18, 7.5%). All subjects suffered from pruritus for at least 6 week, i.e., they were all considered as having chronic pruritus of dermatological subtype.

Study Design

All included patients were asked to assess their pruritus according to several methods in following order: the 5-point Verbal Rating Scale (VRS), the Numeric Rating Scale (NRS) (7, 8), and 12-PSS (3). The 12-PSS is a one-page instrument assessing different aspects of pruritus. The items are grouped into five domains: pruritus intensity, pruritus extent, frequency and duration of pruritus, impact of pruritus on daily activities and mood, and assessment of scratching (3). Patients evaluated their worst peak pruritus within 24 h before entering the study using VRS and NRS. Patients used the following descriptions within VRS: none, mild, moderate, severe, and very severe pruritus which were next translated into scores from 0 to 4. With NRS patients scored their pruritus from 0 (no pruritus) to 10 (worst imaginable pruritus), while with 12-PSS participants answered 12 questions referring to their pruritus and the total scoring ranged from 3 (the lowest pruritus intensity) to 22 points (the highest pruritus intensity). In addition, 202 patients completed the validated Polish version of the Dermatology Life Quality Index (DLQI) to assess their health-related quality of life (9). The scoring ranged from 0 (no impact of the disease on QoL) to 30 points (the worst impact of the disease on QoL). The study was accepted by Bioethics' Committee of Local Physician Chamber in Rzeszów, Poland.

Statistical Analysis

All data were analyzed statistically using Statistica 12.0 (Statsoft, Kraków, Poland). Mean values, standard deviations, minimal, and maximal values, as well as frequencies, were calculated. Paired and unpaired Student's t-test, χ^2 test with Yates correction, analysis of variance (ANOVA) with Scheffé's *post hoc* test and Spearman's rank correlation test were used where appropriate. The weighted κ coefficient of agreement was calculated for VRS, NRS, DLQI, and various sets of bands of 12-PSS total scores. The following assumptions regarding κ coefficient were made: <0 no agreement, 0–0.2—slight, 0.21–0.4—fair, 0.41–0.6—moderate, 0.61–0.8—substantial, and 0.81–1—almost perfect agreement. $P < 0.05$ were considered significant.

RESULTS

Pruritus Intensity

According to VRS, 43 (17.9%) patients assessed their pruritus as mild, 96 (40%) as moderate, 65 (27.1%) as severe, and remaining 36 (15%) as very severe one. The mean pruritus intensity according to NRS was 5.9 ± 2.4 points (range 1–10 points) and according to 12-PSS: 11.1 ± 4.4 points (range 3–22 points; **Table 1**). All scales assessing pruritus intensity significantly correlated between themselves (VRS and NRS: $\rho = 0.92$, $p < 0.001$; VRS and 12-PSS: $\rho = 0.49$, $p < 0.001$; NRS and 12-PSS: $\rho = 0.51$, $p < 0.001$). There were no significant differences regarding pruritus intensity between males and females (**Table 1**), while considering age we observed weak, albeit significant correlation with 12-PSS indicating that older patients had slightly higher pruritus than younger individuals ($\rho = 0.15$, $p = 0.02$), however, such relationship was neither observed for VRS ($\rho = 0.07$, $p = 0.28$) nor for NRS ($\rho = 0.07$, $p = 0.28$). No significant differences were also observed between various skin diseases when itch intensity was assessed with NRS or VRS. However, using 12-PSS we found, that patients suffering from lichen planus or from CLE suffered from significantly less intense pruritus than patients with psoriasis ($p = 0.01$ and $p < 0.0001$, respectively) or AD ($p = 0.002$ and $p < 0.0001$, respectively; **Figure 1**). Patients with CLE experienced also significantly less severe pruritus than subjects with eczema ($p = 0.04$; **Figure 1**). Significant differences between various dermatoses regarding single questions of 12-PSS are demonstrated in **Supplementary Table 1**.

Considering QoL, the mean DLQI scoring was 9.9 ± 7.3 points (range 0–30 points). Based on DLQI total scoring, 15 (7.4%) individuals reported no negative influence of skin disease on their QoL, 56 (27.7%) demonstrated small effect, 51 (25.2%) moderate effect, 58 (28.7%) very large, and remaining 22 (10.9%) extremely

TABLE 1 | Pruritus severity in studied patients.

	VRS	NRS	12-PSS	DLQI
All patients	2.4 ± 0.9 (1–4)	5.9 ± 2.4 (1–10)	11.1 ± 4.4 (0–30)	9.9 ± 7.3 (3–21)
Females	2.4 ± 1.0 (1–4)	6.0 ± 2.5 (1–10)	10.7 ± 4.4 (0–30)	9.3 ± 7.2 (3–20)
Males	2.3 ± 0.9 (1–4)	5.8 ± 2.3 (1–10)	11.8 ± 4.4 (0–28)	11.2 ± 7.5 (4–21)
*p**	0.51	0.47	0.06	0.08
Psoriasis	2.3 ± 0.9 (1–4)	5.8 ± 2.3 (1–9)	13.1 ± 3.8 (3–28)	15.3 ± 7.7 (6–20)
AD	2.4 ± 1.0 (1–4)	6.0 ± 2.4 (1–10)	14.3 ± 4.4 (1–21)	11.8 ± 7.6 (5–21)
Lichen planus	2.7 ± 1.0 (1–4)	6.5 ± 2.7 (1–10)	10.2 ± 4.0 (0–22)	9.2 ± 5.9 (3–20)
CLE	2.2 ± 0.9 (1–4)	5.5 ± 2.3 (2–10)	8.5 ± 3.2 (0–30)	7.1 ± 7.0 (3–17)
Eczema	2.2 ± 1.0 (1–4)	5.3 ± 2.5 (1–9)	12.6 ± 5.1 (1–18)	11.0 ± 6.2 (7–19)
Other dermatoses	2.7 ± 0.8 (1–4)	6.3 ± 2.4 (1–10)	15.0 ± 3.3 (2–25)	13.9 ± 7.2 (5–20)
*p***	0.05	0.21	<0.001	<0.001

*AD, atopic dermatitis; CLE, cutaneous lupus erythematosus; DLQI, Dermatology Life Quality Index; NRS, Numeric Rating Scale; 12-PSS, 12-item Pruritus Severity Scale; VRS, Verbal Rating Scale; *p-values according to Student's T-test, **p-values according to analysis of variance; min-max values provided in brackets.*

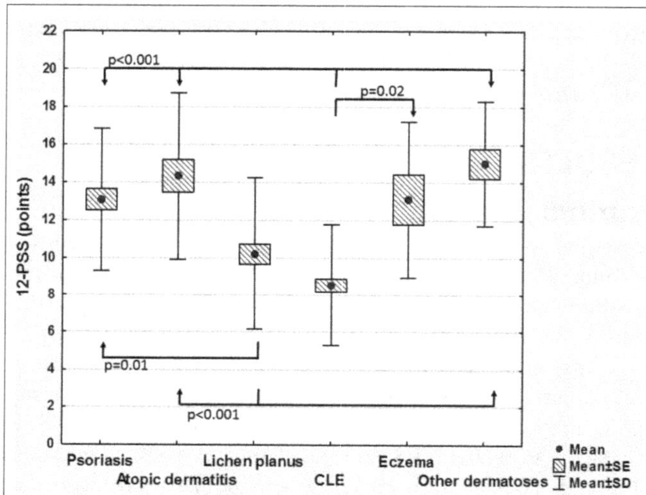

FIGURE 1 | Comparison of 12-item Pruritus Severity Scale scoring (12-PSS) between various skin diseases (CLE, cutaneous lupus erythematosus; SD, standard deviation; SE, standard error).

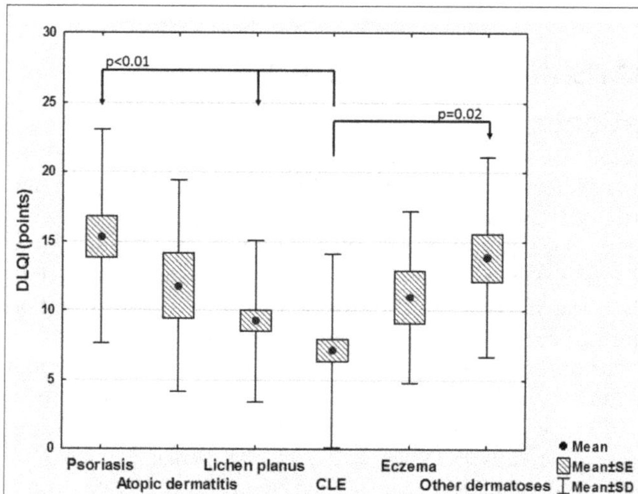

FIGURE 2 | Comparison of Dermatology Life Quality Index scoring (DLQI) between various skin diseases (CLE, cutaneous lupus erythematosus; SD, standard deviation; SE, standard error).

large effect on QoL. No significant differences regarding DLQI scoring was found between women and men (**Table 1**). However, similarly to 12-PSS, we were able to show significant differences between various skin conditions with DLQI ($p < 0.001$; **Figure 2**). DLQI total scoring also demonstrated much better correlation with 12-PSS scoring ($\rho = 0.54$) than with VRS ($\rho = 0.24, p < 0.001$) or NRS ($\rho = 0.25, p < 0.001$).

Determination of Severity Bands

To determine the cut off values for 12-PSS we have used VRS categories as anchor measures. We observed that each VRS category significantly differed from the others regarding the mean 12-PSS scoring ($p < 0.01$ for each between group comparisons), except the mean total scoring in subjects who described their pruritus as severe or very severe (13.0 ± 3.8 vs. 13.9 ± 3.8, $p = 0.72$ according to Scheffe *post hoc* test; **Figure 3**). For that reason, only three pruritus severity categories of 12-PSS were further defined, namely mild, moderate, and severe pruritus. Based on mean and median 12-PSS scores for different VRS categories, several cut off values were proposed, which were next tested with weighted kappa coefficient. Calculation of weighted kappa coefficient for VRS revealed, that two sets of 12-PSS bands best define the categories of mild, moderate and severe pruritus, namely 3–6, 7–12, and 13–22 points ($\kappa = 0.4889 \pm 0.62$, 95% CI 0.3674–0.6104), and 3–6, 7–11, and 12–22 points ($\kappa = 0.4856 \pm 0.622$, 95%CI 0.3638–0.6074; **Supplementary Table 2**). To further elaborate, which set of bands should be chosen for future interpretation of 12-PSS scoring, we have also compared the predefined 12-PSS cut-offs with NRS (**Supplementary Table 3**) and DLQI (**Supplementary Table 4**) (10, 11). With both anchor measures following scoring: 3–6, 7–11, and 12–22 points defined better mild, moderate and severe pruritus ($\kappa = 0.5339 \pm$

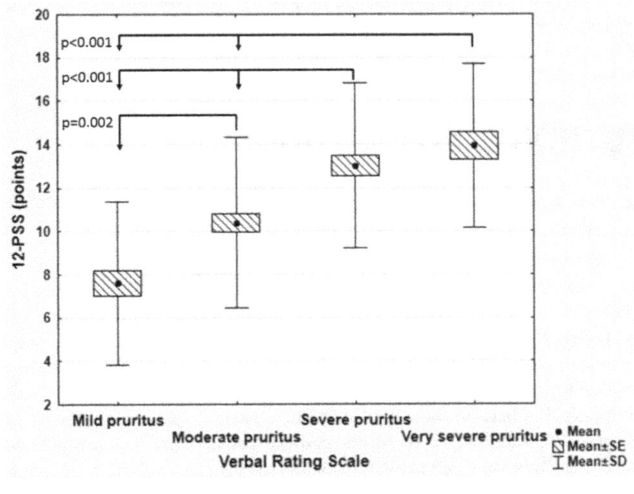

FIGURE 3 | Comparison of 12-item Pruritus Severity Scale scoring (12-PSS) between various categories of the Verbal Rating Scale (SD, standard deviation; SE, standard error).

0.0673, 95%CI: 0.402–0.6658 for NRS, and $\kappa = 0.4115 \pm 0.0633$, 95%CI: 0.2875–0.5355 for DLQI) than 3–6, 7–12, and 13–22 points ($\kappa = 0.5188 \pm 0.0675$, 95%CI: 0.3865–0.6511 for NRS, and $\kappa = 0.4098 \pm 0.0641$, 95%CI: 0.2842–0.5354 for DLQI) (**Supplementary Tables 3, 4**). The proposed set of bands (3–6, 7–11, and 12–22 points) also showed the highest correlation coefficients with VRS, NRS categories, and DLQI categories than any other tested grouping of 12-PSS scoring (**Supplementary Table 5**).

DISCUSSION

The 12-PSS consists of 12 questions, that assess different aspects of pruritus. The items are grouped into several domains related to pruritus: intensity, extent, frequency and duration of pruritus, impact of pruritus on daily activities, and mood and scratching assessment as a response to pruritus (3). As already suggested, 12-PSS is able to catch a more complex influence of pruritus on patient well-being than the Visual Analog Scale, VRS or NRS (6). Our previous study also demonstrated, that 12-PSS shows strong internal consistency, satisfactory convergent validity, as well as does not have a significant ceiling or bottom effect (3). Our current study also documented that 12-PSS is characterized by significant discriminative validity, as it enabled us to find marked differences regarding pruritus severity between various dermatoses. Remarkably, such differences could not be detected with VRS or NRS. Similarly, 12-PSS scoring demonstrated significant correlation with patients' age suggesting that older people may experience slightly more intense pruritus than younger individuals, a finding which could not be observed with VRS or NRS. Again, these findings may support the suggestion, that 12-PSS is able to assess broader aspects of the perception of pruritus intensity by particular patients (6, 12). In addition, results demonstrated by Samhan and Abdelhalim (4) indicated that 12-PSS shows also good responsiveness. These authors have used 12-PSS in patients with burn to assess the impact of low-energy extracorporeal shockwave therapy on pruritus and observed, that the post-treatment improvement of 12-PSS scoring was significantly greater in the study group than in the placebo group (scoring change of 5.9 points in treated patients vs. 1.8 points in control group, $p < 0.001$) (4).

In our current study we have focused on defining the grouping of 12-PSS scoring to provide more data on the interpretability of 12-PSS. Based on calculation of the weighted κ coefficient for different predefined sets of 12-PSS bands against various anchor parameters, we have proposed following 12-PSS scoring in relation to pruritus severity: mild pruritus—3–6 points, moderate pruritus—7–11 points, and severe pruritus—$\geq$12 points. Such score grouping also showed the best correlations with VRS, NRS and DLQI categories. We do hope, that providing the cut offs value of 12-PSS, it will encourage other clinicians and researchers to use this scale more commonly, both in clinical practice as well as for scientific purposes.

However, we also have to mention some limitations of our results. First of all, we have defined the cut off values of 12-PSS only in patients with dermatological pruritus. It is unknown, if the same grouping can be employed for other pruritus subtypes or maybe the scoring should be interpreted in different way. Thus, physicians should use proposed scoring with caution when assessing patients with pruritus subtype other than a dermatological one, and further studies are needed to confirm that proposed set of bands is valid for patients with other pruritus types. As in our study we have analyzed only dermatological patients with pruritus concomitant to skin disorders, we have decided to evaluate QoL impairment with DLQI because this scale is widely used giving the possibility to compare our results with other authors, consists of only 10 questions, and the QoL impairment categories are well-defined. However, when assessing other pruritus subtypes, ItchyQol, an itch-specific QoL measure, would probably be more suitable (13). Nevertheless, it was shown, that DLQI scoring is strongly correlated with ItchyQol scoring (14), suggesting that at least in dermatological condition both scales may be used interchangeably and the use of DLQI in group of patients should not be considered as detrimental. Another aspects is the application of our results to other patient populations and to other languages. To date the questionnaire is available in following languages: English, Turkish, Persian, and Kannada. However, answers to questionnaire items may vary according to languages and current cut-offs, which were defined only using Polish version of 12-PSS, should be applied to another language versions with a great caution. Finally, we have to underline, that we assessed pruritus only once. It would be quite interesting to check, if the evaluation and interpretation of pruritus with 12-PSS changes over time with repeated assessments.

Despite the above mentioned limitations, we do believe that our results are convincing and provide a valid grouping of 12-PSS scoring. We hope, that giving a clear indication, how to interpret the results achieved with 12-PSS we will encourage other physicians and researchers to use this scale more commonly in their routine clinical and scientific work.

Nevertheless, further studies are needed to confirm our results in various patient groups.

ETHICS STATEMENT

The studies involving human participants were reviewed and approved by Komisja Bioetyczna at Okręgowej Izbie Lekarskiej in Rzeszów. The patients/participants provided their written informed consent to participate in this study.

AUTHOR CONTRIBUTIONS

All authors listed have made a substantial, direct and intellectual contribution to the work, and approved it for publication.

REFERENCES

1. Ständer S, Augustin M, Reich A, Blome C, Ebata T, Phan NQ, et al. Pruritus assessment in clinical trials: consensus recommendations from the International forum for the study of Itch (IFSI) special interest group scoring itch in clinical trials. *Acta Derm Venereol.* (2013) 93:509–14. doi: 10.2340/00015555-1620
2. Weisshaar E, Gieler U, Kupfer J, Furue M, Saeki H, Yosipovitch G, et al. Questionnaires to assess chronic itch: a consensus paper of the special interest group of the International forum on the study of itch. *Acta Derm Venereol.* (2012) 92:493–6. doi: 10.2340/00015555-1402
3. Reich A, Bozek A, Janiszewska K, Szepietowski JC. 12-Item Pruritus Severity Scale: development and validation of new itch severity questionnaire. *Biomed Res Int.* (2017) 2017:3896423. doi: 10.1155/2017/3896423
4. Samhan AF, Abdelhalim NM. Impacts of low-energy extracorporeal shockwave therapy on pain, pruritus, and health-related quality of life in patients with burn: a randomized placebo-controlled study. *Burns.* (2019) 45:1094–101. doi: 10.1016/j.burns.2019.02.007
5. Almeida V, Constante D, Leite A, Almeida IF, Rocha JC, Sá R, et al. Influence of disease phase on embitterment and emotional dysregulation in psoriatic patients. *Psychol Health Med.* (2020) 29:1–18. doi: 10.1080/13548506.2020.1741655
6. Dominick F, van Laarhoven A, Evers AWM, Weisshaar E. A systematic review of questionnaires on itch by the special interest group "Questionnaires" of the International forum for the study of itch (IFSI). *Itch.* (2019) 4:e26. doi: 10.1097/itx.0000000000000026
7. Phan NQ, Blome C, Fritz F, Gerss J, Reich A, Ebata T, et al. Assessment of pruritus intensity: prospective study on validity and reliability of the visual analogue scale, numerical rating scale and verbal rating scale in 471 patients with chronic pruritus. *Acta Derm Venereol.* (2012) 92:502–7. doi: 10.2340/00015555-1246
8. Reich A, Heisig M, Phan NQ, Taneda K, Takamori K, Takeuchi S, et al. Visual analogue scale: evaluation of the instrument for the assessment of pruritus. *Acta Derm Venereol.* (2012) 92:497–501. doi: 10.2340/00015555-1265
9. Finlay AY, Khan GK. Dermatology life quality index (DLQI) – a simple practical measure for routine clinical use. *Clin Exp Dermatol.* (1994) 19:210–6. doi: 10.1111/j.1365-2230.1994.tb01167.x
10. Reich A, Chatzigeorkidis E, Zeidler C, Osada N, Furue M, Takamori K, et al. Tailoring the cut-off values of the visual analogue scale and numeric rating scale in itch assessment. *Acta Derm Venereol.* (2017) 97:759–60. doi: 10.2340/00015555-2642
11. Hongbo Y, Thomas CL, Harrison MA, Salek MS, Finlay AY. Translating the science of quality of life into practice: what do dermatology life quality index scores mean? *J Invest Dermatol.* (2005) 125:659–64. doi: 10.1111/j.0022-202X.2005.23621.x
12. Rehman IU Khan TM. Epidemiology of chronic kidney diseases (CKD) in Malaysia and Pakistan, pathophysiology of CKD-associated pruritus and other CKD-associated dermatological disorders. *Prog Microbes Mol Biol.* (2020) 3:a0000063. doi: 10.36877/pmmb.a0000063
13. Zeidler C, Steinke S, Riepe C, Bruland P, Soto-Rey I, Storck M, et al. Cross-European validation of the ItchyQoL in pruritic dermatoses. *J Eur Acad Dermatol Venereol.* (2019) 33:391–7. doi: 10.1111/jdv.15225
14. Stumpf A, Pfleiderer B, Fritz F, Osada N, Chen SC, Ständer S. Assessment of quality of life in chronic pruritus: relationship between ItchyQoL and dermatological life quality index in 1,150 patients. *Acta Derm Venereol.* (2018) 98:142–3. doi: 10.2340/00015555-2782

4

Interleukin-31 as a Clinical Target for Pruritus Treatment

Kenji Kabashima and Hiroyuki Irie*

Department of Dermatology, Graduate School of Medicine, Kyoto University, Kyoto, Japan

Correspondence:
Kenji Kabashima
kaba@kuhp.kyoto-u.ac.jp

In recent years, the published literature has suggested the key involvement of the cytokine interleukin-31 (IL-31) in the symptomatology of pruritus, and both IL-31 and its receptor have become potential therapeutic targets for a range of pruritic diseases. Elevated levels of IL-31 or its receptor have been reported in the tissue or serum of patients with pruritic skin diseases, such as atopic dermatitis, prurigo nodularis, and psoriasis. Pruritus places a heavy burden on patients, and can have a negative impact on daily life, sleep, and mental health. Since current anti-pruritic treatments are often ineffective, affected patients are in urgent need of new therapies. As a result, drug development targeting the IL-31 pathway is evolving rapidly. To date, only nemolizumab, a humanized monoclonal antibody targeting the IL-31 receptor, has successfully completed late-stage clinical studies. This article will highlight our current clinical understanding of the role of IL-31 in pruritic disease, and explore recent progress in drug development as well as the anticipated future advances in this field.

Keywords: interleukin-31, interleukin-31 receptor, pruritus, itch, anti-IL-31, anti-IL-31RA, nemolizumab

INTRODUCTION

The T-cell-derived cytokine interleukin-31 (IL-31) was first identified in 2004 (1). Investigation in animal models suggested a role for IL-31 in the cutaneous and epithelial signs and symptoms observed in pruritus, skin inflammation, and airway hypersensitivity (1). Overexpression of IL-31 has been shown to be associated with promotion of sensory neuronal outgrowth (2) and stimulation (3), providing increased sensitivity to minimal itch-inducing stimuli which can result in sustained pruritus. Expression of IL-31 in skin is also associated with a profound repression of the filaggrin protein, which is critical in the differentiation of keratinocytes and skin barrier maintenance (4).

The receptor for IL-31 is a heterodimeric complex composed of IL-31 receptor A (IL-31RA) and the oncostatin M receptor (OSMR) (1, 5); the binding of IL-31 to its receptor activates cell signaling pathways including Jak/STAT, PI3K/AKT, and MAPK (5). In keratinocytes, IL-31 has been shown to induce cell cycle arrest, resulting in reduced proliferation, which in turn leads to atypical skin development, defects, and barrier dysfunction (4) (**Figure 1**). In other organs and physiologic systems, IL-31 has been linked to hematopoiesis and regulation of the immune response (5).

The recent published literature from both preclinical and clinical studies has suggested the key involvement of IL-31 in the symptomatology of acute and chronic pruritus (6–9). The objectives of this article are to highlight our current clinical understanding of the role of IL-31 in pruritic diseases, and explore recent progress in drug development and the anticipated future advances in this field. Itching is a symptom that greatly impairs quality of life, and is often not well-controlled with current treatments (10, 11). In addition to the induction of itch,

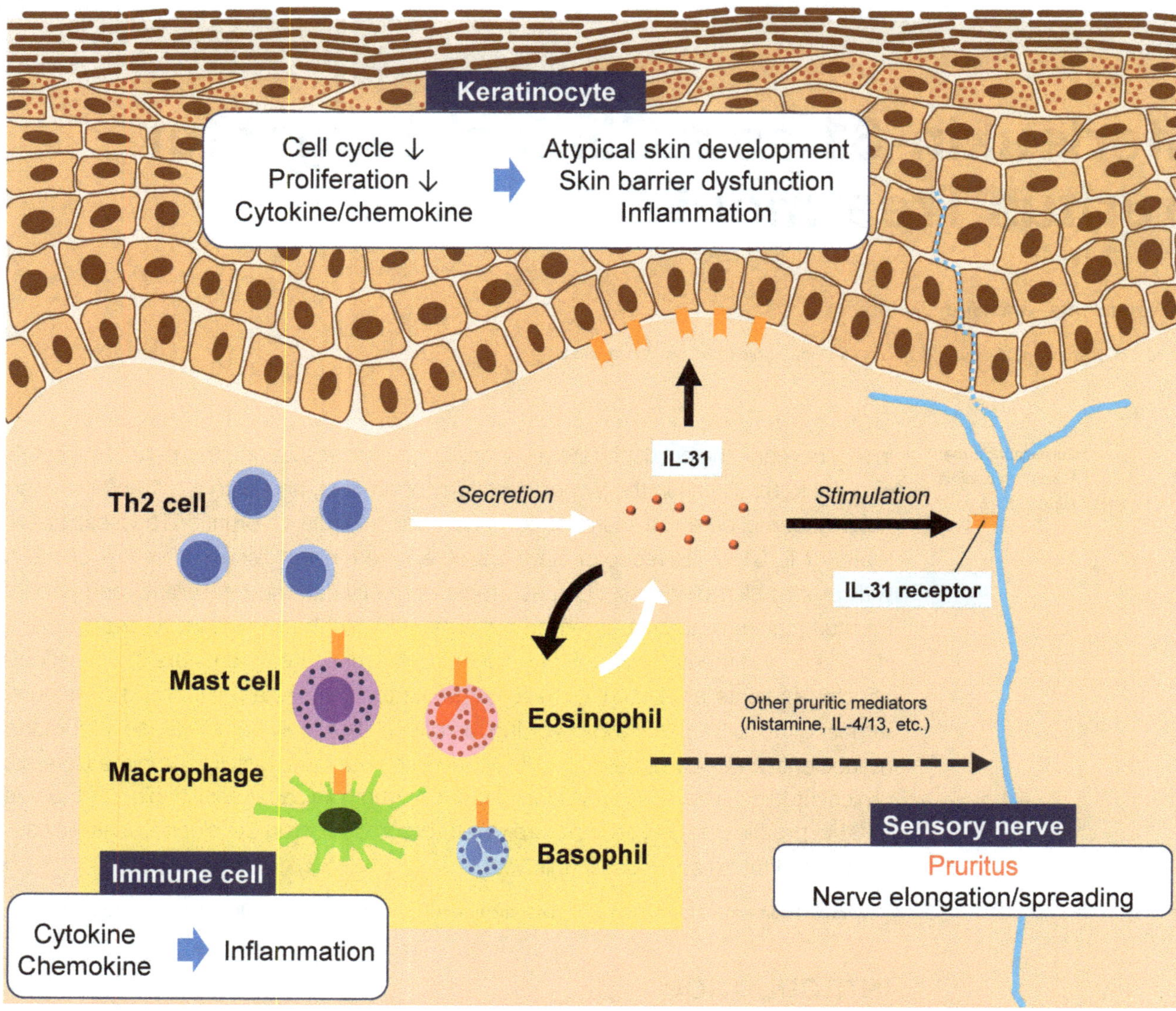

FIGURE 1 | Illustration of the hypothesized roles of interleukin (IL)-31 in pruritic skin diseases. IL-31 is primarily produced by T helper 2 (Th2) cells, although other innate immune cells can also produce IL-31. The IL-31 receptor is widely expressed by various cell types, including peripheral sensory nerves, epidermal keratinocytes, and immune cells. IL-31 binding to its receptor on sensory neurons stimulates the nerve, causing pruritus. IL-31 is also involved skin barrier dysfunction and inflammation.

the IL-31 pathway also stimulates the release of inflammatory mediators and reduces the expression of molecules involved in the skin barrier, resulting in additional skin signs and symptoms (4, 12–14). As a result, both IL-31 and its receptor have become potential therapeutic targets for a range of pruritic diseases (14–18).

THE BURDEN OF PRURITUS

Itch is the most common complaint among patients who attend dermatology clinics, and for many patients, pruritic symptoms are intractable despite medication (19). In one study, 90% of patients with chronic skin diseases reported that they had experienced pruritus, and that the intensity of itch was related to impairment in several areas of daily life, including sleep quality, work productivity, and mental health (20).

Patient Burden

Chronic pruritus has been shown to be as debilitating as chronic pain in terms of its impact on quality of life, with more severe itch having a more profound negative effect on daily life (21). In a recent study of 132 North American adults with chronic pruritus, health performance was found to be significantly reduced compared with normative controls ($p < 0.001$) (22). In a cross-sectional study of 602 US adults with atopic dermatitis, the most burdensome symptom was reported to be itch (54.4%), and severe itch scores (measured using the patient-oriented scoring atopic dermatitis-itch scale) were associated with poor mental health scores (23). Suicidal ideation has been reported to be highly prevalent in patients with chronic pruritus (20), and several studies have shown that patients with pruritus are more likely to have anxiety and depression compared with non-pruritic controls (20, 24, 25).

Pruritus also impairs sleep quality (20, 26–28), likely due to both the effects of scratching and underlying systemic inflammation (29). In one analysis, chronic pruritic dermatoses were found to be associated with increased nighttime awakenings (odds ratio 1.329–1.646) (30), while another study of patients with psoriasis found that pruritus significantly increased the difficulty of falling asleep ($p = 0.031$) (27). Thus, treatments for pruritus that can also improve sleep and quality of life are urgently needed.

Economic Burden

A study in North American adults calculated that chronic pruritus was associated with a mean of −5.5 quality-adjusted life-years per patient, which translated into an individual lifetime economic burden of US$275, and a societal burden of almost US$90 billion (22). Another study calculated median annualized costs of chronic pruritus of US$1067 per patient (31). In addition to the costs of clinic consultations, referrals, laboratory tests, and prescription medication (32), the scratching behavior associated with pruritus may be associated with skin breakdown and increased infection, resulting in increased direct medical costs from attendance at emergency departments and hospitalization (33, 34). Indirect costs associated with pruritus include reduced work or school productivity (absenteeism and presenteeism), over-the-counter treatments, and the time required to apply topical agents or perform other self-treatment (31).

IL-31 IN DISEASE

In the past few years, an increasing number of researchers have postulated a link between IL-31 and the manifestations of various diseases, both dermatologic and non-dermatologic (5, 14, 17, 35). In addition to the development of itch (12), dysregulation of IL-31 and its receptor is thought to underlie alterations in the skin barrier (thickening or breakdown) (13), as well as auto-immune and inflammatory signs and symptoms (14). Individual diseases, and the putative role(s) of IL-31 in these disorders, are summarized below.

Atopic Dermatitis

In preclinical studies, mice treated with IL-31 exhibited skin lesions and scratching behavior similar to those seen in atopic dermatitis (1, 18, 36), and treatments targeting IL-31 were found to reduce scratching (37, 38). In clinical studies, levels of serum IL-31 have been found to be elevated in patients with atopic dermatitis, compared with healthy individuals (39–41), and decreased after cyclosporin treatment (42); furthermore, IL-31 levels were shown to correlate with disease severity and pruritic symptoms (39–41).

IL-31 receptors are expressed constitutively on the surface of keratinocytes, eosinophils and small diameter neurons (43). Keratinocyte levels of IL-31RA expressed in atopic dermatitis lesions have been shown to be higher than those of normal skin in healthy subjects (44, 45), while no difference in levels of OSMR has been observed (44), emphasizing the greater importance of IL-31RA in the pathogenesis of the disease.

Prurigo Nodularis

Prurigo nodularis, a chronic disease presenting as one or more hyperkeratotic papules which are intensely pruritic, results in a difficult to treat itch-scratch cycle, and causes sleep disturbances and psychiatric comorbidities in affected patients (46). An analysis of skin samples from patients with various chronic inflammatory skin diseases revealed that the highest levels of IL-31 were located in lesional skin from individuals with prurigo nodularis, with an elevation of IL-31 mRNA almost 50-fold higher than that of skin from healthy individuals (47).

Psoriasis

Like atopic dermatitis, psoriasis is an inflammatory skin disease affecting millions of people worldwide, and can have a negative impact on the mental health and quality of life of patients (48). A role for IL-31 in the pathogenesis of psoriasis has been suggested (49), with elevated levels of serum IL-31 observed in psoriatic patients compared with controls (8). Patients with early-onset psoriasis have greater levels of Il-31 gene induction compared with healthy controls, and even compared with patients with atopic dermatitis (50). However, the data are inconsistent; other studies have failed to show elevated levels of IL-31 in psoriasis (51), or any association between IL-31 and pruritus intensity in psoriatic patients (52).

Cutaneous T-Cell Lymphoma (CTCL)

CTCL comprises a heterogeneous group of diseases arising from the T cells involved in tumor responses (53). Most patients (around 88%) with CTCL are affected by pruritus (54), and studies have demonstrated elevated levels of IL-31, IL-31RA, and OSMRβ within the epidermis of affected patients (54), as well as increased serum IL-31 levels (55, 56). In one analysis, levels of IL-31 mRNA appeared to be correlated with the severity of pruritus in CTCL patients (57), although data from another study did not support this contention (58). It has been hypothesized that IL-31 may induce epidermal neoplastic T cells and keratinocytes to transmit itch, indirectly affecting sensory nerves (54). Although IL-31 appears to have a role in pruritus in CTCL, there is conflicting evidence as to whether it plays a larger role in the pathogenesis of CTCL itself (56, 58, 59). However, of note, chronic prurigo has also been reported in cases of Hodgkin lymphoma (HL) (60), and a study in HL patients demonstrated elevated IL-31 in HL cells and in the immune cells infiltrating affected lymph nodes (61). Another recent study showed that plasma concentrations of IL-31 decreased in HL patients entering remission (62); taken together, these findings suggest that IL-31 may contribute to immune suppression in HL, and may indicate a similar role in CTCL.

Other Pruritic Disorders

Uremic Pruritus

Uremic pruritus occurs in patients with chronic kidney disease, and is characterized by intractable systemic itching, often without any other obvious cutaneous symptoms (63, 64). IL-31 may play a role in the development and maintenance of uremic pruritus in patients receiving hemodialysis (65). In a study of 178 hemodialysis patients, significantly higher levels of IL-31 were recorded in patients with pruritic symptoms compared with those without ($p = 0.04$) (66).

Cholestatic Pruritus

The development of cholestatic pruritus, which is found in patients with primary biliary cirrhosis, primary sclerosing cholangitis, and intrahepatic cholestasis of pregnancy (ICP) (67, 68), may also be linked to an elevation in levels of IL-31. In a small-scale study, median levels of serum IL-31 were found to be significantly higher in 13 pregnant women with ICP than in the control group of 26 pregnant women without ICP ($p = 0.004$); in addition, levels of IL-31 showed a direct correlation with liver transaminase levels (68). Of note, the IL-31 pathway has also been reported to be involved in the pathogenesis of hepatitis B virus-related liver cirrhosis (69), potentially suggesting a wider role for IL-31 in hepatic health.

Bullous Pemphigoid and Chronic Urticaria

In autoimmune skin diseases, such as bullous pemphigoid and chronic urticaria, IL-31 may be involved in both pruritus and immunomodulation, potentially underpinning the IgE-associated pathophysiology involved in these diseases (35). Skin (70) and serum (71) samples from patients with chronic urticaria have been shown to have high levels of IL-31, and following stimulation, basophils from normal skin also demonstrated increased IL-31 expression, resulting in the release of pro-inflammatory cytokines and the induction of chemotaxis (70). In bullous pemphigoid, it is eosinophils that appear to be the major source of IL-31 (72, 73). Another, related, condition in which IL-31 has been implicated is pemphigus herpetiformis (dermatitis herpetiformis) (74, 75).

Allergic Contact Dermatitis (ACD)

Around 20% of adults worldwide are affected by ACD, either as a result of sensitivity to everyday products (particularly fragrances) or via exposure to allergens within their work environment (76). A role for IL-31 in ACD has been postulated, with elevated serum levels of IL-31 found in ACD patients compared with controls (77). However, the precise details remain to be clarified, as a preclinical study has suggested that IL-31 may be associated only with pruritus, but not inflammation in contact hypersensitivity (78).

Dermatomyositis

Dermatomyositis is a chronic, inflammatory, autoimmune disease characterized by cutaneous involvement (79). Although symptoms can be heterogeneous, pruritus is a common manifestation (80). A recent analysis indicated that gene and protein expression of IL-31 and IL-31RA was increased in dermatomyositis lesions compared with non-lesional skin and normal control skin (81).

Chronic Pruritus of Unknown Origin (CPUO)

CPUO is the nomenclature used to describe the presentation of chronic itch which has no distinct etiology (82). The pathophysiology of CPUO remains unclear (10), but patients with CPUO have been shown to have elevated serum levels of IL-31 compared with healthy subjects (7). In regression analysis the presence of CPUO was found to be independently and significantly associated with serum Il-31 levels ($p < 0.001$) (7).

Other Dermatologic Conditions

Other dermatologic conditions in which IL-31/IL-31R have been implicated include lichen planus (83), cutaneous (lichen) amyloidosis (84–86), statis dermatitis (87), scleroderma (88), and the itch associated with wound healing (89). However, detailed data are lacking, and further studies are necessary to fully determine the role of IL-31 in the pathophysiology and symptomatology of each of these conditions.

Non-pruritic Diseases

Allergic Asthma

Expression of IL-31RA is tightly regulated within the various cells found in the lung (90), and *in vitro* studies have suggested IL-31-stimulation of bronchial cells results in the production of proinflammatory cytokines, growth factors, and chemokines, which could contribute to the inflammation, tissue damage and pulmonary remodeling observed in asthma (91). Studies have shown that levels of IL-31 mRNA and protein are elevated in patients with allergic asthma (92), and expression of both IL-31 and IL-31R are increased in the bronchial tissue of patients with severe asthma (93). Serum IL-31 levels were also found to positively correlate with asthma severity and IgE levels (93).

Inflammatory Bowel Disease (IBD)

Analysis of colonic biopsies from patients with Crohn's disease and ulcerative colitis found that IL-31, IL-31RA, and OSMR mRNA expression was increased in inflamed lesions compared with non-inflamed lesions (94). There has been a great deal of recent interest in the possibility of targeting OSM in IBD (95), but IL-31 does not currently appear to be a drug target for this condition.

Osteoporosis

Numerous inflammatory cytokines have been demonstrated to be involved in bone remodeling, and there are both *in vitro* and clinical observations which suggest a role for IL-31 in the development of osteoporosis (96). In a study in postmenopausal females, patients with osteoporosis exhibited elevated levels of serum IL-31 compared with healthy controls ($p < 0.049$) (97). Notably, higher levels of IL-31 were associated with increased age, suggesting an association between Th2 cytokine overexpression and bone resorption in senile osteoporosis (98).

CURRENT CLINICAL STATUS OF ANTI-IL-31 THERAPIES

Since current anti-pruritic treatments are often ineffective (99, 100), affected patients are in urgent need of new therapies (101, 102). As a result, drug development targeting the IL-31 pathway is evolving rapidly. An overview is provided in **Table 1**.

Anti-IL-31

Two agents targeting IL-31 have been developed thus far, one intended for clinical use and one for veterinary use.

BMS-981164

BMS-981164 was an anti-IL-31 monoclonal antibody targeting circulating IL-31 being developed by Bristol-Myers Squibb. A two-part, phase I, single-dose, dose-escalation study was conducted between 2012 and 2015 to explore the safety and pharmacokinetic profile of BMS-981164 (NCT01614756). The study design was randomized, double-blind, placebo-controlled, and the drug was administered as both SC and IV formulations (0.01 to 3 mg/kg) to healthy volunteers (part 1) and adults with atopic dermatitis (part 2). Adult subjects in part 2 were required to have at least moderate atopic dermatitis (assessed by Physician Global Assessment rating of ≥3 on a scale of 0 to 5) and pruritus severity of at least 7 of 10 on a visual analog scale.

To date, no results from this study have been released. As of 2016, BMS-981164 was no longer listed in the development pipeline of Bristol-Myers Squibb, and no new trials have been announced.

Lokivetmab

The amino acid sequence of IL-31 has been shown to vary across species, with the human sequence showing >80% homology with isoforms isolated from several species of monkey, but decreased similarities with canine (54%) and murine (30–31%) forms (106, 107). Despite this variation, IL-31 has been linked with the development of pruritus in multiple mammalian species (1, 106, 108).

Lokivetmab (ZTS-00103289) is a caninized IL-31 monoclonal antibody that has demonstrated efficacy in reducing pruritus in dogs, in various conditions including atopic dermatitis (109–111), and mastocytosis (112). Although not suitable for use in humans, data accruing from this agent could inform the future development of other novel anti-IL-31 therapeutic agents.

Anti-IL-31RA

To date, the only agent targeting IL-31RA is nemolizumab, a subcutaneously-administered humanized monoclonal antibody manufactured by Chugai Pharmaceutical Co., Ltd., and being developed by Maruho Co., Ltd., in Japan and Galderma SA in Europe and the US (106, 113). This has been the most successful strategy to date, with nemolizumab being the only agent targeting the IL-31 pathway to reach phase 3 development. In addition to its effects on pruritus, nemolizumab has also been evaluated for its effectiveness in improving sleep, daily functioning, and quality of life in patients with atopic dermatitis (103).

Nemolizumab

In early-phase clinical studies involving adults with moderate-to-severe atopic dermatitis, nemolizumab showed efficacy in reducing both pruritus and also the skin signs of atopic dermatitis (113–116). In the first in-human study, a single administration decreased pruritus, sleep disturbance, and use of topical hydrocortisone, and was well tolerated (113).

In a phase 2, double-blind, placebo-controlled, 12-week trial, adults with moderate-to-severe atopic dermatitis that was inadequately controlled by topical treatments were randomly assigned to receive subcutaneous nemolizumab (at a dose of 0.1, 0.5, or 2.0 mg/kg) or placebo every 4 weeks (Q4W), or nemolizumab 2.0 mg/kg Q8W (115). The primary end point was the percentage improvement from baseline in the score on the pruritus visual analog scale (VAS) at Week 12, and nemolizumab Q4W was shown to significantly improve pruritus at Week 12 ($p < 0.01$ for all doses vs. placebo). Adverse events occurred at similar frequencies with nemolizumab and placebo; however, more nemolizumab-treated patients reported exacerbations in atopic dermatitis and peripheral edema.

In the long-term (52-week) double-blind extension of the phase 2 study (114), the improvements in the pruritus VAS and Eczema Area and Severity Index (EASI) scores from baseline to Week 12 were maintained or increased from Week 12 to Week 64 with nemolizumab treatment. No new or late-onset safety concerns were identified. The mean decrease in Work Productivity and Activity Impairment-Atopic Dermatitis questionnaire score from baseline at Week 12 was greater in nemolizumab-treated patients compared with those receiving placebo for work productivity and ability to perform daily activities (117). Improvements were sustained through Week 64 of the study.

In a phase 2b, randomized, double-blind, placebo-controlled, dose-ranging study of 24 weeks' duration, nemolizumab produced rapid improvements in cutaneous inflammation and pruritus, which were maintained throughout the treatment period, and had an acceptable safety profile (116).

A 16-week, double-blind, phase 3 trial in patients with atopic dermatitis and moderate-to-severe pruritus and an inadequate response to topical agents was recently conducted in Japan (103). Patients were randomly assigned 2:1 to receive subcutaneous nemolizumab 60 mg or placebo Q4W plus concomitant topical corticosteroids/topical calcineurin inhibitors (TCS/TCI). The primary end point (mean percent change in pruritus VAS from baseline to week 16) was reduced by −42.8% in the nemolizumab group and −21.4% in the placebo group (difference, −21.5%; $p < 0.001$). Secondary efficacy data indicated that nemolizumab provided additional benefits to patients, with a reduction in the EASI score of −45.9% (vs. −33.2% with placebo), more patients with a score of 4 or less on the Dermatology Life Quality Index (40 vs. 22% with placebo), and more patients with a score of 7 or less on the Insomnia Severity Index (55 vs. 21% with placebo). Rates of adverse events were similar between treatment groups. Cytokine abnormalities (increased thymus and activation-regulated chemokine level) occurred in the nemolizumab group after treatment; however, there was no association with the EASI score.

TABLE 1 | Summary of anti-IL-31 therapies in development.

Agent	Target	Drug attributes	Disease	Highest development stage	Key outcomes
BMS-981164	IL-31	Monoclonal antibody, administered SC and IV	Atopic dermatitis	Phase 1	• Unknown (completed 2015 but unpublished)
Lokivetmab	IL-31	Caninized monoclonal antibody, administered SC	Canine atopic dermatitis, canine mastitis	N/A (veterinary use only)	• Reduces pruritus in dogs
Nemolizumab	IL-31RA	Humanized monoclonal antibody, administered SC	Atopic dermatitis	Phase 3 (administered with concomitant TCS/TCI) (103)	• Mean percent change in pruritus VAS from baseline to week 16: nemolizumab−42.8%, placebo−21.4% (difference, −21.5%; $p < 0.001$) • Reduction in EASI score: nemolizumab −45.9%, placebo −33.2% • Score of ≤ 4 on DLQI: nemolizumab 40%, placebo 22% • Score of ≤ 7 on ISI: nemolizumab 55%, placebo 21% • Rates of adverse events were similar between treatment groups
			Prurigo nodularis	Phase 2 (104)	• Percent change in the mean peak pruritus NRS score from baseline to week 4: nemolizumab−53.0%, placebo −20.2% (difference −32.8%; $p < 0.001$) • Similar trends observed for secondary outcomes • The overall tolerability profiles were comparable between treatment groups
Vixarelimab	OSMR	Monoclonal antibody, administered SC	Prurigo nodularis	Phase 2a (105)	• LSM change in weekly average WI-NRS from baseline at Week 8: vixarelimab−50.6%, placebo−29.4% (difference 21.1%; $p = 0.035$) • No dose-limiting AEs, no serious AEs, no atopic dermatitis flares
			Chronic pruritic diseases[a]	Phase 2 (105)	• Plaque psoriasis: LSM change in WI-NRS from baseline to Week 8: vixarelimab −66.5%, placebo −29.0% ($p = 0.012$). • Chronic idiopathic pruritus: LSM change in WI-NRS from baseline to Week 8: vixarelimab−52.4%, placebo −48.8% ($p = 0.813$). • No formal statistical analysis in lichen simplex chronicus, chronic idiopathic urticaria, and lichen planus due to small patient numbers (<5 per group) • No dose-limiting AEs

[a]Including plaque psoriasis, chronic idiopathic pruritus, lichen simplex chronicus, chronic idiopathic urticaria, or lichen planus.
AE, adverse event; DLQI, dermatology life quality index; EASI, eczema area and severity index; IL-31, interleukin-31; IL-31RA, interleukin 31 receptor A; ISI, insomnia severity index; IV, intravenously; LSM, least squares mean; N/A, not applicable; NRS, numeric rating scale; OSMR, oncostatin M receptor; SC, subcutaneously; TCS/TCI, topical corticosteroids/topical calcineurin inhibitors; VAS, visual analog scale; WI-NRS, worst-itch numeric rating scale.

Nemolizumab has also demonstrated efficacy in the reduction of pruritus in patients with moderate-to-severe prurigo nodularis and severe pruritus (104). A 12-week, randomized, double-blind, placebo-controlled, phase 2 trial of nemolizumab 0.5 mg/kg administered at baseline, week 4, and week 8 was conducted. The primary outcome (percent change from baseline in the mean peak score for pruritus on the numeric rating scale at week 4) was reduced by −53.0% with nemolizumab vs.−20.2% in the placebo group (difference −32.8%; $p < 0.001$). Secondary outcomes followed the same trend as the primary outcome. Nemolizumab was associated with gastrointestinal symptoms (abdominal pain and diarrhea; 21% vs. placebo 14%) and musculoskeletal symptoms (18% vs. placebo 14%); however, the overall tolerability profile was comparable with that of placebo and only 2 patients in each group discontinued treatment due to adverse events.

Anti-OSMR

Although modulation of the oncostatin M receptor is potentially of clinical interest, to date, only one drug which directly targets OSMR has been evaluated in clinical trials, and few published details are available.

Vixarelimab (KPL-716)

Vixarelimab is a monoclonal antibody being developed for the treatment pf prurigo nodularis by Kiniksa Pharmaceuticals Corp; it simultaneously targets both the OSMRβ, which mediates signaling of IL-31, and the oncostatin M pathways (105). It is subcutaneously administered as a loading dose of 720 mg followed by weekly injections of 360 mg.

In a randomized, double-blind, placebo-controlled phase 2a clinical trial of vixarelimab in 49 patients with prurigo nodularis, vixarelimab met its primary efficacy endpoint of the reduction in weekly average Worst-Itch Numeric Rating Scale (WI-NRS)

from baseline at Week 8. At Week 8, the least squares mean change from baseline in weekly average WI-NRS was−50.6% in the vixarelimab treatment group compared with −29.4% in the placebo group (mean difference 21.1%; $p = 0.035$).

In an exploratory phase 2 study, the efficacy of vixarelimab was evaluated in patients with other chronic pruritic diseases, including plaque psoriasis, chronic idiopathic pruritus, lichen simplex chronicus, chronic idiopathic urticaria, or lichen planus. In the plaque psoriasis cohort, the least squares mean change in WI-NRS from baseline to Week 8 was −66.5% in the vixarelimab group and −29.0% in the placebo group ($p = 0.012$). In the chronic idiopathic pruritus cohort, the changes were−52.4% with vixarelimab and−48.8% with placebo ($p = 0.813$). Due to small numbers of patients (<5 per group) with lichen simplex chronicus, chronic idiopathic urticaria, and lichen planus, no formal statistical analysis was performed, but the data were reported to show an encouraging effect of treatment.

In both studies, vixarelimab was said to be well-tolerated, with no dose-limiting adverse events; moreover, no serious adverse events or atopic dermatitis flares were noted in the phase 2a study. However, to date, the only available information has been provided on the manufacturer website (105); no publications are available and the data have not been peer-reviewed. In addition, no phase 3 studies have yet been planned.

DISCUSSION

Pruritus affects patients of all ages, races, and sex, and can have an extremely negative impact on their quality of life (118). Given that many patients are refractory to available treatments (99, 100), it is important to develop new drugs to improve clinical and social outcomes.

Based on its roles in the development of itch, skin deficits, and inflammation (4, 12–14, 119), targeting the IL-31 pathway is a logical step in the development of new pharmacologic agents against pruritus. To date, however, only the anti-IL-31RA antibody nemolizumab has progressed to late-stage clinical trials. Based on the positive results of the recent phase 3 clinical trial of nemolizumab plus concomitant topical agents to treat patients with atopic dermatitis and moderate-to-severe pruritus (103), and the efficacy benefits shown in reducing pruritus in patients with moderate-to-severe prurigo nodularis (104), this drug appears to hold new hope for patients whose treatment options are currently limited. Moreover, the administration of nemolizumab alongside topical agents closely mirrors the likely real-world clinical situation, in which many patients with atopic dermatitis are already treating their conditions, making the addition of nemolizumab into an ongoing treatment regimen relatively straightforward.

For several of the other diseases discussed herein, the underlying role of IL-31 in their pathophysiology remains unclear or unproven. The notable heterogeneity in IL-31 levels, ranging from >1,000 pg/mL among patients with atopic dermatitis (40) to <200 pg/mL in other diseases (7, 65, 93, 97), requires additional explanation, and further research is clearly warranted.

In addition to IL-31, there has been an explosion of recent interest in novel antipruritic drugs targeting other pathways thought to play role in the development or maintenance of itch, including opioid receptor agonists and antagonists, antibodies against various IL family members, and Janus kinase inhibitors (15, 120, 121). It remains to be seen how many of these drugs will successfully demonstrate long-term effectiveness in controlling the signs and symptoms of pruritus, but it seems likely that the current management algorithms for pruritus will undergo extensive modification over the next few years.

In conclusion, IL-31 plays an important role in several inflammatory skin diseases, and treatment targeting IL-31 is expected to contribute meaningfully to the clinical management of a wide range of diseases.

AUTHOR CONTRIBUTIONS

KK and HI were involved in writing and critically reviewing the manuscript and both authors provided final approval of the manuscript for submission and agree to be accountable for the content.

ACKNOWLEDGMENTS

We thank Akihiko Ikoma, MD, Ph.D., of Maruho Co., Ltd., Osaka, Japan and Sally-Anne Mitchell, Ph.D., of McCANN HEALTH CMC, Japan, for providing editorial assistance, which was funded by Maruho Co., Ltd., Osaka, Japan.

REFERENCES

1. Dillon SR, Sprecher C, Hammond A, Bilsborough J, Rosenfeld-Franklin M, Presnell SR, et al. Interleukin 31, a cytokine produced by activated T cells, induces dermatitis in mice. *Nat Immunol.* (2004) 5:752–60. doi: 10.1038/ni1084
2. Feld M, Garcia R, Buddenkotte J, Katayama S, Lewis K, Muirhead G, et al. The pruritus- and TH2-associated cytokine IL-31 promotes growth of sensory nerves. *J Allergy Clin Immunol.* (2016) 138:500–8. doi: 10.1016/j.jaci.2016.02.020
3. Furue M, Ulzii D, Vu YH, Tsuji G, Kido-Nakahara M, Nakahara T. Pathogenesis of atopic dermatitis: current paradigm. *Iran J Immunol.* (2019) 16:97–107. doi: 10.22034/IJI.2019.80253
4. Cornelissen C, Marquardt Y, Czaja K, Wenzel J, Frank J, Lüscher-Firzlaff J, et al. IL-31 regulates differentiation and filaggrin expression in human organotypic skin models. *J Allergy Clin Immunol.* (2012) 129:426–33. doi: 10.1016/j.jaci.2011.10.042
5. Zhang Q, Putheti P, Zhou Q, Liu Q, Gao W. Structures and biological functions of IL-31 and IL-31 receptors. *Cytokine Growth Factor Rev.* (2008) 19:347–56. doi: 10.1016/j.cytogfr.2008.08.003
6. Park K, Mori T, Nakamura M, Tokura Y. Increased expression of mRNAs for IL-4, IL-17, IL-22 and IL-31 in skin lesions of subacute and chronic forms of prurigo. *Eur J Dermatol.* (2011) 21:135–6. doi: 10.1684/ejd.2010.1196
7. Salao K, Sawanyawisuth K, Winaikosol K, Choonhakarn C, Chaowattanapanit S. Interleukin-31 and chronic pruritus of unknown origin. *Biomark Insights.* (2020) 15:1177271920940712. doi: 10.1177/1177271920940712
8. Bodoor K, Al-Qarqaz F, Heis LA, Alfaqih MA, Oweis AO, Almomani R, et al. IL-33/13 axis and IL-4/31 axis play distinct roles in inflammatory process and

itch in psoriasis and atopic dermatitis. *Clin Cosmet Investig Dermatol.* (2020) 13:419–24. doi: 10.2147/CCID.S257647
9. Gonzales AJ, Fleck TJ, Humphrey WR, Galvan BA, Aleo MM, Mahabir SP, et al. IL-31-induced pruritus in dogs: a novel experimental model to evaluate anti-pruritic effects of canine therapeutics. *Vet Dermatol.* (2016) 27:34–e10. doi: 10.1111/vde.12280
10. Andrade A, Kuah CY, Martin-Lopez JE, Chua S, Shpadaruk V, Sanclemente G, et al. Interventions for chronic pruritus of unknown origin. *Cochrane Database Syst Rev.* (2020) 1:CD013128. doi: 10.1002/14651858.CD013128.pub2
11. Pereira MP, Mittal A, Stander S. Current treatment strategies in refractory chronic pruritus. *Curr Opin Pharmacol.* (2019) 46:1–6. doi: 10.1016/j.coph.2018.11.007
12. Furue M, Yamamura K, Kido-Nakahara M, Nakahara T, Fukui Y. Emerging role of interleukin-31 and interleukin-31 receptor in pruritus in atopic dermatitis. *Allergy.* (2018) 73:29–36. doi: 10.1111/all.13239
13. Singh B, Jegga AG, Shanmukhappa KS, Edukulla R, Khurana Hershey GH, Medvedovic M, et al. IL-31-driven skin remodeling involves epidermal cell proliferation and thickening that lead to impaired skin-barrier function. *PLoS ONE.* (2016) 11:e0161877. doi: 10.1371/journal.pone.0161877
14. Bagci IS, Ruzicka T. IL-31: a new key player in dermatology and beyond. *J Allergy Clin Immunol.* (2018) 141:858–66. doi: 10.1016/j.jaci.2017.10.045
15. Erickson S, Heul AV, Kim BS. New and emerging treatments for inflammatory itch. *Ann Allergy Asthma Immunol.* (2020) 1:S1081-206. doi: 10.1016/j.anai.2020.05.028
16. Nygaard U, Vestergaard C, Deleuran M. Emerging treatment options in atopic dermatitis: systemic therapies. *Dermatology.* (2017) 233:344–57. doi: 10.1159/000484406
17. Gangemi S, Quartuccio S, Casciaro M, Trapani G, Minciullo PL, Imbalzano E. Interleukin 31 and skin diseases: a systematic review. *Allergy Asthma Proc.* (2017) 38:401–8. doi: 10.2500/aap.2017.38.4080
18. Nakashima C, Otsuka A, Kabashima K. Interleukin-31 and interleukin-31 receptor: new therapeutic targets for atopic dermatitis. *Exp Dermatol.* (2018) 27:327–31. doi: 10.1111/exd.13533
19. Wong LS, Wu T, Lee CH. Inflammatory and noninflammatory itch: implications in pathophysiology-directed treatments. *Int J Mol Sci.* (2017) 18:1485. doi: 10.3390/ijms18071485
20. Hawro T, Przybylowicz K, Spindler M, PsyM MH, Steć M, Altrichter S, et al. The characteristics and impact of pruritus in adult dermatologic patients: a prospective, cross-sectional study. *J Am Acad Dermatol.* (2020). doi: 10.1016/j.jaad.2020.08.035. [Epub ahead of print].
21. Kini SP, Delong LK, Veledar E, Mckenzie-Brown AM, Schaufele M, Chen SC. The impact of pruritus on quality of life: the skin equivalent of pain. *Arch Dermatol.* (2011) 147:1153–6. doi: 10.1001/archdermatol.2011.178
22. Whang KA, Khanna R, Williams KA, Mahadevan V, Semenov Y, Kwatra SG. Health-related quality of life and economic burden of chronic pruritus. *J Invest Dermatol.* (2020). doi: 10.1016/j.jid.2020.08.020. [Epub ahead of print].
23. Silverberg JI, Gelfand JM, Margolis DJ, Boguniewicz M, Fonacier L, Grayson M, et al. Patient burden and quality of life in atopic dermatitis in US adults: a population-based cross-sectional study. *Ann Allergy Asthma Immunol.* (2018) 121:340–7. doi: 10.1016/j.anai.2018.07.006
24. Jafferany M, Davari ME. Itch and psyche: psychiatric aspects of pruritus. *Int J Dermatol.* (2019) 58:3–23. doi: 10.1111/ijd.14081
25. Lee HG, Stull C, Yosipovitch G. Psychiatric disorders and pruritus. *Clin Dermatol.* (2017) 35:273–80. doi: 10.1016/j.clindermatol.2017.01.008
26. Chee A, Branca L, Jeker F, Vogt DR, Schwegler S, Navarini A, et al. When life is an itch: what harms, helps, and heals from the patients' perspective? Differences and similarities among skin diseases. *Dermatol Ther.* (2020) 33:e13606. doi: 10.1111/dth.13606
27. Hawro T, Hawro M, Zalewska-Janowska A, Weller K, Metz M, Maurer M. Pruritus and sleep disturbances in patients with psoriasis. *Arch Dermatol Res.* (2020) 312:103–11. doi: 10.1007/s00403-019-01998-7
28. Ramirez FD, Chen S, Langan SM, Prather AA, McCulloch CE, Kidd SA, et al. Association of atopic dermatitis with sleep quality in children. *JAMA Pediatr.* (2019) 173:e190025. doi: 10.1001/jamapediatrics.2019.0025
29. Xerfan EMS, Tomimori J, Andersen ML, Tufik S, Facina AS. Sleep disturbance and atopic dermatitis: a bidirectional relationship? *Med Hypotheses.* (2020) 140:109637. doi: 10.1016/j.mehy.2020.109637
30. Patel SP, Khanna R, Choi J, Williams KA, Roh YS, Hong MS, et al. Sleep disturbance in adults with chronic pruritic dermatoses is associated with increased C-reactive protein levels. *J Am Acad Dermatol.* (2020) 84:265–72. doi: 10.1016/j.jaad.2020.08.059
31. Luk KM, Shaw FM, Zhang C, Culler SD, Chen SC. The annual direct and indirect health care costs for patients with chronic pruritus and their determining factors. *J Invest Dermatol.* (2020) 140:699–701. doi: 10.1016/j.jid.2019.07.711
32. Guevara-Sangines E, Perez-Rojas D, Nevárez-Sida A, Aceves MA, Barrón-Tapia MT, Abaroa-Cantú FJ, et al. [The annual cost of medical care for patients with moderate to severe atopic dermatitis in Mexico. *A multicenter study] (In Spanish). Rev Alerg Mex.* (2020) 67:9–18. doi: 10.29262/ram.v67i1.700
33. Whang KA, Gabriel S, Chavda R, Kwatra SG. Emergency department utilization by patients with prurigo nodularis in the United States. *J Am Acad Dermatol.* (2020). doi: 10.1016/j.jaad.2020.06.1002. [Epub ahead of print].
34. Whang KA, Kang S, Kwatra SG. Inpatient burden of prurigo nodularis in the United States. *Medicines.* (2019) 6:88. doi: 10.3390/medicines6030088
35. Gibbs BF, Patsinakidis N, Raap U. Role of the pruritic cytokine IL-31 in autoimmune skin diseases. *Front Immunol.* (2019) 10:1383. doi: 10.3389/fimmu.2019.01383
36. Arai I, Tsuji M, Miyagawa K, Takeda H, Akiyama N, Saito S. Repeated administration of IL-31 upregulates IL-31 receptor A (IL-31RA) in dorsal root ganglia and causes severe itch-associated scratching behaviour in mice. *Exp Dermatol.* (2015) 24:75–8. doi: 10.1111/exd.12587
37. Grimstad O, Sawanobori Y, Vestergaard C, Bisborough J, Oslen UB, Grønhøj-Larsen C, et al. Anti-interleukin-31-antibodies ameliorate scratching behaviour in NC/Nga mice: a model of atopic dermatitis. *Exp Dermatol.* (2009) 18:35–43. doi: 10.1111/j.1600-0625.2008.00766.x
38. Kasutani K, Fujii E, Ohyama S, Adachi H, HasegawanM, Kitamura H, et al. Anti-IL-31 receptor antibody is shown to be a potential therapeutic option for treating itch and dermatitis in mice. *Br J Pharmacol.* (2014) 171:5049–58. doi: 10.1111/bph.12823
39. Byeon JH, Yoon W, Ahn SH, Lee HS, Kim S, Yoo Y. Correlation of serum interleukin-31 with pruritus and blood eosinophil markers in children with atopic dermatitis. *Allergy Asthma Proc.* (2020) 41:59–65. doi: 10.2500/aap.2020.41.190016
40. Ezzat MH, Hasan ZE, Shaheen KY. Serum measurement of interleukin-31 (IL-31) in paediatric atopic dermatitis: elevated levels correlate with severity scoring. *J Eur Acad Dermatol Venereol.* (2011) 25:334–9. doi: 10.1111/j.1468-3083.2010.03794.x
41. Lu J, Wu K, Zeng Q, Xiang Y, Gao L, Huang J. Serum interleukin-31 level and pruritus in atopic dermatitis: a meta-analysis. *Zhong Nan Da Xue Xue Bao Yi Xue Ban.* (2018) 43:124–30. doi: 10.11817/j.issn.1672-7347.2018.02.003
42. Otsuka A, Tanioka M, Nakagawa Y, Honda T, Ikoma A, Miyachi Y, et al. Effects of cyclosporine on pruritus and serum IL-31 levels in patients with atopic dermatitis. *Eur J Dermatol.* (2011) 21:816–7. doi: 10.1684/ejd.2011.1470
43. Saleem MD, Oussedik E, D'amber V, Feldman SR. Interleukin-31 pathway and its role in atopic dermatitis: a systematic review. *J Dermatol Treat.* (2017) 28:591–9. doi: 10.1080/09546634.2017.1290205
44. Cevikbas F, Wang X, Akiyama T, Kempkes C, Savinko T, Antal A, et al. A sensory neuron-expressed IL-31 receptor mediates T helper cell-dependent itch: Involvement of TRPV1 and TRPA1. *J Allergy Clin Immunol.* (2014) 133:448–60. doi: 10.1016/j.jaci.2013.10.048
45. Bilsborough J, Leung DY, Maurer M, Howell M, Boguniewicz M, Yao L, et al. IL-31 is associated with cutaneous lymphocyte antigen-positive skin homing T cells in patients with atopic dermatitis. *J Allergy Clin Immunol.* (2006) 117:418–25. doi: 10.1016/j.jaci.2005.10.046
46. Zeidler C, Tsianakas A, Pereira M, Stander H, Yosipovitch G, Stander S. Chronic prurigo of nodular type: a review. *Acta Derm Venereol.* (2018) 98:173–9. doi: 10.2340/00015555-2774
47. Sonkoly E, Muller A, Lauerma AI, Pivarcsi A, Soto H, Kemeny L, et al. IL-31: a new link between T cells and pruritus in atopic skin inflammation. *J Allergy Clin Immunol.* (2006) 117:411–7. doi: 10.1016/j.jaci.2005.10.033
48. Armstrong AW, Read C. Pathophysiology, clinical presentation, and treatment of psoriasis: a review. *JAMA.* (2020) 323:1945–60. doi: 10.1001/jama.2020.4006

49. Narbutt J, Olejniczak I, Sobolewska-Sztychny D, Sysa-Jedrzejowska A, Słowik-Kwiatkowska I, Howro T, et al. Narrow band ultraviolet B irradiations cause alteration in interleukin-31 serum level in psoriatic patients. *Arch Dermatol Res.* (2013) 305:191–5. doi: 10.1007/s00403-012-1293-6
50. Chen J, Li C, Li H, Yu H, Zhang X, Yan M, et al. Identification of a TH 2-high psoriasis cluster based on skin biomarker analysis in a Chinese psoriasis population. *J Eur Acad Dermatol Venereol.* (2020). doi: 10.1111/jdv.16563. [Epub ahead of print].
51. Neis MM, Peters B, Dreuw A, Wenzel J, Bieber T, Mauch C, et al. Enhanced expression levels of IL-31 correlate with IL-4 and IL-13 in atopic and allergic contact dermatitis. *J Allergy Clin Immunol.* (2006) 118:930–7. doi: 10.1016/j.jaci.2006.07.015
52. Czarnecka-Operacz M, Polańska A, Klimańska M, Teresiak-Mikołajczak E, Molińska-Glura M, Adamski Z, et al. Itching sensation in psoriatic patients and its relation to body mass index and IL-17 and IL-31 concentrations. *Postepy Dermatol Alergol.* (2015) 32:426–30. doi: 10.5114/pdia.2015.56097
53. Bobrowicz M, Fassnacht C, Ignatova D, Chang YT, Dimitriou F, Guenova E. Pathogenesis and therapy of primary cutaneous T-cell lymphoma: Collegium Internationale Allergologicum (CIA) update 2020. *Int Arch Allergy Immunol.* (2020) 181:733–45. doi: 10.1159/000509281
54. Nattkemper LA, Martinez-Escala ME, Gelman AB, Singer EM, Rook AH, Guitart J, et al. Cutaneous T-cell lymphoma and pruritus: the expression of IL-31 and its receptors in the skin. *Acta Derm Venereol.* (2016) 96:894–8. doi: 10.2340/00015555-2417
55. Ohmatsu H, Sugaya M, Suga H, Morimura S, Miyagaki T, Kai H, et al. Serum IL-31 levels are increased in patients with cutaneous T-cell lymphoma. *Acta Derm Venereol.* (2012) 92:282–3. doi: 10.2340/00015555-1345
56. Mobs M, Gryzik S, Haidar A, Humme D, Beyer M, Vandersee S. Analysis of the IL-31 pathway in Mycosis fungoides and Sezary syndrome. *Arch Dermatol Res.* (2015) 307:479–85. doi: 10.1007/s00403-014-1527-x
57. Singer EM, Shin DB, Nattkemper LA, Benoit BM, Klein RS, Didigu CA, et al. IL-31 is produced by the malignant T-cell population in cutaneous T-cell lymphoma and correlates with CTCL pruritus. *J Invest Dermatol.* (2013) 133:2783–5. doi: 10.1038/jid.2013.227
58. Malek M, Glen J, Rebala K, Kowalczyk A, Sobjanek M, Nowicki R, et al. Il-31 does not correlate to pruritus related to early stage cutaneous T-cell lymphomas but is involved in pathogenesis of the disease. *Acta Derm Venereol.* (2015) 95:283–8. doi: 10.2340/00015555-1958
59. Olszewska B, Sokolowska-Wojdylo M, Lakomy J, Nowicki RJ. The ambiguous pruritogenic role of interleukin-31 in cutaneous T-cell lymphomas in comparison to atopic dermatitis: a review. *Postepy Dermatol Alergol.* (2020) 37:319–25. doi: 10.5114/ada.2020.96260
60. Dumont S, Péchère M, Toutous Trellu L. Chronic prurigo: an unusual presentation of Hodgkin lymphoma. *Case Rep Dermatol.* (2018) 10:122–6. doi: 10.1159/000489161
61. Ferretti E, Hohaus S, Di Napoli A, Belmonte B, Cuccaro A, Cupelli E, et al. Interleukin-31 and thymic stromal lymphopoietin expression in plasma and lymph node from Hodgkin lymphoma patients. *Oncotarget.* (2017) 8:85263–75. doi: 10.18632/oncotarget.19665
62. Zeng Q, Gupta A, Xin L, Poon M, Schwarz H. Plasma factors for the differentiation of Hodgkin's lymphoma and diffused large B cell lymphoma and for monitoring remission. *J Hematol.* (2019) 8:47–54. doi: 10.14740/jh499
63. Kfoury LW, Jurdi MA. Uremic pruritus. *J Nephrol.* (2012) 25:644–52. doi: 10.5301/jn.5000039
64. Mettang T, Kremer AE. Uremic pruritus. *Kidney Int.* (2015) 87:685–91. doi: 10.1038/ki.2013.454
65. Oweis AO, Al-Qarqaz F, Bodoor K, Heis L, Alfaqih MA, Almomani R, et al. Elevated interleukin 31 serum levels in hemodialysis patients are associated with uremic pruritus. *Cytokine.* (2020) 138:155369. doi: 10.1016/j.cyto.2020.155369
66. Ko MJ, Peng YS, Chen HY, Hsu SP, Pai MF, Yang JY, et al. Interleukin-31 is associated with uremic pruritus in patients receiving hemodialysis. *J Am Acad Dermatol.* (2014) 71:1151–9 e1151. doi: 10.1016/j.jaad.2014.08.004
67. Kremer AE, Namer B, Bolier R, Fischer MJ, Oude Elferink RP, Beuers U. Pathogenesis and management of pruritus in PBC and PSC. *Dig Dis.* (2015) 33 Suppl 2:164–75. doi: 10.1159/000440829
68. Basile F, Santamaria A, Mannucci C, Rizzo L, Gangemi S, D'anna R, et al. Interleukin 31 is involved in intrahepatic cholestasis of pregnancy. *J Matern Fetal Neonatal Med.* (2017) 30:1124–7. doi: 10.1080/14767058.2016.1205025
69. Ming D, Yu X, Guo R, Deng Y, Li J, Lin C, et al. Elevated TGF-beta1/IL-31 pathway is associated with the disease severity of hepatitis B virus-related liver cirrhosis. *Viral Immunol.* (2015) 28:209–16. doi: 10.1089/vim.2014.0142
70. Raap U, Gehring M, Kleiner S, Rüdrich U, Eiz-Vesper B, Haas H, et al. Human basophils are a source of - and are differentially activated by - IL-31. *Clin Exp Allergy.* (2017) 47:499–508. doi: 10.1111/cea.12875
71. Raap U, Wieczorek D, Gehring M, Pauls I, Ständer S, Kapp A, et al. Increased levels of serum IL-31 in chronic spontaneous urticaria. *Exp Dermatol.* (2010) 19:464–6. doi: 10.1111/j.1600-0625.2010.01067.x
72. Rüdrich U, Gehring M, Papakonstantinou E, Illerhaus A, Engmann J, Kapp A, et al. Eosinophils are a major source of interleukin-31 in bullous pemphigoid. *Acta Derm Venereol.* (2018) 98:766–71. doi: 10.2340/00015555-2951
73. Salz M, Haeberle S, Hoffmann J, Enk AH, Hadaschik EN. Elevated IL-31 serum levels in bullous pemphigoid patients correlate with eosinophil numbers and are associated with BP180-IgE. *J Dermatol Sci.* (2017) 87:309–11. doi: 10.1016/j.jdermsci.2017.07.019
74. Kulczycka-Siennicka L, Cynkier A, Waszczykowska E, Wozniacka A, Zebrowska A. The role of interleukin-31 in pathogenesis of itch and its intensity in a course of bullous pemphigoid and dermatitis herpetiformis. *Biomed Res Int.* (2017) 2017:5965492. doi: 10.1155/2017/5965492
75. Morais KL, Miyamoto D, Orfali RL, Maruta CW, Santi CG, Sotto MN, et al. Increased expression of in situ IL-31RA and circulating CXCL8 and CCL2 in pemphigus herpetiformis suggests participation of the IL-31 family in the pathogenesis of the disease. *J Eur Acad Dermatol Venereol.* (2020) 34:2890–97. doi: 10.1111/jdv.16730
76. Martin SF, Rustemeyer T, Thyssen JP. Recent advances in understanding and managing contact dermatitis. *F1000Res.* (2018) 7:810. doi: 10.12688/f1000research.13499.1
77. Guarneri F, Minciullo PL, Mannucci C, Calapai F, Saitta S, Cannavò SP, et al. IL-31 and IL-33 circulating levels in allergic contact dermatitis. *Eur Ann Allergy Clin Immunol.* (2015) 47:156–8.
78. Takamori A, Nambu A, Sato K, Yamaguchi S, Matsuda K, Numata T, et al. IL-31 is crucial for induction of pruritus, but not inflammation, in contact hypersensitivity. *Sci Rep.* (2018) 8:6639. doi: 10.1038/s41598-018-25094-4
79. Dewane ME, Waldman R, Lu J. Dermatomyositis: clinical features and pathogenesis. *J Am Acad Dermatol.* (2020) 82:267–81. doi: 10.1016/j.jaad.2019.06.1309
80. Shirani Z, Kucenic MJ, Carroll CL, Fleischer AB Jr, Feldman SR, Yosipovitch G, et al. Pruritus in adult dermatomyositis. *Clin Exp Dermatol.* (2004) 29:273–6. doi: 10.1111/j.1365-2230.2004.01510.x
81. Kim HJ, Zeidi M, Bonciani D, Pena SM, Tiao J, Sahu S, et al. Itch in dermatomyositis: the role of increased skin interleukin-31. *Br J Dermatol.* (2018) 179:669–78. doi: 10.1111/bjd.16498
82. Kim BS, Berger TG, Yosipovitch G. Chronic pruritus of unknown origin (CPUO): uniform nomenclature and diagnosis as a pathway to standardized understanding and treatment. *J Am Acad Dermatol.* (2019) 81:1223–4. doi: 10.1016/j.jaad.2019.06.038
83. Welz-Kubiak K, Kobuszewska A, Reich A. IL-31 is overexpressed in lichen planus but its level does not correlate with pruritus severity. *J Immunol Res.* (2015) 2015:854747. doi 10.1155/2015/854747
84. Dousset L, Seneschal J, Boniface K, Charreau S, Ezzedine K, Milpied B, et al. A Th2 cytokine interleukin-31 signature in a case of sporadic lichen amyloidosis. *Acta Derm Venereol.* (2015) 95:223–4. doi: 10.2340/00015555-1829
85. Tey HL, Cao T, Nattkemper LA, Tan VW, Pramono ZA, Yosipovitch G. Pathophysiology of pruritus in primary localized cutaneous amyloidosis. *Br J Dermatol.* (2016) 174:1345–50. doi: 10.1111/bjd.14391
86. Fawzi MMT, Gawdat HI, Mahmoud SB, El-Hawary MS, Rashed LA, Esmat SM. Fractional carbon dioxide laser is effective in amelioration of pruritus in primary cutaneous amyloidosis: a clinical and biochemical study. *Lasers Surg Med.* (2020). doi: 10.1002/lsm.23313. [Epub ahead of print].
87. Hashimoto T, Kursewicz CD, Fayne RA, Nanda S, Shah SM, Nattkemper L, et al. Mechanisms of itch in stasis dermatitis: significant role of IL-31 from macrophages. *J Invest Dermatol.* (2020) 140:850–9 e853. doi: 10.1016/j.jid.2019.09.012

88. Yaseen B, Lopez H, Taki Z, Zafar S, Rosario H, Abdi BA, et al. Interleukin-31 promotes pathogenic mechanisms underlying skin and lung fibrosis in scleroderma. *Rheumatology.* (2020) 59:2625–36. doi: 10.1093/rheumatology/keaa195
89. Xu J, Zanvit P, Hu L, Tseng PY, Liu N, Wang F, et al. The cytokine TGF-beta induces interleukin-31 expression from dermal dendritic cells to activate sensory neurons and stimulate wound itching. *Immunity.* (2020) 53:371–83. doi: 10.1016/j.immuni.2020.06.023
90. Jawa RS, Chattopadhyay S, Tracy E, Wang Y, Huntoon K, Dayton MT, et al. Regulated expression of the IL-31 receptor in bronchial and alveolar epithelial cells, pulmonary fibroblasts, and pulmonary macrophages. *J Interferon Cytokine Res.* (2008) 28:207–19. doi: 10.1089/jir.2007.0057
91. Ip WK, Wong CK, Li ML, Li PW, Cheung PF, Lam CW. Interleukin-31 induces cytokine and chemokine production from human bronchial epithelial cells through activation of mitogen-activated protein kinase signalling pathways: Implications for the allergic response. *Immunology.* (2007) 122:532–41. doi: 10.1111/j.1365-2567.2007.02668.x
92. Lei Z, Liu G, Huang Q, Lv M, Zu R, Zhang GM, et al. SCF and IL-31 rather than IL-17 and BAFF are potential indicators in patients with allergic asthma. *Allergy.* (2008) 63:327–32. doi: 10.1111/j.1398-9995.2007.01566.x
93. Lai T, Wu D, Li W, Chen M, Yi Z, Huang D, et al. Interleukin-31 expression and relation to disease severity in human asthma. *Sci Rep.* (2016) 6:22835. doi: 10.1038/srep22835
94. Dambacher J, Beigel F, Seiderer J, Haller D, Göke B, Auernhammer CJ, et al. Interleukin 31 mediates MAP kinase and STAT1/3 activation in intestinal epithelial cells and its expression is upregulated in inflammatory bowel disease. *Gut.* (2007) 56:1257–65. doi: 10.1136/gut.2006.118679
95. Verstockt S, Verstockt B, Vermeire S. Oncostatin M as a new diagnostic, prognostic and therapeutic target in inflammatory bowel disease (IBD). *Expert Opin Ther Targets.* (2019) 23:943–54. doi: 10.1080/14728222.2019.1677608
96. De Martinis M, Sirufo MM, Suppa M, Ginaldi L. IL-33/IL-31 axis in osteoporosis. *Int J Mol Sci.* (2020) 21:1239. doi: 10.3390/ijms21041239
97. Ginaldi L, De Martinis M, Ciccarelli F, Saitta S, Imbesi S, Mannucci C, et al. Increased levels of interleukin 31 (IL-31) in osteoporosis. *BMC Immunol.* (2015) 16:60. doi: 10.1186/s12865-015-0125-9
98. Mannucci C, Calapai G, Gangemi S. Commentary: circulatory pattern of cytokines, adipokines and bone markers in postmenopausal women with low BMD. *Front Immunol.* (2019) 10:2666. doi: 10.3389/fimmu.2019.02666
99. He A, Feldman SR, Fleischer AB Jr. An assessment of the use of antihistamines in the management of atopic dermatitis. *J Am Acad Dermatol.* (2018) 79:92–6. doi: 10.1016/j.jaad.2017.12.077
100. Yang TB, Kim BS. Pruritus in allergy and immunology. *J Allergy Clin Immunol.* (2019) 144:353–60. doi: 10.1016/j.jaci.2019.06.016
101. Metz M. Treatments for chronic pruritus outside of the box. *Exp Dermatol.* (2019) 28:1476–81. doi: 10.1111/exd.14007
102. Pereira MP, Zeidler C, Storck M, Agelopoulos K, Philipp-Dormston WG, Zink A, et al. Challenges in clinical research and care in pruritus. *Acta Derm Venereol.* (2020) 100:adv00028. doi: 10.2340/00015555-3348
103. Kabashima K, Matsumura T, Komazaki H, Kawashima M, Nemolizumab-Jp01 Study Group. Trial of nemolizumab and topical agents for atopic dermatitis with pruritus. *N Engl J Med.* (2020) 383:141–50. doi: 10.1056/NEJMoa1917006
104. Ständer S, Yosipovitch G, Legat FJ, Lacour JP, Paul C, Narbutt J, et al. Trial of nemolizumab in moderate-to-severe prurigo nodularis. *N Engl J Med.* (2020) 382:706–16. doi: 10.1056/NEJMoa1908316
105. Vixarelimab. *Kiniksa Pharmaceuticals Corp.* Lexington, MA (2020). Available online at: https://www.kiniksa.com/our-pipeline/vixarelimab/ (accessed November 2020).
106. Oyama S, Kitamura H, Kuramochi T, Higuchi Y, Matsushita H, Suzuki T, et al. Cynomolgus monkey model of interleukin-31-induced scratching depicts blockade of human interleukin-31 receptor A by a humanized monoclonal antibody. *Exp Dermatol.* (2018) 27:14–21. doi: 10.1111/exd.13236
107. Mizuno T, Kanbayashi S, Okawa T, Maeda S, Okuda M. Molecular cloning of canine interleukin-31 and its expression in various tissues. *Vet Immunol Immunopathol.* (2009) 131:140–3. doi: 10.1016/j.vetimm.2009.03.014
108. Gonzales AJ, Humphrey WR, Messamore JE, Fleck TJ, Fici GJ, Shelly JA, et al. Interleukin-31: Its role in canine pruritus and naturally occurring canine atopic dermatitis. *Vet Dermatol.* (2013) 24:48–53. doi: 10.1111/j.1365-3164.2012.01098.x
109. Michels GM, Walsh KF, Kryda KA, Martinon OM, Mahabir SP, Hoevers JD, et al. A blinded, randomized, placebo-controlled trial of the safety of lokivetmab (ZTS-00103289), a caninized anti-canine IL-31 monoclonal antibody in client-owned dogs with atopic dermatitis. *Vet Dermatol.* (2016) 27:505–e136. doi: 10.1111/vde.12364
110. Souza CP, Rosychuk RaW, Contreras ET, Schissler JR, Simpson AC. A retrospective analysis of the use of lokivetmab in the management of allergic pruritus in a referral population of 135 dogs in the western USA. *Vet Dermatol.* (2018) 29:489–e164. doi: 10.1111/vde.12682
111. Szczepanik MP, Popiel J, Cekiera A, Pomorska-Handwerker D, Karaś-Tecza J, Sciskalska M, et al. Evaluation of the clinical efficiency of lokivetmab in client privately owned atopic dogs - multicenter study. *Pol J Vet Sci.* (2020) 23:191–5. doi: 10.24425/pjvs.2020.132765
112. Meichner K, Kiupel M, Kasantikul T, Rakich P, Banovic F. Lokivetmab therapy for pruritus in a dog with cutaneous mastocytosis. *Vet Dermatol.* (2019) 30:73–e22. doi: 10.1111/vde.12702
113. Nemoto O, Furue M, Nakagawa H, Shiramoto M, Hanada R, Matsuki S, et al. The first trial of CIM331, a humanized antihuman interleukin-31 receptor A antibody, in healthy volunteers and patients with atopic dermatitis to evaluate safety, tolerability and pharmacokinetics of a single dose in a randomized, double-blind, placebo-controlled study. *Br J Dermatol.* (2016) 174:296–304. doi: 10.1111/bjd.14207
114. Kabashima K, Furue M, Hanifin JM, Pulka G, Wollenberg A, Galus R, et al. Nemolizumab in patients with moderate-to-severe atopic dermatitis: randomized, phase II, long-term extension study. *J Allergy Clin Immunol.* (2018) 142:1121–30. doi: 10.1016/j.jaci.2018.03.018
115. Ruzicka T, Hanifin JM, Furue M, Pulka G, Mlynarczyk I, Wollenberg A, et al. Anti-interleukin-31 receptor A antibody for atopic dermatitis. *N Engl J Med.* (2017) 376:826–35. doi: 10.1056/NEJMoa1606490
116. Silverberg JI, Pinter A, Pulka G, Poulin Y, Bouaziz JD, Wollenberg A, et al. Phase 2b randomized study of nemolizumab in adults with moderate-severe atopic dermatitis and severe pruritus. *J Allergy Clin Immunol.* (2020) 145:173–82. doi: 10.1016/j.jaci.2019.08.013
117. Mihara R, Kabashima K, Furue M, Nakano M, Ruzicka T. Nemolizumab in moderate to severe atopic dermatitis: an exploratory analysis of work productivity and activity impairment in a randomized phase II study. *J Dermatol.* (2019) 46:662–71. doi: 10.1111/1346-8138.14934
118. Silverberg JI, Hinami K, Trick WE, Cella D. Itch in the general internal medicine setting: a cross-sectional study of prevalence and quality-of-life effects. *Am J Clin Dermatol.* (2016) 17:681–90. doi: 10.1007/s40257-016-0215-3
119. Furue M, Chiba T, Tsuji G, Ulzii D, Kido-Nakahara M, Nakahara T, et al. Atopic dermatitis: immune deviation, barrier dysfunction, IgE autoreactivity and new therapies. *Allergol Int.* (2017) 66:398–403. doi: 10.1016/j.alit.2016.12.002
120. Puar N, Chovatiya R, Paller AS. New treatments in atopic dermatitis. *Ann Allergy Asthma Immunol.* (2021) 126:21–31. doi: 10.1016/j.anai.2020.08.016
121. Reszke R, Krajewski P, Szepietowski JC. Emerging therapeutic options for chronic pruritus. *Am J Clin Dermatol.* (2020) 21:601–18. doi: 10.1007/s40257-020-00534-y

5

How Do Neurons Signal Itch?

*Martin Schmelz**

Department of Experimental Pain Research, Medical Faculty Mannheim, University of Heidelberg, Mannheim, Germany

Correspondence:
Martin Schmelz
martin.schmelz@
medma.uni-heidelberg.de

Mechanistic theories of itch are based on neuronal specificity, stimulus intensity, and temporal or spatial discharge patterns. Traditionally, these theories are conceptualized as mutually exclusive, assuming that finding evidence for one theory would exclude the others and could sufficiently explain itch. Current experimental data primarily support the specificity or pattern theory of itch. However, in contrast to an assumed inherent exclusivity, recent results have shown that even within itch-specific pathways in the spinal cord, temporal discharge patterns are important as sustained pruriceptor is required to allow successful transsynaptic signal progression. Also, optogenetic activation of pruriceptors suggest that the combination of neuronal specificity and temporal pattern determines the sensory effect: tonic activation of pruriceptors is required to induce scratching behavior whereas short-lasting stimulation rather causes withdrawal. In addition to the mere duration of discharge, also the temporal pattern or spatial aspects could critically contribute to elicit pruritus instead of pain. Basic neurophysiological studies trying to validate neuronal theories for pruritus in their pure form provide unitary concepts leading from neuronal discharge to the itch sensation. However, the crucial clinical questions have the opposite perspective: which mechanisms explain the chronic itch in a given patient or a given disease? In trying to solve these clinical problems we should not feel bound to the mutual exclusive nature of itch theories, but rather appreciate blending several theories and also accept combinations of itch and pain. Thus, blended versions of itch theories might better suffice for an explanation of chronic itch in patients and will improve the basis for mechanistic treatment options.

Keywords: itch theories, temporal pattern, specificity, spatial contrast, pruriceptor, pain

INTRODUCTION

Several neurophysiological theories have been proposed to explain itch based on neuronal specificity ("labeled line"), stimulus intensity, or temporal & spatial discharge patterns (1). Assuming that these theories are mutually exclusive, authors are tempted to generalize their finding when providing evidence for one theory that could sufficiently explain itch (2). Evidence for the "labeled line" processing of itch via histamine sensitive fibers exist for human and cat (2, 3), but not for monkey (4). Clinically, it is obvious that most chronic itch conditions in patients cannot be sufficiently treated with anti-histamines shedding doubts on the clinical importance of a histamine-dependent itch pathway. More recent data from rodents have identified specific non-histaminergic pathways and thus, one might easily switch to a specificity theory of itch based on non-histaminergic pathways. However, it has become obvious that even supposedly itch-specific pathways have complex interactions with pain-processing in the spinal cord "leaky gate." We might follow up on the traditional neurophysiologic approach that tests certain isolated neuronal activation pattern for their ability to cause the itch sensation (**Figure 1A**). In this review we will try to change perspective and start with the complex clinical condition (**Figure 1B**). We focus on the question: how can we explain a complex clinical combination of chronic itch and pain based on the divergent neurophysiological determinants: intensity, pattern and specificity of primary afferent neurons. The complex processing of noxious and pruritic information in the spinal cord (5–7) and more central circuits (8) have been targeted excellently (9–11) and will not be part of this review.

Experimental protocols often are designed along the lines of the intensity-, pattern- or specificity theory of itch suggesting mutual exclusivity. Here we suggest that combinations of the pure theories are providing a framework that might be more adequate to explain clinical itch conditions.

CLASSIC THEORIES OF PRURITUS AND EVIDENCE FOR INTERACTIONS BETWEEN THEM

Specificity

More than 20 years ago, mechanoinsensitive ("silent") histamine-sensitive C-nociceptors in human (2) and spino-thalamic projection neurons in the cat (12) have been identified as part of a specific pruritic pathway. More recently, molecular markers of non-histaminergic itch-specific neurons were identified in rodent, such as B-type natriuretic peptide (BNP) (13, 14) and members of the mas-related G-protein receptor family (mrgprA3, C11) (15–17) in primary afferent neurons, but also gastrin releasing peptide (GRP) (18–20) in dorsal horn neurons. Non-histaminergic itch signaling has received major interest when mas-related G-protein coupled receptors (Mrgprs) were identified on presumably itch-related neurons in the mouse, i.e., MrgprA3 (21), MrgprD (22), and MrgprC11 (23). For humans, BAM8-22, an activator of MrgrpC11 (24) and beta-alanine–an activator of MrgprD—provoke itch in humans (22, 25). Chloroquine has often been used in mice to elicit itch-behavior via activation of MrgprA3 (21, 26, 27). Thus, the plethora of new information on pathways and mediators for itch have been found and summarized in excellent reviews (8, 10, 28). All the itch-specific markers and pathways might imply that among the competing itch theories the "labeled line" theory has finally been validated.

However, not necessarily these pruritic mediators are part of a labeled line. In mice, peripheral nerve injuries provoke a broad *de-novo* GRP expression in DRG neurons (29). Thus, upon activation or via spontaneous activity such a "phenotypic switch" might convert nociceptors that typically inhibit itch into neurons that by releasing GRP spinally actively contribute to chronic itch. It is important to note that no direct synaptic contact might be required to get access to the spinal itch pathway, but volume transmission (30) might suffice. Single cell expression patterns have been used to define pruriceptive subpopulations of primary afferent neurons in mouse revealing the key marker proteins Mrgpr A3 (often co-expressing MrgprA1 and MrgprC11), B-type natriuretic peptide / Somatostatin, and MrgprD (31–33). In humans, classification of primary afferent nociceptors is classically based on their sensory characteristics obtained from single fiber recordings (34–38), such as mechanical thresholds and temperature sensitivity (**Table 1**). Currently, important work is being performed to reduce the translational gaps between rodent and human single cell expression patterns (39, 40), but also to link functional characteristics and expression pattern within a single neuron (41). This ongoing work will provide a much more detailed basis for the differentiation between itch and pain processing neurons and the extent of overlap in mediators and receptors.

Temporal and Spatial Pattern

Electrophysiological data from rodents and monkey did not support a "labeled line" for itch (28, 42–44) as no specific subpopulation of itch neurons was found. The results rather support the pattern theory of itch according to which nociceptors can signal itch or pain based on the combination of activated fibers resulting in a population coding (1) or based on specific discharge patterns that might differentiate between itch and pain (1).

Very focal activation of nociceptors in the skin has been suggested as a spatial discharge pattern that could explain itch without a "labeled line:" noxious stimulation that is directed only to few cells within the epidermis elicits itch in human skin (45), even when the stimulus is the algogen capsaicin known to activate most human C-nociceptors (46). It has been suggested that local activation of only few epidermal nociceptors can cause itch by a "mismatch signal" (47) or "spatial contrast" (48), provided by few activated and many non-activated nociceptive endings innervating the same skin site, for example by a minute glass wool fiber. Such a discharge pattern indicates that a noxious event is minute and localized within the epidermis. Teleologically, one might conclude that scratching off a part of the epidermis is an adequate response as it will eliminate the threat in this situation. Moreover, scratching will elicit a consistent response of all mechanosensitive polymodal nociceptors innervating this skin and might thereby terminate the "spatial contrast" itch pattern. As shown in **Figure 2** such a spatial contrast can not only result from a very focal stimulation in the epidermis, but may also result from strong activation of only a subpopulation of the nociceptors at the stimulation site. Importantly, this activated subpopulation not necessarily belongs to an itch-selective class of nociceptors, it is rather the resulting "spatial contrast" of their response that is responsible for the interpretation as itch on a spinal level.

When the temporal aspects of neuronal discharge are considered, primary afferents activated by the pruritogen histamine are characterized by lower frequencies as compared to discharges to the algogen capsaicin and periods of bursting have longer intervals (49). However, this difference does not allow a clear separation. New data have found differential temporal discharge pattern to heat stimuli between potential primary afferents linked to pain or itch processing: polymodal nociceptors were differentiated according to their response to a step-like

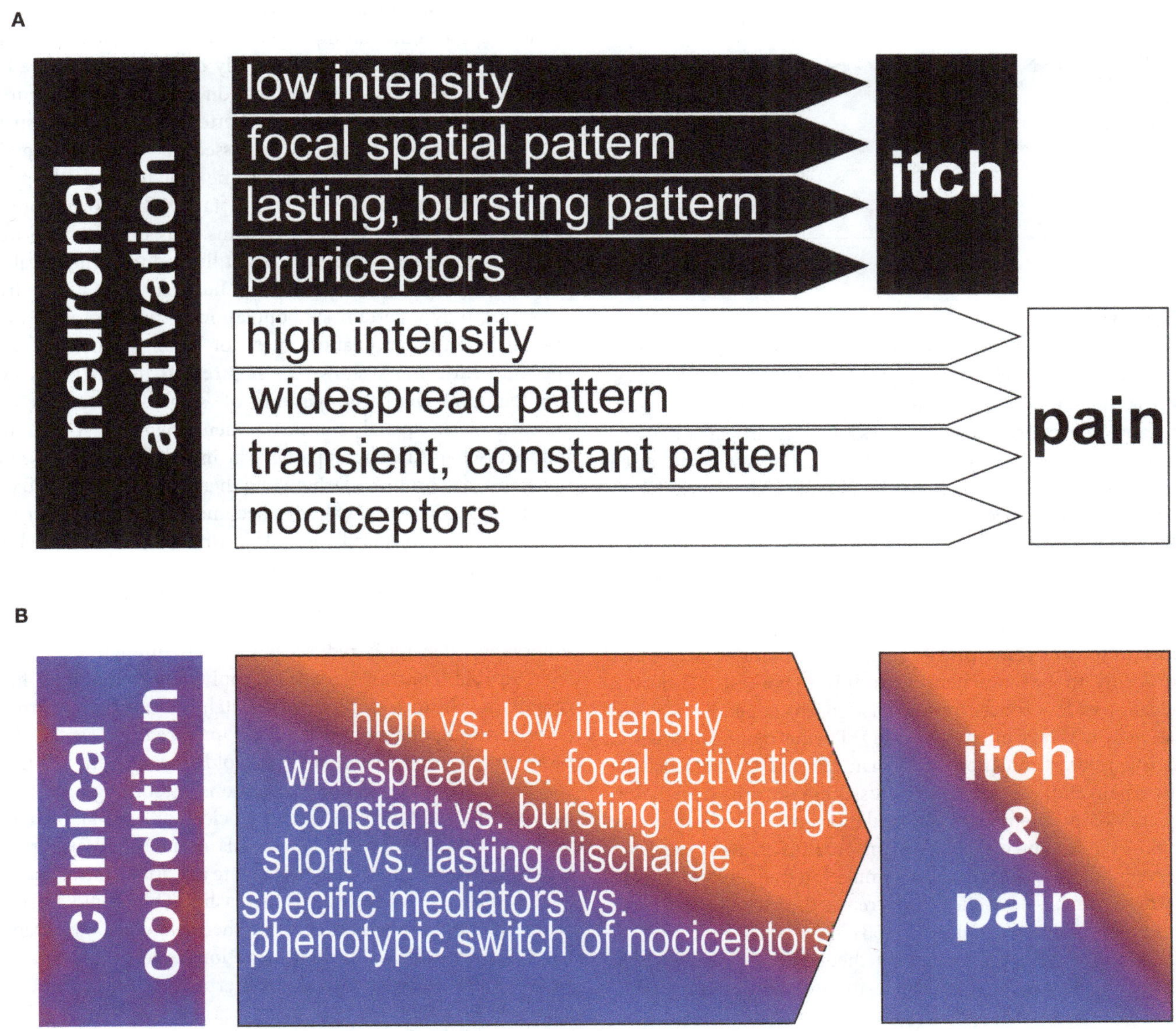

FIGURE 1 | (A) Traditional view of neurophysiologic itch theories: Based on low intensity, focal spatial and bursting temporal pattern or to activation of a specific population of pruriceptors itch is generated. In contrast, higher intensity, widespread or constant discharge patterns or the activation of a specific population of nociceptors is generating the sensation of itch. Note, that the different theories are often assumed to be mutually exclusive and binary. **(B)** Reversed perspective is shown: how can the clinical neuronal discharge patterns lead to itch and pain in the patients? We propose that a combination of the different factors intensity, spatial/temporal pattern and specific pathways is required to produce the observed complex combination of clinical itch and pain.

noxious heat stimulus into quick ("QC") or delayed/slow fibers ("SC") in the monkey (25). C-nociceptors with immediate phasic heat responses were particularly responsive to the pruritogen β-alanine, suggesting that the QC/SC classification might be helpful to characterize a pruriceptive subpopulation (25). Beyond such a characterization, it does is not obvious how this acute response pattern might be linked to a differential signal in itch or pain processing.

As noted above another important temporal aspect is duration and intensity of the discharge: longer lasting activation and higher frequency of GRP-positive neurons were required to finally allow transsynaptic activation of the tertiary GRP-receptor neurons (30). Thus, even when stimulating the itch-specific pathway via optogenetic stimulation of GRP-positive neurons single pulses were inefficient and repetitive lasting stimulation was required (30). Such a temporal pattern of delayed starting of itch after pruritogen application resonates with the psychophysics observed in humans (2). Moreover, in accordance with these considerations optogenetic studies investigating scratching upon specific stimulation generally use prolonged activation periods for example to show disinhibition via dynorphin spinal neurons (30 min at 20 Hz) (50).

TABLE 1 | Translational challenges in pruriceptor classification.

Mouse DRG neurons		Human DRG neurons		Human fibers, in-vivo
single neuron expression pattern	⟷	**single neuron expression pattern**	⟷	**single fiber functional classification**
NP1 / MrgprD		?		polymodal nociceptors
NP2 /MrgprA3		?		very high threshold (VHT)
NP3 / SSt, nppb	······	itch nociceptors		silent nociceptors
TRPM8	······	cold nociceptors	······	cold nociceptors
				C-touch fibers
				warm fibers

Intensity

According to the intensity hypothesis of itch (51) low level activation of unspecific nociceptors would induce pruritus, whereas higher discharge frequencies would provoke pain. Clinically, impairment of pain processing in neuropathy allowed to provoke itch in some patients (52): in patients with impaired nociception, but intact touch system painful stimuli were felt as itch whereas more specific stimulation using "itch powder" was ineffective (52). Thus, the authors concluded that low intensity of slow nociceptive input provokes itch, whereas increasing the intensity of noxious input by scratching would inhibit itch. Also, the observation that intradermal application of high concentrations of some pruritogens, e.g., histamine, may cause pain seems to be consistent with this hypothesis. However, application of low concentrations of algogens generally does not cause itch, just less intense pain (1). Furthermore, intraneural electrical microstimulation of human afferent C-fibers usually induces pain and, very rarely, pruritus. Increasing the stimulation frequency of intraneural microstimulation enhances the intensity of pain or itch, but no switch from pruritus to pain has been observed. Likewise, a decrease of stimulation frequency at a nerve site where pain has been elicited, decreases the magnitude of pain; but at no point does it induce itch (53).

In summary, the pure intensity theory according to which pruritus is gradually converted to itch upon increasing stimulation without change of quality can be regarded as rejected. Yet, as will be discussed below, there might also be indirect evidence for "unmasking" of itch when the pain input is impaired or treated. Thus, it might not be adequate to leave out all possible aspects of the intensity theory.

COMBINATIONS OF TEMPORAL AND SPATIAL PATTERNS INTERACTING WITH SPECIFIC PATHWAY

Basic itch mechanisms are generally discussed in their "pure" form. However, as shown above, there is evidence that itch processing—in particular under pathophysiologic conditions–may combine elements from different basic theories traditionally regarded as mutually exclusive (see **Figure 1**).

Under experimental conditions, such combinations may be required to consistently explain experimental data: activation of subpopulations of C-afferents with traditional algogens such as capsaicin or endothelin or even populations, such as MrgprA3 positive nociceptors (54, 55), might generate itch not only via the assumed specificity, but will also activate only a subset of nociceptors innervating a given skin site. Broad activation of nociceptors frequency-dependently causes pain (**Figure 2A**). However, when only a subpopulation of these nociceptors is activated the resulting discharge pattern resembles a "spatial contrast" pattern (**Figure 2B**) discussed above. Assuming that such an itch signal might require some time to "open the spinal gate" (30) the itch sensation might start with a corresponding delay (dotted box in **Figure 2B**). Thus, it is important to note, that the term "spatial contrast" is not limited to highly localized stimulation within the epidermis, but can also result from activating only a certain subpopulation of nociceptors. This is even true if this population does not belong to the dedicated specific pruriceptors shown in **Figure 2D**. Interestingly, even the temporal discharge pattern of single nociceptors may generate such spatial contrast: when chemical stimulations induce discharge in a burst pattern the initial broad response may occur in a synchronized fashion and thereby mainly induced pain (**Figure 2C**). However, as bursts become less frequent over time there will be stochastically periods in which only few fibers burst in synchrony whereas neighboring fibers are silent thereby again creating the pattern of spatial contrast (**Figure 2C**).

Under pathophysiological conditions such as neuropathy innervation density is reduced and local stimulation may lead to a spatial contrast based on only few remaining fibers resembling historical reports on itch induced by normally painful stimulation in patients with impaired nociceptors (52). Moreover, another element of the old intensity theory might still be useful under clinical conditions: Assuming that a high number of spontaneously active nociceptors signal pain in a given patient; upon reduction of this number, for example by analgesic therapy, the chances to create a spatial contrast pattern by the still active nociceptors is increasing. This would represent a combination of a spatial contrast theory and the old intensity theory. Interestingly, clinical observations indeed support such a development: in patients with postherpetic neuralgia, resolving pain may be combined with an increase in itch (56, 57). Thus, based on defined experimental models, we have successfully developed basic theories that can explain differentiation between itch and pain based on specificity in a "labeled line" or the discharge pattern in its temporal or spatial expression (**Figure 2**, lower part). These approaches provide us with powerful tools when trying to explain clinical neuropathic itch. However, rather than assuming that in pathological conditions there is a mutually exclusive explanation for itch purely based on one theory of itch, we rather might adapt our conceptual framework and include mechanisms that borrow aspects from different theories.

In summary, discharge of subpopulations of primary afferent sensory neurons can contribute to the itch generation via their specific spinal connection to pruriceptive pathways and via their spatial and temporal pattern including to some extent also the intensity of discharge. Thus, even on the relatively simple level of primary afferents we find a clear overlap between traditionally separated and mutually exclusive concepts of itch (see **Figure 1A**). Therefore, it appears adequate to allow combinations of itch theories for the explanation of complex

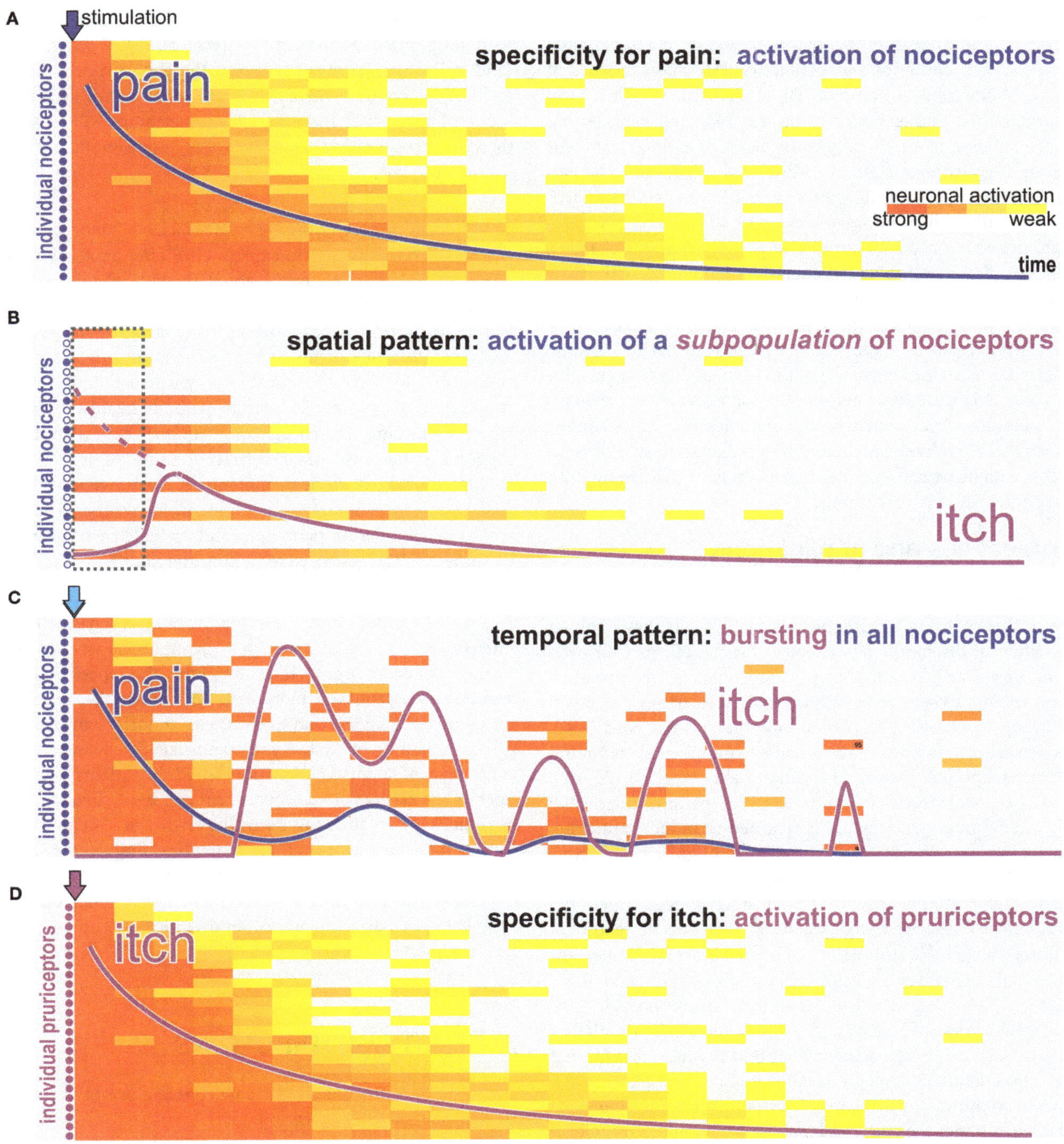

FIGURE 2 | How can nociceptors signal itch? Schematic view of activation intensity (weak to strong indicated by yellow to red color) of single neurons over time after stimulation with algogens (blue arrows **A–C**) or a pruritogen (purple arrow **D**). **(A)** Classic activation of nociceptors by stimulation with a pure algogen: activation of nociceptors in a decrescendo pattern is felt as gradually declining pain sensation (blue line). **(B)** In case of algogens that provoke lasting activation only of a selective subpopulation of nociceptors the activation pattern resembles a "spatial contrast" with silent and highly active nociceptors innervating the same stimulation site. Such a spatial activation pattern is interpreted on spinal level as itch. However, the itch sensation (purple line) will start with some delay required to allow spinally released gastrin releasing peptide to allow activation of the itch pathway (dotted interval in gray; dotted purple line indicates the magnitude of the peripheral input). **(C)** For algogens that provoke prolonged bursting activation patterns there may be an initial phasic activation of all nociceptors leading to a transient pain sensation (blue line). However, in the ensuing phase randomly bursting neurons will stochastically provoke a pattern that resembles the "spatial contrast" shown in B and that is interpreted as itch (purple line) on a spinal level. **(D)** Classic pruritogens are activating specific pruriceptors that will provoke an itch sensation (purple line) according to the specificity theory.

clinical itch conditions (see **Figure 1B**). However, this rather theoretic aspect does not sufficiently capture the complexity inherent in the clinical setting: pathophysiologic changes linked to chronic itch conditions may affect crucial characteristics of peripheral and central neurons. These changes my affect even well-established markers such as gastrin releasing peptide that has been shown to be broadly upregulated in primary afferent neurons after axotomy (29). In addition to such specific changes of pruriceptive processing, there are broader consequences of neuropathy that impinge on itch processing, such as partial denervation of nociceptors, expression pattern changes, Wallerian degeneration & regeneration, and glial activation. These processes can fundamentally change neuronal excitability leading to modified discharge patterns and spontaneous activity that will generate an even more complex scenario. Chronic inflammation can lead to corresponding excitability changes with and without concomitant neuropathic or neuroplastic changes and therefore even increases the complexity under clinical conditions. Therefore, our ability to predict sensory effects in patients with neuropathy or chronic inflammation differentiating between itch and pain are limited.

Perspectives and Implications

Implications for basic experimental approaches. Current experimental data primarily support the specificity and pattern theory of itch. However, recent results have shown that temporal discharge patterns have crucial effects (49) even within itch-specific pathways in the spinal cord: sustained peripheral input via pruriceptors is required to enable successful transsynaptic signal progression in the spinal cord (30). Optogenetic techniques have enabled unmatched temporal control of specific classes of primary afferents (50, 58–61). Again, neuronal specificity and temporal pattern interacted: tonic activation of pruriceptors is required to induce scratching behavior whereas short-lasting stimulation might be ineffective or may even cause withdrawal (30). Thus, the implications of temporal patterns need to be considered even when the experimental approach is focused on an itch-specific pathway, i.e., upon optogenetic stimulation of pruriceptors it is important to compare responses to acute phasic stimulation and tonic discharge. Moreover, the spatial aspect of activation might play a role even for specific activation using optogenetic stimulation in particular for transcutaneous stimulus when the limited penetration depth of blue light is taken into consideration.

When analyzing the discharge of primary afferents we usually analyze area under the curve and maximum discharge frequency. However, considering the importance of other temporal patterns such as lasting and bursting discharge we might expand our analysis accordingly as bursting discharge patterns of nociceptors with long silent periods in between can also generate some kind of spatial contrast pattern thereby merging temporal and spatial contrast theory. On the other hand, synchronous input of high discharge of many nociceptors will cause pain thereby incorporating aspects of the intensity theory to the overall outcome.

Implications for clinical approaches: The "phenotypic switch" of nociceptors that start to express GRP after axotomy (29) not only adds to the controversy about the role of this peptide in primary afferents (62, 63), but may have major implications for clinical pruritus. Beyond the direct involvement of GRP in the generation of pruritus it may render the spinal cord more susceptible for evoked pruritus: in particular acute electrical stimulation may provoke mainly pain in healthy volunteers. However, in chronic itch patients it might also evoke itch (64) suggesting that the spinal cord processing of itch has been facilitated in these patients potentially be previous release of GRP. For experimental stimulation protocols therefore phasic and tonic stimulation paradigms and possible carry-over effects by spinal GRP release need to be considered.

Animal models have been optimized to separately assess intensity of itch and pain, for example via scratching vs. wiping behavior upon injection into the cheek has been successfully established in rodents (65). However, even under these experimental conditions these models can also elicit a combination of itch- and pain-like behaviors (65, 66) suggestive of a mixed sensation. Indeed, patients with small fiber neuropathy often report concomitant itch and pain sensations (67) such as "burning itch" or "itching sting." Rather than separating itch and pain according to the involved discipline (pain for anesthesiologists/neurologists vs. itch for dermatologists) we need to further our translational efforts not only between basic researchers and clinical scientists, but also between pain and itch specialists.

AUTHOR CONTRIBUTIONS

The author confirms being the sole contributor of this work and has approved it for publication.

REFERENCES

1. Handwerker HO. Itch hypotheses: from pattern to specificity and to population coding. In: Carstens E, Akiyama T, editors. *Itch: Mechanisms and Treatment.* Boca Raton (FL): CRC Press (2014). p. 1–8. doi: 10.1201/b16573-2
2. Schmelz M, Schmidt R, Bickel A, Handwerker HO, Torebjörk HE. Specific C-receptors for itch in human skin. *J Neurosci.* (1997) 17:8003–8. doi: 10.1523/JNEUROSCI.17-20-08003.1997
3. Andrew D, Craig AD. Histamine-selective lamina I Spinothalamic tract neurons. *Soc Neurosci Abstr.* (1999) 25:149.
4. Davidson S, Zhang X, Khasabov SG, Moser HR, Honda CN, Simone DA, et al. Pruriceptive spinothalamic tract neurons: physiological properties and projection targets in the primate. *J Neurophysiol.* (2012) 108:1711–23. doi: 10.1152/jn.00206.2012
5. Ross SE, Hachisuka J, Todd AJ. Spinal microcircuits and the regulation of itch. In: Carstens E, Akiyama T, editors. *Itch: Mechanisms and Treatment.* Boca Raton (FL): CRC Press (2014). p. 339–58.

6. Koch SC, Acton D, Goulding M. Spinal circuits for touch, pain, and itch. *Annu Rev Physiol.* (2018) 80:189–217. doi: 10.1146/annurev-physiol-022516-034303
7. Nguyen E, Lim G, Ding H, Hachisuka J, Ko MC, Ross SE. Morphine acts on spinal dynorphin neurons to cause itch through disinhibition. *Sci Transl Med.* 13:579. doi: 10.1126/scitranslmed.abc3774
8. Chen XJ, Sun YG. Central circuit mechanisms of itch. *Nat Commun.* (2020) 11:3052. doi: 10.1038/s41467-020-16859-5
9. Carstens E, Akiyama T. Central mechanisms of itch. *Curr Probl Dermatol.* (2016) 50:11–7. doi: 10.1159/000446011
10. Cevikbas F, Lerner EA. Physiology and pathophysiology of itch. *Physiol Rev.* (2020) 100:945–82. doi: 10.1152/physrev.00017.2019
11. Lay M, Dong X. Neural mechanisms of itch. *Annu Rev Neurosci.* (2020) 43:187–205. doi: 10.1146/annurev-neuro-083019-024537
12. Andrew D, Craig AD. Spinothalamic lamina 1 neurons selectively sensitive to histamine: a central neural pathway for itch. *Nat Neurosci.* (2001) 4:72–7. doi: 10.1038/82924
13. Mishra SK, Hoon MA. The cells and circuitry for itch responses in mice. *Science.* (2013) 340:968–71. doi: 10.1126/science.1233765
14. Aresh B, Freitag FB, Perry S, Blumel E, Lau J, Franck MCM, et al. Spinal cord interneurons expressing the gastrin-releasing peptide receptor convey itch through VGLUT2-mediated signaling. *Pain.* (2017) 158:945–61. doi: 10.1097/j.pain.0000000000000861
15. Reddy VB, Iuga AO, Shimada SG, LaMotte RH, Lerner EA. Cowhage-evoked itch is mediated by a novel cysteine protease: a ligand of protease-activated receptors. *J Neurosci.* (2008) 28:4331–5. doi: 10.1523/JNEUROSCI.0716-08.2008
16. Buddenkotte J, Steinhoff M. Pathophysiology and therapy of pruritus in allergic and atopic diseases. *Allergy.* (2010) 65:805–21. doi: 10.1111/j.1398-9995.2010.01995.x
17. Bader M, Alenina N, Andrade-Navarro MA, Santos RA. MAS and its related G protein-coupled receptors, Mrgprs. *Pharmacol Rev.* (2014) 66:1080–105. doi: 10.1124/pr.113.008136
18. Sun YG, Zhao ZQ, Meng XL, Yin J, Liu XY, Chen ZF. Cellular basis of itch sensation. *Science.* (2009) 325:1531–4. doi: 10.1126/science.1174868
19. Mu D, Deng J, Liu KF, Wu ZY, Shi YF, Guo WM, et al. A central neural circuit for itch sensation. *Science.* (2017) 357:695–9. doi: 10.1126/science.aaf4918
20. Sun S, Xu Q, Guo C, Guan Y, Liu Q, Dong X. Leaky gate model: intensity-dependent coding of pain and itch in the spinal cord. *Neuron.* (2017) 93:840–53 e845. doi: 10.1016/j.neuron.2017.01.012
21. Liu Q, Tang Z, Surdenikova L, Kim S, Patel KN, Kim A, et al. Sensory neuron-specific GPCR Mrgprs are itch receptors mediating chloroquine-induced pruritus. *Cell.* (2009) 139:1353–65. doi: 10.1016/j.cell.2009.11.034
22. Liu Q, Sikand P, Ma C, Tang Z, Han L, Li Z, et al. Mechanisms of itch evoked by beta-alanine. *J Neurosci.* (2012) 32:14532–7. doi: 10.1523/JNEUROSCI.3509-12.2012
23. Liu Q, Weng HJ, Patel KN, Tang Z, Bai H, Steinhoff M, et al. The distinct roles of two GPCRs, MrgprC11 and PAR2, in itch and hyperalgesia. *Sci Signal.* (2011) 4:ra45. doi: 10.1126/scisignal.2001925
24. Sikand P, Dong X, LaMotte RH. BAM8-22 peptide produces itch and nociceptive sensations in humans independent of histamine release. *J Neurosci.* (2011) 31:7563–7. doi: 10.1523/JNEUROSCI.1192-11.2011
25. Wooten M, Weng HJ, Hartke TV, Borzan J, Klein AH, Turnquist B, et al. Three functionally distinct classes of C-fibre nociceptors in primates. *Nat Commun.* (2014) 5:4122. doi: 10.1038/ncomms5122
26. Akiyama T, Tominaga M, Davoodi A, Nagamine M, Blansit K, Horwitz A, et al. Cross-sensitization of histamine-independent itch in mouse primary sensory neurons. *Neuroscience.* (2012) (12):10. doi: 10.1016/j.neuroscience.2012.09.019
27. Ru F, Sun H, Jurcakova D, Herbstsomer RA, Meixong J, Dong X, et al. Mechanisms of pruritogen-induced activation of itch nerves in isolated mouse skin. *J Physiol.* (2017) 595:3651–66. doi: 10.1113/JP273795
28. Carstens E, Follansbee T, Iodi Carstens M. The challenge of basic itch research. *Acta Derm Venereol.* (2020) 100:adv00023. doi: 10.2340/00015555-3343
29. Solorzano C, Villafuerte D, Meda K, Cevikbas F, Braz J, Sharif-Naeini R, et al. Primary afferent and spinal cord expression of gastrin-releasing peptide: message, protein, and antibody concerns. *J Neurosci.* (2015) 35:648–57. doi: 10.1523/JNEUROSCI.2955-14.2015
30. Pagani M, Albisetti GW, Sivakumar N, Wildner H, Santello M, Johannssen HC, et al. How gastrin-releasing peptide opens the spinal gate for itch. *Neuron.* (2019) 103:102–17.e5. doi: 10.1016/j.neuron.2019.04.022
31. Usoskin D, Furlan A, Islam S, Abdo H, Lonnerberg P, Lou D, et al. Unbiased classification of sensory neuron types by large-scale single-cell RNA sequencing. *Nat Neurosci.* (2015) 18:145–53. doi: 10.1038/nn.3881
32. Zeisel A, Hochgerner H, Lonnerberg P, Johnsson A, Memic F, van der Zwan J, et al. Molecular architecture of the mouse nervous system. *Cell.* (2018) 174:999–1014 e1022. doi: 10.1016/j.cell.2018.06.021
33. Sharma N, Flaherty K, Lezgiyeva K, Wagner DE, Klein AM, Ginty DD. The emergence of transcriptional identity in somatosensory neurons. *Nature.* (2020) 577:392–8. doi: 10.1038/s41586-019-1900-1
34. Hallin RG, Torebjörk HE, Wiesenfeld Z. Nociceptors and warm receptors innervated by C fibres in human skin. *J Neurol Neurosurg Psychiatry.* (1982) 45:313–9. doi: 10.1136/jnnp.45.4.313
35. Vallbo AB, Olausson H, Wessberg J, Norrsell U. A system of unmyelinated afferents for innocuous mechanoreception in the human skin. *Brain Res.* (1993) 628:301–4. doi: 10.1016/0006-8993(93)90968-S
36. Campero M, Serra J, Ochoa JL. C-polymodal nociceptors activated by noxious low temperature in human skin. *J Physiol.* (1996) 497:565–72. doi: 10.1113/jphysiol.1996.sp021789
37. Serra J, Campero M, Ochoa J, Bostock H. Activity-dependent slowing of conduction differentiates functional subtypes of C fibres innervating human skin. *J Physiol.* (1999) 515:799–811. doi: 10.1111/j.1469-7793.1999.799ab.x
38. Werland F, Hirth M, Rukwied R, Ringkamp M, Turnquist B, Jorum E, et al. Maximum axonal following frequency separates classes of cutaneous unmyelinated nociceptors in the pig. *J Physiol.* (2021) 599:1595–1610. doi: 10.1113/JP280269
39. Kupari J, Usoskin D, Lou D, Parisien M, Hu Y, Fatt M, et al. Single cell transcriptomics of primate sensory neurons identifies cell types associated with human chronic pain. *bioRxiv [Preprint].* (2020). doi: 10.1101/2020.12.07.414193
40. Tavares-Ferreira D, Shiers S, Ray PR, Wangzhou A, Jeevakumar V, Sankaranarayanan I, et al. Spatial transcriptomics reveals unique molecular fingerprints of human nociceptors. *bioRxiv [Preprint].* (2021). doi: 10.1101/2021.02.06.430065
41. Adelman PC, Baumbauer KM, Friedman R, Shah M, Wright M, Young E, et al. Single-cell q-PCR derived expression profiles of identified sensory neurons. *Mol Pain.* (2019) 15:1744806919884496. doi: 10.1177/1744806919884496
42. Akiyama T, Iodi CM, Carstens E. Transmitters and pathways mediating inhibition of spinal itch-signaling neurons by scratching and other counterstimuli. *PLoS ONE.* (2011) 6:e22665. doi: 10.1371/journal.pone.0022665
43. Davidson S, Moser H, Giesler G. Ascending Pathways for Itch. In: Carstens E, Akiyama T, editors. *Itch: Mechanisms and Treatment.* Boca Raton (FL): CRC Press (2014). p. 373–90.
44. Ringkamp M, Meyer R. Pruriceptors. In: Carstens E, Akiyama T, editors. *Itch: Mechanisms and Treatment.* Boca Raton (FL): CRC Press (2014). p. 129–42.
45. Sikand P, Shimada SG, Green BG, LaMotte RH. Similar itch and nociceptive sensations evoked by punctate cutaneous application of capsaicin, histamine and cowhage. *Pain.* (2009) 144:66–75. doi: 10.1016/j.pain.2009.03.001
46. Rostock C, Schrenk-Siemens K, Pohle J, Siemens J. Human vs. mouse nociceptors - similarities and differences. *Neuroscience.* (2018) 387:13–27. doi: 10.1016/j.neuroscience.2017.11.047
47. Schmelz M. Itch and pain. *Neurosci Biobehav Rev.* (2010) 34:171–6. doi: 10.1016/j.neubiorev.2008.12.004
48. Namer B, Reeh P. Scratching an itch. *Nat Neurosci.* (2013) 16:117–8. doi: 10.1038/nn.3316
49. LaMotte RH, Dong X, Ringkamp M. Sensory neurons and circuits mediating itch. *Nat Rev Neurosci.* (2014) 15:19–31. doi: 10.1038/nrn3641
50. Huang J, Polgar E, Solinski HJ, Mishra SK, Tseng PY, Iwagaki N, et al. Circuit dissection of the role of somatostatin in itch and pain. *Nat Neurosci.* (2018) 21:707–16. doi: 10.1038/s41593-018-0119-z
51. v.Frey M. Zur Physiologie der Juckempfindung. *Arch Neerl Physiol.* (1922) 7:142–5.
52. Rothmann S. Beiträge zur Physiologie der Juckempfindung. *Arch f Dermat.* (1922) 139:227–34. doi: 10.1007/BF01828928
53. Torebjörk HE, Ochoa J. Pain and itch from C fiber stimulation. *Soc Neurosci Abstr.* (1981) 7:228.

54. Huang CC, Yang W, Guo C, Jiang H, Li F, Xiao M, et al. Anatomical and functional dichotomy of ocular itch and pain. *Nat Med.* (2018) 24:1268–76. doi: 10.1038/s41591-018-0083-x
55. Albisetti GW, Pagani M, Platonova E, Hosli L, Johannssen HC, Fritschy JM, et al. Dorsal horn gastrin-releasing peptide expressing neurons transmit spinal itch but not pain signals. *J Neurosci.* (2019) 39:2238–50. doi: 10.1523/JNEUROSCI.2559-18.2019
56. Ishikawa R, Iseki M, Koga R, Inada E. Investigation of the correlation between postherpetic itch and neuropathic pain over time. *Pain Res Manag.* (2018) 2018:9305126. doi: 10.1155/2018/9305126
57. Kramer S, Baeumler P, Geber C, Fleckenstein J, Simang M, Haas L, et al. Somatosensory profiles in acute herpes zoster and predictors of postherpetic neuralgia. *Pain.* (2019) 160:882–94. doi: 10.1097/j.pain.00000000000 01467
58. Yuan L, Liang TY, Deng J, Sun YG. Dynamics and functional role of dopaminergic neurons in the ventral tegmental area during itch processing. *J Neurosci.* (2018) 38:9856–69. doi: 10.1523/JNEUROSCI.1483-18.2018
59. Sanders KM, Sakai K, Henry TD, Hashimoto T, Akiyama T. A subpopulation of amygdala neurons mediates the affective component of itch. *J Neurosci.* (2019) 39:3345–56. doi: 10.1523/JNEUROSCI.2759-18.2019
60. Sakai K, Sanders KM, Lin SH, Pavlenko D, Funahashi H, Lozada T, et al. Low-threshold mechanosensitive VGLUT3-lineage sensory neurons mediate spinal inhibition of itch by touch. *J Neurosci.* (2020) 40:7688–701. doi: 10.1523/JNEUROSCI.0091-20.2020
61. Sharif B, Ase AR, Ribeiro-da-Silva A, Seguela P. Differential coding of itch and pain by a subpopulation of primary afferent neurons. *Neuron.* (2020) 106:940–51 e944. doi: 10.1016/j.neuron.2020.03.021
62. Barry DM, Liu XT, Liu B, Liu XY, Gao F, Zeng X, et al. Exploration of sensory and spinal neurons expressing gastrin-releasing peptide in itch and pain related behaviors. *Nat Commun.* (2020) 11:1397. doi: 10.1038/s41467-020-15230-y
63. Bell AM, Gutierrez-Mecinas M, Stevenson A, Casas-Benito A, Wildner H, West SJ, et al. Expression of green fluorescent protein defines a specific population of lamina II excitatory interneurons in the GRP::eGFP mouse. *Sci Rep.* (2020) 10:13176. doi: 10.1038/s41598-020-69711-7
64. Rukwied R, Schnakenberg M, Solinkski HJ, Schmelz M, Weisshaar E. Transcutaneous slowly depolarizing currents elicit pruritus in patients with atopic dermatitis. *Acta Derm Venereol.* (2020) 100:adv00302. doi: 10.2340/00015555-3658
65. Shimada SG, LaMotte RH. Behavioral differentiation between itch and pain in mouse. *Pain.* (2008) 139:681–7. doi: 10.1016/j.pain.2008.08.002
66. Qu L, Fan N, Ma C, Wang T, Han L, Fu K, et al. Enhanced excitability of MRGPRA3- and MRGPRD-positive nociceptors in a model of inflammatory itch and pain. *Brain.* (2014) 137:1039–50. doi: 10.1093/brain/awu007
67. Brenaut E, Marcorelles P, Genestet S, Menard D, Misery L. Pruritus: an underrecognized symptom of small-fiber neuropathies. *J Am Acad Dermatol.* (2015) 72:328–32. doi: 10.1016/j.jaad.2014.10.034

6

The Role of Gut Microbiota in Chronic Itch-Evoked Novel Object Recognition-Related Cognitive Dysfunction in Mice

Yujuan Li [1], Wencui Zhang [1], Tainning Sun [1], Baowen Liu [1], Anne Manyande [2], Weiguo Xu [3] and Hong-Bing Xiang [1*]*

[1] Department of Anesthesiology, Tongji Hospital, Tongji Medical College, Huazhong University of Science and Technology, Wuhan, China, [2] School of Human and Social Sciences, University of West London, London, United Kingdom, [3] Department of Orthopedics, Tongji Hospital of Tongji Medical College, Huazhong University of Science and Technology, Wuhan, China

***Correspondence:**
Weiguo Xu
xuweiguo@tjh.tjmu.edu.cn
Hong-Bing Xiang
hbxiang@tjh.tjmu.edu.cn

The high incidence of patients with chronic itch highlights the importance of fundamental research. Recent advances in the interface of gut microbiota have shed new light into exploring this phenomenon. However, it is unknown whether gut microbiota plays a role in chronic itch in rodents with or without cognitive dysfunction. In this study, the role of gut microbiota in diphenylcyclopropenone (DCP)-evoked chronic itch was investigated in mice and hierarchical cluster analysis of novel object recognition test (ORT) results were used to classify DCP-evoked itch model in mice with or without cognitive dysfunction (CD)-like phenotype and 16S ribosomal RNA (rRNA) gene sequencing was used to compare gut bacterial composition between CD (Susceptible) and Non-CD phenotypes (Unsusceptible) in chronic itch mice. Results showed that the microbiota composition was significantly altered by DCP-evoked chronic itch and chronic itch induced novel object recognition-related CD. However, abnormal gut microbiota composition induced by chronic itch may not be correlated with novel object recognition-related CD.

Keywords: chronic itch, gut microbiota, novel object recognition, cognitive dysfunction, metabolites

INTRODUCTION

Everyone has experienced symptoms of pain and itching stress. According to present studies, pain and itching share close associations in sensory perceptions and neural pathways (1–3). Similar to pain, itching is classified into two forms. Acute itching is easily reduced by scratching or anti-allergic drugs whereas chronic repetitive itching remains a challenge to clinic cure (4–7). It has been reported that the itch-scratch cycle plays an important role in the maintenance of the chronic itch (8–11). Furthermore, the itch-scratch cycle is centered around three key points of itch neurobiology and skin immunology (12): the epithelial barrier, the peripheral nervous system and the immune system dysfunction (13, 14). While well-known clinically, its mechanisms have historically lacked in-depth understanding, possibly due to the complexity of the chronic itch.

Several studies have reported that gut microbiota and their dependent metabolites are associated with the development of chronic diseases (15, 16). Cani et al. (17) demonstrated that changes in gut microbiota control metabolic endotoxemia-induced inflammation in high-fat diet-induced obesity and diabetes in mice. Ke et al. (18) observed a change in gut flora-dependent metabolite Trimethylamine-N-oxide (TMAO) during the aging process and the effects of TMAO on chronic cardiovascular diseases, and reported that TMAO accelerated endothelial cell senescence and vascular aging and increased oxidative stress through the activation of the p53/p21/Rb pathway. Thus, we speculate that gut microbiota may affect the development of chronic itch.

Increasing evidence has further demonstrated an important association between gut flora-derived metabolites and the maintenance of cognitive function impairment (19–23). Findings of Yu et al. (20) showed that abnormal gut microbiota composition contributed to the onset of diabetes-induced cognitive dysfunction, suggesting that improving gut microbiota composition may be a potential therapeutic strategy for diabetes and related comorbidities. Yang et al. (21) used hierarchical cluster analysis of sucrose preference test to classify the spared nerve injury (SNI) model rats with or without anhedonia-like phenotype and found that gut microbiota plays a key role in pain as well as depression-like phenotypes including anhedonia in rodents with neuropathic pain. Nevertheless, whether chronic itch-related cognitive function dysfunction is implicated in gut microbiota remains unclear.

In this study, we first investigated the role of gut microbiota in diphenylcyclopropenone (DCP)-evoked chronic itch in mice. Next, we used hierarchical cluster analysis of novel object recognition test (ORT) results to classify the chronic itch in mice with or without cognitive dysfunction (CD)-like phenotype and 16S ribosomal RNA (rRNA) gene sequencing was used to compare gut bacterial composition between CD (Susceptible) and Non-CD phenotypes (Unsusceptible) in chronic itch mice. Furthermore, we examined the effects of fecal bacteria transplantation from chronic itch-induced CD and Non-CD phenotypes on novel object recognition and scratching behaviors of host pseudo-germ-free mice.

MATERIALS AND METHODS

Animals

Male C57/BL6 mice aged 8–10 weeks were supplied by the Experimental Animal Research Center of Hubei Province (Hubei, China). All animals were adapted to their environment 7 days before the experiment. Animals were humanely treated according to the National Institutes of Health Guide for the Care and Use of Laboratory Animals (revised 2011) and the Guide for the Care and Use of Laboratory Animals (National Academic Press, USA; revised 2011). Animals were housed in a temperature-controlled holding room (22 ± 1°C) on a 12-h light/dark cycle and given food and water *ad libitum*. Experimental protocols were approved by the Institutional Animal Care and Use Committee of Tongji Hospital, Tongji Medical College, Huazhong University of Science and Technology, Wuhan, China (IRB ID:TJ-A0803).

Experimental Design

Experiment A: Mice were randomly assigned to two groups: (1) control group (n = 6); (2) DCP group ($n = 14$). Pruritic behaviors were video-recorded and 16S rRNA sequencing was used to analyze the change of gut microbiota.

Experiment B: After hierarchical cluster analysis of novel object recognition test was used, mice were divided into the control group (control, $n = 6$), DCP-CD phenotypes (Susceptible, $n = 6$) and DCP-Non-CD phenotypes (Unsusceptible, $n = 8$). Pruritic behaviors were measured and fecal samples were collected for 16S rRNA gene sequencing.

Experiment C: Mice were assigned to one of four groups: (1) control group ($n = 6$), mice were given food and water *ad libitum*; (2) PBS group ($n = 5$); (3) Susceptible group ($n = 7$); (4) Unsusceptible group ($n = 7$). PBS (PBS group), fecal suspension of DCP-CD (susceptible group) and DCP-Non-CD (unsusceptible group) were transplanted into pseudo-germ-free mice intragastrically for 14 consecutive days. A novel object recognition test was performed.

DCP-Evoked Chronic Itch

Mice were shaved on the back of the neck and divided into the DCP group ($n = 14$) and control group ($n = 6$). 0.1 ml 1% DCP (Shanghai Aladdin Biochem Technology Co., Ltd.) dissolved in acetone was painted on the neck skin of mice in the DCP group on day 1 and day 7 under conventional conditions. The neck skin of mice in the control group was painted with 0.1 ml acetone (24). Scratching behaviors were video-recorded on the day before the DCP treatment and day 9 following DCP application.

Scratching Behaviors in Mice

Mice were habituated in a plastic chamber (9 ×9 ×13 cm) for 15 min before the experiment. The scratching behaviors were video-recorded through a transparent glass under the plastic chamber in the absence of any observer for 30 min. According to our previous research (5, 6, 9, 25, 26), a scratching bout is defined as lifting a hind paw toward the shaved region and returning the hind paw back to the floor or mouth for licking (27). Analyses of the videotapes were carried out in a blinded manner.

Novel Object Recognition Test

In an open field, two identical objects were placed at two corners 6 cm from each border as previously described (28–30). During the first stage, the animal was allowed free exploration for 5 min and the exploration time around each object was recorded. The next day, the experiment was the same as before except that one of the two objects was replaced by a novel object same in size but different in appearance. The exploration time around the novel object was recorded. The apparatus was wiped with 75% ethanol to eliminate odor after each experiment.

Feces Sample Collection

Mice were placed in a clean cage with sterile paper on the bottom. The feces were immediately collected in a sterilized centrifuge tube after mice defecated. Fecal samples were stored in −80°C freezer till 16S rRNA gene sequencing analysis. 1 g fecal samples obtained from DCP-CD or DCP-Non-CD mice were diluted in 10 mL aseptic PBS to prepare for fecal transplantation.

16S rRNA Gene Sequencing for Fecal Sampling

Based on a previous report (20, 21, 31–33), 16S rRNA gene sequencing was used to perform bioinformatics analysis. Detailed methods are provided in **Supplementary Information.**

Pseudo-Germ-Free Mice Modeling and Fecal Transplantation

The pseudo-germ-free mice modeling was prepared as previously reported (20, 21, 34). Briefly, C57BL/6 mice drunk special water containing broad-spectrum antibiotics (ampicillin 1 g/L, neomycin sulfate 1 g/L, metronidazole 1 g/L, Sigma-Aldrich Co. Ltd, USA) *ad libitum* for 14 consecutive days. The drinking solutions were renewed every 2 days.

The fecal material was suspended and each recipient pseudo-germ-free mouse was intragastrically infused with 0.2 mL suspension for 14 consecutive days.

Statistical Analysis

All quantification data are expressed as means ± SEM, and error bars represent SEM. Statistical analyzes were performed using SPSS software version 17.0 (SPSS Inc., Armonk, New York, USA) and GraphPad Prism software (GraphPad Software, Inc.). Z scores were standardized in Hierarchical cluster analysis. Then, by using the Ward method and Euclidean distance square as distance measurement, ORT results were Hierarchically clustered, and mice were divided into two groups: DCP-CD (susceptible) and DCP-Non-CD (unsusceptible) mice. Behavioral tests were analyzed by one-way or two-way analysis of variance (ANOVA), followed by post hoc Bonferroni's test. $P < 0.05$ was considered to indicate a statistically significant difference.

RESULTS

DCP-Evoked Scratching Behaviors in Mice

Mice assigned to the DCP group showed a greater number of spontaneous scratching bouts (SSBs) compared to the control group within 30 min of observation. As depicted in **Figure 1A**, the number of SSBs in the DCP-treated mice (SSB $= 85.77 \pm 15.56$, $n = 14$) showed a significant distinction between the acetone-treated mice at day 10 (SSB $= 3.33 \pm 0.42$, $n = 6$, $P < 0.0001$). **Figures 1C,E** shows the H&E staining of the skin in the control group and the DCP group. The skin of the control group was smooth and soft while the skin of mice in the DCP group (**Figure 1D**) was rough and sclerotic, accompanied by scratches and scabs. Compared with the control group (**Figure 1B**), there was significant epidermal hyperplasia in the DCP group.

Comparisons of Differential Profiles in Gut Microbiota Among Control, Susceptible and Unsusceptible Mice

We used 16S rRNA gene sequencing to compare differential profiles of gut microbiota in the two groups. A large number of gut bacteria were altered in three groups (**Figure 2A**). DCP mice showed a significant decrease in α-diversity value compared with control mice (**Figures 2B–D**). As depicted in the three-dimensional PCoA picture (**Figure 2E**), the dots of the DCP group were far apart from the control group. **Figure 2F** displays the circular tree data, which suggests that the composition of gut microbiota was pretty distinct between the two groups.

Alterations in the Gut Microbiota Composition Between the DCP and Control Mice

The results of 16S rRNA gene sequencing demonstrate that the alterations of the gut microbiota composition between the DCP and control mice were distinct (**Figures 3E–H** and **Supplementary Figures 1–3**). The analysis depicts that 52 bacteria differed between the fecal samples of the DCP and control mice. The relative abundance of 48 bacteria at six phylogenetic levels (phylum, class, order, etc.) was significantly decreased in the DCP mice compared with control mice. On the contrary, the relative abundance of 4 bacteria at genus, phylum and species level increased in the DCP mice compared with control mice. The heat maps of the gut microbiota composition at 6 phylogenetic levels (phylum, class, order, family, genus, and species) outlined specific differences between the control and DCP groups (**Supplementary Figures 4, 5**).

Comparisons of Gut Microbiota Among the Control, DCP-CD and DCP-Non-CD Mice

Timeline of the chronic itch model and behavior tests were showed in Figure 3A. Hierarchical cluster analysis was used to classify the result of the novel object recognition test (**Figure 3B**). The schematic presentation for the protocol of novel-object recognition test was showed in **Figure 3C**. There was a significant difference in recognition index between susceptible (DCP-CD) or unsusceptible (DCP-Non-CD) mice (**Figure 3D**). Based on this result, the DCP mice were divided into either the cognition impairment susceptible (DCP-CD) or unsusceptible (DCP-Non-CD) mice. The Chao1 and Simpson indices indicated no significant difference between DCP-CD (Susceptible) and DCP-NCD (Unsusceptible) mice (**Figures 2E,F**). Moreover, the unweighted unifrac PCoA analysis showed that the DCP-CD and DCP-Non-CD mice might have similar gut microbiota composition (**Figure 2G**). A Binary Jaccard circular tree suggested there were similarities between the DCP-CD and DCP-Non-CD mice (**Figure 2H**).

Effects of Fecal Microbiota Transplantation From DCP-CD or DCP-Non-CD Mice on Short-Term Memory in Pseudo-Germ-Free Mice

Pseudo-germ-free mice were established by adding a large dose of antibiotics into the drinking water for 14 consecutive days. For another consecutive 14 days, fecal microbiotas were transplanted on pseudo-germ-free mice by intragastric administration (**Figure 4A**). Recognition index between mice receiving transplantation of fecal samples from susceptible or unsusceptible mice showed no significant difference (**Figure 4B**).

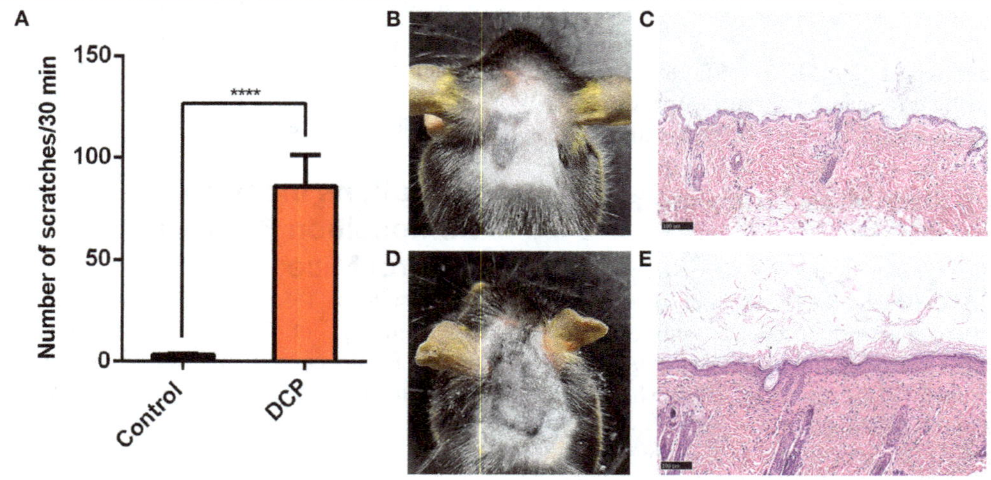

FIGURE 1 | Scratching behaviors and Hematoxylin and eosin (H&E) staining of the neck skin in the control and DCP group. 0.1 ml 1% DCP dissolved in acetone or acetone was painted on the neck skin of the mice on day 1 and day 7 under conventional conditions. Scratching behaviors **(A)** were observed on day 9. Each value represents the mean ± SEM ($n = 6–14$ mice per group). H&E-stained sections from the neck skins treated with **(B,C)** acetone, **(D,E)** DCP. **(B)** A representative image of the neck skin from an acetone treated mouse. The skin was smooth and soft. **(D)** A representative image of the DCP application site from the DCP group. The skin manifested as rough and sclerotic, accompanied by scratches and scabs. ****$P < 0.0001$ vs. the mice treated with acetone. DCP, diphenylcyclopropenone.

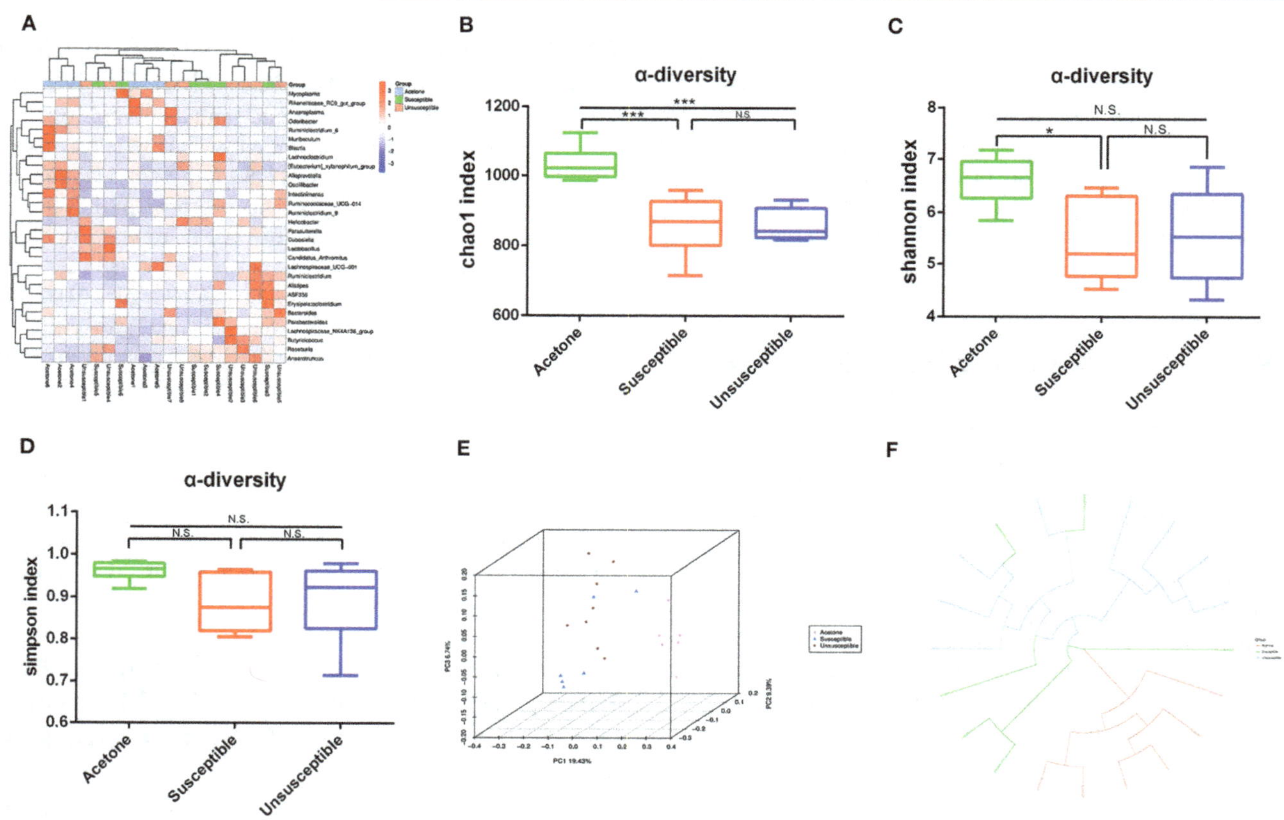

FIGURE 2 | Differential profiles of the gut microbiota among control (acetone), DCP-CD (Susceptible) and DCP-Non-CD (Unsusceptible) mice. **(A)** Heat map of differential levels of bacteria among three groups. **(B)** Chao 1 index between control and susceptible mice (t-test, $P < 0.0001$). **(C)** Simpson index between control and susceptible mice (t-test, $P < 0.01$). **(D)** Shannon index (t-test, $P < 0.05$). **(E)** Chao 1 index. **(F)** Simpson index. PCoA, principal coordinates analysis. *$P < 0.05$, ***$P < 0.0001$.

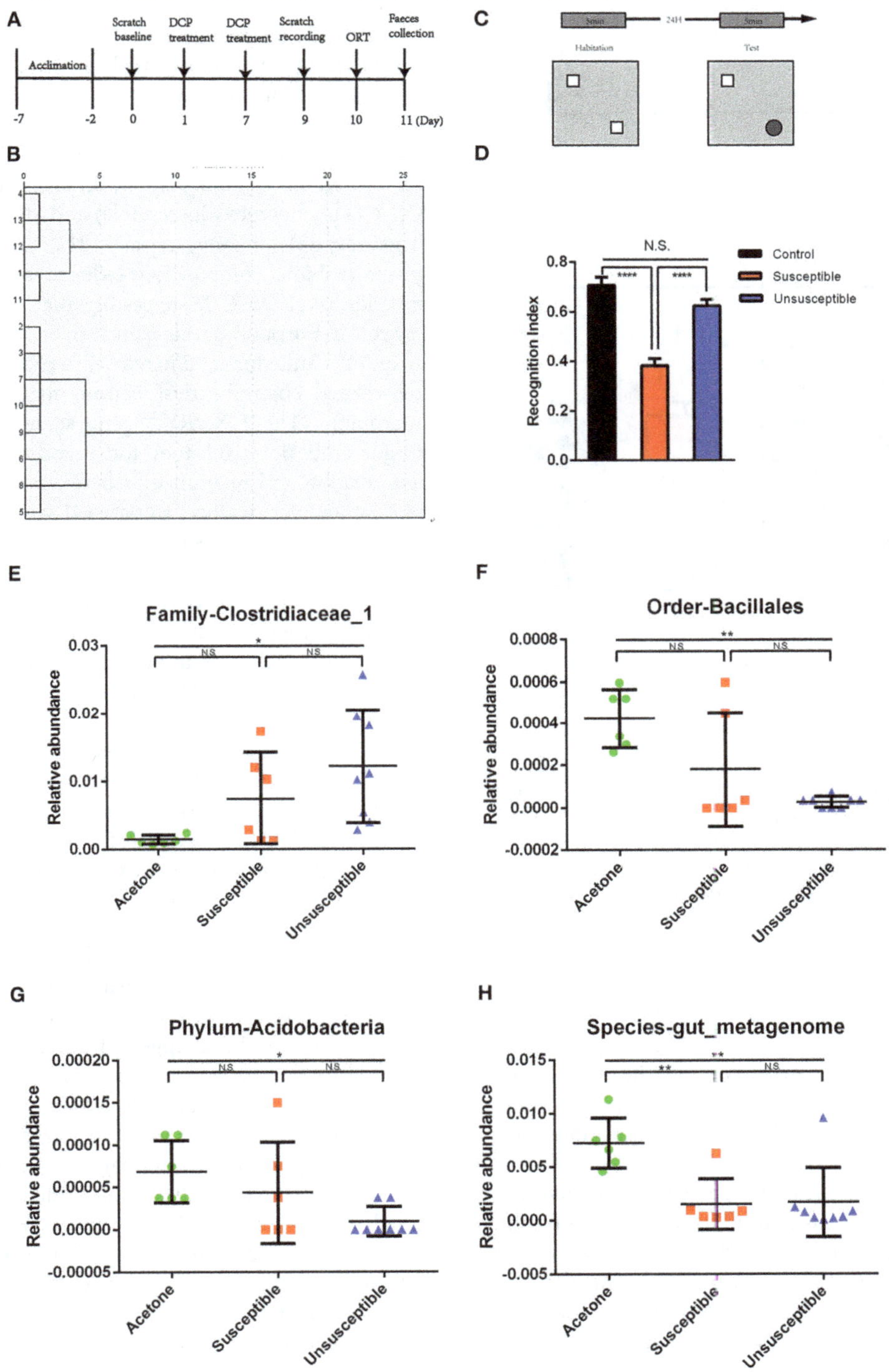

FIGURE 3 | Differences of relative abundance in the gut microbiota among control (acetone), DCP-CD (Susceptible) and DCP-Non-CD (Unsusceptible) mice. **(A)** Timeline of the chronic itch model and behavior tests. Administration of DCP started on day 1 and day 7 after acclimation. Scratching behavior was recorded on day 9. Object recognition test was performed on day 10. Feces was collected on day 11. **(B)** Dendrogram of hierarchical clustering analysis. 14 DCP mice were divided into cognitive dysfunction susceptible and unsusceptible groups by ORT results of hierarchical clustering analysis. **(C)** The schematic presentation for the protocol of novel-object recognition test. **(D)** ORT recognition index [$F_{(2, 16)} = 29.30$, $P < 0.0001$]. **(E)** Family-Clostridiaceae_1 between control and susceptible mice. **(F)** Order-Bacillales. **(G)** Phylum-Acidobacteria. **(H)** Species-gut_metagenome. N.S., not significant; DCP, diphenylcyclopropenone; ORT, Object recognition test. $^{*}P < 0.05$, $^{**}P < 0.001$, $^{****}P < 0.0001$.

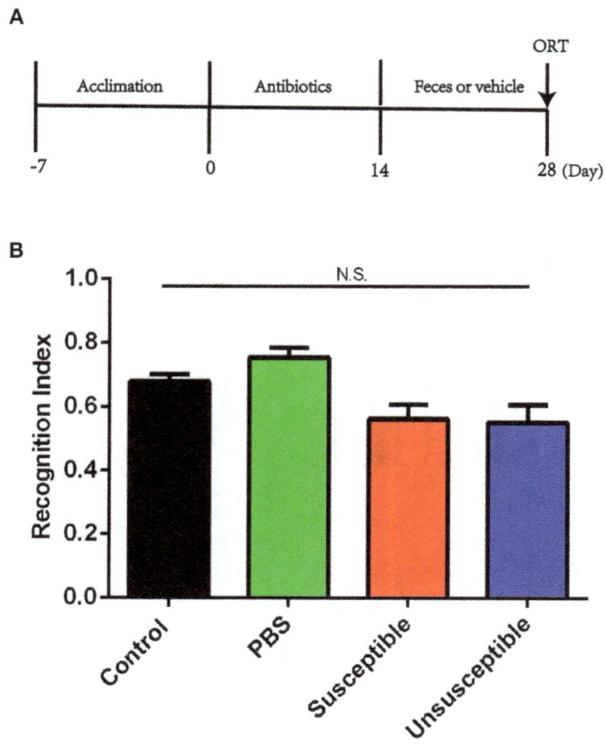

FIGURE 4 | Effects of fecal microbiota transplantation from DCP-CD or DCP-Non-CD mice on cognitive dysfunction in pseudo-germ-free mice. **(A)** Timeline of the establishment of pseud-germ-free mice and fecal transplantation. Antibiotics were dissolved in drinking water for 14 consecutive days. Fecal transplantation was performed for the other 14 consecutive days. ORT was performed on day 28. **(B)** ORT recognition index. N.S., not significant; ORT, Object recognition test.

DISCUSSION

This study provides novel insights into the vital role of gut microbiota in the process of chronic itch. Our findings are as follows: (1) There are abnormal compositions of gut microbiota in DCP-evoked chronic itch mice; (2) chronic itch may induce novel object recognition-related CD; (3) There are no differential alterations for abnormal gut microbiota compositions between chronic itch mice with and without CD; (4) Fecal microbiota transplantation from chronic itch mice with or without CD do not induce ORT-related CD in the pseudo-germ-free mice. Chronic itch is a common manifestation of a number of inflammatory skin diseases including contact dermatitis. Clinical studies have reported that DCP, an immunotherapy agent for patients with alopecia areata, induces eczematous skin diseases including contact dermatitis and severe pruritus. Contact dermatitis evoked by DCP has become a model system for studying chronic itch (27, 35). We successfully established DCP-evoked chronic itch model in C57BL/6J mice and found persistent scratching behavior and skin histopathological data. These results are in line with previous reports (9, 36). A vast array of clinical data show that chronic itch can cause the alteration of cognitive schemas (37, 38), for example, more negative memories and expectations with regard to itch. Our behavior evidences in mice strongly support that DCP-induced chronic itch can lead to novel object recognition-related cognitive dysfunction.

It is well-known that the impact of the wide variety of intestinal microbiota on numerous functions of the central nervous system has been increasingly recognized (39, 40). After the spared nerve injury (SNI) model rats were divided into SNI-CD phenotypes (Susceptible) and SNI-Non-CD phenotypes (Unsusceptible), Yang et al. (21) showed that abnormal gut microbiota composition induced by SNI correlated with anhedonia-related CD, suggesting that gut microbiota plays a key role in the neuropathic pain with depression-like phenotypes including anhedonia. Therefore, we speculate that chronic itch-related cognitive dysfunction may be implicated in gut microbiota. The 16S rRNA gene sequencing technology is a unique and powerful tool for revealing the gut microbiota composition and relationships between physiological functions and pathological features to date (41–44). α-diversity is defined as the degree of the species diversity in a biological environment and is mainly concerned with the number of bacteria or species therein (45). The Chao 1, Shannon, and Simpson indices are commonly used to evaluate the α-diversity of microbiota. In the present study, all three indices showed a significant decrease in fecal samples from the DCP mice than from control mice. PcoA demonstrated the differences between individuals or groups. The closer the distance is, the greater the biological repetition is within the same group. The distance of different groups represents their similarity or difference. As depicted in the three-dimensional PCoA picture, the dots of the DCP group were far apart from the control group. Circular tree data also illustrates that the composition of gut microbiota was pretty distinct between the two groups.

In our previous research, using diphenylcyclopropenone (DCP)- and acetone/ether/water (AEW)-induced chronic itch models, we showed that chronic itch did (not DCP or AEW) result in the changes of multiple mediators, such as chemokines in the spinal cord (9). In our other study, we demonstrated that alpha-Me-5-HT- and histamine-evoked acute pruritus induced specific patterns of spinal metabolites assessed by proton nuclear magnetic resonance spectroscopy, not alpha-Me-5-HT or histamine induced specific patterns of spinal metabolites (5). Thereby, we think that the alteration of gut microbiota is due to DCP-induced chronic itch, but not DCP treatment *per se* (Reviewer's suggestion). We used this method to reveal that 52 bacteria were altered at 6 levels in the DCP group compared to the control mice. At the genus level, *uncultured_bacterium, Mycoplasma, Alloprevotella, Rikenellaceae_RC9_gut_group, Anaeroplasma, Muribaculum, Ruminiclostridium_6, Blautia, uncultured_organism, Prevotellaceae_UCG-001, Ruminococcus_1, Ruminiclostridium_5, Prevotella, Azospirillum_sp._47_25, Dialister* were significantly decreased in DCP mice compared with control group. On the contrary, *Helicobacter, Roseburia, Anaerotruncus, ASF356, Candidatus_Arthromitus, Erysipelato-clostridium, Clostridium_sensu_stricto_1, GCA-900066225, Negativibacillus, Lactococcs, Ru-minococcaceae_UCG-004, Romboutsia, [Clostridium]_innocuum_group, Prevotella_9, Fusobact-erium* were significantly increased in DCP mice. These results suggest that gut microbiota may play an important role in DCP-evoked chronic itch in mice. At the species level, *uncultured_bacterium, Lachnospiraceae_bacterium_28-4, gut_metagenome, Lachnospiraceae_bacterium_COE1, Bacteroides_fragilis, Azospirillum_sp._47_25, uncultured_Ali-stipes_sp.* were significantly decreased in the DCP mice compared with the control group. In contrast, *uncultured_Clostridiales_bacterium, Lactobacillus_murinus, Clostridium_butyricum, Clostridium_sp._ND2, Lactococcus_lactis* were significantly increased in DCP mice. It seems that abnormal composition of these microbiota may play a role in DCP-evoked chronic itch.

It has been reported that the alterations in the composition of gut microbes may effect cognitive function (46–49). We adopted hierarchical cluster analysis of novel object recognition performance indices to classify the chronic itch model in mice into the DCP-CD (Susceptible) and DCP-Non-CD (Unsusceptible) phenotypes. In the present study, we observed no significant difference in α-diversity (consisting of Shannon and Simpson indices) among the Susceptible and Unsusceptible groups, suggesting little change in bacterial numbers in the two groups. In addition, the separation of groups according to β-diversity (PCoA) indicates that the microbiota composition was not significantly altered by the novel object recognition-related CD. These results are consistent with our findings that gut bacteria were not significantly different in the fecal samples between Control, Susceptible and Unsusceptible groups using 16S rRNA gene sequencing (**Supplementary Figure 6**). We, therefore, propose that gut bacteria might be not correlated with novel object recognition-related CD in the chronic itch mice.

Using large doses of antibiotics to establish pseudo-germ-free mice has become a common approach of fecal microbiota transplant studies (50, 51). In the present study, we observed that fecal microbiota transplant from DCP-CD (Susceptible) and DCP-Non-CD (Unsusceptible) mice did not induce novel object recognition-related CD, supporting the notion that regulating gut microbiota composition cannot improve chronic itch-induced CD.

In conclusion, these findings suggest that the microbiota composition was significantly altered by DCP-evoked chronic itch and that chronic itch may induce novel object recognition-related CD. However, abnormal gut microbiota composition induced by chronic itch may not be correlated with novel object recognition-related CD.

ETHICS STATEMENT

The animal study was reviewed and approved by Experimental protocols were approved by Institutional Animal Care and Use Committee of Tongji Hospital, Tongji Medical College, Huazhong University of Science and Technology, Wuhan, China (IRB ID:TJ-A0803).

AUTHOR CONTRIBUTIONS

All authors listed have made a substantial, direct and intellectual contribution to the work, and approved it for publication.

ACKNOWLEDGMENTS

We thank the OEbiotech Co. Ltd. (Shanghai, China) for providing assistance with the data analysis of 16S rRNA sequencing.

SUPPLEMENTARY MATERIAL

Supplementary Information | 16S rRNA analysis of fecal samples: The 16S rRNA analysis of fecal samples was performed at OEbiotech Co. Ltd. (Shanghai, China). DNA extraction was performed using DNA Extraction Kit following the manufacturer's instructions. V3-V4 (or V4-V5) variable regions of 16S rRNA genes were amplified with universal primers 343 F and 798 R. PCR products were then purified for further sequencing. Clean reads were subjected to primer sequences removal and clustering to generate operational taxonomic units (OTUs) using Vsearch software with 97% similarity cutoff (27). All representative reads were annotated and blasted against Silva database Version 123 (or Greengens) using RDP classifier (confidence threshold was 70%) (32). All representative reads were annotated and blasted against Unite database (ITSs rDNA) using blast (33).

Supplementary Figure 1 | Differences in the relative abundance of various gut microbes between control and DCP mice. **(A)** Cla2ss-Mollicutes (*t*-test. $P = 0.0117$). **(B)** Class-Alphaproteobacteria (*t*-test, $P = 0.0109$). **(C)** Class-Other (*t*-test. $P = 0.0297$). **(D)** Class-Fus-obacteriia (*t*-test. $P = 0.0029$). **(E)** Class-Negativicutes (*t*-test, $P = 0.0401$). **(F)** Class-Melainabacteria (*t*-test, $P = 0.0051$). **(G)** Class-Thermoanaerobaculia (*t*-test, $P = 0.0089$). **(H)** Class-Gemmatimona-detes (*t*-test, $P = 0.0139$). **(I)** Family-Prevotellaceae (*t*-test, $P = 0.0244$). **(J)** Family-Prevotellaceae (*t*-test, $P = 0.0064$). **(K)** Family-Other (*t*-test, $P < 0.0001$). **(L)** Family-Flavobacteriaceae (*t*-test, $P = 0.0031$). **(M)** Family-Fusobacteriaceae (*t*-test, $P = 0.0017$). **(N)** Family-Staphylococcaceae (*t*-test, $P = 0.0011$). **(O)** Genus-Mycoplasma (*t*-test, $P = 0.0061$). **(P)** Genus-Alloprevotella (*t*-test, $P = 0.0326$). **(Q)** Genus-Roseburia (*t*-test, $P = 0.0021$). **(R)** Genus-Anaerotruncus (*t*-test, $P = 0.0086$). **(S)** Genus-Riken-ellaceae_RC9_gut_group (*t*-test, $P < 0.0001$). **(T)** Genus-ASF356 (*t*-test, $P = 0.0341$).

Supplementary Figure 2 | Differences in the relative abundance of various gut microbes between control and DCP mice. **(A)** Genus-Anaeroplasma (*t*-test, $P = 0.0304$). **(B)** Genus-Ruminiclostridium_6 (*t*-test, $P = 0.0002$). **(C)** Genus-Blautia (*t*-test, $P = 0.0256$). **(D)** Genus-uncultured_organism (*t*-test, $P = 0.0198$). **(E)** Genus-Prevotellaceae_UCG-001 (*t*-test, $P = 0.0209$). **(F)** Genus-Ruminococcus_1 (*t*-test, $P < 0.0001$). **(G)** Genus-GCA-900066225 (*t*-test, $P = 0.0213$). **(H)** Genus-Negativibacillus (*t*-test, $P = 0.0342$). **(I)** Genus-Ruminiclostridium_5 (*t*-test, $P = 0.0425$). **(J)** Genus-Ruminococcaceae_UCG-004 (*t*-test, $P = 0.0478$). **(K)** Genus-Lactococcus (*t*-test, $P < 0.0001$). **(L)** Genus-Prevotella (*t*-test, $P = 0.0006$). **(M)** Genus-Romboutsia (*t*-test, $P = 0.0301$). **(N)**

Genus-[Clostridium]_innocuum_group (t-test, $P = 0.0158$). **(O)** Genus-Prevotella_9 (t-test, $P = 0.0219$). **(P)** Genus-Azospirillum_sp._47_25 (t-test, $P = 0.0034$). **(Q)** Genus-Dialister (t-test, $P = 0.0401$). **(R)** Genus-Fusobacterium (t-test, $P = 0.0017$). **(S)** Order-Anaeroplasmatales (t-test, $P = 0.0304$). **(T)** Order-Rhodospirillales (t-test, $P = 0.0124$).

Supplementary Figure 3 | Differences in the relative abundance of various gut microbes between control and DCP mice. **(A)** Order-Other (t-test, $P = 0.0076$). **(B)** Order-Fusobacteriales (t-test, $P = 0.0029$). **(C)** Order-Gastranaerophilales (t-test, $P = 0.0051$). **(D)** Order-Thermoanaerobaculales (t-test, $P = 0.0089$). **(E)** Order-Bacillales (t-test, $P = 0.0027$). **(F)** Phylum-Tenericutes (t-test, $P = 0.0117$). **(G)** Phylum-Other ($P = 0.0142$). **(H)** Phylum-Fusobacteria (t-test, $P = 0.0029$). **(I)** Phylum-Cyanobacteria (t-test, $P = 0.0051$). **(J)** Phylum-Acidobacteria (t-test, $P = 0.0109$). **(K)** Phylum-Gemmatimonadetes (t-test, $P = 0.0139$). **(L)** Species-uncultured_Clostridiales_bacterium (t-test, $P = 0.0227$). **(M)** Species-Lachnospiraceae_bacterium_28-4 (t-test, $P = 0.0092$). **(N)** Species-Lachnospiraceae_bacterium_COE1 (t-test, $P = 0.0022$). **(O)** Species-Bacteroides_fragilis (t-test, $P = 0.0272$). **(P)** Species-Clostridium_butyricum (t-test, $P = 0.0018$). **(Q)** Species-Clostridium_sp._ND2 (t-test, $P = 0.0141$). **(R)** Species-Azospirillum_sp._47_25 (t-test, $P = 0.0034$). **(S)** Species-uncultured_Alistipes_sp (t-test, $P = 0.0009$). **(T)** Species-Lac-tococcus_lactis (t-test, $P = 0.0393$).

Supplementary Figure 4 | Heatmaps of gut microbiota composition at class, family, and genus levels for control and DCP mice. **(A)** Heatmap (class level). **(B)** Heatmap (family level). **(C)** Heatmap (genus level).

Supplementary Figure 5 | Heatmaps of gut microbiota composition at order, phylum, and species levels for control and DCP mice. **(A)** Heatmap (order level). **(B)** Heatmap (phylum level). **(C)** Heatmap (species level).

Supplementary Figure 6 | Differences in relative abundance of gut microbiota at various phylogenetic levels among control (acetone), DCP-CD (Susceptible) and DCP-Non-CD (Unsusceptible) mice. **(A)** Class-Bacteroidia (one-way ANOVA, $F_{(2, 17)} = 7.894$, $P = 0.0038$). **(B)** Class-Fusobacteriia (one-way ANOVA, $F_{(2, 17)} = 8.708$, $P = 0.0025$). **(C)** Family-Muribaculaceae (one-way ANOVA, $F_{(2, 17)} = 9.514$, $P = 0.0017$). **(D)** Family-Prevotellaceae (one-way ANOVA, $F_{(2, 17)} = 4.296$, $P = 0.0309$). **(E)** Family-Rikenellaceae (one-way ANOVA, $F_{(2, 17)} = 5.805$, $P = 0.0120$). **(F)** Family-Clostridiaceae_1 (one-way ANOVA, $F_{(2, 17)} = 4.723$, $P = 0.0234$). **(G)** Genus-Blautia (one-way ANOVA, $F_{(2, 17)} = 5.117$, $P = 0.0182$). **(H)** Genus-uncultured_organism (one-way ANOVA, $F_{(2, 17)} = 5.396$, $P = 0.0153$). **(I)** Genus-uncultured_organism (one-way ANOVA, $F_{(2, 17)} = 4.168$, $P = 0.0336$). **(J)** Genus-Clostridium_sensu_stricto_1 (one-way ANOVA, $F_{(2, 17)} = 4.168$, $P = 0.0336$). **(K)** Genus-Prevotella (one-way ANOVA, $F_{(2, 17)} = 14.52$, $P = 0.0002$). **(L)** Genus-Az-ospirillum_sp._47_25 (one-way ANOVA, $F_{(2, 17)} = 4.208$, $P = 0.0328$). **(M)** Order-Bacteroidales (one-way ANOVA, $F_{(2, 17)} = 7.623$, $P = 0.0043$). **(N)** Order-Flavobacteriales (one-way ANOVA, $F_{(2, 17)} = 8.464$, $P = 0.0028$). **(O)** Order-Fusobacteriales (one-way ANOVA, $F_{(2, 17)} = 8.708$, $P = 0.0025$). **(P)** Phylum-B-acteroidetes (one-way ANOVA, $F_{(2, 17)} = 7.894$, $P = 0.0038$). **(Q)** Phylum-Bacteroidetes (one-way A-NOVA, $F_{(2, 17)} = 4.180$, $P = 0.0334$). **(R)** Phylum-Fusobacteria (one-way ANOVA, $F_{(2, 17)} = 8.708$, $P = 0.0025$). **(S)** Species-Lactobacillus_murinus (one-way ANOVA, $F_{(2, 17)} = 4.184$, $P = 0.0333$). **(T)** Species-gut_metagenome (one-way ANOVA, $F_{(2, 17)} = 8.906$, $P = 0.0023$).

REFERENCES

1. Ji RR, Donnelly CR Nedergaard M. Astrocytes in chronic pain and itch. *Nat Rev Neurosci.* (2019) 20:667–85. doi: 10.1038/s41583-019-0218-1
2. Ji RR. Neuroimmune interactions in itch: Do chronic itch, chronic pain, and chronic cough share similar mechanisms? *Pulm Pharmacol Ther.* (2015) 35:81–6. doi: 10.1016/j.pupt.2015.09.001
3. Feng J Hu H. A novel player in the field: Merkel disc in touch, itch and pain. *Exp Dermatol.* (2019) 28:1412–5. doi: 10.1111/exd.13945
4. Yosipovitch G, Rosen JD Hashimoto T. Itch: From mechanism to (novel) therapeutic approaches. *J Allergy Clin Immunol.* (2018) 142:1375–90. doi: 10.1016/j.jaci.2018.09.005
5. Liu T, He Z, Tian X, Kamal GM, Li Z, Liu Z, et al. Specific patterns of spinal metabolites underlying alpha-Me-5-HT-evoked pruritus compared with histamine and capsaicin assessed by proton nuclear magnetic resonance spectroscopy. *Biochim Biophys Acta Mol Basis Dis.* (2017) 1863:1222–30. doi: 10.1016/j.bbadis.2017.03.011
6. Chen YL, He ZG, Wang Q, Xiang HB, Fan L Xiong J. Specific patterns of spinal metabolite ratio underlying alpha-me-5-ht-evoked pruritus compared with compound 48/80 based on proton nuclear magnetic resonance spectroscopy. *Curr Med Sci.* (2020) 40:761–6. doi: 10.1007/s11596-020-2233-x
7. Geng X, Shi H, Ye F, Du H, Qian L, Gu L, et al. Matrine inhibits itching by lowering the activity of calcium channel. *Sci Rep.* (2018) 8:11328. doi: 10.1038/s41598-018-28661-x
8. Cevikbas F Lerner EA. Physiology and pathophysiology of itch. *Physiol Rev.* (2020) 100:945–82. doi: 10.1152/physrev.00017.2019
9. Liu BW, Li ZX, He ZG, Wang Q, Liu C, Zhang XW, et al. Altered expression of itch-related mediators in the lower cervical spinal cord in mouse models of two types of chronic itch. *Int J Mol Med.* (2019) 44:835–46. doi: 10.3892/ijmm.2019.4253
10. Zhao ZQ, Huo FQ, Jeffry J, Hampton L, Demehri S, Kim S, et al., Zhong J Chen ZF. Chronic itch development in sensory neurons requires BRAF signaling pathways. *J Clin Invest.* (2013) 123:4769–80. doi: 10.1172/JCI70528
11. Chen S, Gao XF, Zhou Y, Liu BL, Liu XY, Zhang Y, et al. A spinal neural circuitry for converting touch to itch sensation. *Nat Commun.* (2020) 11:5074. doi: 10.1038/s41467-020-18895-7
12. Gao ZR, Chen WZ, Liu MZ, Chen XJ, Wan L, Zhang XY, et al. Tac1-expressing neurons in the periaqueductal gray facilitate the itch-scratching cycle via descending regulation. *Neuron.* (2019) 101:45. doi: 10.1016/j.neuron.2018.11.010
13. Mack MR Kim BS. The itch-scratch cycle: a neuroimmune perspective. *Trends Immunol.* (2018) 39:980–91. doi: 10.1016/j.it.2018.10.001
14. Fowler E Yosipovitch G. Chronic itch management: therapies beyond those targeting the immune system. *Ann Allergy Asthma Immunol.* (2019) 123:158–65. doi: 10.1016/j.anai.2019.01.016
15. Tremaroli V Backhed F. Functional interactions between the gut microbiota and host metabolism. *Nature.* (2012) 489:242–9. doi: 10.1038/nature11552
16. Shen S, Lim G, You Z, Ding W, Huang P, Ran C, et al. Gut microbiota is critical for the induction of chemotherapy-induced pain. *Nat Neurosci.* (2017) 20:1213–216. doi: 10.1038/nn.4606
17. Cani PD, Bibiloni R, Knauf C, Waget A, Neyrinck AM, Delzenne NM Burcelin R. Changes in gut microbiota control metabolic endotoxemia-induced inflammation in high-fat diet-induced obesity and diabetes in mice. *Diabetes.* (2008) 57:1470–81. doi: 10.2337/db07-1403
18. Ke Y, Li D, Zhao M, Liu C, Liu J, Zeng A, et al. Gut flora-dependent metabolite Trimethylamine-N-oxide accelerates endothelial cell senescence and vascular aging through oxidative stress. *Free Radic Biol Med.* (2018) 116:88–100. doi: 10.1016/j.freeradbiomed.2018.01.007
19. Ticinesi A, Tana C, Nouvenne A, Prati B, Lauretani F Meschi T. Gut microbiota, cognitive frailty and dementia in older individuals: a systematic review. *Clin Interv Aging.* (2018) 13:1497–511. doi: 10.2147/CIA.S139163
20. Yu F, Han W, Zhan G, Li S, Xiang S, Zhu B, et al. Abnormal gut microbiota composition contributes to cognitive dysfunction in streptozotocin-induced diabetic mice. *Aging.* (2019) 11:3262–79. doi: 10.18632/aging.101978
21. Yang C, Fang X, Zhan G, Huang N, Li S, Bi J, et al. Key role of gut microbiota in anhedonia-like phenotype in rodents with neuropathic pain. *Transl Psychiatry.* (2019) 9:57. doi: 10.1038/s41398-019-0379-8
22. Codagnone MG, Spichak S, O'Mahony SM, O'Leary OF, Clarke G, Stanton C, et al. Programming bugs: microbiota and the developmental origins of brain health and disease. *Biol Psychiatry.* (2019) 85:150–63. doi: 10.1016/j.biopsych.2018.06.014
23. Arnoriaga-Rodriguez M Fernandez-Real JM. Microbiota impacts on chronic inflammation and metabolic syndrome - related cognitive dysfunction. *Rev Endocr Metab Disord.* (2019) 20:473–80. doi: 10.1007/s11154-019-09537-5
24. Kiguchi N, Uta D, Ding H, Uchida H, Saika F, Matsuzaki S, et al. GRP receptor and AMPA receptor cooperatively regulate itch-responsive neurons in the spinal dorsal horn. *Neuropharmacology.* (2020) 170:108025. doi: 10.1016/j.neuropharm.2020.108025

25. Chen M, Li ZX, Wang Q Xiang HB. Altered expression of differential genes in thoracic spinal cord involved in experimental cholestatic itch mouse model. *Curr Med Sci.* (2018) 38:679–83. doi: 10.1007/s11596-018-1930-1
26. Liu BW, Li ZX, He ZG, Liu C, Xiong J Xiang HB. Altered expression of target genes of spinal cord in different itch models compared with capsaicin assessed by RT-qPCR validation. *Oncotarget.* (2017) 8:74423–33. doi: 10.18632/oncotarget.20148
27. Sun YG, Zhao ZQ, Meng XL, Yin J, Liu XY Chen ZF. Cellular basis of itch sensation. *Science.* (2009) 325:1531–4. doi: 10.1126/science.1174868
28. Xiong B, Zhang W, Zhang L, Huang X, Zhou W, Zou Q, et al. Hippocampal glutamatergic synapses impairment mediated novel-object recognition dysfunction in rats with neuropathic pain. *Pain.* (2020) 161:1824–36. doi: 10.1097/j.pain.0000000000001878
29. Lueptow LM. Novel object recognition test for the investigation of learning and memory in mice. *J Vis Exp.* (2017) 126:e55718. doi: 10.3791/55718
30. Zhu L, Wang Z, Du Z, Qi X, Shu H, Liu D, et al. Impaired parahippocampal gyrus-orbitofrontal cortex circuit associated with visuospatial memory deficit as a potential biomarker and interventional approach for Alzheimer disease. *Neurosci Bull.* (2020) 36:831–44. doi: 10.1007/s12264-020-00498-3
31. Yang C, Fujita Y, Ren Q, Ma M, Dong C Hashimoto K. Bifidobacterium in the gut microbiota confer resilience to chronic social defeat stress in mice. *Sci Rep.* (2017) 7:45942. doi: 10.1038/srep45942
32. Wang Q, Garrity GM, Tiedje JM Cole JR. Naive Bayesian classifier for rapid assignment of rRNA sequences into the new bacterial taxonomy. *Appl Environ Microbiol.* (2007) 73:5261–7. doi: 10.1128/AEM.00062-07
33. Altschul SF, Gish W, Miller W, Myers EW Lipman DJ. Basic local alignment search tool. *J Mol Biol.* (1990) 215:403–10. doi: 10.1016/S0022-2836(05)80360-2
34. Ge X, Zhao W, Ding C, Tian H, Xu L, Wang H, et al. Potential role of fecal microbiota from patients with slow transit constipation in the regulation of gastrointestinal motility. *Sci Rep.* (2017) 7:441. doi: 10.1038/s41598-017-00612-y
35. Zhang TT, Shen FY, Ma LQ, Wen W, Wang B, Peng YZ, et al. Potentiation of synaptic transmission in Rat anterior cingulate cortex by chronic itch. *Mol Brain.* (2016) 9:73. doi: 10.1186/s13041-016-0251-1
36. Liu Y, Liu J, Li M, Dai S, Liang J Ji W. The effect of kinin B1 receptor on chronic itching sensitization. *Mol Pain.* (2015) 11:70. doi: 10.1186/s12990-015-0070-x
37. Rosen JD, Fostini AC Yosipovitch G. Diagnosis and management of neuropathic itch. *Dermatol Clin.* (2018) 36:213–224. doi: 10.1016/j.det.2018.02.005
38. Bartels DJP, van Laarhoven AIM, Heijmans N, Hermans D, Debeer E, van de Kerkhof PCM Evers AWM. Cognitive schemas in placebo and nocebo responding: role of autobiographical memories and expectations. *Clin Ther.* (2017) 39:502–12 e1. doi: 10.1016/j.clinthera.2017.02.004
39. Sharon G, Sampson TR, Geschwind DH Mazmanian SK. The central nervous system and the gut microbiome. *Cell.* (2016) 167:915–32. doi: 10.1016/j.cell.2016.10.027
40. Chevalier G, Siopi E, Guenin-Mace L, Pascal M, Laval T, Rifflet A, et al. Effect of gut microbiota on depressive-like behaviors in mice is mediated by the endocannabinoid system. *Nat Commun.* (2020) 11:6363. doi: 10.1038/s41467-020-19931-2
41. Watts GS, Youens-Clark K, Slepian MJ, Wolk DM, Oshiro MM, Metzger GS, et al. 16S rRNA gene sequencing on a benchtop sequencer: accuracy for identification of clinically important bacteria. *J Appl Microbiol.* (2017) 123:1584–96. doi: 10.1111/jam.13590
42. Klindworth A, Pruesse E, Schweer T, Peplies J, Quast C, Horn M Glockner FO. Evaluation of general 16S ribosomal RNA gene PCR primers for classical and next-generation sequencing-based diversity studies. *Nucleic Acids Res.* (2013) 41:e1. doi: 10.1093/nar/gks808
43. Louca S, Doebeli M Parfrey LW. Correcting for 16S rRNA gene copy numbers in microbiome surveys remains an unsolved problem. *Microbiome.* (2018) 6:41. doi: 10.1186/s40168-018-0420-9
44. Whelan FJ Surette MG. A comprehensive evaluation of the sl1p pipeline for 16S rRNA gene sequencing analysis. *Microbiome.* (2017) 5:100. doi: 10.1186/s40168-017-0314-2
45. Feng Y, Duan Y, Xu Z, Lyu N, Liu F, Liang S Zhu B. An examination of data from the American Gut Project reveals that the dominance of the genus Bifidobacterium is associated with the diversity and robustness of the gut microbiota. *MicrobiologyOpen.* (2019) 8:e939. doi: 10.1002/mbo3.939
46. Al-Asmakh M, Anuar F, Zadjali F, Rafter J Pettersson S. Gut microbial communities modulating brain development and function. *Gut Microbes.* (2012) 3:366–73. doi: 10.4161/gmic.21287
47. Fujimura KE, Slusher NA, Cabana MD Lynch SV. Role of the gut microbiota in defining human health. *Expert Rev Anti Infect Ther.* (2010) 8:435–54. doi: 10.1586/eri.10.14
48. Ochoa-Reparaz J Kasper LH. The second brain: is the gut microbiota a link between obesity and central nervous system disorders? *Curr Obes Rep.* (2016) 5:51–64. doi: 10.1007/s13679-016-0191-1
49. Petra AI, Panagiotidou S, Hatziagelaki E, Stewart JM, Conti P Theoharides TC. Gut-microbiota-brain axis and its effect on neuropsychiatric disorders with suspected immune dysregulation. *Clin Ther.* (2015) 37:984–95. doi: 10.1016/j.clinthera.2015.04.002
50. Hernandez-Chirlaque C, Aranda CJ, Ocon B, Capitan-Canadas F, Ortega-Gonzalez M, Carrero JJ, et al. Germ-free and antibiotic-treated mice are highly susceptible to epithelial injury in DSS colitis. *J Crohns Colitis.* (2016) 10:1324–35. doi: 10.1093/ecco-jcc/jjw096
51. Zhan G, Yang N, Li S, Huang N, Fang X, Zhang J, et al. Abnormal gut microbiota composition contributes to cognitive dysfunction in SAMP8 mice. *Aging (Albany NY).* (2018) 10:1257–67. doi: 10.18632/aging.101464

7

Chronic Prurigo: Similar Clinical Profile and Burden Across Clinical Phenotypes

Claudia Zeidler, Manuel Pedro Pereira and Sonja Ständer*

Department of Dermatology and Center for Chronic Pruritus, University Hospital Münster, Münster, Germany

***Correspondence:**
Claudia Zeidler
claudia.zeidler@ukmuenster.de

Chronic prurigo is a debilitating skin disease characterized by the presence of chronic pruritus and scratching-related pruriginous lesions. The pruriginous lesions can differ in their clinics what has recently been categorized into different clinical phenotypes. The most common one is chronic nodular prurigo (syn. prurigo nodularis); other phenotypes are papular, plaque, umbilicated, and linear prurigo. A comparison between these phenotypes regarding similarities and differences has not yet been performed. In this explorative analysis, itch characteristics, scratching behavior, and disease burden of the nodular, papular, plaque, and umbilicated prurigo were investigated in 1,128 patients. Patients with nodular and plaque prurigo were younger than patients with papular and umbilicated prurigo. The shortest duration of the underlying pruritus was found in papular and umbilicated prurigo, the longest in plaque prurigo. Itch intensity, impairment of sleep, mood and the quality of life did not differ. These findings confirm that the clinical phenotypes of chronic prurigo belong to a spectrum of one disease with similar disease characteristics and can be categorized under the umbrella term of chronic prurigo. Future clinical trials should include all phenotypes of chronic prurigo.

Keywords: prurigo nodularis, pruritus, burden, quality of life, itch characteristics

INTRODUCTION

Chronic prurigo (CPG) is a rare but worldwide occurring disease (1, 2). It is characterized by the presence of chronic pruritus (CP), history, and/or evidence of repeated scratching (e.g., excoriations, scars) as well as localized or generalized pruriginous lesions (3). The clinical picture differs in the number, distribution and the type of the pruriginous lesions such as papules, nodules, and/or plaques (3, 9, 10). However, multiple types of pruriginous lesions can be present in the same patient. These lesions dot not allow a conclusion to the underlying etiology of CPG. Depending on the predominant pruriginous lesion in one patient (**Figure 1**), the CPG is divided into the following clinical phenotypes according to the disease definition (3): chronic nodular prurigo (nodules predominate), chronic papular prurigo (papules predominate), chronic plaque prurigo (plaques predominate), and chronic umbilicated prurigo (ulcerated pruriginous lesions predominate) (3). As these phenotypes fulfill the definition of CPG, it was proposed that CPG is an umbrella term for the various clinical presentations (3).

In the past, studies in CPG focused on analyzing itch characteristics and disease burden exclusively in chronic nodular prurigo. From these studies it is known that patients with chronic nodular prurigo have a high burden and a substantial impairment of the quality of life, even when compared to patients with CP on non-lesional skin (4, 5). Sleep quality can be severely limited in

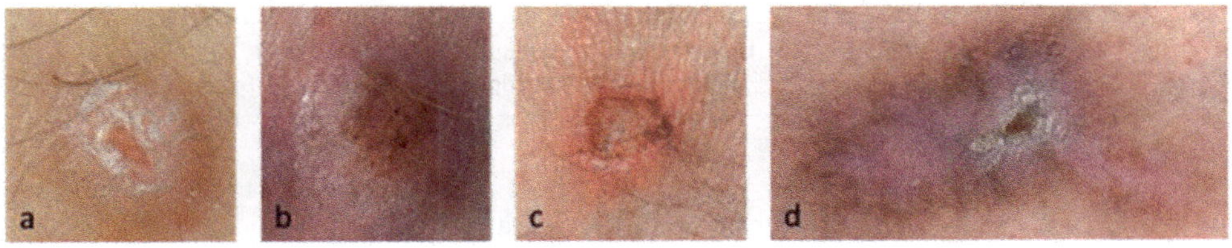

FIGURE 1 | Different types of pruriginous lesions. **(a)** papules (<1 cm), **(b)** nodules (≥1 cm), **(c)** ulcerated pruriginous lesions, **(d)** plaques.

these patients and the presence of psychological comorbidities can frequently occur in patients with chronic nodular prurigo (5, 6). However, until now, no study included the other clinical phenotypes of CPG (papular, plaque, and umbilicated type) and it is unknown if the aggregation of these phenotypes under one disease is justified and if there are biological differences between the clinical phenotypes of CPG.

Therefore, this study aims detecting possible differences between the CPG phenotypes regarding clinical characteristics using a retrospective approach and to verify the suggestion that the clinical phenotypes can categorized under the umbrella term of CPG.

MATERIALS AND METHODS

Data Source

Data from routine care were used to perform this retrospective analysis. All data from patients of the Center for Chronic Pruritus were transferred into a biomedical data base. After written informed consent, data were collected by the physicians (i.e., medical history and physical examination), and from several patient reported outcome tools (e.g., pruritus questionnaire, quality of life). Afterwards the data were reviewed by the physician-in-chief and transferred to the research database of the Center for Chronic Pruritus at the University Hospital Münster, which is approved by the Ethics Committee of the Medical Faculty of the University of Münster (2007-413-f-S) (7). For this analysis, data of the first consultation of patients with CPG, who presented between October 2004 and February 2018, were included.

Etiology of CPG

According to the International Forum for the Study of Itch (IFSI) (8) the etiology of CPG was diagnosed and classified by a physician.

Patient Reported Outcome Tools

The numerical rating scale (NRS), ranging from 0 (no pruritus) to 10 (worst imaginable pruritus) was used to assess itch intensity of the previous 24 h (worst itch intensity in the last 24 h = WI-NRS/24 h; average itch intensity of the last 24 h = AI-NRS/24 h). The "Neuroderm" questionnaire, a pruritus questionnaire, was used to assess the scratching behavior and the impact on sleep (9). The impairment of the quality of life was assessed by using the "Dermatology Life Quality Index (DLQI)" (10) and the possible presence of an anxiety and/or a depression was investigated using the screening questionnaire "Hospital Anxiety and Depression Scale (HADS)" (11).

Statistical Analyses

For each metric endpoint, the Hodges-Lehmann estimate of the median with two-sided 95% confidence interval (CI) was calculated by using the R function wilcox.exact from the R package exactRankTests. For each binary endpoint, the absolute numbers and percentages per category were calculated for each group. For a chosen reference, an exact Clopper-Pearson 95% CI for the percentage was calculated by using the R function exactci from the R package PropCIs. All analyses are of explorative character. No adjustments for multiple testing were performed. If the CIs of the groups did not differ considerably, it was interpreted as an indication of equivalence. All statistical analyses were predetermined in a statistical analysis plan and were performed by R 3.4.4.

RESULTS

1,128 patients with CPG [692 (61.4%) female] were included in this study. Most of them suffered from chronic nodular prurigo [n = 908 (80.5%)] (**Table 1**). Patients with nodular prurigo and plaque prurigo were younger than patients with papular or umbilicated prurigo (**Table 1**). Nodular, popular, and plaque prurigo predominantly affected women (60.6-66.7%); in the group of patients suffering from umbilicated prurigo, men were more affected (66.7%).

Duration and Cause of Chronic Prurigo

Overall, the patients suffered from CP for a median duration of 2.9 years (CI 2.6-3.1) before presenting in our center. A comparison of the groups showed that patients with papular prurigo and umbilicated prurigo had the shortest, patients with nodular prurigo an intermediate and patients with plaque prurigo the longest duration from CP (**Table 1**).

The etiology of pruritus classified according to the IFSI classification (8) was most frequently found to be of multifactorial origin in nodular and umbilicated prurigo. The patients with papular and plaque prurigo showed most common a dermatosis as the cause of CP (**Table 1**). Dermatological diseases were the second most frequently found origins in patients with nodular prurigo, while in umbilicated prurigo the second most frequent origin was a systemic disease.

TABLE 1 | Demographics, duration and origin of chronic pruritus and burden of disease in the different clinical phenotypes.

	Nodular Prurigo	Popular prurigo	Umbilicated prurigo	Plaque prurigo	Differences
Number					
N	908	193	24	3	Plaque < umbilicated < papular < nodular prurigo
%	80.5	17.1	2.1	0.3	
Age (yrs)					
Median	64.3	71	73	60.3	Plaque < nodular < papular < umbilicated prurigo
95% CI	62.8-65.8	66-73.4	66.8-77.8	52.2-64.7	
Sex					
Male, *n* (%)	343 (37.8)	76 (39.4)	16 (66.7)	1 (33.3)	More females affected except in umbilicated prurigo.
Female, *n* (%)	565 (62.2)	117 (60.6)	8 (33.3)	2 (66.7)	
Duration of pruritus (yrs)					
Median	3.5	1.86	1.64	6	Umbilicated < papular < nodular < plaque prurigo
95% CI	3.03-4.11	1.59-2.05	1.08-3.04	6.4-10.2	
Origin of pruritus (%)					
Dermatologic	22.8	36.7	12.5	66.7	Most frequent origin per phenotype is highlighted in gray.
Systemic	9.0	8.8	20.8	0	
Neurologic	6.5	12.8	12.5	0	
Psychiatric	1.2	2.4	4.2	0	
Multifactorial	54.4	36.2	50	33.3	
Unknown	6.1	3.1	0	0	
Intensity of pruritus					
WI-NRS/24h					
Median	8.5	8.5	8.75	8	No differences according to 95% CI.
95% CI	8.5-9.0	8-9.0	7.5-9.0	6.5-8.0	
AI-NRS/24h					
Median	6.5	6.5	7.75	6.5	
95% CI	6.0-7.0	6.0-7.0	5.0-8.5	5.2-6.8	
Scratching behavior (%)					
Scratching only when itching	71.0	81.3	82.4	66.6	Positive outliers are highlighted in dark gray, negative outliers in light gray.
Scratching causes itch relief	68.8	47.0	47.1	33.3	
Scratching injures the skin	63.0	51.5	64.7	33.3	
Scratching is done unconsciously	51.2	29.5	29.4	33.3	
Scratching causes itch aggravation	49.3	36.6	23.5	33.3	
Scratching provides satisfaction	30.5	27.1	17.6	33.3	
Rubbing	64.9	67.9	41.1	66.6	
Chafing	25.6	20.1	5.9	33.3	
Pinching	16.5	10.5	17.6	33.3	
Kneading	7.8	9.0	5.9	33.3	
Quality of life					
DLQI					
Median	13.0	10.0	12.0	8.0	No differences according to 95% CI.
95% CI	11.0-15.5	9.2-13.5	9-12.7	7.4-12.0	
Anxiety and depressions					
HADS-A					
Median	7.0	7.0	8.0	7.0	No differences according to 95% CI.
95% CI	6.4-9.3	5.9-8.7	6.6-9.0	5.8-8.4	

(Continued)

TABLE 1 | Continued

	Nodular Prurigo	Popular prurigo	Umbilicated prurigo	Plaque prurigo	Differences
HADS-D					
Median	7.0	6.0	8.5	5.0	
95% CI	7.0-9.2	6.0-8.1	8.5-9.4	5.0-7.4	
Loss of slept hours/day					
Median	3	3	3.5	2	No differences.
Mean	3.2	3	3	2.6	
SD(±)	2	1.8	1.8		

Yrs, years; WI-NRS/24h, worst pruritus intensity in the last 24 h; AI-NRS/24 h, average pruritus intensity in the last 24 h; DLQI, Dermatology Life Quality Index; HADS-A, Hospital Anxiety and Depressions Scale for Anxiety; HADS-D, Hospital Anxiety and Depressions Scale for Depressions; SD, standard deviation.

Itch Intensity

The median AI-NRS/24h was 6.5/10, whereas the median WI-NRS/24h was 8.5 for the whole patient population. No differences between the phenotypes were found when comparing the pruritus intensity (**Table 1**).

Scratching Behavior

Almost all patients (over 90%) reported that they scratch themselves, and that they were aware that scratching injures the skin (60.7%). Interestingly, 42.4% of all patients stated scratching can cause itch aggravation. Divided into the phenotypes, some differences could be found: Patients with nodular prurigo stated more frequently "scratching causes itch relief," "scratching is done unconsciously," and "scratching causes itch aggravation" (**Figure 2**).

There were no differences in the kind of scratching between patients with nodular and papular prurigo. Whereas in contrast to all other phenotypes patients with plaque prurigo reported more frequent to pinch and knead and patients with umbilicated prurigo do less rub and chafe their skin (**Table 1**).

Burden of CPG

Patients reported sleep problems independent of the clinical phenotype. The loss of sleeping hours did not differ between the phenotypes. All patients achieved comparable values in the total score of the DLQI and the subscores for anxiety and depression in the HADS (**Table 1**).

DISCUSSION

The aim of this explorative study was to investigate the demographic profile, itch intensity, scratching behavior, and burden of the different clinical phenotypes of CPG. We found more similarities in the analyzed parameter than differences between phenotypes. For example, pruritus characteristics, the impact on sleep, quality of life and mood did not differ between the groups. Regarding pruritus intensity at baseline, the median of the average pruritus intensity in the last 24 h was classified as moderate to severe; the median of the worst pruritus intensity in the last 24 h as severe in all phenotypes. These results confirm analyzes of previous studies examining the pruritus intensity of patients with chronic nodular prurigo (4, 5). It can be speculated that as soon as the CPG has developed due to neuronal sensitization processes and the development of a vicious circle of experiencing pruritus and continuously scratching independent of the origin, the severity of the itch intensity in the different phenotypes is similar.

Differences were identified regarding the categorized etiology of CPG. A multifactorial etiolgy was prominent in nodular and umbilicated prurigo whereas more dermatological diseases were found in papular and plaque prurigo. Despite these differences in the categories, no conclusion is justified based on these data to make a differential diagnosis regarding the individual etiology of CPG in affected patients.

Another descriptive difference was found regarding the duration of the underlying pruritus in CPG. Patients with plaque prurigo suffered the longest, followed by patients with nodular prurigo and then papular and umbilicated type. It can thus be assumed that the duration of the CPG and the associated prolonged scratching contributes to different clinical phenotypes. This supports the assumption that some clinical phenotypes of CPG are a continuous spectrum of the disease and can merge. Also another earlier study suggested that the various pruriginous lesions such as papules, nodules and plaques represent stages of the development in CPG (12).

All patients have in common a severe scratching behavior with some differences which might be relevant for development of the different phenotypes. More than half of the patients with nodular prurigo scratch themselves unconsciously, while only a third of patients suffering from the other CPG phenotypes made this statement. Patients with umbilicated prurigo less often chafe or rub compared to all other phenotypes. However, there are also patients in these group who do chafing or rubbing their skin. This observation does not disambiguate that the way of scratching leads to a particular phenotype of CPG.

It was also noticeable that scratching was reported to cause both pruritus relief and aggravation. These statements, contradicting at first glance, reflect the vicious circle of itching

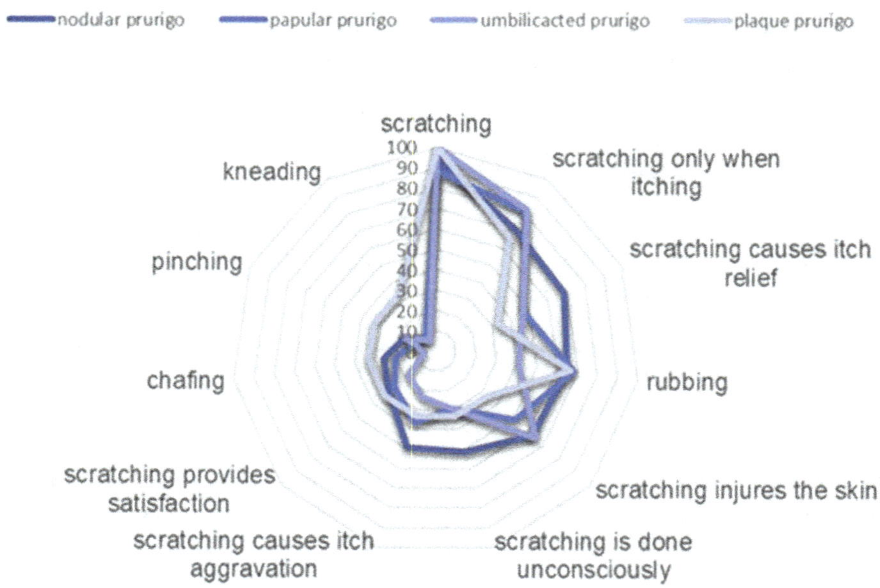

FIGURE 2 | Comparison of scratching behavior in patients with different clinical phenotypes of chronic prurigo (in %).

and scratching that is a typical characteristic of CPG. Satisfaction and pruritus control by scratching may directly occur while or shortly after scratching, but the pruritus recurs again afterwards.

Comparing the burden of patients, the phenotypes of CPG showed no differences in the impairment of the quality of life, in the scores for screening for anxiety and depression and in restriction of sleep. The median values from the DLQI for nodular prurigo, umbilicated prurigo, and plaque prurigo were in the range that indicate a strong impairment of the quality of life, for papular prurigo with one point below the cut-off value in the range for moderate impairment. However, all confidence intervals are comparable, therefore no important differences can be assumed here. In the past, the use of DLQI in patients with nodular prurigo showed also a strong impairment of the quality of life (13–15). Compared to these analyses of the quality of life in patients with nodular prurigo, our findings in patients of different clinical phenotypes are identical.

CONCLUSIONS

Overall, differences could be found in the age of the patients, in the duration and origin of the underlying CP and, though minimal, the scratching behavior. However, the itch intensity and the burden did not differ across the different clinical phenotypes of CPG. These findings confirm that clinical phenotypes of CPG are a spectrum and a part of the same disease, supporting the proposed term CPG as an umbrella term including all phenotypes of CPG. Based on these data and the assumed identical pathogenesis of the phenotypes, we suppose that the treatment response of patients with CPG is equal, regardless of the clinical phenotype. In the future, further studies should be carried out to confirm this statement and in order to find out whether new antipruritic treatments should be tested in each individual phenotype or in a cohort of CPG independent from its phenotype.

LIMITATIONS

Since data were not normally distributed, we did not perform comparisons of distributions to calculate *p*-values in this exploratory analysis. We rather examined if the 95% CI's differed from each other for each variable. If this was not the case, it was interpreted as an indication of equivalence. The differences to plaque prurigo should be interpreted carefully, as very few patients suffered from it.

AUTHOR CONTRIBUTIONS

All authors listed have made a substantial, direct and intellectual contribution to the work, and approved it for publication.

REFERENCES

1. Williams KA, Huang AH, Belzberg M, Kwatra SG. Prurigo nodularis: pathogenesis and management. *J Am Acad Dermatol.* (2020) 83:1567–75. doi: 10.1016/j.jaad.2020.04.182
2. Ständer S, Ketz M, Kossack N, Akumo D, Pignot M, Gabriel S, et al. Epidemiology of prurigo nodularis compared with psoriasis in Germany: a claims database analysis. *Acta Derm Venereol.* (2020) 100:adv00309. doi: 10.2340/00015555-3655
3. Pereira MP, Steinke S, Zeidler C, Forner C, Riepe C, Augustin M, et al. European academy of dermatology and venereology European prurigo project: expert consensus on the definition, classification and terminology of chronic prurigo. *J Eur Acad Dermatol Venereol.* (2018) 32:1059–65. doi: 10.1111/jdv.14570
4. Gründel S, Pereira MP, Storck M, Osada N, Schneider G, Ständer S, et al. Analysis of 325 patients with chronic nodular prurigo: clinics, burden of disease and course of treatment. *Acta Derm Venereol.* (2020) 100:adv00269. doi: 10.2340/00015555-3571
5. Pereira MP, Hoffmann V, Weisshaar E, Wallengren J, Halvorsen JA, Garcovich S, et al. Chronic nodular prurigo: clinical profile and burden. A European cross-sectional study. *J Eur Acad Dermatol Venereol.* (2020) 34:2373–83. doi: 10.1111/jdv.16309
6. Gwillim EC, Janmohamed SR, Yousaf M, Patel KR, Silverberg JI. The impact of prurigo nodularis on sleep disturbance and related impact: a systematic review. *J Eur Acad Dermatol Venereol.* (2020). 34:e815-7. doi: 10.1111/jdv.16696
7. Bruland P, Forster C, Breil B, Ständer S, Dugas M, Fritz F. Does single-source create an added value? Evaluating the impact of introducing x4T into the clinical routine on workflow modifications, data quality and cost-benefit. *Int J Med Inform.* (2014) 83:915–28. doi: 10.1016/j.ijmedinf.2014.08.007
8. Ständer S. Classification of Itch. *Curr Probl Dermatol.* (2016) 50:1–4. doi: 10.1159/000446009
9. Ständer S, Pogatzki-Zahn E, Stumpf A, Fritz F, Pfleiderer B, Ritzkat A, et al. Facing the challenges of chronic pruritus: a report from a multi-disciplinary medical itch centre in Germany. *Acta Derm Venereol.* (2015) 95:266–71. doi: 10.2340/00015555-1949
10. Finlay AY, Khan GK. Dermatology Life Quality Index (DLQI)– a simple practical measure for routine clinical use. *Clin Exp Dermatol.* (1994) 19:210–6. doi: 10.1111/j.1365-2230.1994.tb01167.x
11. Zigmond AS, Snaith RP. The hospital anxiety and depression scale. *Acta Psychiatr Scand.* (1983) 67:361–70. doi: 10.1111/j.1600-0447.1983.tb09716.x
12. Schedel F, Schürmann C, Metze D, Ständer S. Prurigo. Clinical definition and classification. *Hautarzt.* (2014) 65:684–90. doi: 10.1007/s00105-014-2753-z
13. Ferrucci S, Tavecchio S, Berti E, Angileri L. Dupilumab and prurigo nodularis-like phenotype in atopic dermatitis: our experience of efficacy. *J Dermatolog Treat.* (2021) 32:453–4. doi: 10.1080/09546634.2019.1659479
14. Brenaut E, Halvorsen JA, Dalgard FJ, Lien L, Balieva F, Sampogna F, et al. The self-assessed psychological comorbidities of prurigo in European patients: a multicentre study in 13 countries. *J Eur Acad Dermatol Venereol.* (2019) 33:157–62. doi: 10.1111/jdv.15145
15. Steinke S, Zeidler C, Riepe C, Bruland P, Soto-Rey I, Storck M, et al. Humanistic burden of chronic pruritus in patients with inflammatory dermatoses: results of the European Academy of Dermatology and Venereology Network on Assessment of Severity and Burden of Pruritus (PruNet) cross-sectional trial. *J Am Acad Dermatol.* (2018) 79:457-63.e5. doi: 10.1016/j.jaad.2018.04.044

8

Itch Matrixes

Peyman Najafi[1,2], *Laurent Misery*[1,3*], *Jean-Luc Carré*[1], *Douraied Ben Salem*[4,5] *and Olivier Dufor*[1,6]

[1] *Univ Brest, LIEN, Brest, France,* [2] *Paris-Saclay Institute of Neuroscience, Centre National de la Recherche Scientifique/ Université Paris-Saclay, Gif-sur-Yvette, France,* [3] *University Hospital of Brest, Department of Dermatology, Brest, France,* [4] *Univ Brest, LATIM, INSERM UMR, Brest, France,* [5] *University Hospital of Brest, Department of Radiology, Brest, France,* [6] *L@bISEN Yncréa Ouest, ISEN, Brest, France*

Keywords: itch, matrix, pain, brain, imaging

Correspondence:
Laurent Misery
laurent.misery@chu-brest.fr

INTRODUCTION

In a recent meta-analysis from our group based on a systematic review we have identified brain regions reported to be responsible for central mechanisms of itch processing (1). We also have discussed the central mechanisms of itch proceeding in the brain more in depth in a review paper (2). The research papers that have studied central mechanism of itch are presented in **Table 1** while their results are presented in **Table 2**. Here in this paper, we are exploring a new idea in which we categorize the itch matrix in the brain into three matrixes that each of them is contributing to a specific aspect of itch perception. This conceptualizes the processing of itch signals into different itch matrices could be useful in order to model different aspects of itch. For example, it is possible, that an overactivity in second matrix cause a higher susceptivity to contagious itch.

Unlike the visual system pain and itch can evoke multitude of regions in the brain, which we call pain matrix and itch matrix respectively. Recent studies have proposed that the pain matrix can be categorized into three different pain matrixes (40, 41): one contributing to perception and the location of pain; another matrix responsible for the affective aspect of the pain; and a third involving decoding the cognitive aspect of pain. In the same manner, we guardedly propose that the itch processing network can be broken down into three main matrixes although many data are still lacking. These three matrixes have been presented in **Figure 1**.

FIRST ITCH MATRIX

The first itch matrix includes but is not restricted to the primary sensorimotor cortex, the parietal/central operculum, and the posterior insular cortex (**Figure 2A**).

Among these three regions the primary sensorimotor cortex is involved in the encoding of the recognition, localization, and intensity of painful stimuli (42). In pain studies, activation in this region bears a linear relationship with pain intensity (43–47). In a positron emission tomography (PET) study by Drzezga et al. (5) the authors reported that SI activity, is positively correlated with itch intensity. Six years after Drzezga, in 2007, Mochizuki et al. added the secondary somatosensory cortex (SII) demonstrating an increase of activity in this region after itch induction with histamine (10). The increase was statistically not different than the proven one observed in the painful condition (pain vs. itch) but did not reach a statistically corrected threshold when comparing itch against no itch.

In another study which includes both AD patients and healthy controls, itch was found to activate the post-central gyrus in the right hemisphere (12). This study together with Drzezga study in 2001 are reported in the meta-analysis on Itch from Lee et al. (48). Out of 56 regions listed in the parietal cortex (31 Left and 25 Right) from 18 studies (**Table 1**). Brain activity upon itch stimulation, in (48), left SI appears to be activated eight times against two only in the right hemisphere. On the contrary, right SII is reported five times against two only in the left hemisphere. The other regions mentioned ($n = 39$) are in both left and right parietal cortices sometime very near to the SI/SII regions (i.e., SMG, SPL, IPL, anterior parietal cortex).

In the meta-analysis from Roberts et al. (49), the authors suggest the possibility of a specificity of these regions for the itching process as they appear to be better activated by itching than by pain. Interestingly, they also group these regions with the central operculum. In a recent meta-analysis of our group (1), SI/SII region was not clearly identified but we discussed this point regarding the diversity of studies we included. Our results on correlations with itch intensity also showed two important clusters in bilateral insular cortices (5068 voxels right 4589 voxels left) that spread to a great extent on the post-central gyri.

The co-activation of the central operculum together with SI/SII cortex is widely reported in itch literature both in healthy subjects and patients. Indeed, central operculum corresponding to the junction of pre- and post-central gyri accompanied with the region located laterally to the posterior convolution of the insula is often confounded with insula itself or even SI. In the regions abbreviated OPC, also named rolandic operculum elsewhere, itch intensity was also correlated with PET signal both in healthy subjects and AD patients (4, 33).

Finally, we propose that the insular cortex, and especially its posterior portion, takes part into this first matrix. As a common point between these regions, their gradual response with itch intensity seems important to highlight. In Leknes et al. bilateral insular and left posterior insular activity (BOLD) is correlated with histamine-induced itch intensity (9). Following Craig (50, 51), Mochizuki et al. postulate that the posterior part of insula plays a different role than its anterior part (52, 53). A distinction that can also find its basis on cytoarchitectural composition of these structures and their connectives with other brain areas (50, 54).

Despite weak evidences in itch literature, other evidences can help to understand the insula role in processing the sensations which are common to itch and pain. Mazzola et al. explain that the two thirds of posterior insula submitted to low electrical stimulation (SEEG) directly translate these stimulations as pain sensations (55). Another study from Frot et al. showed that once pain feeling is reached, the posterior insular cortex activity still correlates with noxious thermal stimulation intensity (47).

In summary, all these regions encode the feeling of itchy sensation and are somewhat translating its intensity level as well as their location following a somatotopic representation. When compared to Xiang et al. study (41), this first matrix includes all already reported regions for pain. However, studies reporting activities in those regions only for itch are rare and some studies need to be carefully interpreted given approximations inherent to main peak reporting. Effectively, secondary peaks of wide clusters or percentage of anatomical regions covered by these clusters are most often not indicated. As an example, the absence of parietal operculum in Roberts et al. study (49) needs to be put in perspective. Indeed, the point that the contrast pain—itch shows an increased activity in the parietal operculum does not mean that this region is silent in itch. Moreover, in the same study, the opposite contrast itch—pain, which reveals an implication of both right supramarginal gyrus and central operculum, could have led us to add more parietal areas to this first matrix.

So far, we have dealt with the membership of each of these brain regions in the matrix separately. However, interesting arguments reside in the fact that new pathological conditions can appear when these regions grouped and malfunction together. Hence, some studies reported that SI/SII together with the insular cortex participate in creating the allodynia phenomenon (56–59). Consecutively, these regions once activated lead to an ignition of the pain network inducing activity in the PAG, the prefrontal cortex, the thalamus, the amygdala, the ACC and many other regions within the pain network. Allodynia has repercussions on the way normal brain areas react to tactile stimuli and authors do not only consider the condition through the scope of pain matrix. Many brain areas are those involved in tactile or thermal sensitivity and this allows more faithful comparison with itch perception. The difficulty with allodynia is that even when it is spontaneous, painful sensation is quickly reached and its intensity then depends on other brain region listed above.

To illustrate this phenomenon, we adduce together both Ducreux et al. study (60) and an article from Geuter et al. (61) about predictive coding. In Ducreux et al. authors demonstrated with noxious and non-noxious cold stimulation (4° and 22°C) that while non-noxious cold in control subjects activates SII and the insular cortex (mostly its anterior part), the same non-noxious stimulation did activates SII and mid-posterior insula in allodynic patients together with other regions of the pain network (60). In Geuter et al. work, the authors used the predictive coding theory of brain functioning to demonstrate a difference within the anterior and the posterior part of the insula. While the anterior part would be dedicated to pain feelings as a prediction error on perceived sensations, the posterior part only responds to pain intensity with no comparisons to any predicted sensation (61). We propose that in Ducreux et al. even if the feeling is non-noxious in control subjects, it remains unpredictable and then activates the anterior part of the insula. However, allodynic patients are prepared to feel painful

Abbreviations: ACC, Anterior Cingulate Cortex; AD, Atopic Dermatitis; aIC, Anterior part of the Insular Cortex; aMCC, Anterior part of the Middle Cingulate Cortex; BOLD, Blood Oxygenation Level Dependent; dACC, Dorsal part of the Anterior Cingulate Cortex; DLPFC, Dorso-Lateral Pre-Frontal Cortex; IPL, Inferior Parietal Lobule; OPC, Operculum Central; PAG, Peri-Aqueductal Gray matter; PCC, Posterior Cingulate Cortex; PET, Positron Emission Tomography; pIC, Posterior Insular Cortex; pMCC, Posterior part of the Middle Cingulate Cortex; SI, Primary Somatosensory cortex; SII, Secondary Somatosensory cortex; SEEG, Stereo-Electro-Encephalo-Graphy; SMG, Supra-Marginal Gyrus; SPL, Superior Parietal Lobule.

TABLE 1 | Papers and methods which have been used in order to study central mechanism of itch.

#	References	Scanner	Neuroimaging analysis	Itch induction	Itch stimulus	Number of subjects	Pathology	Comments
1	Hsieh et al. (3)	PET	Subtraction	Intracutaneous injection	Histamine	10	Healthy	
2	Darsow et al. (4)	PET	Subtraction	Skin prick	Histamine	6	Healthy	
3	Darsow et al. (4)	PET	Correlation	Skin prick	Histamine	6	Healthy	
4	Drzezga et al. (5)	PET	Correlation	Skin prick	Histamine	6	Healthy	
5	Mochizuki et al. (6)	PET	Subtraction	Iontophoresis	Histamine	15	Healthy	
6	Walter et al. (7)	fMRI	Correlation	Skin prick	Histamine	6	Healthy	
7	Herde et al. (8)	fMRI	Subtraction	Intracutaneous microdialysis	Histamine	10	Healthy	
8	Leknes et al. (9)	fMRI	Correlation	Skin prick	Histamine	8	Healthy	
9	Leknes et al. (9)	fMRI	Correlation		Allergan	8	Atopic cohort	
10	Mochizuki et al. (10)	fMRI	Correlation	Iontophoresis	Histamine	14	Healthy	
11	Mochizuki et al. (10)	fMRI	Subtraction	Iontophoresis	Histamine	14	Healthy	
12	Valet et al. (11)	fMRI	Subtraction	Skin prick	Histamine	12	Healthy	
13	Valet et al. (11)	fMRI	Subtraction	Skin prick	Histamine	12	Healthy	Temperature modeling
14	Schneider et al. (12)	PET	Subtraction	Iontophoresis	Histamine	6	Healthy	
15	Schneider et al. (12)	PET	Subtraction	Iontophoresis	Histamine	8	Atopic dermatitis	
16	Schneider et al. (12)	PET	Subtraction	Iontophoresis	Histamine	8	Healthy <> AD	
17	Yosipovitch et al. (13)	fMRI	Subtraction	Scratching		13	Healthy	
18	Ishiuji et al. (14)	fMRI	ASL	Iontophoresis	Histamine	8	Atopic dermatitis	
19	Ishiuji et al. (14)	fMRI	ASL	Iontophoresis	Histamine	7	Healthy	
20	Ishiuji et al. (14)	fMRI	ASL	Iontophoresis	Histamine	7	Healthy <> AD	
21	Mochizuki et al. (15)	fMRI	Subtraction	Electrically induced itch		10	Healthy	
22	Mochizuki et al. (15)	MEG	Subtraction	Electrically induced itch		10	Healthy	
23	Vierow et al. (16)	fMRI	Subtraction	Scratching		15	Healthy	
24	Vierow et al. (16)	fMRI	Subtraction	Scratching in presence of itch		15	Healthy	
25	Pfab et al. (17)	fMRI	Subtraction	Skin prick non lesion skin	Histamine	13	Atopic dermatitis	Thermal modulation
26	Pfab et al. (17)	fMRI	Subtraction	Skin prick lesion skin	Histamine	13	Atopic dermatitis	Thermal modulation
27	Bergeret et al. (18)	PET	Subtraction	Iontophoresis	Histamine	28	Healthy	
28	Bergeret et al. (18)	PET	Correlation	Iontophoresis	Histamine	29	Healthy	Itch sensation
29	Holle et al. (19)	fMRI	Subtraction	Audiovisual itch		18	Healthy	
30	Holle et al. (19)	fMRI	Correlation	Audiovisual itch		19	Healthy	
31	Kleyn et al. (20)	fMRI	Subtraction	Skin prick	Histamine	16	Healthy	
32	Kleyn et al. (20)	fMRI	Correlation	Skin prick	Histamine	16	Healthy	
33	Papoiu et al. (21)	fMRI	ASL	Iontophoresis	Histamine	15	Healthy	
34	Papoiu et al. (21)	fMRI	ASL	Spicules rubbing	Cowhage	15	Healthy	

(Continued)

TABLE 1 | Continued

#	References	Scanner	Neuroimaging analysis	Itch induction	Itch stimulus	Number of subjects	Pathology	Comments
35	Papoiu et al. (21)	fMRI	ASL			15	Healthy	Cowhage <>Histamine
36	Papoiu et al. (21)	fMRI	Subtraction	Audiovisual pain		18	Healthy	
37	Papoiu et al. (21)	fMRI	Subtraction	Itch & Pain		18	Healthy	Itch & Pain
38	Papoiu et al. (22)	fMRI	ASL-correlation	Scratching		14	Healthy	Correlated with the pleasurability
39	Papoiu et al. (22)	fMRI	ASL-correlation	Scratching		14	Healthy	Correlated with itch relief
40	Stumpf et al. (23)	fMRI	Subtraction	Microdialysis	Histamine	33	Healthy	Female>Males
41	Stumpf et al. (23)	fMRI	Subtraction	Microdialysis	Histamine	33	Healthy	Female>Males (with stroop task)
42	Napadow et al. (24)	fMRI	Subtraction	Skin prick	Allergen-induced	14	Atopic dermatitis	Temperature modeling
43	Napadow et al. (24)	fMRI	Subtraction	Skin prick	Allergen-induced	14	Atopic dermatitis	Temperature modeling and acupuncture intervention
44	Desbordes et al. (25)	fMRI	Connectivity	Skin prick	Allergen-induced	14	Atopic dermatitis	Right premotor as seed
45	Desbordes et al. (25)	fMRI	Connectivity	Skin prick	Allergen-induced	14	Atopic dermatitis	Right insula as seed
46	Desbordes et al. (25)	fMRI	Connectivity	Skin prick	Allergen-induced	14	Atopic dermatitis	Right putamen as seed
47	Desbordes et al. (25)	fMRI	Connectivity	Skin prick	Allergen-induced	14	Atopic dermatitis	Left superior parietal lobule as seed
48	Desbordes et al. (25)	fMRI	Connectivity	Skin prick	Allergen-induced	14	Atopic dermatitis	Right anterior mid-cingulate cortex as seed
49	Desbordes et al. (25)	fMRI	Connectivity	Skin prick	Allergen-induced	14	Atopic dermatitis	Right caudate as seed
50	Desbordes et al. (25)	fMRI	Connectivity	Skin prick	Allergen-induced	14	Atopic dermatitis	Right globus pallidus
51	Mochizuki et al. (26)	fMRI	Subtraction	Electrically induced itch		16	Healthy	
52	Mochizuki et al. (26)	fMRI	Subtraction	Electrically induced itch	Passive scratching	16	Healthy	Scratching itch
53	Mochizuki et al. (26)	fMRI	Subtraction	Electrically induced itch	Passive scratching	16	Healthy	Scratching itch> scratching another region
54	Mochizuki et al. (26)	fMRI	Subtraction	Electrically induced itch	Passive scratching	16	Healthy	Deactivation scratching itch region
55	Mochizuki et al. (26)	fMRI	Subtraction	Electrically induced itch	Passive scratching	16	Healthy	Scratching another region
56	Papoiu et al. (27)	fMRI	ASL	Iontophoresis	Histamine	13	End-stage renal disease	

(Continued)

TABLE 1 | Continued

#	References	Scanner	Neuroimaging analysis	Itch induction	Itch stimulus	Number of subjects	Pathology	Comments
57	Papoiu et al. (27)	fMRI	ASL	Spicules rubbing	Cowhage	13	End-stage renal disease	
58	Kim et al. (28)	fMRI	Subtraction	Audiovisual itch		14	Neurodermatosis	Stress-induced pruritus
59	Kim et al. (28)	fMRI	Subtraction	Audiovisual itch		14	Neurodermatosis	Stress-induced pruritus (after sedating antihistamine treatment)
60	Kim et al. (28)	fMRI	Subtraction	Audiovisual itch		14	Neurodermatosis	Stress-induced pruritus (after non-sedating antihistamine treatment)
61	Mochizuki et al. (29)	fMRI	ASL	Spicules rubbing	Cowhage	10	Healthy	Scratching
62	Mochizuki et al. (29)	fMRI	ASL	Spicules rubbing	Cowhage	10	Chronic itch patients	Scratching
63	Mochizuki et al. (29)	fMRI	ASL	Spicules rubbing	Cowhage	20	Patients>Healthy	Scratching
64	Mochizuki et al. (29)	fMRI	ASL	Spicules rubbing	Cowhage	10	Healthy	Scratching
65	Mochizuki et al. (29)	fMRI	ASL	Spicules rubbing	Cowhage	10	Chronic itch patients	Scratching
66	Mochizuki et al. (29)	fMRI	ASL	Spicules rubbing	Cowhage	20	Patients>Healthy	Scratching
67	Napadow et al. (30)	fMRI		Skin prick	Allergan	14	Atopic dermatitis	Nocebo > open saline
68	Papoiu et al. (31)	fMRI	ASL	Iontophoresis	Histamine	24	Healthy	Areas significantly activated during the suppression of histamine itch by butorphanol
69	Papoiu et al. (31)	fMRI	ASL	Spicules rubbing	Cowhage	25	Healthy	Deactivation areas significantly correlated with the reduction in cowhage itch
70	Vierow et al. (32)	fMRI	Subtraction	Spicules rubbing	Capsaicin	16	Healthy	Placebo
71	Vierow et al. (32)	fMRI	Subtraction	Spicules rubbing	Capsaicin	16	Healthy	Naltrexone
72	Vierow et al. (32)	fMRI	Subtraction	Spicules rubbing	Histamine	16	Healthy	Placebo
73	Vierow et al. (32)	fMRI	Subtraction	Spicules rubbing	Histamine	16	Healthy	Naltrexone
74	Schut et al. (33)	fMRI	ASL-Subtraction	Audiovisual		11	Atopic dermatitis	
75	Schut et al. (33)	fMRI	ASL-correlation	Audiovisual		11	Atopic dermatitis	

(Continued)

TABLE 1 | Continued

#	References	Scanner	Neuroimaging analysis	Itch induction	Itch stimulus	Number of subjects	Pathology	Comments
76	Stumpf et al. (34)	fMRI	Subtraction	Microdialysis	Histamine	33	Healthy	Itch modulation by distraction (Itch>stroop)
77	van de Sand et al. (35)	fMRI	Subtraction	Skin patch	Histamine	30	Healthy	Nocebo modulation Itch-nocebo > itch only (temperature modulating)
78	van de Sand et al. (35)	fMRI	Connectivity with insula	Skin patch	Histamine	30	Healthy	Nocebo modulation Itch-nocebo > itch only (temperature modulating)
79	Wang et al. (36)	fMRI	Resting state			40+40	Chronic urticaria +Healthy	CSU > HC (amplitude of low frequency fluctuations)
80	Wang et al. (36)	fMRI	Resting state			40+40	Chronic urticaria +Healthy	CSU > HC (functional connectivity with right ventral striatum)
81	Wang et al. (36)	fMRI	Resting state			40+40	Chronic urticaria +Healthy	CSU > HC (functional connectivity with right putamen)
82	Wang et al. (37)	fMRI	Resting state			40+40	Chronic urticaria +Healthy	CSU > HC (regional homogeneity)
83	Wang et al. (37)	fMRI	Resting state			40	Chronic urticaria	After intervention > Before intervention (regional homogeneity)
84	Wang et al. (37)	fMRI	Resting state			40+40	Chronic urticaria +Healthy	CSU > HC (functional connectivity with Cerebellum)
85	Wang et al. (37)	fMRI	Resting state			40	Chronic urticaria	After intervention > Before intervention (functional connectivity with Cerebellum)

(Continued)

TABLE 1 | Continued

#	References	Scanner	Neuroimaging analysis	Itch induction	Itch stimulus	Number of subjects	Pathology	Comments
86	Wang et al. (37)	fMRI	Resting state			40	Chronic urticaria	After intervention > Before intervention (functional connectivity with SI/MI/SMA)
87	Min et al. (38)	fMRI	Resting state	Skin prick	Histamine	20	Healthy	Acupuncture (itch-baseline)> Non-responder (itch-baseline) (functional connectivity with left Putamen)
88	Min et al. (38)	fMRI	Resting state	Skin prick	Histamine	20	Healthy	Acupuncture (itch-baseline)> Non-responder (itch-baseline) (functional connectivity with right Putamen)
89	Min et al. (38)	fMRI	Resting state	Skin prick	Histamine	20	Healthy	Acupuncture (itch-baseline)> Non-responder (itch-baseline) (functional connectivity with Pallidum)
90	Mochizuki et al. (39)	fMRI	Subtraction	Electrically induced itch		25	Healthy	
91	Mochizuki et al. (39)	fMRI	Connectivity	Electrically induced itch		25	Healthy	

stimulation and then, the anterior part shut down as painful sensation are correctly predicted. Meanwhile, the posterior part of the insula starts to encode its intensity like it was demonstrated by Frot et al. (47) in implanted subjects when stimulation becomes noxious.

SECOND ITCH MATRIX

The second itch matrix could consist of the ACC, aMCC, aIC, amygdala, striatum and hippocampus (**Figure 2B**). This network could encode the affective and motivational aspects of itch. Significant activation in the ACC, especially dorsal, extending to the anterior part of the middle cingulate cortex (aMCC), has been linked to the reward network and the positive or negative emotional response (40). Noteworthy, Vogt has reported that the aMCC reflects emotional awareness and fear leading to the questioning of the enrolment of the aMCC to the ACC gross function (62, 63). Considering the anterior insula, it is reported to be involved in the awareness of emotions and subjective feelings (50) as well as errors of predictions like mentioned above. Another literature about lesions in the aIC would cause deficits in emotional awareness (e.g., alexithymia) (64). Several studies have reported that activity in the aIC is significantly correlated with the unpleasantness of itch (8–10, 18, 21). For the hippocampus, it has been also shown that this structure is fully integrated in the itch network (13, 21, 22). For example, only active scratching can relief activity in ipsi-hippocampal structure (53). The role of hippocampus together with amygdala, dACC and insular cortex are well-documented in Sanders and Akiyama (65). The authors noticed and argued that "amygdala and hippocampus activation appears to go hand-in-hand in most studies of itch, suggesting that the memory of previous itch experiences may be a significant factor in itch-related anxiety." Stratum possibly

TABLE 2 | Results of the all the papers studied the central mechanism of itch.

#	Parts of which matrix	1	1				1/2	3	2	3	3	3				2	1		2			2									2		2	
	Regions	**Primary somatosensory cortex (BA 1, 2, 3)**	**Somatosensory associated/parietal cortex (BA 5, 7)**	**Primary motor cortex (BA 4)**	**Pre- motor and supplementary motor cortex (BA 6)**	**Cerebellum**	**Insular cortex (BA 13, 16)**	**Posterior cingulate cortex (BA 23,31)**	**Anterior cingulate cortex (BA 24, 32, 33)**	**Prefrontal cortex (BA 9)**	**Frontopolar and orbifrontal area (BA 8, 10, 11, 12)**	**Inferior and dorsolateral prefrontal cortex (BA 44, 45, 46, 47)**	**Temporal gyrus (BA 20, 21, 22, 38) + fusiform**	**Prietal pole/Wernicke's area (BA 39, 40) Inferior parietal, supramarginal**	**Thalamus**	**Basal ganglia**	**Secondary somatosensory cortex (BA 40, 43) OPC**	**Precuneus (BA 7, 31)**	**Putamen**	**Visual association gyrus (BA 17, 18, 19) ocipital**	**Anterior entorhinal cortex (BA 34)**	**Hippocampus**	**Parahippocampal gyrus**	**Ventral tegmental area cum om Ventral tegmental area**	**Raphé nucleus**	**Red Nucleus**	**PAG**	**Substantia nigra**	**Clastrum**	**Midbrain**	**Amygdala**	**Brain steem**	**Lentiform nucleus**	**Pons**
#	**Author**																																	
1	(3)				B	B			C	B																								
2	Darsow et al. (4)	B		C	B				C	C		C	C																					
3	Darsow et al. (4)	B	B	B	C		C		B	C	C	C	C	B			I			C														
4	Drzezga et al., (5)																																	
5	Mochizuki et al. (6)		I		I				C			B		I	C																			
6	Walter et al. (7)					C			C		B		C																					
7	Herde et al. (8)	C	C		B	B	B		B (m)	B	C	B	B	B	B	B																		
8	Leknes et al. (9)						B		B						B	I																		
9	Leknes et al. (9)	C		C	C				B		B			C	B	B																		
10	Mochizuki et al. (10)				I		B	C	C							I																		
11	Mochizuki et al. (10)				I		B		C							I																		
12	Valet et al. (11)	B-		C-	I		C		I-		B-	B		B	B																			
13	Valet et al. (11)			C-	I		B				I-			B																				
14	Schneider et al. (12)	C	C		C			C		I																								
15	Schneider et al. (12)				B	B	I			I	B	C		C	C	I																		
16	Schneider et al. (12)														C	I																		
17	Yosipovitch et al. (13)	B-		B-	B,B-	B	B	B-	I,D-		I,B-	B	R	B			B	B-																
18	Ishiuji et al. (14)		B		B		I	B	B	B	B	B		I		C		B	C	B	C													
19	Ishiuji et al. (14)	C	C	C										C				C																
20	Ishiuji et al. (14)							C										C		C														
21	Mochizuki et al. (15)				C	I	B	I	I			C		B	B		B	C																
22	Mochizuki et al. (15)						B										B	C																
23	Vierow et al. (16)	B		B	B	B	B	B	B	B		B			I		B		B															
24	Vierow et al. (16)	B		B	B	B	B	B	B	B	B	B			B		B		B															
25	Pfab et al. (17)	B-		B-			B-		B-	B		B	B-		B	I																		
26	Pfab et al. (17)	B-	B-		B-		B		B-	B-					B																			
27	Bergeret et al. (18)	I	I			I	C	I					I	B				C		B														

(Continued)

TABLE 2 | Continued

#	Parts of which matrix	1	1				1/2	3	2	3	3	3				2	1		2			2									2		2	
#	Regions / Author	Primary somatosensory cortex (BA 1, 2, 3)	Somatosensory associated/parietal cortex (BA 5, 7)	Primary motor cortex (BA 4)	Pre- motor and supplementary motor cortex (BA 6)	Cerebellum	Insular cortex (BA 13, 16)	Posterior cingulate cortex (BA 23,31)	Anterior cingulate cortex (BA 24, 32, 33)	Prefrontal cortex (BA 9)	Frontopolar and orbifrontal area (BA 8, 10, 11, 12)	Inferior and dorsolateral prefrontal cortex (BA 44, 45, 46, 47)	Temporal gyrus (BA 20, 21, 22, 38) + fusiform	Prietal pole/Wernicke's area (BA 39, 40) Inferior parietal, supramarginal	Thalamus	Basal ganglia	Secondary somatosensory cortex (BA 40, 43) OPC	Precuneus (BA 7, 31)	Putamen	Visual association gyrus (BA 17, 18, 19) ocipital	Anterior entorhinal cortex (BA 34)	Hippocampus	Parahippocampal gyrus	Ventral tegmental area cum om Ventral tegmental area	Raphé nucleus	Red Nucleus	PAG	Substantia nigra	Clastrum	Midbrain	Amygdala	Brain steem	Lentiform nucleus	Pons
28	Bergeret et al. (18)						C		I																									
29	Holle et al. (19)	L	L		L	B	B					L			B					B														
30	Holle et al. (19)	L			L							L																						
31	Kleyn et al. (20)			I		B			B				C																					
32	Kleyn et al. (20)						C					B	B																					
33	Papoiu et al. (21)																																	
34	Papoiu et al. (21)	C			C	B	C	B	B				C	B	B	B	B	C		B		C	C											
35	Papoiu et al. (21)						B				C	B	C	I			C																	
36	Papoiu et al. (21)				L	B	B			L	L		B		L	B				R														
37	Papoiu et al. (21)				L	B	L			L	L				B	L																		
38	Papoiu et al. (22)							I	B			C	C		B		I	I	I	B		C	C	B	B	B	B	C						
39	Papoiu et al. (22)							C							C	I			I	I														
40	Stumpf et al. (23)				B	B				C	C	B		I		B	C			C, I-														
41	Stumpf et al. (23)				I	C-					C	B	I																					
42	Napadow et al. (24)		I		B		C	C				C				B			B															
43	Napadow et al. (24)	B		B	C		C	I		C						C	C		C	C									C					
44	Desbordes et al. (25)													R				L																
45	Desbordes et al. (25)							L	L				L										L											
46	Desbordes et al. (25)	L			L			B									L (42)																	
47	Desbordes et al. (25)						R				L			L					R															
48	Desbordes et al. (25)						R							R					R															
49	Desbordes et al. (25)											L								L														
50	Desbordes et al. (25)							L				R																						
51	Mochizuki et al. (26)	L		R	R		B	B	R			L			B	B	B	B												B				
52	Mochizuki et al. (26)	B		B	B	B		B	B			B	B	B	B	B	B													B				

(Continued)

TABLE 2 | Continued

#	Parts of which matrix	1	1				1/2	3	2	3	3	3				2	1		2			2									2		2	
	Regions	**Primary somatosensory cortex (BA 1, 2, 3)**	**Somatosensory associated/parietal cortex (BA 5, 7)**	**Primary motor cortex (BA 4)**	**Pre- motor and supplementary motor cortex (BA 6)**	**Cerebellum**	**Insular cortex (BA 13, 16)**	**Posterior cingulate cortex (BA 23,31)**	**Anterior cingulate cortex (BA 24, 32, 33)**	**Prefrontal cortex (BA 9)**	**Frontopolar and orbifrontal area (BA 8, 10, 11, 12)**	**Inferior and dorsolateral prefrontal cortex (BA 44, 45, 46, 47)**	**Temporal gyrus (BA 20, 21, 22, 38) + fusiform**	**Prietal pole/Wernicke's area (BA 39, 40) Inferior parietal, supramarginal**	**Thalamus**	**Basal ganglia**	**Secondary somatosensory cortex (BA 40, 43) OPC**	**Precuneus (BA 7, 31)**	**Putamen**	**Visual association gyrus (BA 17, 18, 19) ocipital**	**Anterior entorhinal cortex (BA 34)**	**Hippocampus**	**Parahippocampal gyrus**	**Ventral tegmental area cum om Ventral tegmental area**	**Raphé nucleus**	**Red Nucleus**	**PAG**	**Substantia nigra**	**Clastrum**	**Midbrain**	**Amygdala**	**Brain steem**	**Lentiform nucleus**	**Pons**
#	**Author**																																	
53	Mochizuki et al. (26)	B		B	L	L	B		R						L	B		L												L				
54	Mochizuki et al. (26)			B	B	L		L			B							L		B		B												
55	Mochizuki et al. (26)			B	B			R			B							R		B		B												
56	Papoiu et al. (27)	I	I					B	L	B	B	B	B	B				B		I		C	I			B	B	B		I				
57	Papoiu et al. (27)	C		I	B		C	I	B					C	I	C	C	B	C	C		I								C				
58	Kim et al. (28)					R							R	R						L		L												
59	Kim et al. (28)					B			R	L	L		B						L	R			R						L					
60	Kim et al. (28)									B	B		B																					
61	Mochizuki et al. (29)	B	B	B	B	I	B	B	I	B		I			B	B	B										C			C				
62	Mochizuki et al. (29)	C	B	C	B		B	I	I	B		C			B	B	C	I		B										C				
63	Mochizuki et al. (29)			C,I-	B,I-	B-	I-	C				B	C				I-	C																
64	Mochizuki et al. (29)	C	B	C	I	B	B	B	B		B	B			B	I	B	C									B			B				
65	Mochizuki et al. (29)		B	B	B		B	I			I	I	C		B	B	B																	
66	Mochizuki et al. (29)	I	I	C	B	C	C,I-	I			C	I	C		I-	C				I-														
67	Napadow et al. (30)											C		I		C																		
68	Papoiu et al. (31)								I							B																		
69	Papoiu et al. (31)	C				B	I	C					I		I	C						B	B	I		C		I	I					
70	Vierow et al. (32)	B		I-			B	B	B,C-					B	B		B		C			B-									B-			
71	Vierow et al. (32)	B		I-			B	B	B					B	B		B		C			C-												
72	Vierow et al. (32)	B		I-			B	B	B					B	B	C	B		C			C-									B-			
73	Vierow et al. (32)	B		I-			B	B	I					B	B	C	B		C			C-												
74	Schut et al. (33)				B						I					C																		
75	Schut et al. (33)												I				I	I		I														
76	Stumpf et al. (34)				B-		C	C		B-		B-	I-	I	I-			I		B-			C-						I-			I-	B-	
77	van de Sand et al. (35)				C	I					I-					C	I,C-														C			B

(Continued)

TABLE 2 | Continued

#	Regions / Author	Primary somatosensory cortex (BA 1, 2, 3)	Somatosensory associated/parietal cortex (BA 5, 7)	Primary motor cortex (BA 4)	Pre- motor and supplementary motor cortex (BA 6)	Cerebellum	Insular cortex (BA 13, 16)	Posterior cingulate cortex (BA 23,31)	Anterior cingulate cortex (BA 24, 32, 33)	Prefrontal cortex (BA 9)	Frontopolar and orbifrontal area (BA 8, 10, 11, 12)	Inferior and dorsolateral prefrontal cortex (BA 44, 45, 46, 47)	Temporal gyrus (BA 20, 21, 22, 38) + fusiform	Prietal pole/Wernicke's area (BA 39, 40) Inferior parietal, supramarginal	Thalamus	Basal ganglia	Secondary somatosensory cortex (BA 40, 43) OPC	Precuneus (BA 7, 31)	Putamen	Visual association gyrus (BA 17, 18, 19) ocipital	Anterior entorhinal cortex (BA 34)	Hippocampus	Parahippocampal gyrus	Ventral tegmental area cum om Ventral tegmental area	Raphé nucleus	Red Nucleus	PAG	Substantia nigra	Clastrum	Midbrain	Amygdala	Brain steem	Lentiform nucleus	Pons
	Parts of which matrix	1	1				1/2	3	2	3	3	3				2	1		2			2									2		2	
78	van de Sand et al. (35)				C-	C	I	I,C-	C				I														I							
79	Wang et al. (36)															R			R															
80	Wang et al. (36)																			R-														
81	Wang et al. (36)				L-																													
82	Wang et al. (37)					B																												
83	Wang et al. (37)	B		B	B																													
84	Wang et al. (37)								B	B	R	R		R		B				R														
85	Wang et al. (37)			R-	R-					R-	R-																							
86	Wang et al. (37)								B-			L-	R-		L-	L-			L-															
87	Min et al. (38)							L															L											
88	Min et al. (38)							L																										
89	Min et al. (38)								C		L	C																						
90	Mochizuki et al. (39)	C	C		C		B	L	B		B	B	B	B		B	B																	

If laterality applicable: B, Bilateral; C, Contralateral to stimulus; I, Ipsilateral to stimulus. If laterality not applicable: B, Bilateral; L, Left; R, Right.
When only the peak locations were reported the sprout022 tool (Dept. of Radiology and Biomedical Imaging, Yale School of Medicine) was used to identify the regions.

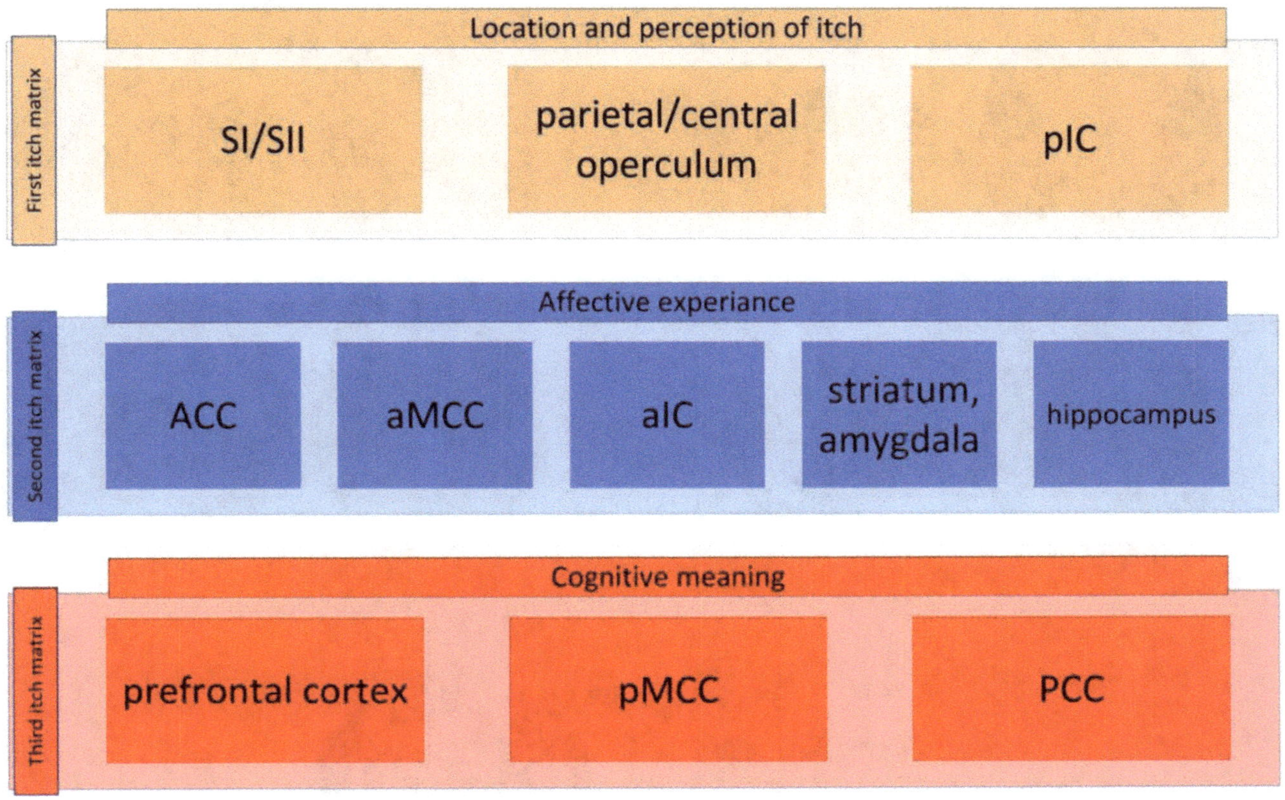

FIGURE 1 | The itch matrix categorized into three itch matrixes. First itch matrix consisted of primary and secondary sensorimotor cortex (SI and SII, respectively), the parietal/central operculum, and the posterior insular cortex (pIC) (here presented in brown, this matrix is also presented in **Figure 2A**). The second itch matrix consisting of anterior singular cortex (ACC), anterior part of the middle cingulate cortex (aMCC), anterior part of the insular cortex (aIC), amygdala, striatum and hippocampus (here presented in blue, this matrix is also presented in **Figure 2B**). The third matrix contains prefrontal cortex, posterior part of the middle cingulate cortex (pMCC), and posterior cingulate cortex (PCC) (here presented in red, this matrix is also presented in **Figure 2C**).

involved with motivation aspects of itch and/or the carving for scratching.

According to original paradigms, two other studies have reported diminished activation of these regions in tasks that change the nature of pain perception with context variations (66) or with analgesia induced by meditation (67). While the first of these shows a diminished activation in dorsal ACC and insula as the subjects switch their perception from unpleasant to pleasant (or less unpleasant) revealing the link between emotional and motivational function. The second demonstrate that experienced Zen meditators can reduce activity of their prefrontal medial cortex, amygdala and hippocampus regions at the expense of an increased activity in dorsal ACC or insula which still belong to this second matrix but are more related to mindfulness. These articles suggest that making things more conscious by bringing activities closer to the awareness matrix (with insula as a common region) putatively lead to less harmful psychological consequences. This second matrix is more robust than the first one. Many arguments in the itch literature exist and converge about its functional role.

THIRD ITCH MATRIX

The third itch matrix would include parts of the prefrontal cortex, pMCC, and PCC (**Figure 2C**). This network should be involved in the subjective perception of itch. The cognitive state of the mind can affect the itch sensation e.g., emotions, obsessions, religious beliefs, disgusts, expectations, and past experiences. This pattern of activation is also present in the distraction from itch caused by the Stroop task (e.g., in the DLPFC) (14, 30, 34). The third matrix receives and integrates information from the foregoing two and triggers behavioral response.

CONCLUSION

Knowledge of itch processing in the brain is growing thanks to brain imaging (2, 68). A better understanding of interactions between itch matrixes would allow a better understanding

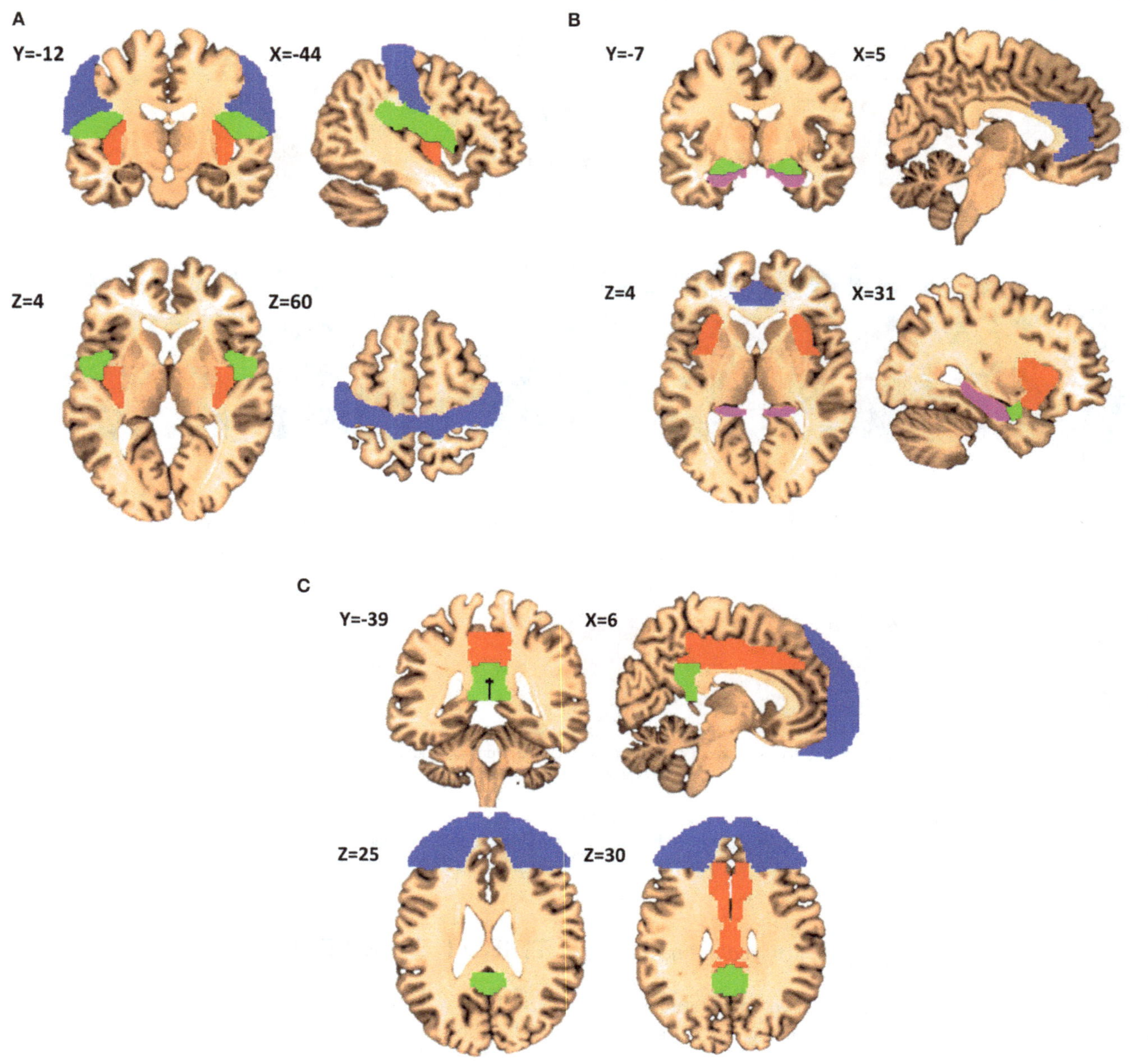

FIGURE 2 | Proposals for itch matrixes (X,Y,Z denotes the location of the corresponding slice in Montreal Neurological Institute (MNI) coordinate system). **(A)** Elements of the first matrix contributing to encoding of the recognition, localization, and intensity of itch. Primary sensorimotor cortex is presented in Blue, parietal operculum in Green, and posterior insular cortex in Red (Regions have been extracted from Automated Anatomical Labeling and Harvard-Oxford atlases). **(B)** The second matrix itch processing matrix consenting of anterior cingulate cortex (Blue), anterior insular cortex (Red), amygdala (Green) and hippocampus (Violet). This matrix is in charge of affective and motivational aspects of itch. **(C)** The third matrix consists of frontal cortex (Blue), middle cingulate cortex (Red), and posterior cingulate cortex (Green), and it is involved in the interpretation of the cognitive meaning of itch.

of pruritus in different cutaneous or extra-cutaneous etiologies (69).

AUTHOR CONTRIBUTIONS

LM, J-LC, DB, and OD contributed to conception and design of the study. PN organized the database and wrote the first draft of the manuscript. OD wrote sections of the manuscript. All authors contributed to manuscript revision, read, and approved the submitted version.

ACKNOWLEDGMENTS

We thank the French Society of Dermatology for providing a grant.

REFERENCES

1. Najafi P, Carré JL, Ben Salem D, Brenaut E, Misery L, Dufor O. Central mechanisms of itch: a systematic literature review and meta-analysis. *J Neuroradiol.* (2020) 47:450–7. doi: 10.1016/j.neurad.2019.11.005
2. Najafi P, Dufor O, Ben Salem D, Misery L, Carré JL. Itch processing in the brain. *J Eur Acad Dermatol Venereol.* (2020) 47:400–1. doi: 10.1111/jdv.17029
3. Hsieh JC, Hagermark O, Stahle-Backdahl M, Ericson K, Eriksson L, Stone-Elander S, et al. Urge to scratch represented in the human cerebral cortex during itch. *J Neurophysiol.* (1994) 72:3004–8. doi: 10.1152/jn.1994.72.6.3004
4. Darsow U, Drzezga A, Frisch M, Munz F, Weilke F, Bartenstein P, et al. Processing of histamine-induced itch in the human cerebral cortex: a correlation analysis with dermal reactions. *J Invest Dermatol.* (2000) 115:1029–33. doi: 10.1046/j.1523-1747.2000.00193.x
5. Drzezga A, Darsow U, Treede RD, Siebner H, Frisch M, Munz F, et al. Central activation by histamine-induced itch: analogies to pain processing: a correlational analysis of O-15 H2O positron emission tomography studies. *Pain.* (2001) 92:295–305. doi: 10.1016/S0304-3959(01)00271-8
6. Mochizuki H, Tashiro M, Kano M, Sakurada Y, Itoh M, Yanai K. Imaging of central itch modulation in the human brain using positron emission tomography. *Pain.* (2003) 105:339–46. doi: 10.1016/S0304-3959(03)00249-5
7. Walter B, Sadlo MN, Kupfer J, Niemeier V, Brosig B, Stark R, et al. Brain activation by histamine prick test-induced itch. *J Gen Intern Med.* (2005) 20:380–2. doi: 10.1111/j.0022-202X.2005.23817.x
8. Herde L, Forster C, Strupf M, Handwerker HO. Itch induced by a novel method leads to limbic deactivations— a functional MRI study. *J Neurophysiol.* (2007) 98:2347–56. doi: 10.1152/jn.00475.2007
9. Leknes SG, Bantick S, Willis CM, Wilkinson JD, Wise RG, Tracey I. Itch and motivation to scratch: an investigation of the central and peripheral correlates of allergen- and histamine-induced itch in humans. *J Neurophysiol.* (2007) 97:415–22. doi: 10.1152/jn.00070.2006
10. Mochizuki H, Sadato N, Saito DN, Toyoda H, Tashiro M, Okamura N, et al. Neural correlates of perceptual difference between itching and pain: A human fMRI study. *Neuroimage.* (2007) 36:706–17. doi: 10.1016/j.neuroimage.2007.04.003
11. Valet M, Pfab F, Sprenger T, Wöller A, Zimmer C, Behrendt H, et al. Cerebral Processing of histamine-induced itch using short-term alternating temperature modulation - an fMRI study. *J Invest Dermatol.* (2007) 128:426–33. doi: 10.1038/sj.jid.5701002
12. Schneider G, Stander S, Burgmer M, Driesch G, Heuft G, Weckesser M. Significant differences in central imaging of histamine-induced itch between atopic dermatitis and healthy subjects. *Eur J Pain.* (2008) 12:834–41. doi: 10.1016/j.ejpain.2007.12.003
13. Yosipovitch G, Ishiuji Y, Patel TS, Hicks MI, Oshiro Y, Kraft RA, et al. The brain processing of scratching. *J Invest Dermatol.* (2008) 128:1806–11. doi: 10.1038/jid.2008.3
14. Ishiuji Y, Coghill R, Patel T, Oshiro Y, Kraft R, Yosipovitch G. Distinct patterns of brain activity evoked by histamine-induced itch reveal an association with itch intensity and disease severity in atopic dermatitis. *Br J Dermatol.* (2009) 161:1072–80. doi: 10.1111/j.1365-2133.2009.09308.x
15. Mochizuki H, Inui K, Tanabe HC, Akiyama LF, Otsuru N, Yamashiro K, et al. Time course of activity in itch-related brain regions: a combined MEG -fMRI study. *J Neurophysiol.* (2009) 102:2657–66. doi: 10.1152/jn.00460.2009
16. Vierow V, Fukuoka M, Ikoma A, Dörfler A, Handwerker HO, Forster C. Cerebral representation of the relief of itch by scratching. *J Neurophysiol.* (2009) 102:3216–24. doi: 10.1152/jn.00207.2009
17. Pfab F, Valet M, Sprenger T, Huss-Marp J, Athanasiadis GI, Baurecht HJ, et al. Temperature modulated histamine-itch in lesional and nonlesional skin in atopic eczema - a combined psychophysical and neuroimaging study. *Allergy.* (2010) 65:84–94. doi: 10.1111/j.1398-9995.2009.02163.x
18. Bergeret L, Black D, Theunis J, Misery L, Chauveau N, Aubry F, et al. Validation of a model of itch induction for brain positron emission tomography studies using histamine iontophoresis. *Acta Derm Venereol.* (2011) 91:504–10. doi: 10.2340/00015555-1067
19. Holle H, Warne K, Seth AK, Critchley HD, Ward J. Neural basis of contagious itch and why some people are more prone to it. *PNAS.* (2012) 109:19816–21. doi: 10.1073/pnas.1216160109
20. Kleyn C e., McKie S, Ross A, Elliott R, Griffiths CEM. A temporal analysis of the central neural processing of itch. *Br J Dermatol.* (2012) 166:994–1001. doi: 10.1111/j.1365-2133.2012.10849.x
21. Papoiu AD, Coghill RC, Kraft RA, Wang H, Yosipovitch G. A tale of two itches. *Common features and notable differences in brain activation evoked by cowhage and histamine induced itch. Neuroimage.* (2012) 59:3611–23. doi: 10.1016/j.neuroimage.2011.10.099
22. Papoiu AD, Nattkemper LA. Sanders KM, Kraft RA, Chan YH, Coghill RC, et al. Brain's reward circuits mediate itch relief: *a functional MRI study of active scratching. PLoS ONE.* (2013) 8:e82389. doi: 10.1371/journal.pone.0082389
23. Stumpf A, Burgmer M, Schneider G, Heuft G, Schmelz M, Phan NQ, et al. Sex differences in itch perception and modulation by distraction - an fMRI pilot study in healthy volunteers. *PLoS ONE.* (2013) 8:e0079123. doi: 10.1371/journal.pone.0079123
24. Napadow V, Li A, Loggia ML, Kim J, Schalock PC, Lerner E, et al. The brain circuitry mediating antipruritic effects of acupuncture. *Cereb Cortex.* (2014) 24:873–82. doi: 10.1093/cercor/bhs363
25. Desbordes G, Li A, Loggia ML, Kim J, Schalock PC, Lerner E, et al. Evoked itch perception is associated with changes in functional brain connectivity. *Neuroimage Clin.* (2014) 7:213–21. doi: 10.1016/j.nicl.2014.12.002
26. Mochizuki H, Tanaka S, Morita T, Wasaka T, Sadato N, Kakigi R. The cerebral representation of scratching-induced pleasantness. *J Neurophysiol.* (2014) 111:488–98. doi: 10.1152/jn.00374.2013
27. Papoiu ADP, Emerson NM, Patel TS, Kraft RA, Valdes-Rodriguez R, Nattkemper LA, et al. Voxel-based morphometry and arterial spin labeling fMRI reveal neuropathic and neuroplastic features of brain processing of itch in end-stage renal disease. *J Neurophysiol.* (2014) 112:1729–38. doi: 10.1152/jn.00827.2013
28. Kim HJ, Park JB, Lee JH, Kim I-H. How stress triggers itch: a preliminary study of the mechanism of stress-induced pruritus using fMRI. *Int J Dermatol.* (2015) 55:434–42. doi: 10.1111/ijd.12864
29. Mochizuki H, Papoiu ADP, Nattkemper LA, Lin AC, Kraft RA, Coghill RC, et al. Scratching induces overactivity in motor-related regions and reward system in chronic itch patients. *J Invest Dermatol.* (2015) 135:2814–23. doi: 10.1038/jid.2015.223
30. Napadow V, Li A, Loggia ML, Kim J, Mawla I, Desbordes G, et al. The imagined itch: brain circuitry supporting nocebo-induced itch in atopic dermatitis patients *Allergy.* (2015) 70:1485–92. doi: 10.1111/all.12727
31. Papoiu ADP, Kraft RA, Coghill RC, Yosipovitch G. Butorphanol suppression of histamine itch is mediated by nucleus accumbens and septal nuclei: a pharmacological fMRI study. *J Invest Dermatol.* (2015) 135:560–8. doi: 10.1038/jid.2014.398
32. Vierow V, Forster C, Vogelgsang R, Dörfler A, Handwerker H. Cerebral networks linked to itch-related sensations induced by Histamine and Capsaicin. *Acta Dermato Venereologica.* (2015) 95:645–52. doi: 10.2340/00015555-2006
33. Schut C, Mochizuki H, Grossman SK, Lin AC, Conklin CJ, Mohamed FB, et al. Brain processing of contagious itch in patients with atopic dermatitis. *Front Psychol.* (2017) 8:1267. doi: 10.3389/fpsyg.2017.01267
34. Stumpf A, Pfleiderer B, Schneider G, Heuft G, Schmelz M, Phan NQ, et al. Distraction from itch shows brainstem activation without reduction in experimental itch sensation. *Acta Derm Venereol.* (2017) 97:1074–80. doi: 10.2340/00015555-2732
35. van de Sand MF, Menz MM, Sprenger C, Büchel C. Nocebo-induced modulation of cerebral itch processing - an fMRI study. *NeuroImage.* (2018) 166:209–18. doi: 10.1016/j.neuroimage.2017.10.056
36. Wang Y, Fang J-L, Cui B, Liu J, Song P, Lang C, et al. The functional and structural alterations of the striatum in chronic spontaneous urticarial. *Sci Rep.* (2018) 8:1725. doi: 10.1038/s41598-018-19962-2
37. Wang Y, Fang J, Song P, Bao Y, Song W, Liu J, et al. The dysfunction of the cerebellum and its cerebellum-reward-sensorimotor loops in chronic spontaneous urticaria. *Cerebellum.* (2018) 17:507–16. doi: 10.1007/s12311-018-0933-6

38. Min S, Kim K-W, Jung W-M, Lee M-J, Kim Y-K, Chae Y, et al. Acupuncture for histamine-induced itch: association with increased parasympathetic tone and connectivity of putamen-midcingulate cortex. *Front Neurosci.* (2019) 13:215. doi: 10.3389/fnins.2019.00215
39. Mochizuki H, Hernandez LE, Yosipovitch G, Sadato N, Kakigi R. The functional network processing acute electrical itch stimuli in humans. *Front Physiol.* (2019) 10:555. doi: 10.3389/fphys.2019.00555
40. Fenton BW, Shih E, Zolton J. The neurobiology of pain perception in normal and persistent pain. *Pain Manage.* (2015) 5:297–317. doi: 10.2217/pmt.15.27
41. Xiang Y, Wang Y, Gao S, Zhang X, Cui R. Neural mechanisms with respect to different paradigms and relevant regulatory factors in empathy for pain. *Front Neurosci.* (2018) 12:507. doi: 10.3389/fnins.2018.00507
42. Apkarian AV, Bushnell MC, Treede RD, Zubieta JK. Human brain mechanisms of pain perception and regulation in health and disease. *Eur J Pain.* (2005) 9:463–84. doi: 10.1016/j.ejpain.2004.11.001
43. Dong WK, Salonen LD, Kawakami Y, Shiwaku T, Kaukoranta EM, Martin RF. Nociceptive responses of trigeminal neurons in SII-7b cortex of awake monkeys. *Brain Res.* (1989) 484:314–24. doi: 10.1016/0006-8993(89)90375-2
44. Dong WK, Chudler EH, Sugiyama K, Roberts VJ, Hayashi T. Somatosensory, multisensory, and task-related neurons in cortical area 7b (PF) of unanesthetized monkeys. *J Neurophysiol.* (1994) 72:542–64. doi: 10.1152/jn.1994.72.2.542
45. Timmermann L, Ploner M, Haucke K, Schmitz F, Baltissen R, Schnitzler A. Differential coding of pain intensity in the human primary and secondary somatosensory cortex. *J Neurophysiol.* (2001) 86:1499–503. doi: 10.1152/jn.2001.86.3.1499
46. Bornhövd K, Quante M, Glauche V, Bromm B, Weiller C, Büchel C. Painful stimuli evoke different stimulus–response functions in the amygdala, prefrontal, insula and somatosensory cortex: a singletrial fMRI study. *Brain.* (2002) 125:1226–36. doi: 10.1093/brain/awf137
47. Frot M, Magnin M, Mauguière F, Garcia-Larrea L. Human SII and posterior insula differently encode thermal laser stimuli. *Cereb Cortex.* (2007) 17:610–20. doi: 10.1093/cercor/bhk007
48. Lee JS, Han JS, Lee K, Bang J, Lee H. The peripheral and central mechanisms underlying itch. *BMB Rep.* (2016) 49:474–96. doi: 10.5483/BMBRep.2016.49.9.108
49. Roberts CA, Stancak A, Fallon N, Thomas A, Kirkham TC. Where is itch represented in the brain, and how does it differ from pain? *An* activation likelihood estimation meta-analysis of experimentally-induced itch. *J Invest Dermatol.* (2019) 139:2245–8. doi: 10.1016/j.jid.2019.04.007
50. Craig AD. The sentient self. *Brain Struct Funct.* (2010) 214:563–77. doi: 10.1007/s00429-010-0248-y
51. Craig AD. Significance of the insula for the evolution of human awareness of feelings from the body. *Ann N Y Acad Sci.* (2011) 1225:72–82. doi: 10.1111/j.1749-6632.2011.05990.x
52. Mochizuki H, Kakigi R. Central mechanisms of itch *Clin Neurophysiol.* (2015) 126:1650–60. doi: 10.1016/j.clinph.2014.11.019
53. Mochizuki H, Yosipovitch G. Neuroimaging of itch as a tool of assessment of chronic itch and its management. *Handb Exp Pharmacol.* (2015) 226:57–70. doi: 10.1007/978-3-662-44605-8_4
54. Kurth F, Eickhoff SB, Schleicher A, Hoemke L, Zilles K, Amunts K. Cytoarchitecture and probabilistic maps of the human posterior insular cortex. Cereb Cortex. (2010) 20:1448–61. doi: 10.1093/cercor/bhp208
55. Mazzola L, Isnard J, Peyron R, Guenot M, Mauguiere F. Somatotopic organization of pain responses to direct electrical stimulation of the human insular cortex. *Pain.* (2009) 146:99–104. doi: 10.1016/j.pain.2009.07.014
56. Iadarola MJ, Berman KF, Zeffiro TA, Byas-Smith MG, Gracely RH, Max MB, et al. Neural activation during acute capsaicin-evoked pain and allodynia assessed with PET. *Brain.* (1998) 121:931–47. doi: 10.1093/brain/121.5.931
57. Peyron R, Schneider F, Faillenot I, Convers P, Barral FG, Garcia-Larrea L, et al. An fMRI study of cortical representation of mechanical allodynia in patients with neuropathic pain. *Neurology.* (2004) 63:1838–46. doi: 10.1212/01.WNL.0000144177.61125.85
58. Schweinhardt P, Glynn C, Brooks J, Mcquay H, Jack T, Chessell I, et al. An fMRI study of cerebral processing of brush-evoked allodynia in neuropathic pain patients. *Neuroimage.* (2006) 32:256–65. doi: 10.1016/j.neuroimage.2006.03.024
59. Seifert F, Maihöfner C. Representation of cold allodynia in the human brain—a functional MRI study. *Neuroimage.* (2007) 35:1168–80. doi: 10.1016/j.neuroimage.2007.01.021
60. Ducreux D, Attal N, Parker F, Bouhassira D. Mechanisms of central neuropathic pain: a combined psychophysical and fMRI study in syringomyelia. *Brain.* (2006) 129:963–76. doi: 10.1093/brain/awl016
61. Geuter S, Boll S, Eippert F, Büchel C. Functional dissociation of stimulus intensity encoding and predictive coding of pain in the insula. *eLife.* (2017) 6:e24770. doi: 10.7554/eLife.24770.016
62. Vogt BA. Pain and emotion interactions in subregions of the cingulate gyrus. *Nat Neurosci.* (2005) 6:533–44. doi: 10.1038/nrn1704
63. Vogt BA. Midcingulate cortex: Structure, connections, homologies, functions and diseases. *J Chem Neuroanat.* (2016) 74:28–46. doi: 10.1016/j.jchemneu.2016.01.010
64. Gu X, Hof PR, Friston KJ, Fan J. Anterior insular cortex and emotional awareness. *J Comp Neurol.* (2013) 521:3371–88. doi: 10.1002/cne.23368
65. Sanders KM, Akiyama T. The vicious cycle of itch and anxiety. *Neurosci Biobehav Rev.* (2018) 87:17–26. doi: 10.1016/j.neubiorev.2018.01.009
66. Leknes S, Berna C, Lee MC, Snyder GD, Biele G, Tracey I. The importance of context: when relative relief renders pain pleasant. *Pain.* (2013) 154:402–10. doi: 10.1016/j.pain.2012.11.018
67. Grant J, Courtemanche J, Rainville P. A non-elaborative mental stance and decoupling of executive and pain-related cortices predicts low pain sensitivity in Zen meditators. *Pain.* (2011) 152:150–6. doi: 10.1016/j.pain.2010.10.006
68. Cheddad El Aouni M, Ben Salem D, Misery L. Functional MRI of pruritus. *J Neuroradiol.* (2020) 47:400–1. doi: 10.1016/j.neurad.2020.09.001
69. Najafi P, Ben Salem D, Carré JL, Misery L, Dufor O. Functional and anatomical brain connectivity in psoriasis patients and healthy controls: a pilot brain imaging study after exposure to mentally induced itch. *J Eur Acad Dermatol Venereol.* (2020) 34:2557–65. doi: 10.1111/jdv.16441

9

Involvement of Neuro-Immune Interactions in Pruritus with Special Focus on Receptor Expressions

Aylin Ruppenstein[1], *Maren M. Limberg*[1], *Karin Loser*[2], *Andreas E. Kremer*[3], *Bernhard Homey*[4] *and Ulrike Raap*[1,5*]

[1] Division of Experimental Allergy and Immunodermatology, Faculty of Medicine and Health Sciences, University of Oldenburg, Oldenburg, Germany, [2] Division of Immunology, Faculty of Medicine and Health Sciences, University of Oldenburg, Oldenburg, Germany, [3] Department of Medicine 1, University Hospital Erlangen and Friedrich-Alexander-University Erlangen-Nürnberg, Erlangen, Germany, [4] Department of Dermatology, Heinrich-Heine-University of Düsseldorf, Düsseldorf, Germany, [5] University Clinic of Dermatology and Allergy, Oldenburg Clinic, Oldenburg, Germany

***Correspondence:**
Ulrike Raap
raap.ulrike@klinikum-oldenburg.de

Pruritus is a common, but very challenging symptom with a wide diversity of underlying causes like dermatological, systemic, neurological and psychiatric diseases. In dermatology, pruritus is the most frequent symptom both in its acute and chronic form (over 6 weeks in duration). Treatment of chronic pruritus often remains challenging. Affected patients who suffer from moderate to severe pruritus have a significantly reduced quality of life. The underlying physiology of pruritus is very complex, involving a diverse network of components in the skin including resident cells such as keratinocytes and sensory neurons as well as transiently infiltrating cells such as certain immune cells. Previous research has established that there is a significant crosstalk among the stratum corneum, nerve fibers and various immune cells, such as keratinocytes, T cells, basophils, eosinophils and mast cells. In this regard, interactions between receptors on cutaneous and spinal neurons or on different immune cells play an important role in the processing of signals which are important for the transmission of pruritus. In this review, we discuss the role of various receptors involved in pruritus and inflammation, such as TRPV1 and TRPA1, IL-31RA and OSMR, TSLPR, PAR-2, NK1R, H1R and H4R, MRGPRs as well as TrkA, with a focus on interaction between nerve fibers and different immune cells. Emerging evidence shows that neuro-immune interactions play a pivotal role in mediating pruritus-associated inflammatory skin diseases such as atopic dermatitis, psoriasis or chronic spontaneous urticaria. Targeting these bidirectional neuro-immune interactions and the involved pruritus-specific receptors is likely to contribute to novel insights into the underlying pathogenesis and targeted treatment options of pruritus.

Keywords: pruritus, inflammation, neuro-immune, sensory neurons, skin disease, atopic dermatitis (AD), psoriasis, chronic spontaneous urticaria (CSU)

INTRODUCTION

The complex symptom of pruritus shows up in several diseases which ranges from numerous inflammatory skin diseases, metabolic disorders, liver and kidney diseases, or lymphoproliferative and myeloproliferative disorders (1). The most common chronic inflammatory skin diseases include atopic dermatitis (AD), psoriasis and chronic spontaneous urticaria (CSU). These patients often suffer from moderate to severe pruritus and experience a reduced quality of life (2, 3). Chronic pruritus in these patients remains a challenge regarding effective anti-pruritic treatments (4). The physiology of pruritus is transmitted by a complex interaction network of cutaneous and neuronal cells (5–7). Thus, it is very important to understand this network and dynamic processes to identify novel signaling pathways and pruritus mediators. Particularly, immune and neuronal systems are not acting separately, but interact rather closely with each other. Neurons modulate the function of immune cells by releasing neurotransmitters and neuropeptides leading to the transmission of pruritus and inflammation. In turn, activation of immune cells leads to the production and release of proinflammatory mediators including several cytokines, chemokines and neuropeptides that trigger neuronal pruritus response and inflammation in the skin (8, 9). These neuro-immune interactions arise not only from an intense biochemical crosstalk between immune cells and neurons, but also from sharing many properties, including receptor and ligand expression, which enables efficient communication between these two systems (10, 11). Thus, linking immune and neuronal systems provides a powerful way to gain insight into complex interactions associated with the neuro-immune interaction mechanism in pruritus. In this review, we highlight recent discoveries and approaches concerning interaction of pruritus receptors and channels in a neuro-immune manner in the field of pruritus research. We set our focus on transient receptor potential (TRP) channels, such as TRP vanilloid 1 (TRPV1) and ankyrin 1 (TRPA1), the heterodimer IL-31 receptor A (IL-31RA) and oncostatin-M receptor (OSMR), thymic stromal lymphopoietin receptor (TSLPR) and different G protein-coupled receptors (GPCR). These GPCRs comprise protease-activated receptor-2 (PAR-2), neurokinin-1 receptor (NK1R), histamine receptors H1 and H4 (H1R/H4R) and mas-related G-protein coupled receptors (MRGPRs) as well as tropomyosin receptor kinase A (TrkA) receptor (**Figure 1**, **Table 1**). These receptors and channels have been found on sensory neurons and play a crucial role in pruritus and neuro-immune pathways as well as pruritus associated inflammatory skin diseases (4, 12, 13). Here, we put emphasis on inflammatory skin diseases including AD, psoriasis and CSU that are highly in context with symptom of pruritus. In previous research, several treatment options for patients suffering from these pruritus-associated disorders were described (14–17). Additionally, we outline current therapeutic options in correspondence with these pruritus-associated receptors and channels (**Table 2**). Targeting neuro-immune pathways may open up new perspectives in terms of the development of more effective pharmacological treatment options for patients suffering from chronic pruritus.

RECEPTORS IN NEURO-IMMUNE INTERACTIONS

Transient Receptor Potential Channels TRPV1 and TRPA1

TRP channels are non-selective calcium-permeable cation channels comprising 28 members in mammals that can be categorized in six related protein families including TRPA, TRPC, TRPM, TRPML, TRPP, and TRPV (18, 19). TRP channels are involved in various sensory functions, such as mechanosensation, olfaction, osmolarity, pain, taste and thermoception (20–22). Several studies presented evidence showing that TRPV1 and TRPA1 play crucial roles in pruritus transmission (23–27). TRPA1 is essential in the signaling pathways that promote histamine-independent pruritus (22, 24), whereas TRPV1 is presumed to be required for both histaminergic and non-histaminergic pruritus (23, 28–31). These recent studies used knockout (KO) mice models and corresponding inhibitors and led to the conclusion that TRP channels are necessary in the pruritus pathways initiated by GPCR agonists like chloroquine and histamine (24, 29, 31). On the other hand, Ru et al. (32) demonstrated that TRPV1 and TRPA1 channels are not required for chloroquine activation of nerves by using dorsal skin-nerve preparation of healthy mice. This indicated that these TRP channels could affect other than primary afferent terminals (32). However, both ion channels are well-expressed in primary afferent sensory neurons, but also in non-neuronal cells like keratinocytes (33, 34), monocytes and macrophages (35–38), mast cells (39, 40), neutrophils (41, 42) and T cells (25, 43–45). TRPV1 is additionally expressed in dendritic cells (46, 47) and eosinophils (48). Besides neuro-immune interactions, crosstalk between the channels TRPV1 and TRPA1 and other receptors has been established in previous studies (5, 24, 47, 49, 50). An experimental study of Oh et al. (40) has described a case of complex interactions among nerve fibers and mast cells with the TRPA1 channel. The study demonstrated a neural TRPA1 dependent mechanism comprising interactions between TRPA1+ dermal mast cells and TRPA1+ dermal afferent nerves in a T_H2-dominated inflammatory environment, which is responsible for the pruritogenesis of chronic pruritus in AD (40). Another example of neuro-immune interactions highlights the involvement of TRPV1 in the crosstalk between neurons and T-lymphocytes (25). Experiments revealed that IL-31 induces pruritus by binding to IL-31RA that is exclusively expressed on TRPV1+/TRPA1+ DRG neurons indicating TRP channels as key mediators of T-cell mediated IL-31-induced pruritus. Interestingly, only around 4% of DRG neurons were observed to be IL-31RA+ (25, 51). Surprisingly, IL-31 was shown to be a potential pruritogen, since injection of IL-31 into the cheek of mice induced profound pruritus, but not pain. This implicates that pruritus and pain may be induced by different subsets of unmyelinated afferents and pruritus specific afferents might exist (25). Interestingly, several studies reported a delayed pruritus after IL-31 injection in mice (52) as well as in patients with AD and healthy volunteers (53). These studies have led to great interest in targeting TRPV1 and developing potential drugs to treat pruritus, especially in AD. In that regard, a topical TRPV1 antagonist termed asivatrep, has shown to significantly improve symptoms (e.g., pruritus, sleep disturbance) of patients with mild-to-moderate AD (54, 55). Further investigations will be needed to unravel the neuro-immune axis involving TRP channels TRPA1 and TRPV1, neurons and different immune cells for new anti-pruritic therapeutic options.

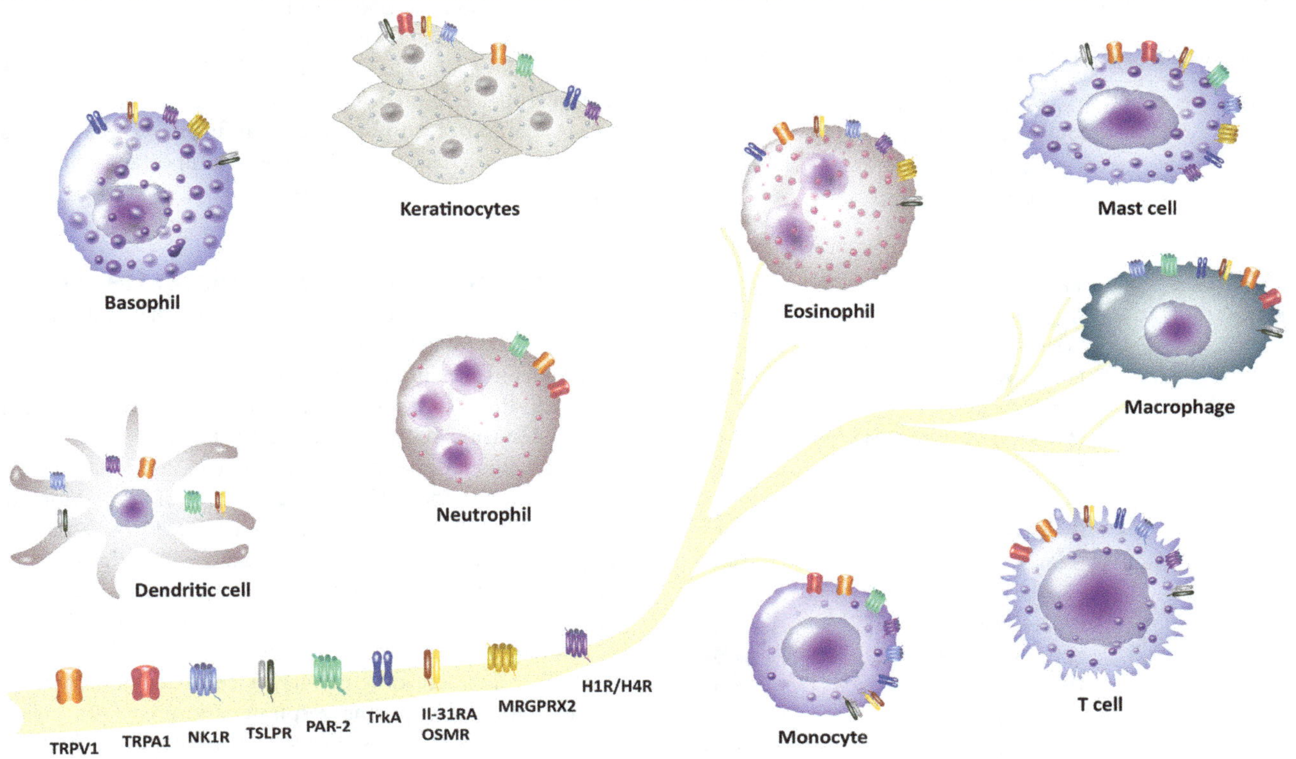

FIGURE 1 | Involvement of different receptors/channels in neuro-immune interactions in pruritus. There is a complex interplay between neurons and immune cells in transmission of pruritus and inflammation. Several receptors act as a bridge between the neuronal and immune network and function as pruritus mediators. These receptors are located on neurons, but also expressed by different non-neuronal cells (e.g., basophils, dendritic cells, eosinophils, keratinocytes, mast cells, macrophages and monocytes, neutrophils or T cells): Transient receptor potential vanilloid 1 (TRPV1) and ankyrin 1 (TRPA1), IL-31 receptor A (IL-31RA) and the oncostatin-M receptor (OSMR), thymic stromal lymphopoietin receptor (TSLPR), protease-activated receptor 2 (PAR-2), neurokinin-1 receptor (NK1R), histamine receptors H1/H4 (H1R/H4R), mas-related G-protein coupled receptor X2 (MRGPRX2), tropomyosin receptor kinase A (TrkA).

IL-31 Receptor A and Oncostatin-M Receptor

The novel cytokine IL-31 signals through a heterodimeric receptor composed of IL-31RA and the OSMR. IL-31 is a T_H2-cell-derived cytokine and the only known ligand for IL-31RA (56–58). It has previously been observed by Cevikbas et al. (25) that T_H2 cells are main producers of IL-31. Besides T_H2 cells, other immune cells like basophils, eosinophils or mast cells can produce and release IL-31 (59–62). The IL-31 receptor complex is not only expressed by DRG neurons (63), but also located on non-neuronal cells, such as basophils (62), eosinophils (61, 64), monocytes and macrophages (65–67), mast cells (13), dendritic cells (68), keratinocytes (69, 70), and T cells (25, 57, 71). IL-31/IL-31RA interaction activates signal transduction pathways leading to expression and release of various chemokines, proinflammatory cytokines, regulation of cell proliferation and stimulation of DRG neurons that play important role in pruritus induction and inflammatory diseases (72–74). A number of researchers observed an association between IL-31 and inflammatory skin diseases with severe pruritus including AD (61, 75), bullous pemphigoid (76), cutaneous T-cell lymphoma (77), CSU (78) and psoriasis (79). Regarding treatment approaches, a successful therapy of urticaria using omalizumab led to decreased serum levels of IL-31 (80). Previous research has established a neuro-immune crosstalk between IL-31 receptor, T cells and sensory nerves in pruritus (25). Cevikbas et al. (25) have shown that T_H2-derived IL-31 is able to activate IL-31RA on TRPV1+/TRPA1+ sensory nerves in the skin causing the pruritus associated with AD. Furthermore, it was shown that the T_H2-related and atopy-associated cytokine IL-31 directly induces nerve fiber elongation *in vitro* and *in vivo* in mice, suggesting that IL-31-associated nerve fiber elongation could be involved in skin hypersensitivity of AD patients (57). In this regard, IL-31 has been shown to correlate with disease severity and pruritus in AD patients (75). More recent findings have demonstrated that nemolizumab, an anti-IL-31RA antibody that binds to IL-31RA with subsequent inhibition of IL-31 signaling effectively relieves AD-associated pruritus (81, 82). The first clinical study revealed a statistically significant reduced pruritus visual analog scale (VAS) score to about 50% at week 4 compared with 20% with placebo in patients with AD (81). In a subsequent phase II study 264 adults with moderate to severe AD were treated every 4 weeks with nemolizumab in doses of 0.1, 0.5, or 2.0 mg/kg. Treatment led to decrease of pruritus VAS by 43.7% to 63.1% in a dose-dependent manner over a 12-week period compared with a 20.9% decrease with placebo

TABLE 1 | Expression of receptors/channels on various non-neuronal cells.

Receptors/channels	Non-neuronal cells	References
TRPV1/TRPA1	Dendritic cells (only TRPV1)	(46, 47)
	Eosinophils (only TRPV1)	(48)
	Keratinocytes	(33, 34)
	Macrophages and monocytes	(35–37)
	Mast cells	(39, 40)
	Neutrophils	(41, 42)
	T cells	(25, 43–45)
IL-31RA/OSMR	Basophils	(62)
	Dendritic cells	(68)
	Eosinophils	(61, 64)
	Keratinocytes	(69, 70)
	Macrophages and monocytes	(65–67)
	Mast cells	(13)
	T cells	(25, 57, 71)
TSLPR	Basophils	(89)
	Eosinophils	(90)
	Dendritic cells	(91)
	Keratinocytes	(92)
	Macrophages and monocytes	(94, 95)
	Mast cells	(93)
	T and B cells	(96, 97)
PAR-2	Dendritic cells	(125, 126)
	Keratinocytes	(124)
	Macrophages and monocytes	(125–127)
	Mast cells	(128, 129)
	Neutrophils	(130)
NK1R	Dendritic cells	(148)
	Eosinophils	(149)
	Keratinocytes	(154, 155)
	Macrophages and monocytes	(151)
	Mast cells	(150)
	T and B cells	(152, 153)
H1R/H4R	Basophils	(185)
	Dendritic cells	(186, 187)
	Eosinophils	(13)
	Keratinocytes	(183, 184)
	Monocytes	(187)
	Mast cells	(188)
	T cells	(28, 189–191)
MRGPRX2	Basophils	(206)
	Eosinophils	(206)
	Mast cells	(205)
TrkA	Basophils	(238)
	Eosinophils	(233)
	Keratinocytes	(228)
	Macrophages and monocytes	(239)
	Mast cells	(231, 232)
	T and B cells	(240, 241)

(82). Further, a long-term extension study based on phase II trial resulted in reduced pruritus up to 90%, whereby it was limited by a placebo group (83). Another approach is provided by a human monoclonal antibody KPL-716, which specifically targets the OSMRβ chain and simultaneously inhibits both IL-31 and OSM signaling. Therefore, blocking OSMRβ with KPL-716 may be a potential treatment option of inflammatory skin diseases (e.g., AD) and needs to be clarified in further experiments (84). These studies indicate that IL-31 is an important cytokine for regulating pruritus and AD disease activity.

Thymic Stromal Lymphopoietin Receptor

TSLP is a four-helix bundle, IL-7-like cytokine, and a member of the IL-2 cytokine family that contributes to the initiation of type-2 inflammation. It is primarily produced by epithelial cells including keratinocytes, fibroblasts and stromal cells, but also by dendritic cells and mast cells (85, 86). TSLP signaling requires a heterodimeric receptor complex that consists of the IL-7 receptor α-chain (IL-7Rα) and the TSLP receptor chain (TSLPR) (87, 88). TSLP receptor is expressed by a variety of cell populations including non-neuronal cells, such as basophils (89), eosinophils (90), dendritic cells (91), keratinocytes (92), mast cells (93), macrophages and monocytes (94, 95), B and T cells (96, 97), but also by neurons (11, 98). The expression of TSLP from these different target cells can be triggered by various stimuli comprising respiratory viruses (99), cigarette smoke extracts (100) as well as several cytokines, such as TNF-α and IL-1β (101). TSLP is known to be involved in various allergic diseases such as AD (102, 103), bronchial asthma (104) and eosinophilic esophagitis (105). There is a growing evidence indicating that TSLP may also play role in other diseases including autoimmune, chronic inflammatory disorders and cancer (86, 106, 107). In terms of AD several studies show that TSLP serum level as well as TSLP level in the skin of AD patients is elevated (102, 103, 108). An overexpression of TSLP in mice models resulted in the development of AD (109, 110). Wilson et al. (98) have demonstrated that intradermal injection of TSLP led to scratching behavior in mice. Additionally, their data confirmed that TSLP released from keratinocytes acts directly on sensory neurons to induce itch-evoked scratching that was depended on TSLPR. Further it was evidenced that both functional TSLPRs and TRPA1 channels are required for TSLP-induced pruritus. A crosstalk between TSLP and PAR-2 was also observed. PAR-2 activation by its agonists SLIGLR and tryptase induced scratching behavior and Ca^{2+}-dependent release of TSLP (98). However, the mechanism behind the TSLP-induced pruritus remains to be elucidated in further experimental studies. Targeting TSLP-TSLPR signaling via anti-TSLP therapy like with tezepelumab, a human monoclonal antibody targeting circulating TSLP, might be a promising tool to prevent and treat several diseases associated with elevated TSLP such as AD (111, 112). Contrarily, a phase II clinical trial tezepelumab treatment of patient with moderate to severe AD showed limited efficacy and insignificant pruritus reduction (111). More recently, Fitoussi et al. (113) demonstrated that a topical spray containing *Tambourissa trichophylla* leaf extract (TTLE) and 18β-glycyrrhetinic acid (GA), which inhibits TSLP secretion, efficiently decreases pruritus in AD patients and improves their quality of life.

TABLE 2 | Emerging therapeutic targets for treatment of pruritus associated inflammatory skin diseases in humans.

Receptors/channels	Therapeutic agents	Indications	References
TRPV1/TRPA1	Asivatrep/PAC-14028 (TRPV1 antagonist)	Atopic dermatitis	(54, 55)
IL-31RA/OSMR	Nemolizumab/CIM331 (IL-31RA antagonist)	Atopic dermatitis	(83)
	Vixarelimab/KPL-716 (OSMR antagonist)	Atopic dermatitis	(84)
TSLPR	Tezepelumab/AMG-157/MEDI9929 (anti-TSLP antibody)	Atopic dermatitis	(111)
	Topical spray containing TTLE and GA (TSLP inhibitor)	Atopic dermatitis	(113)
PAR-2	currently not available in humans	–	–
NK1R	Aprepitant (NK1R antagonist)	Atopic dermatitis	(168, 169)
	Serlopitant/VPD-737 (NK1R antagonist)	Atopic dermatitis, Psoriasis	(173)
	Tradipitant/VLY-688 (NK1R antagonist)	Atopic dermatitis	(174)
H1R/H4R	Bilastine (H1R antagonist)	Chronic spontaneous urticaria	(195)
	Adriforant/ZPL-3893787 (H4R antagonist)	Atopic dermatitis	(193)
	JNJ-39758979 (H4R antagonist)	Atopic dermatitis	(202)
MRGPRs	currently not available	–	–
TrkA	Pegcantratinib/CT327 (TrkA inhibitor)	Psoriasis	(255)

Protease-Activated Receptor-2

The PAR family consists of four members, PAR-1, PAR-2, PAR-3, and PAR-4. All together they belong to G-protein coupled receptors activated by proteolytic cleavage of amino-terminal exodomain (114–117). Furthermore, an activation by different proteases generated by endogenous (e.g., proteases from endothelium, epithelium, fibroblast or immune cells) or exogenous sources (e.g., allergens, dust mite and various plants) is possible (118, 119). Existing research recognizes the critical role played by PAR-2 in skin neurogenic inflammation and in pruritic skin diseases such as AD (119–123). PAR-2 is expressed by various cell types including endothelial cells and keratinocytes (124), dendritic cells, monocytes and macrophages (125–127), mast cells (128, 129), neutrophils (130) and sensory nerve fibers (123, 131, 132). Steinhoff et al. (120) reported an increased signaling through PAR-2 that comprises an increased release of endogenous PAR-2 agonist mast cell tryptase followed by a higher occurrence of PAR-2+ nerve fibers in AD patients (120, 133). In addition to the crosstalk between nerve fibers, mast cells and PAR-2, it was shown that PAR-2 synergistically interact with TRPV1 channel resulting in pruritus sensation (134, 135). A key role of TRPV1 channel in PAR2-evoked Ca^{2+} release in differentiated human primary keratinocytes was shown by Gouin et al. (136). They demonstrated that TRPV1 independently regulate the production of inflammatory mediators, such as IL-1β, TNF-α, and TSLP via Ca^{2+} and NF-kB signaling (136). Overexpression of these inflammatory mediators is in connection with inflammatory skin diseases, such as AD or psoriasis (137–141). In a very recent follow-up study Buhl et al. (119) found that PAR-2 regulates neuro-epidermal communication in AD using a mouse model with epidermal overexpression of PAR-2. The research results indicate that PAR-2 signaling in keratinocytes causes epidermal responses leading to neuronal sensory and inflammatory responses in their AD model (119). A promising therapeutic approach presents a PAR-2 pepducin, termed PZ-235. Barr et al. (142) examined the capacity of PZ-235 to suppress skin lesion thickening, inflammation, and pruritus in acute and chronic models of AD. For this, MA-1, a mast cell-degranulating peptide from wasp venom, was utilized to induce severe scratching in mice. Subsequent PZ-235 treatment significantly reduced scratching behavior in mice up to 50%. Further results demonstrated that targeting PAR-2 via PZ-235 application attenuated production of inflammatory factors, leukocyte infiltration, skin thickening as well as severity of skin lesions. Therefore, PZ-235 may have potential in the effective treatment of patients with AD (142). More studies and clinical trials in humans are currently lacking and needs to be investigated.

Neurokinin-1 Receptor

Neurokinin receptors belong to G protein-coupled receptors and consists of three members, neurokinin-1-3 receptors (NK1-3R) that are implicated in afferent neuronal signal transduction. There are various ligands for these receptors like neurokinin A (NKA), neurokinin B (NKB), neuropeptide K (NPK), neuropeptide-γ (NKγ), endokinin, hemokinin 1 as well as substance P (SP), belonging to tachykinin family, whereas SP binds with high affinity to the NK1R (143–146). Especially, NK1R is known to mainly contribute to transmission of pruritus (4, 12, 147). NK1R is widely expressed by different immune cells, such as dendritic cells (148), eosinophils (149), mast cells (150), macrophages and monocytes (151) and T and B cells (152, 153), but also by keratinocytes (154, 155) and sensory nerve endings (11, 156, 157). Activation of NK1R via SP leads to multiple signaling cascades involving mast cell degranulation and release of proinflammatory mediators, such as histamine, nerve growth factor expression and leukotriene B4 in keratinocytes and neurogenic inflammation resulting in induction of inflammation and pruritus (145, 146, 158). Several studies investigated the role of SP and NK1R in the pathogenesis of pruritus in various diseases like AD, psoriasis and CSU (7, 159–163). Recently, it was reported that SP and its receptor NK1R are overexpressed in pruritic AD and psoriatic lesional skin (164). A previous study demonstrated that increased serum levels of SP in AD patients correlate with pruritus intensity (165, 166). Interestingly, oral treatment with the NK1R antagonist aprepitant led to reduced serum levels of immunoglobulin E (IgE) and SP levels in tissue as well as decreased cutaneous infiltration of regulatory T cells in an NC/Nga mouse model (167). In contrast, clinical studies revealed no significant differences between aprepitant treatment and placebo concerning reduction in pruritus, improvement in pruriginous lesions or quality of life (168, 169). However, another clinical study has shown that the NK1R antagonist serlopitant has potential as a therapeutic agent for the treatment of patients with chronic pruritus by significantly reducing the pruritus symptom (170–172). A phase II clinical study concluded that serlopitant reduced pruritus in patients with mild to moderate psoriasis (173). Another NK1R antagonist, tradipitant, was examined in terms of reduction of pruritus associated with AD through inhibition of SP-mediated itch signaling. Tradipitant treatment improved pruritus and sleep in mild AD (174). Several NK1R antagonists that potentially reduce pruritus activity in dermatological diseases are reviewed by Pojawa-Goła et al. (146) and Reszke et al. (172). Thus, targeting SP and/or NK1R with regard to neuro-immune crosstalk seems to be a promising approach in the treatment of pruritus. In a previous research it was established that Mas-related GPCR X2, which is also activated by SP, induced inflammation (175). Further, it was suggested that SP-induced pruritus may be mediated by MRGPRs rather than NK1R, since SP-induced pruritus was not decreased in *Nk1r* KO mice. Co-injection of QWF and SP in both *Nk1r* KO and wild-type mice led to significantly decreased SP-induced pruritus. Interestingly, an NK1R antagonist termed QWF was shown to have a dual action on MRGPRX2 (176). However, not only the crosstalk between different immune cells, neurons and NK1R, but also the interaction of NK1R with other receptors is an interesting approach for a better understanding of the pathogenesis of pruritic diseases.

Histamine Receptors H1 and H4

One of the well-characterized pruritogens is histamine. Histamine is released from mast cells and basophils via activation of histamine receptors, which belong to the G protein-coupled receptor superfamily. While four histamine receptor subtypes (H1–H4) exist, notably histamine receptors H1 and H4 are known to modulate pruritus (13, 177–181). Both histamine receptors (H1R and H4R) are extensively expressed in a wide range of cell types involving sensory neurons (182), epithelial cells like keratinocytes (183, 184), but also immune cells, such as basophils (185), dendritic cells (186, 187), eosinophils (13), monocytes (187), mast cells (188) and T cells (28, 189–191). Especially, the H4R is predominantly expressed by immune cells and is in conjunction with lots of functional histamine-mediated inflammatory responses like modulation of cytokine and chemokine release, chemotaxis and cell recruitment as well as upregulation of adhesion molecule expression (192, 193). However, both the H1 and the H4 histamine receptors play pivotal roles in various pruritic skin diseases, such as AD or CSU (188, 194–196). Various H1R antihistamines like ebastine, cetirizine, and levocetirizine were shown to decrease pruritus symptom of patients with CSU by 60–70% (197). A very recent clinical study presented a switch to bilastine, a H1R antagonist, as an optional treatment for patients with CSU, who are unresponsive to H1R antihistamines at the licensed doses (195). Although H1R antihistamines demonstrated convincing anti-pruritic effects in urticaria, they show limited efficiency in other pruritic skin diseases such as AD (11, 197, 198). In the study of Gutzmer et al. (190), it was demonstrated that AD patients express increased levels of H4R on T cells. Upon stimulation of the H4 receptor pruritogenic IL-31 is up-regulated leading to pruritic response (190). H4R antagonists were shown to reduce T_H2 cytokine production, pruritus and skin inflammation in AD-associated animal models (199, 200). Therefore, new clinical trials using novel H4R antagonists might a promising treatment for patients with AD such as the H4R antagonist JNJ-39758979, which led to an improvement of inflammatory skin lesions in AD patients (193, 201). In addition, marked effects against pruritus in Japanese patients with AD could be observed in a phase II clinical trial, but the development of agranulocytosis by 2 subjects resulted in early trial termination (202). More recently, H4R antagonist adriforant was shown to improve inflammatory skin lesions in patients with AD. Although adriforant treatment cause a 3-point reduction (scale, 1–10) in pruritus, there was no significant difference in comparison to reduced pruritus with placebo (193). Interestingly, a combined treatment of both H1R and H4R antagonists demonstrated an anti-inflammatory effect in an AD mice model that might be a good strategy to treat patients with AD (203).

Mas-Related G-Protein Coupled Receptors

MRGPRs are G-protein coupled receptors that comprise at least 50 family members in mice, divided into subgroups MRGPRA-H and 8 members in humans named MRGPRX1-X4, D, E, F, and G. Several members of MRGPRs have emerged as critically important receptors in histamine-independent pruritus. They are mainly expressed by sensory neurons and some also by mast cells (5, 8, 204, 205). Recently, human basophils and eosinophils were reported to express MRGPRX2 (206). However, the MRGPRs can be activated by various endogenous and exogenous peptides or molecules, such as antimicrobial host defense or opioid peptides, SP or eosinophilic granules, but also by drugs like vancomycin or chloroquine (CQ) (12, 207). Particularly, MRGPRA3 and MRGPRC11 in mice as well as the human ortholog MRGPRX1 got into the focus of pruritus researchers over the past decade (12, 208). It was shown that CQ activated MRGPRA3 leading to a pruritus signal via the activation of TRPA1 (24). Furthermore, it was demonstrated that expression of MRGPRA3 establishes a subset of nociceptors that specifically mediate pruritus, but not pain in a mouse model. In addition, a deletion of MRGPRA3+ sensory neurons significantly inhibits scratching behavior (209, 210). A recent study by Lee et al. (211) determined that Korean Red Ginseng water extract (KRGE) inhibits CQ-induced pruritus by blocking the MRGPRA3/TRPA1 pathway. Interestingly, KRGE has also anti-pruritic effects on the histamine-dependent H1R/TRPV1 pathway, which might provide a dual anti-pruritic candidate agent for the treatment of pruritus patients (211, 212). Moreover, KRGE treatment significantly decreased hyperplasia and hyperkeratosis in the epidermis, infiltration of inflammatory cells and suppressed the overexpression of cytokines in the AD-like skin lesions of AD mice model (167). MRGPRC11 is in addition to MRGPRA3 co-localized and expressed in a subset of TRPV1+ afferents and mediates pruritus induced by BAM8-22 (24, 209, 213). Liu et al. (204) has proven that activation through MRGPRC11-specific agonist BAM8-22 induces scratching in murine models. In a following clinical study, BAM8-22 triggered pruritus and nociceptive sensations in humans in a histamine-independent manner as topical antihistamine-containing cream did not attenuate scratching behavior (214). This indicates BAM8-22 as an endogenous pruritus mediator and MRGPRX1 antagonists may present potential anti-pruritic therapies. The synthetic peptide SLIGRL was long believed to mediate scratching behavior via the PAR-2. However, intradermal injected SLIGRL caused scratching behavior in PAR-2 KO mice similar to that of wild-type mice. Liu and colleagues (215) proved that the pruritus induction of SLIGRL was mediated by MRGPRC11 while its hyperalgesic mode of action was derived from PAR-2 (2, 215). Furthermore, MRGPRX1 is responsible for neuronal activation and scratching behavior induced by both CQ and BAM8-22 (204, 213, 216). To date, there is a lack of knowledge about the involvement of MRGPRX1 in the pathology in chronic pruritic diseases such as AD and the potential role of MRGPRX1 antagonists in affected patients. Recently, researchers have shown an increased interest in MRGPRX2 in terms of pruriceptive receptor and its involvement in pruritic diseases like AD or psoriasis (164, 176, 217, 218). MRGPRX2 is expressed in mast cells and an activation of MRGPRX2 by peptides such as SP results in mast cell degranulation leading to release of proinflammatory factors as well as modulation of neurogenic inflammation and pruritus (219, 220). Previous research has established that both the percentage of MRGPRX2+ mast cells and MRGPRX2+ skin mast cells of patients with CSU were significantly higher in comparison to non-chronic urticaria subjects. It was further shown that SP-induced histamine release from human skin mast cells through MRGPRX2 contributing to neurogenic inflammation (221). Interestingly, Green et al. (222) found out that SP-mediated inflammatory responses were independent of its canonical receptor NK1R and identified MRGPRX2 and its mouse homolog MRGPRB2 as an important neuro-immune modulator and a potential target for treating inflammatory pain. Involvement in pruritus transmission and anti-pruritic treatment therapies remain elusive and needs to be clarified in further studies (222). In a recent study, increased MRGPRX2 mRNA expression in pruritic skin of patients with AD and psoriasis was demonstrated as well (164). However, research has consistently shown that only few endogenous agonists for most of these receptors are known so far and their role in the pathogenesis chronic pruritus diseases such as AD remains still unclear.

Tropomyosin Receptor Kinase A

Trk receptors were firstly described in 1986 and three members of the tyrosine kinase receptor family, TrkA, TrkB, and TrkC, have been identified so far. Trk receptors are activated by various neurotrophins including nerve-growth factor (NGF), brain-derived neurotrophic factor (BDNF), neurotrophin-3 (NT-3) and neurotrophin-4 (NT-4) (223–226). The main source of NGF are keratinocytes in the skin (227, 228), but it is also expressed and secreted by other immune cells, such as basophils (229), monocytes and macrophages (230), mast cells (231, 232) and eosinophils (233) as well as by neurons (234, 235) during inflammation. NGF binds with high affinity to its receptor TrkA as well as the low-affinity neurotrophin receptor p75NTR. TrkA is widely expressed across the airway smooth muscles, the lung epithelium and sensory neurons (236, 237), but also located on various non-neuronal cells like basophils (238), eosinophils (233), keratinocytes (228), monocytes and macrophages (239), mast cells (231, 232) as well as B and T cells (240, 241). Both NGF and its receptor TrkA are suggested to play important roles in pruritus and allergic inflammation. Several studies reported that NGF in the skin and NGF serum levels of AD and psoriatic patients as well as serum levels of patients with asthma are increased (227, 242–245). Additionally, an increased TrkA expression in keratinocytes of patients with AD has been observed during inflammation (228). In AD it was shown, that increased peripheral serum levels of BDNF significantly correlate with disease severity and pruritus (246, 247). Also scratching activities were significantly correlated to increased levels of BDNF as shown by Hon and colleagues (248) which used a DigiTrac model to assess scratching activities in children with AD. In this regard, it has been shown that eosinophils are a source of BDNF and release BDNF and are functionally activated by BDNF with induction of chemotaxis (246–248). Thus, the question arises if BDNF which is released by eosinophils of AD patients is also capable to stimulate nerves. This has recently been shown in a study by us in which we could see that BDNF released by peripheral blood eosinophils of patients with AD led to a significant sprouting of peripheral nerves derived from spinal neurons of mice (247). Thus, also BDNF seems to have an important impact in neuro-immune interaction mechanisms and pruritus. However, NGF affects neurite outgrowth and neuronal survival (236, 249). Interestingly, sprouting of itch-sensitive nerve fibers, promoted by increased NGF levels, has been observed in the skin of patients with AD (242) and in AD-associated mice models (250, 251). Since NGF is known to increase cutaneous innervation in AD models and might contribute to the development of chronic pruritus, NGF and its receptor TrkA could be targets for future treatment of pruritus and allergic inflammation in pruritic diseases like AD or psoriasis. A clinical study demonstrated a promising treatment of AD by neutralizing antibodies against NGF that inhibited the development of skin lesions and epidermal innervation as well as scratching behavior in AD mice model (252). In human sensory neurons, NGF up-regulated the expression and sensitivity of TRPV1 channels by activating TrkA (253, 254). Interestingly, TrkA inhibitor CT327 was shown to significantly reduce chronic pruritus in patients with psoriasis as measured by VAS in a phase II clinical study. The results demonstrated that 62, 46, and 61% of patients treated with CT327 0.05, 0.1, and 0.5%, respectively, had at least a 50% decrease in pruritus VAS in comparison to 32% on vehicle (255). Further trials are necessary to prove the anti-pruritic effects of CT327 in AD. There is growing evidence that cutaneous NGF-TrkA-TRPV1 signaling might be a key mechanism contributing to neurogenic inflammation and pruritus in different dermatological diseases (147, 255).

CONCLUSION

Our understanding of the pathogenesis of pruritus has significantly evolved in recent years. There is a growing body of literature on the complex crosstalk between neuronal and immune cells that are involved in the development of acute and chronic pruritus. Neurons directly communicate with and regulate the function of various immune cells, such as mast cells, dendritic cells, eosinophils and T cells in pruritus transmission and inflammation. Immune cells release proinflammatory mediators including cytokines, chemokines, neurotrophins, and neuropeptides that activate sensory neurons to mediate pruritus. Activation of these neurons leads to a release of neurotransmitters and neuropeptides that vice versa have a direct impact on the functional activity of immune cells. The literature on neuro-immune crosstalk has emphasized several key mediators and neuronal pathways involved in the transmission of pruritus. Potential mediator and promising receptor therapeutic targets in the skin as well as in peripheral nerves comprises TRPV1, TRPA1, IL-31RA, TSLPR, PAR-2, NK1R, H1R and H4R, MRGPRs and TrkA, which are highlighted in this review (**Figure 1**, **Tables 1**, **2**). Future studies targeting neuro-immune interactions will help to unravel the underlying mechanisms of pruritus and to develop specific therapies.

AUTHOR CONTRIBUTIONS

AR has performed the literature research and wrote the manuscript including the tables. MML designed the figure and revised the manuscript. UR, KL, AEK, and BH critically revised the manuscript. All authors read and approved the final version of the submitted manuscript.

REFERENCES

1. Raap U, Ständer S, Metz M. Pathophysiology of itch and new treatments. *Curr Opin Allergy Clin Immunol.* (2011) 11:420–7. doi: 10.1097/ACI.0b013e32834a41c2
2. Han L, Dong X. Itch mechanisms and circuits. *Annu Rev Biophys.* (2014) 43:331–55. doi: 10.1146/annurev-biophys-051013-022826
3. Silverberg JI, Hinami K, Trick WE, Cella D. Itch in the general internal medicine setting: a cross-sectional study of prevalence and quality-of-life effects. *Am J Clin Dermatol.* (2016) 17:681–90. doi: 10.1007/s40257-016-0215-3
4. Mack MR, Kim BS. The itch-scratch cycle: a neuroimmune perspective. *Trends Immunol.* (2018) 39:980–91. doi: 10.1016/j.it.2018.10.001
5. Mollanazar NK, Smith PK, Yosipovitch G. Mediators of chronic pruritus in atopic dermatitis: getting the itch out? *Clin Rev Allergy Immunol.* (2016) 51:263–92. doi: 10.1007/s12016-015-8488-5
6. Pereira MP, Agelopoulos K, Kremer AE, Schmelz M. [New findings regarding the neurobiology of pruritus]. *Hautarzt.* (2018) 69:620–5. doi: 10.1007/s00105-018-4210-x
7. Yosipovitch G, Berger T, Fassett MS. Neuroimmune interactions in chronic itch of atopic dermatitis. *J Eur Acad Dermatol Venereol.* (2020) 34:239–50. doi: 10.1111/jdv.15973
8. Voisin T, Bouvier A, Chiu IM. Neuro-immune interactions in allergic diseases: novel targets for therapeutics. *Int Immunol.* (2017) 29:247–61. doi: 10.1093/intimm/dxx040
9. Kabata H, Artis D. Neuro-immune crosstalk and allergic inflammation. *J Clin Invest.* (2019) 129:1475–82. doi: 10.1172/JCI124609
10. Lopez-Requena A, Boonen B, Van Gerven L, Hellings PW, Alpizar YA, Talavera K. Roles of neuronal TRP channels in neuroimmune interactions. In: Emir TLR, editor. *Neurobiology of TRP Channels.* Boca Raton, FL: Frontiers in Neuroscience. (2017). p. 277–94. doi: 10.4324/9781315152837-15
11. Oetjen LK, Kim BS. Interactions of the immune and sensory nervous systems in atopy. *FEBS J.* (2018) 285:3138–51. doi: 10.1111/febs.14465
12. Ständer S, Raap U, Weisshaar E, Schmelz M, Mettang T, Handwerker H, et al. Pathogenesis of pruritus. *J Dtsch Dermatol Ges.* (2011) 9:456–63. doi: 10.1111/j.1610-0387.2011.07585.x
13. Nakashima C, Ishida Y, Kitoh A, Otsuka A, Kabashima K. Interaction of peripheral nerves and mast cells, eosinophils, and basophils in the development of pruritus. *Exp Dermatol.* (2019) 28:1405–11. doi: 10.1111/exd.14014
14. Misery L, Huet F, Gouin O, Ständer S, Deleuran M. Current pharmaceutical developments in atopic dermatitis. *Curr Opin Pharmacol.* (2019) 46:7–13. doi: 10.1016/j.coph.2018.12.003
15. McEwen MW, Fite EM, Yosipovitch G, Patel T. Drugs on the horizon for chronic pruritus. *Dermatol Clin.* (2018) 36:335–44. doi: 10.1016/j.det.2018.02.016
16. Pereira MP, Ständer S. Chronic pruritus: current and emerging treatment options. *Drugs.* (2017) 77:999–1007. doi: 10.1007/s40265-017-0746-9
17. Golpanian RS, Yosipovitch G. Current and emerging systemic treatments targeting the neural system for chronic pruritus. *Expert Opin Pharmacother.* (2020) 21:1629–36. doi: 10.1080/14656566.2020.1775815
18. Clapham DE. TRP channels as cellular sensors. *Nature.* (2003) 426:517–24. doi: 10.1038/nature02196
19. Montell C. The TRP superfamily of cation channels. *Sci STKE.* (2005) 2005:re3. doi: 10.1126/stke.2722005re3
20. Sun S, Dong X. Trp channels and itch. *Semin Immunopathol.* (2016) 38:293–307. doi: 10.1007/s00281-015-0530-4
21. Kittaka H, Tominaga M. The molecular and cellular mechanisms of itch and the involvement of TRP channels in the peripheral sensory nervous system and skin. *Allergol Int.* (2017) 66:22–30. doi: 10.1016/j.alit.2016.10.003
22. Xie Z, Hu H. TRP channels as drug targets to relieve itch. *Pharmaceuticals.* (2018) 11:4. doi: 10.3390/ph11040100
23. Shim WS, Tak MH, Lee MH, Kim M, Kim M, Koo JY, et al. TRPV1 mediates histamine-induced itching via the activation of phospholipase A2 and 12-lipoxygenase. *J Neurosci.* (2007) 27:2331–7. doi: 10.1523/JNEUROSCI.4643-06.2007
24. Wilson SR, Gerhold KA, Bifolck-Fisher A, Liu Q, Patel KN, Dong X, et al. TRPA1 is required for histamine-independent, Mas-related G protein-coupled receptor-mediated itch. *Nat Neurosci.* (2011) 14:595–602. doi: 10.1038/nn.2789
25. Cevikbas F, Wang X, Akiyama T, Kempkes C, Savinko T, Antal A, et al. A sensory neuron-expressed IL-31 receptor mediates T helper cell-dependent itch: Involvement of TRPV1 and TRPA1. *J Allergy Clin Immunol.* (2014) 133:448–60. doi: 10.1016/j.jaci.2013.10.048

26. Hojland CR, Andersen HH, Poulsen JN, Arendt-Nielsen L, Gazerani P. A human surrogate model of itch utilizing the TRPA1 agonist trans-cinnamaldehyde. *Acta Derm Venereol.* (2015) 95:798–803. doi: 10.2340/00015555-2103
27. Jian T, Yang N, Yang Y, Zhu C, Yuan X, Yu G, et al. TRPV1 and PLC participate in histamine H4 receptor-induced itch. *Neural Plast.* (2016) 2016:1682972. doi: 10.1155/2016/1682972
28. Brennan F. The pathophysiology of pruritus – a review for clinicians. *Progress in Palliative Care.* (2016) 24:133–46. doi: 10.1179/1743291X14Y.0000000110
29. Imamachi N, Park GH, Lee H, Anderson DJ, Simon MI, Basbaum AI, et al. TRPV1-expressing primary afferents generate behavioral responses to pruritogens via multiple mechanisms. *Proc Natl Acad Sci USA.* (2009) 106:11330–5. doi: 10.1073/pnas.0905605106
30. Kim SJ, Park GH, Kim D, Lee J, Min H, Wall E, et al. Analysis of cellular and behavioral responses to imiquimod reveals a unique itch pathway in transient receptor potential vanilloid 1 (TRPV1)-expressing neurons. *Proc Natl Acad Sci USA.* (2011) 108:3371–6. doi: 10.1073/pnas.1019755108
31. Wilson SR, Bautista DM. Role of transient receptor potential channels in acute and chronic itch. In: Carstens E, Akiyama T, editors. *Itch: Mechanisms and Treatment.* Boca Raton, FL: Frontiers in Neuroscience (2014).
32. Ru F, Sun H, Jurcakova D, Herbstsomer RA, Meixong J, Dong X, et al. Mechanisms of pruritogen-induced activation of itch nerves in isolated mouse skin. *J Physiol.* (2017) 595:3651–66. doi: 10.1113/JP273795
33. Denda M, Fuziwara S, Inoue K, Denda S, Akamatsu H, Tomitaka A, et al. Immunoreactivity of VR1 on epidermal keratinocyte of human skin. *Biochem Biophys Res Commun.* (2001) 285:1250–2. doi: 10.1006/bbrc.2001.5299
34. Biro T, Kovacs L. An "ice-cold" TR(i)P to skin biology: the role of TRPA1 in human epidermal keratinocytes. *J Invest Dermatol.* (2009) 129:2096–9. doi: 10.1038/jid.2009.179
35. Billeter AT, Galbraith N, Walker S, Lawson C, Gardner SA, Sarojini H, et al. TRPA1 mediates the effects of hypothermia on the monocyte inflammatory response. *Surgery.* (2015) 158:646–54. doi: 10.1016/j.surg.2015.03.065
36. Parenti A, De Logu F, Geppetti P, Benemei S. What is the evidence for the role of TRP channels in inflammatory and immune cells? *Br J Pharmacol.* (2016) 173:953–69. doi: 10.1111/bph.13392
37. Omari SA, Adams MJ, Geraghty DP. TRPV1 channels in immune cells and hematological malignancies. *Adv Pharmacol.* (2017) 79:173–98. doi: 10.1016/bs.apha.2017.01.002
38. Khalil M, Alliger K, Weidinger C, Yerinde C, Wirtz S, Becker C, et al. Functional role of transient receptor potential channels in immune cells and epithelia. *Front Immunol.* (2018) 9:174. doi: 10.3389/fimmu.2018.00174
39. Ständer S, Moormann C, Schumacher M, Buddenkotte J, Artuc M, Shpacovitch V, et al. Expression of vanilloid receptor subtype 1 in cutaneous sensory nerve fibers, mast cells, and epithelial cells of appendage structures. *Exp Dermatol.* (2004) 13:129–39. doi: 10.1111/j.0906-6705.2004.0178.x
40. Oh MH, Oh SY, Lu J, Lou H, Myers AC, Zhu Z, et al. TRPA1-dependent pruritus in IL-13-induced chronic atopic dermatitis. *J Immunol.* (2013) 191:5371–82. doi: 10.4049/jimmunol.1300300
41. Heiner I, Eisfeld J, Luckhoff A. Role and regulation of TRP channels in neutrophil granulocytes. *Cell Calcium.* (2003) 33:533–40. doi: 10.1016/S0143-4160(03)00058-7
42. Zhou Y, Han D, Follansbee T, Wu X, Yu S, Wang B, et al. Transient receptor potential ankyrin 1 (TRPA1) positively regulates imiquimod-induced, psoriasiform dermal inflammation in mice. *J Cell Mol Med.* (2019) 23:4819–28. doi: 10.1111/jcmm.14392
43. Bertin S, Aoki-Nonaka Y, de Jong PR, Nohara LL, Xu H, Stanwood SR, et al. The ion channel TRPV1 regulates the activation and proinflammatory properties of CD4(+) T cells. *Nat Immunol.* (2014) 15:1055–63. doi: 10.1038/ni.3009
44. Bertin S, Aoki-Nonaka Y, Lee J, de Jong PR, Kim P, Han T, et al. The TRPA1 ion channel is expressed in CD4+ T cells and restrains T-cell-mediated colitis through inhibition of TRPV1. *Gut.* (2017) 66:1584–96. doi: 10.1136/gutjnl-2015-310710
45. Sahoo SS, Majhi RK, Tiwari A, Acharya T, Kumar PS, Saha S, et al. Transient receptor potential ankyrin1 channel is endogenously expressed in T cells and is involved in immune functions. *Biosci Rep.* (2019) 39:BSR20191437. doi: 10.1042/BSR20191437
46. Toth BI, Benko S, Szollosi AG, Kovacs L, Rajnavolgyi E, Biro T. Transient receptor potential vanilloid-1 signaling inhibits differentiation and activation of human dendritic cells. *FEBS Lett.* (2009) 583:1619–24. doi: 10.1016/j.febslet.2009.04.031
47. Gouin O, L'Herondelle K, Lebonvallet N, Le Gall-Ianotto C, Sakka M, Buhe V, et al. TRPV1 and TRPA1 in cutaneous neurogenic and chronic inflammation: pro-inflammatory response induced by their activation and their sensitization. *Protein Cell.* (2017) 8:644–61. doi: 10.1007/s13238-017-0395-5
48. Zhu X, Learoyd J, Butt S, Zhu L, Usatyuk PV, Natarajan V, et al. Regulation of eosinophil adhesion by lysophosphatidylcholine via a non-store-operated Ca2+ channel. *Am J Respir Cell Mol Biol.* (2007) 36:585–93. doi: 10.1165/rcmb.2006-0391OC
49. Patricio ES, Costa R, Figueiredo CP, Gers-Barlag K, Bicca MA, Manjavachi MN, et al. Mechanisms underlying the scratching behavior induced by the activation of proteinase-activated receptor-4 in mice. *J Invest Dermatol.* (2015) 135:2484–91. doi: 10.1038/jid.2015.183
50. Zhang X. Targeting TRP ion channels for itch relief. *Naunyn Schmiedebergs Arch Pharmacol.* (2015) 388:389–99. doi: 10.1007/s00210-014-1068-z
51. Li YR, Gupta P. Immune aspects of the bi-directional neuroimmune facilitator TRPV1. *Mol Biol Rep.* (2019) 46:1499–510. doi: 10.1007/s11033-018-4560-6
52. Kasutani K, Fujii E, Ohyama S, Adachi H, Hasegawa M, Kitamura H, et al. Anti-IL-31 receptor antibody is shown to be a potential therapeutic option for treating itch and dermatitis in mice. *Br J Pharmacol.* (2014) 171:5049–58. doi: 10.1111/bph.12823
53. Hawro T, Saluja R, Weller K, Altrichter S, Metz M, Maurer M. Interleukin-31 does not induce immediate itch in atopic dermatitis patients and healthy controls after skin challenge. *Allergy.* (2014) 69:113–7. doi: 10.1111/all.12316
54. Lim KM, Park YH. Development of PAC-14028, a novel transient receptor potential vanilloid type 1 (TRPV1) channel antagonist as a new drug for refractory skin diseases. *Arch Pharm Res.* (2012) 35:393–6. doi: 10.1007/s12272-012-0321-6
55. Lee YW, Won CH, Jung K, Nam HJ, Choi G, Park YH, et al. Efficacy and safety of PAC-14028 cream - a novel, topical, nonsteroidal, selective TRPV1 antagonist in patients with mild-to-moderate atopic dermatitis: a phase IIb randomized trial. *Br J Dermatol.* (2019) 180:1030–8. doi: 10.1111/bjd.17455
56. Dillon SR, Sprecher C, Hammond A, Bilsborough J, Rosenfeld-Franklin M, Presnell SR, et al. Interleukin 31, a cytokine produced by activated T cells, induces dermatitis in mice. *Nat Immunol.* (2004) 5:752–60. doi: 10.1038/ni1084
57. Feld M, Garcia R, Buddenkotte J, Katayama S, Lewis K, Muirhead G, et al. The pruritus- and TH2-associated cytokine IL-31 promotes growth of sensory nerves. *J Allergy Clin Immunol.* (2016) 138:500–8.e24. doi: 10.1016/j.jaci.2016.02.020
58. Nakashima C, Otsuka A, Kabashima K. Interleukin-31 and interleukin-31 receptor: New therapeutic targets for atopic dermatitis. *Exp Dermatol.* (2018) 27:327–31. doi: 10.1111/exd.13533
59. Ishii T, Wang J, Zhang W, Mascarenhas J, Hoffman R, Dai Y, et al. Pivotal role of mast cells in pruritogenesis in patients with myeloproliferative disorders. *Blood.* (2009) 113:5942–50. doi: 10.1182/blood-2008-09-179416
60. Niyonsaba F, Ushio H, Hara M, Yokoi H, Tominaga M, Takamori K, et al. Antimicrobial peptides human beta-defensins and cathelicidin LL-37 induce the secretion of a pruritogenic cytokine IL-31 by human mast cells. *J Immunol.* (2010) 184:3526–34. doi: 10.4049/jimmunol.0900712
61. Kunsleben N, Rudrich U, Gehring M, Novak N, Kapp A, Raap U. IL-31 Induces Chemotaxis, Calcium Mobilization, Release of Reactive Oxygen Species, and CCL26 in Eosinophils, Which Are Capable to Release IL-31. *J Invest Dermatol.* (2015) 135:1908–11. doi: 10.1038/jid.2015.106
62. Raap U, Gehring M, Kleiner S, Rudrich U, Eiz-Vesper B, Haas H, et al. Human basophils are a source of - and are differentially activated by - IL-31. *Clin Exp Allergy.* (2017) 47:499–508. doi: 10.1111/cea.12875
63. Bando T, Morikawa Y, Komori T, Senba E. Complete overlap of interleukin-31 receptor A and oncostatin M receptor beta in the adult dorsal root ganglia with distinct developmental expression patterns. *Neuroscience.* (2006) 142:1263–71. doi: 10.1016/j.neuroscience.2006.07.009
64. Cheung PF, Wong CK, Ho AW, Hu S, Chen DP, Lam CW. Activation of human eosinophils and epidermal keratinocytes by Th2 cytokine IL-31:

implication for the immunopathogenesis of atopic dermatitis. *Int Immunol.* (2010) 22:453–67. doi: 10.1093/intimm/dxq027

65. Bilsborough J, Leung DY, Maurer M, Howell M, Boguniewicz M, Yao L, et al. IL-31 is associated with cutaneous lymphocyte antigen-positive skin homing T cells in patients with atopic dermatitis. *J Allergy Clin Immunol.* (2006) 117:418–25. doi: 10.1016/j.jaci.2005.10.046
66. Kasraie S, Niebuhr M, Werfel T. Interleukin (IL)-31 induces pro-inflammatory cytokines in human monocytes and macrophages following stimulation with staphylococcal exotoxins. *Allergy.* (2010) 65:712–21. doi: 10.1111/j.1398-9995.2009.02255.x
67. Edukulla R, Singh B, Jegga AG, Sontake V, Dillon SR, Madala SK. Th2 cytokines augment IL-31/IL-31RA Interactions via STAT6-dependent IL-31RA expression. *J Biol Chem.* (2015) 290:13510–20. doi: 10.1074/jbc.M114.622126
68. Horejs-Hoeck J, Schwarz H, Lamprecht S, Maier E, Hainzl S, Schmittner M, et al. Dendritic cells activated by IFN-gamma/STAT1 express IL-31 receptor and release proinflammatory mediators upon IL-31 treatment. *J Immunol.* (2012) 188:5319–26. doi: 10.4049/jimmunol.1101044
69. Heise R, Neis MM, Marquardt Y, Joussen S, Heinrich PC, Merk HF, et al. IL-31 receptor alpha expression in epidermal keratinocytes is modulated by cell differentiation and interferon gamma. *J Invest Dermatol.* (2009) 129:240–3. doi: 10.1038/jid.2008.183
70. Kasraie S, Niebuhr M, Baumert K, Werfel T. Functional effects of interleukin 31 in human primary keratinocytes. *Allergy.* (2011) 66:845–52. doi: 10.1111/j.1398-9995.2011.02545.x
71. Cevikbas F, Kempkes C, Buhl T, Mess C, Buddenkotte J, Steinhoff M. Role of interleukin-31 and oncostatin M in itch and neuroimmune communication. In: Carstens E, Akiyama T, editors. *Itch: Mechanisms and Treatment.* Boca Raton, FL: Frontiers in Neuroscience (2014).
72. Sonkoly E, Muller A, Lauerma AI, Pivarcsi A, Soto H, Kemeny L, et al. IL-31: a new link between T cells and pruritus in atopic skin inflammation. *J Allergy Clin Immunol.* (2006) 117:411–7. doi: 10.1016/j.jaci.2005.10.033
73. Stott B, Lavender P, Lehmann S, Pennino D, Durham S, Schmidt-Weber CB. Human IL-31 is induced by IL-4 and promotes TH2-driven inflammation. *J Allergy Clin Immunol.* (2013) 132:446–54.e5. doi: 10.1016/j.jaci.2013.03.050
74. Gibbs BF, Patsinakidis N, Raap U. Role of the pruritic cytokine IL-31 in autoimmune skin diseases. *Front Immunol.* (2019) 10:1383. doi: 10.3389/fimmu.2019.01383
75. Raap U, Wichmann K, Bruder M, Ständer S, Wedi B, Kapp A, et al. Correlation of IL-31 serum levels with severity of atopic dermatitis. *J Allergy Clin Immunol.* (2008) 122:421–3. doi: 10.1016/j.jaci.2008.05.047
76. Salz M, Haeberle S, Hoffmann J, Enk AH, Hadaschik EN. Elevated IL-31 serum levels in bullous pemphigoid patients correlate with eosinophil numbers and are associated with BP180-IgE. *J Dermatol Sci.* (2017) 87:309–11. doi: 10.1016/j.jdermsci.2017.07.019
77. Ohmatsu H, Sugaya M, Suga H, Morimura S, Miyagaki T, Kai H, et al. Serum IL-31 levels are increased in patients with cutaneous T-cell lymphoma. *Acta Derm Venereol.* (2012) 92:282–3. doi: 10.2340/00015555-1345
78. Raap U, Wieczorek D, Gehring M, Pauls I, Ständer S, Kapp A, et al. Increased levels of serum IL-31 in chronic spontaneous urticaria. *Exp Dermatol.* (2010) 19:464–6. doi: 10.1111/j.1600-0625.2010.01067.x
79. Bodoor K, Al-Qarqaz F, Heis LA, Alfaqih MA, Oweis AO, Almomani R, et al. IL-33/13 axis and IL-4/31 axis play distinct roles in inflammatory process and itch in psoriasis and atopic dermatitis. *Clin Cosmet Investig Dermatol.* (2020) 13:419–24. doi: 10.2147/CCID.S257647
80. Altrichter S, Hawro T, Hanel K, Czaja K, Luscher B, Maurer M, et al. Successful omalizumab treatment in chronic spontaneous urticaria is associated with lowering of serum IL-31 levels. *J Eur Acad Dermatol Venereol.* (2016) 30:454–5. doi: 10.1111/jdv.12831
81. Nemoto O, Furue M, Nakagawa H, Shiramoto M, Hanada R, Matsuki S, et al. The first trial of CIM331, a humanized antihuman interleukin-31 receptor A antibody, in healthy volunteers and patients with atopic dermatitis to evaluate safety, tolerability and pharmacokinetics of a single dose in a randomized, double-blind, placebo-controlled study. *Br J Dermatol.* (2016) 174:296–304. doi: 10.1111/bjd.14207
82. Ruzicka T, Mihara R. Anti-interleukin-31 receptor A antibody for atopic dermatitis. *N Engl J Med.* (2017) 376:2093. doi: 10.1056/NEJMoa1606490
83. Kabashima K, Furue M, Hanifin JM, Pulka G, Wollenberg A, Galus R, et al. Nemolizumab in patients with moderate-to-severe atopic dermatitis: randomized, phase II, long-term extension study. *J Allergy Clin Immunol.* (2018) 142:1121–30.e7. doi: 10.1016/j.jaci.2018.03.018
84. Richards CD, Gandhi R, Botelho F, Ho L, Paolini JF. Oncostatin M induction of monocyte chemoattractant protein 1 is inhibited by anti-oncostatin M receptor beta monoclonal antibody KPL-716. *Acta Derm Venereol.* (2020) 100:adv00197. doi: 10.2340/00015555-3505
85. He R, Geha RS. Thymic stromal lymphopoietin. *Ann N Y Acad Sci.* (2010) 1183:13–24. doi: 10.1111/j.1749-6632.2009.05128.x
86. Ziegler SF, Roan F, Bell BD, Stoklasek TA, Kitajima M, Han H. The biology of thymic stromal lymphopoietin (TSLP). *Adv Pharmacol.* (2013) 66:129–55. doi: 10.1016/B978-0-12-404717-4.00004-4
87. Zhong J, Sharma J, Raju R, Palapetta SM, Prasad TS, Huang TC, et al. TSLP signaling pathway map: a platform for analysis of TSLP-mediated signaling. *Database.* (2014) 2014:bau007. doi: 10.1093/database/bau007
88. Park LS, Martin U, Garka K, Gliniak B, Di Santo JP, Muller W, et al. Cloning of the murine thymic stromal lymphopoietin (TSLP) receptor: Formation of a functional heteromeric complex requires interleukin 7 receptor. *J Exp Med.* (2000) 192:659–70. doi: 10.1084/jem.192.5.659
89. Sokol CL, Barton GM, Farr AG, Medzhitov R. A mechanism for the initiation of allergen-induced T helper type 2 responses. *Nat Immunol.* (2008) 9:310–8. doi: 10.1038/ni1558
90. Cook EB, Stahl JL, Schwantes EA, Fox KE, Mathur SK. IL-3 and TNFalpha increase thymic stromal lymphopoietin receptor (TSLPR) expression on eosinophils and enhance TSLP-stimulated degranulation. *Clin Mol Allergy.* (2012) 10:8. doi: 10.1186/1476-7961-10-8
91. Kashyap M, Rochman Y, Spolski R, Samsel L, Leonard WJ. Thymic stromal lymphopoietin is produced by dendritic cells. *J Immunol.* (2011) 187:1207–11. doi: 10.4049/jimmunol.1100355
92. Kubo T, Kamekura R, Kumagai A, Kawata K, Yamashita K, Mitsuhashi Y, et al. DeltaNp63 controls a TLR3-mediated mechanism that abundantly provides thymic stromal lymphopoietin in atopic dermatitis. *PLoS ONE.* (2014) 9:e105498. doi: 10.1371/journal.pone.0105498
93. Allakhverdi Z, Comeau MR, Jessup HK, Yoon BR, Brewer A, Chartier S, et al. Thymic stromal lymphopoietin is released by human epithelial cells in response to microbes, trauma, or inflammation and potently activates mast cells. *J Exp Med.* (2007) 204:253–8. doi: 10.1084/jem.20062211
94. Hirano R, Hasegawa S, Hashimoto K, Haneda Y, Ohsaki A, Ichiyama T. Human thymic stromal lymphopoietin enhances expression of CD80 in human CD14+ monocytes/macrophages. *Inflamm Res.* (2011) 60:605–10. doi: 10.1007/s00011-011-0310-0
95. Ying S, O'Connor B, Ratoff J, Meng Q, Fang C, Cousins D, et al. Expression and cellular provenance of thymic stromal lymphopoietin and chemokines in patients with severe asthma and chronic obstructive pulmonary disease. *J Immunol.* (2008) 181:2790–8. doi: 10.4049/jimmunol.181.4.2790
96. Tatsuno K, Fujiyama T, Yamaguchi H, Waki M, Tokura Y. TSLP directly interacts with skin-homing Th2 cells highly expressing its receptor to enhance IL-4 production in atopic dermatitis. *J Invest Dermatol.* (2015) 135:3017–24. doi: 10.1038/jid.2015.318
97. Astrakhan A, Omori M, Nguyen T, Becker-Herman S, Iseki M, Aye T, et al. Local increase in thymic stromal lymphopoietin induces systemic alterations in B cell development. *Nat Immunol.* (2007) 8:522–31. doi: 10.1038/ni1452
98. Wilson SR, The L, Batia LM, Beattie K, Katibah GE, McClain SP, et al. The epithelial cell-derived atopic dermatitis cytokine TSLP activates neurons to induce itch. *Cell.* (2013) 155:285–95. doi: 10.1016/j.cell.2013.08.057
99. Tu HY, Chen X, Li J. [Signal transduction in respiratory syncytial virus infection-induced thymic stromal lymphopoietin expression in human epithelial cells]. *Nan Fang Yi Ke Da Xue Xue Bao.* (2007) 27:1581–3.
100. Nakamura Y, Miyata M, Ohba T, Ando T, Hatsushika K, Suenaga F, et al. Cigarette smoke extract induces thymic stromal lymphopoietin expression, leading to T(H)2-type immune responses and airway inflammation. *J Allergy Clin Immunol.* (2008) 122:1208–14. doi: 10.1016/j.jaci.2008.09.022
101. Lee HC, Ziegler SF. Inducible expression of the proallergic cytokine thymic stromal lymphopoietin in airway epithelial cells is controlled by NFkappaB. *Proc Natl Acad Sci USA.* (2007) 104:914–9. doi: 10.1073/pnas.0607305104
102. Lee EB, Kim KW, Hong JY, Jee HM, Sohn MH, Kim KE. Increased serum thymic stromal lymphopoietin in children with atopic dermatitis. *Pediatr*

Allergy Immunol. (2010) 21:e457–60. doi: 10.1111/j.1399-3038.2009.00919.x

103. Nygaard U, Hvid M, Johansen C, Buchner M, Folster-Holst R, Deleuran M, et al. TSLP, IL-31, IL-33 and sST2 are new biomarkers in endophenotypic profiling of adult and childhood atopic dermatitis. *J Eur Acad Dermatol Venereol.* (2016) 30:1930–8. doi: 10.1111/jdv.13679
104. Uller L, Leino M, Bedke N, Sammut D, Green B, Lau L, et al. Double-stranded RNA induces disproportionate expression of thymic stromal lymphopoietin versus interferon-beta in bronchial epithelial cells from donors with asthma. *Thorax.* (2010) 65:626–32. doi: 10.1136/thx.2009.125930
105. Sherrill JD, Gao PS, Stucke EM, Blanchard C, Collins MH, Putnam PE, et al. Variants of thymic stromal lymphopoietin and its receptor associate with eosinophilic esophagitis. *J Allergy Clin Immunol.* (2010) 126:160–5.e3. doi: 10.1016/j.jaci.2010.04.037
106. Fang C, Siew LQ, Corrigan CJ, Ying S. The role of thymic stromal lymphopoietin in allergic inflammation and chronic obstructive pulmonary disease. *Arch Immunol Ther Exp.* (2010) 58:81–90. doi: 10.1007/s00005-010-0064-3
107. Varricchi G, Pecoraro A, Marone G, Criscuolo G, Spadaro G, Genovese A, et al. Thymic stromal lymphopoietin isoforms, inflammatory disorders, and cancer. *Front Immunol.* (2018) 9:1595. doi: 10.3389/fimmu.2018.01595
108. Alysandratos KD, Angelidou A, Vasiadi M, Zhang B, Kalogeromitros D, Katsarou-Katsari A, et al. Increased affected skin gene expression and serum levels of thymic stromal lymphopoietin in atopic dermatitis. *Ann Allergy Asthma Immunol.* (2010) 105:403–4. doi: 10.1016/j.anai.2010.09.017
109. Yoo J, Omori M, Gyarmati D, Zhou B, Aye T, Brewer A, et al. Spontaneous atopic dermatitis in mice expressing an inducible thymic stromal lymphopoietin transgene specifically in the skin. *J Exp Med.* (2005) 202:541–9. doi: 10.1084/jem.20041503
110. Li M, Messaddeq N, Teletin M, Pasquali JL, Metzger D, Chambon P. Retinoid X receptor ablation in adult mouse keratinocytes generates an atopic dermatitis triggered by thymic stromal lymphopoietin. *Proc Natl Acad Sci USA.* (2005) 102:14795–800. doi: 10.1073/pnas.0507385102
111. Simpson EL, Parnes JR, She D, Crouch S, Rees W, Mo M, et al. Tezepelumab, an anti-thymic stromal lymphopoietin monoclonal antibody, in the treatment of moderate to severe atopic dermatitis: A randomized phase 2a clinical trial. *J Am Acad Dermatol.* (2019) 80:1013–21. doi: 10.1016/j.jaad.2018.11.059
112. Nakajima S, Kabata H, Kabashima K, Asano K. Anti-TSLP antibodies: targeting a master regulator of type 2 immune responses. *Allergol Int.* (2020) 69:197–203. doi: 10.1016/j.alit.2020.01.001
113. Fitoussi J, Virassamynaik S, Callejon S, Weber S, Collet E, Scalia J, et al. Inhibition of thymic stromal lymphopoietin production to improve pruritus and quality of life in infants and children with atopic dermatitis. *J Cosmet Dermatol.* (2020) 19:2061–9. doi: 10.1111/jocd.13515
114. Kawabata A, Kuroda R, Hollenberg MD. [Physiology of protease-activated receptors (PARs): involvement of PARs in digestive functions]. *Nihon Yakurigaku Zasshi.* (1999) 114(Suppl. 1):173P–9. doi: 10.1254/fpj.114.supplement_173
115. Compton SJ, Renaux B, Wijesuriya SJ, Hollenberg MD. Glycosylation and the activation of proteinase-activated receptor 2 [PAR(2)] by human mast cell tryptase. *Br J Pharmacol.* (2001) 134:705–18. doi: 10.1038/sj.bjp.0704303
116. Adams MN, Ramachandran R, Yau MK, Suen JY, Fairlie DP, Hollenberg MD, et al. Structure, function and pathophysiology of protease activated receptors. *Pharmacol Ther.* (2011) 130:248–82. doi: 10.1016/j.pharmthera.2011.01.003
117. Akiyama T, Lerner EA, Carstens E. Protease-activated receptors and itch. *Handb Exp Pharmacol.* (2015) 226:219–35. doi: 10.1007/978-3-662-44605-8_13
118. Gieseler F, Ungefroren H, Settmacher U, Hollenberg MD, Kaufmann R. Proteinase-activated receptors (PARs) - focus on receptor-receptor-interactions and their physiological and pathophysiological impact. *Cell Commun Signal.* (2013) 11:86. doi: 10.1186/1478-811X-11-86
119. Buhl T, Ikoma A, Kempkes C, Cevikbas F, Sulk M, Buddenkotte J, et al. Protease-activated receptor-2 regulates neuro-epidermal communication in atopic dermatitis. *Front Immunol.* (2020) 11:1740. doi: 10.3389/fimmu.2020.01740
120. Steinhoff M, Neisius U, Ikoma A, Fartasch M, Heyer G, Skov PS, et al. Proteinase-activated receptor-2 mediates itch: a novel pathway for pruritus in human skin. *J Neurosci.* (2003) 23:6176–80. doi: 10.1523/JNEUROSCI.23-15-06176.2003
121. Steinhoff M, Buddenkotte J, Shpacovitch V, Rattenholl A, Moormann C, Vergnolle N, et al. Proteinase-activated receptors: transducers of proteinase-mediated signaling in inflammation and immune response. *Endocr Rev.* (2005) 26:1–43. doi: 10.1210/er.2003-0025
122. Lee SE, Jeong SK, Lee SH. Protease and protease-activated receptor-2 signaling in the pathogenesis of atopic dermatitis. *Yonsei Med J.* (2010) 51:808–22. doi: 10.3349/ymj.2010.51.6.808
123. Kempkes C, Buddenkotte J, Cevikbas F, Buhl T, Steinhoff M. Role of PAR-2 in neuroimmune communication and itch. In: Carstens E, Akiyama T, editors. *Itch: Mechanisms and Treatment.* Boca Raton, FL: Frontiers in Neuroscience (2014).
124. Steinhoff M, Corvera CU, Thoma MS, Kong W, McAlpine BE, Caughey GH, et al. Proteinase-activated receptor-2 in human skin: tissue distribution and activation of keratinocytes by mast cell tryptase. *Exp Dermatol.* (1999) 8:282–94. doi: 10.1111/j.1600-0625.1999.tb00383.x
125. Colognato R, Slupsky JR, Jendrach M, Burysek L, Syrovets T, Simmet T. Differential expression and regulation of protease-activated receptors in human peripheral monocytes and monocyte-derived antigen-presenting cells. *Blood.* (2003) 102:2645–52. doi: 10.1182/blood-2002-08-2497
126. Shrestha Palikhe N, Nahirney D, Laratta C, Gandhi VD, Vethanayagam D, Bhutani M, et al. Increased Protease-activated receptor-2 (PAR-2) expression on CD14++CD16+ peripheral blood monocytes of patients with severe asthma. *PLoS ONE.* (2015) 10:e0144500. doi: 10.1371/journal.pone.0144500
127. Ge S, Li T, Yao Q, Yan H, Huiyun Z, Zheng Y, et al. Expression of proteinase-activated receptor (PAR)-2 in monocytes from allergic patients and potential molecular mechanism. *Cell Biol Toxicol.* (2016) 32:529–42. doi: 10.1007/s10565-016-9353-x
128. D'Andrea MR, Rogahn CJ, Andrade-Gordon P. Localization of protease-activated receptors-1 and−2 in human mast cells: indications for an amplified mast cell degranulation cascade. *Biotech Histochem.* (2000) 75:85–90. doi: 10.3109/10520290009064152
129. He SH, Xie H, He YS. [Effect of a proteinase-activated receptor-2 (PAR-2) agonist on tryptase release from human mast cells]. *Sheng Li Xue Bao.* (2002) 54:531–4.
130. Wang H, He S. Induction of lactoferrin and IL-8 release from human neutrophils by tryptic enzymes via proteinase activated receptor-2. *Cell Biol Int.* (2006) 30:688–97. doi: 10.1016/j.cellbi.2006.04.007
131. Steinhoff M, Vergnolle N, Young SH, Tognetto M, Amadesi S, Ennes HS, et al. Agonists of proteinase-activated receptor 2 induce inflammation by a neurogenic mechanism. *Nat Med.* (2000) 6:151–8. doi: 10.1038/72247
132. Shpacovitch V, Feld M, Bunnett NW, Steinhoff M. Protease-activated receptors: novel PARtners in innate immunity. *Trends Immunol.* (2007) 28:541–50. doi: 10.1016/j.it.2007.09.001
133. Steinhoff M, Ständer S, Seeliger S, Ansel JC, Schmelz M, Luger T. Modern aspects of cutaneous neurogenic inflammation. *Arch Dermatol.* (2003) 139:1479–88. doi: 10.1001/archderm.139.11.1479
134. Amadesi S, Nie J, Vergnolle N, Cottrell GS, Grady EF, Trevisani M, et al. Protease-activated receptor 2 sensitizes the capsaicin receptor transient receptor potential vanilloid receptor 1 to induce hyperalgesia. *J Neurosci.* (2004) 24:4300–12. doi: 10.1523/JNEUROSCI.5679-03.2004
135. Davidson S, Giesler GJ. The multiple pathways for itch and their interactions with pain. *Trends Neurosci.* (2010) 33:550–8. doi: 10.1016/j.tins.2010.09.002
136. Gouin O, L'Herondelle K, Buscaglia P, Le Gall-Ianotto C, Philippe R, Legoux N, et al. Major role for TRPV1 and InsP3R in PAR2-elicited inflammatory mediator production in differentiated human keratinocytes. *J Invest Dermatol.* (2018) 138:1564–72. doi: 10.1016/j.jid.2018.01.034
137. Schön M, Behmenburg C, Denzer D, Schon MP. Pathogenic function of IL-1 beta in psoriasiform skin lesions of flaky skin (fsn/fsn) mice. *Clin Exp Immunol.* (2001) 123:505–10. doi: 10.1046/j.1365-2249.2001.01421.x
138. Sereflican B, Goksugur N, Bugdayci G, Polat M, Haydar Parlak A. Serum visfatin, adiponectin, and tumor necrosis factor alpha (TNF-alpha) levels in patients with psoriasis and their correlation with disease severity. *Acta Dermatovenerol Croat.* (2016) 24:13–9.
139. Hebert HL, Bowes J, Smith RL, McHugh NJ, Barker J, Griffiths CEM, et al. Polymorphisms in IL-1B distinguish between psoriasis of early and late onset. *J Invest Dermatol.* (2014) 134:1459–62. doi: 10.1038/jid.2013.485

140. Moniaga CS, Jeong SK, Egawa G, Nakajima S, Hara-Chikuma M, Jeon JE, et al. Protease activity enhances production of thymic stromal lymphopoietin and basophil accumulation in flaky tail mice. *Am J Pathol.* (2013) 182:841–51. doi: 10.1016/j.ajpath.2012.11.039
141. Indra AK. Epidermal TSLP: a trigger factor for pathogenesis of atopic dermatitis. *Expert Rev Proteomics.* (2013) 10:309–11. doi: 10.1586/14789450.2013.814881
142. Barr TP, Garzia C, Guha S, Fletcher EK, Nguyen N, Wieschhaus AJ, et al. PAR2 pepducin-based suppression of inflammation and itch in atopic dermatitis models. *J Invest Dermatol.* (2019) 139:412–21. doi: 10.1016/j.jid.2018.08.019
143. Pennefather JN, Lecci A, Candenas ML, Patak E, Pinto FM, Maggi CA. Tachykinins and tachykinin receptors: a growing family. *Life Sci.* (2004) 74:1445–63. doi: 10.1016/j.lfs.2003.09.039
144. Steinhoff MS, von Mentzer B, Geppetti P, Pothoulakis C, Bunnett NW. Tachykinins and their receptors: contributions to physiological control and the mechanisms of disease. *Physiol Rev.* (2014) 94:265–301. doi: 10.1152/physrev.00031.2013
145. Ständer S, Luger TA. NK-1 antagonists and itch. *Handb Exp Pharmacol.* (2015) 226:237–55. doi: 10.1007/978-3-662-44605-8_14
146. Pojawa-Golab M, Jaworecka K, Reich A. NK-1 receptor antagonists and pruritus: review of current literature. *Dermatol Ther.* (2019) 9:391–405. doi: 10.1007/s13555-019-0305-2
147. Yosipovitch G, Rosen JD, Hashimoto T. Itch: From mechanism to (novel) therapeutic approaches. *J Allergy Clin Immunol.* (2018) 142:1375–90. doi: 10.1016/j.jaci.2018.09.005
148. Marriott I, Bost KL. Expression of authentic substance P receptors in murine and human dendritic cells. *J Neuroimmunol.* (2001) 114:131–41. doi: 10.1016/S0165-5728(00)00466-5
149. Raap M, Rudrich U, Ständer S, Gehring M, Kapp A, Raap U. Substance P activates human eosinophils. *Exp Dermatol.* (2015) 24:557–9. doi: 10.1111/exd.12717
150. van der Kleij HP, Ma D, Redegeld FA, Kraneveld AD, Nijkamp FP, Bienenstock J. Functional expression of neurokinin 1 receptors on mast cells induced by IL-4 and stem cell factor. *J Immunol.* (2003) 171:2074–9. doi: 10.4049/jimmunol.171.4.2074
151. Ho WZ, Lai JP, Zhu XH, Uvaydova M, Douglas SD. Human monocytes and macrophages express substance P and neurokinin-1 receptor. *J Immunol.* (1997) 159:5654–60.
152. Lai JP, Douglas SD, Ho WZ. Human lymphocytes express substance P and its receptor. *J Neuroimmunol.* (1998) 86:80–6. doi: 10.1016/S0165-5728(98)00025-3
153. Morelli AE, Sumpter TL, Rojas-Canales DM, Bandyopadhyay M, Chen Z, Tkacheva O, et al. Neurokinin-1 receptor signaling is required for efficient Ca(2+) flux in T-cell-receptor-activated T cells. *Cell Rep.* (2020) 30:3448–65.e8. doi: 10.1016/j.celrep.2020.02.054
154. Liu JY, Hu JH, Zhu QG, Li FQ, Sun HJ. Substance P receptor expression in human skin keratinocytes and fibroblasts. *Br J Dermatol.* (2006) 155:657–62. doi: 10.1111/j.1365-2133.2006.07408.x
155. Roggenkamp D, Kopnick S, Stab F, Wenck H, Schmelz M, Neufang G. Epidermal nerve fibers modulate keratinocyte growth via neuropeptide signaling in an innervated skin model. *J Invest Dermatol.* (2013) 133:1620–8. doi: 10.1038/jid.2012.464
156. Schmelz M, Schmidt R, Bickel A, Handwerker HO, Torebjork HE. Specific C-receptors for itch in human skin. *J Neurosci.* (1997) 17:8003–8. doi: 10.1523/JNEUROSCI.17-20-08003.1997
157. Scholzen T, Armstrong CA, Bunnett NW, Luger TA, Olerud JE, Ansel JC. Neuropeptides in the skin: interactions between the neuroendocrine and the skin immune systems. *Exp Dermatol.* (1998) 7:81–96. doi: 10.1111/j.1600-0625.1998.tb00307.x
158. Ständer S, Yosipovitch G. Substance P and neurokinin 1 receptor are new targets for the treatment of chronic pruritus. *Br J Dermatol.* (2019) 181:932–8. doi: 10.1111/bjd.18025
159. Chang SE, Han SS, Jung HJ, Choi JH. Neuropeptides and their receptors in psoriatic skin in relation to pruritus. *Br J Dermatol.* (2007) 156:1272–7. doi: 10.1111/j.1365-2133.2007.07935.x
160. Amatya B, El-Nour H, Holst M, Theodorsson E, Nordlind K. Expression of tachykinins and their receptors in plaque psoriasis with pruritus. *Br J Dermatol.* (2011) 164:1023–9. doi: 10.1111/j.1365-2133.2011.10241.x
161. Akiyama T, Nguyen T, Curtis E, Nishida K, Devireddy J, Delahanty J, et al. A central role for spinal dorsal horn neurons that express neurokinin-1 receptors in chronic itch. *Pain.* (2015) 156:1240–6. doi: 10.1097/j.pain.0000000000000172
162. Zheng W, Wang J, Zhu W, Xu C, He S. Upregulated expression of substance P in basophils of the patients with chronic spontaneous urticaria: induction of histamine release and basophil accumulation by substance P. *Cell Biol Toxicol.* (2016) 32:217–28. doi: 10.1007/s10565-016-9330-4
163. Zhang Z, Zheng W, Xie H, Chai R, Wang J, Zhang H, et al. Up-regulated expression of substance P in CD8(+) T cells and NK1R on monocytes of atopic dermatitis. *J Transl Med.* (2017) 15:93. doi: 10.1186/s12967-017-1196-6
164. Nattkemper LA, Tey HL, Valdes-Rodriguez R, Lee H, Mollanazar NK, Albornoz C, et al. The genetics of chronic itch: gene expression in the skin of patients with atopic dermatitis and psoriasis with severe itch. *J Invest Dermatol.* (2018) 138:1311–7. doi: 10.1016/j.jid.2017.12.029
165. Salomon J, Baran E. The role of selected neuropeptides in pathogenesis of atopic dermatitis. *J Eur Acad Dermatol Venereol.* (2008) 22:223–8. doi: 10.1111/j.1468-3083.2007.02399.x
166. Hosokawa C, Takeuchi S, Furue M. Severity scores, itch scores and plasma substance P levels in atopic dermatitis treated with standard topical therapy with oral olopatadine hydrochloride. *J Dermatol.* (2009) 36:185–90. doi: 10.1111/j.1346-8138.2009.00621.x
167. Lee JH, Cho SH. Korean red ginseng extract ameliorates skin lesions in NC/Nga mice: an atopic dermatitis model. *J Ethnopharmacol.* (2011) 133:810–7. doi: 10.1016/j.jep.2010.11.020
168. Tsianakas A, Zeidler C, Riepe C, Borowski M, Forner C, Gerss J, et al. Aprepitant in anti-histamine-refractory chronic nodular prurigo: a multicentre, randomized, double-blind, placebo-controlled, cross-over, phase-II trial (APREPRU). *Acta Derm Venereol.* (2019) 99:379–85. doi: 10.2340/00015555-3120
169. Lönndahl L, Holst M, Bradley M, Killasli H, Heilborn J, Hall MA, et al. Substance P Antagonist Aprepitant Shows No Additive Effect Compared With Standardized Topical Treatment Alone In Patients With Atopic Dermatitis. *Acta Derm Venereol.* (2018) 98:324–8. doi: 10.2340/00015555-2852
170. Yosipovitch G, Ständer S, Kerby MB, Larrick JW, Perlman AJ, Schnipper EF, et al. Serlopitant for the treatment of chronic pruritus: results of a randomized, multicenter, placebo-controlled phase 2 clinical trial. *J Am Acad Dermatol.* (2018) 78:882–91.e10. doi: 10.1016/j.jaad.2018.02.030
171. Ständer S, Spellman MC, Kwon P, Yosipovitch G. The NK1 receptor antagonist serlopitant for treatment of chronic pruritus. *Expert Opin Investig Drugs.* (2019) 28:659–66. doi: 10.1080/13543784.2019.1638910
172. Reszke R, Krajewski P, Szepietowski JC. Emerging therapeutic options for chronic pruritus. *Am J Clin Dermatol.* (2020) 21:601–18. doi: 10.1007/s40257-020-00534-y
173. Pariser DM, Bagel J, Lebwohl M, Yosipovitch G, Chien E, Spellman MC. Serlopitant for psoriatic pruritus: a phase 2 randomized, double-blind, placebo-controlled clinical trial. *J Am Acad Dermatol.* (2020) 82:1314–20. doi: 10.1016/j.jaad.2020.01.056
174. Welsh SE, Xiao C, Kaden AR, Brzezynski JL, Mohrman MA, Wang J, et al. Neurokinin-1 receptor antagonist tradipitant has mixed effects on itch in atopic dermatitis: results from EPIONE, a randomized clinical trial. *J Eur Acad Dermatol Venereol.* (2020). doi: 10.1101/2020.06.21.20136911. [Epub ahead of print].
175. McNeil BD, Pundir P, Meeker S, Han L, Undem BJ, Kulka M, et al. Identification of a mast-cell-specific receptor crucial for pseudo-allergic drug reactions. *Nature.* (2015) 519:237–41. doi: 10.1038/nature14022
176. Azimi E, Reddy VB, Shade KC, Anthony RM, Talbot S, Pereira PJS, et al. Dual action of neurokinin-1 antagonists on Mas-related GPCRs. *JCI Insight.* (2016) 1:e89362. doi: 10.1172/jci.insight.89362
177. Bischoff SC, Zwahlen R, Stucki M, Mullner G, de Weck AL, Stadler BM, et al. Basophil histamine release and leukotriene production in response to anti-IgE and anti-IgE receptor antibodies. Comparison of normal subjects and patients with urticaria, atopic dermatitis or bronchial

asthma. *Int Arch Allergy Immunol.* (1996) 110:261–71. doi: 10.1159/000237297
178. Ikoma A, Rukwied R, Ständer S, Steinhoff M, Miyachi Y, Schmelz M. Neuronal sensitization for histamine-induced itch in lesional skin of patients with atopic dermatitis. *Arch Dermatol.* (2003) 139:1455–8. doi: 10.1001/archderm.139.11.1455
179. Parsons ME, Ganellin CR. Histamine and its receptors. *Br J Pharmacol.* (2006) 147(Suppl. 1):S127–35. doi: 10.1038/sj.bjp.0706440
180. Rossbach K, Nassenstein C, Gschwandtner M, Schnell D, Sander K, Seifert R, et al. Histamine H1, H3 and H4 receptors are involved in pruritus. *Neuroscience.* (2011) 190:89–102. doi: 10.1016/j.neuroscience.2011.06.002
181. Toth BI, Szallasi A, Biro T. Transient receptor potential channels and itch: how deep should we scratch? *Handb Exp Pharmacol.* (2015) 226:89–133. doi: 10.1007/978-3-662-44605-8_6
182. Connelly WM, Shenton FC, Lethbridge N, Leurs R, Waldvogel HJ, Faull RL, et al. The histamine H4 receptor is functionally expressed on neurons in the mammalian CNS. *Br J Pharmacol.* (2009) 157:55–63. doi: 10.1111/j.1476-5381.2009.00227.x
183. Giustizieri ML, Albanesi C, Fluhr J, Gisondi P, Norgauer J, Girolomoni G. H1 histamine receptor mediates inflammatory responses in human keratinocytes. *J Allergy Clin Immunol.* (2004) 114:1176–82. doi: 10.1016/j.jaci.2004.07.054
184. Glatzer F, Gschwandtner M, Ehling S, Rossbach K, Janik K, Klos A, et al. Histamine induces proliferation in keratinocytes from patients with atopic dermatitis through the histamine 4 receptor. *J Allergy Clin Immunol.* (2013) 132:1358–67. doi: 10.1016/j.jaci.2013.06.023
185. Mommert S, Kleiner S, Gehring M, Eiz-Vesper B, Stark H, Gutzmer R, et al. Human basophil chemotaxis and activation are regulated via the histamine H4 receptor. *Allergy.* (2016) 71:1264–73. doi: 10.1111/all.12875
186. Idzko M, la Sala A, Ferrari D, Panther E, Herouy Y, Dichmann S, et al. Expression and function of histamine receptors in human monocyte-derived dendritic cells. *J Allergy Clin Immunol.* (2002) 109:839–46. doi: 10.1067/mai.2002.124044
187. Damaj BB, Becerra CB, Esber HJ, Wen Y, Maghazachi AA. Functional expression of H4 histamine receptor in human natural killer cells, monocytes, and dendritic cells. *J Immunol.* (2007) 179:7907–15. doi: 10.4049/jimmunol.179.11.7907
188. Thangam EB, Jemima EA, Singh H, Baig MS, Khan M, Mathias CB, et al. The role of histamine and histamine receptors in mast cell-mediated allergy and inflammation: the hunt for new therapeutic targets. *Front Immunol.* (2018) 9:1873. doi: 10.3389/fimmu.2018.01873
189. Jutel M, Watanabe T, Klunker S, Akdis M, Thomet OA, Malolepszy J, et al. Histamine regulates T-cell and antibody responses by differential expression of H1 and H2 receptors. *Nature.* (2001) 413:420–5. doi: 10.1038/35096564
190. Gutzmer R, Mommert S, Gschwandtner M, Zwingmann K, Stark H, Werfel T. The histamine H4 receptor is functionally expressed on T(H)2 cells. *J Allergy Clin Immunol.* (2009) 123:619–25. doi: 10.1016/j.jaci.2008.12.1110
191. Mahapatra S, Albrecht M, Behrens B, Jirmo A, Behrens G, Hartwig C, et al. Delineating the role of histamine-1- and−4-receptors in a mouse model of Th2-dependent antigen-specific skin inflammation. *PLoS ONE.* (2014) 9:e87296. doi: 10.1371/journal.pone.0087296
192. Panula P, Chazot PL, Cowart M, Gutzmer R, Leurs R, Liu WL, et al. International Union of basic and clinical pharmacology. XCVIII. Histamine receptors. *Pharmacol Rev.* (2015) 67:601–55. doi: 10.1124/pr.114.010249
193. Werfel T, Layton G, Yeadon M, Whitlock L, Osterloh I, Jimenez P, et al. Efficacy and safety of the histamine H4 receptor antagonist ZPL-3893787 in patients with atopic dermatitis. *J Allergy Clin Immunol.* (2019) 143:1830–7 e4. doi: 10.1016/j.jaci.2018.07.047
194. Novak N, Peng WM, Bieber T, Akdis C. FcepsilonRI stimulation promotes the differentiation of histamine receptor 1-expressing inflammatory macrophages. *Allergy.* (2013) 68:454–61. doi: 10.1111/all.12109
195. Fukunaga A, Oda Y, Washio K, Omori T, Kakei Y, Hide M, et al. Efficacy of switching to bilastine, a histamine H1 receptor antagonist, in patients with chronic spontaneous urticaria (H1-SWITCH): study protocol for a randomized controlled trial. *Trials.* (2020) 21:23. doi: 10.1186/s13063-019-3878-2
196. Schaper-Gerhardt K, Rossbach K, Nikolouli E, Werfel T, Gutzmer R, Mommert S. The role of the histamine H4 receptor in atopic dermatitis and psoriasis. *Br J Pharmacol.* (2020) 177:490–502. doi: 10.1111/bph.14550
197. Thurmond RL, Kazerouni K, Chaplan SR, Greenspan AJ. Antihistamines and itch. *Handb Exp Pharmacol.* (2015) 226:257–90. doi: 10.1007/978-3-662-44605-8_15
198. Yamaura K, Oda M, Suwa E, Suzuki M, Sato H, Ueno K. Expression of histamine H4 receptor in human epidermal tissues and attenuation of experimental pruritus using H4 receptor antagonist. *J Toxicol Sci.* (2009) 34:427–31. doi: 10.2131/jts.34.427
199. Suwa E, Yamaura K, Oda M, Namiki T, Ueno K. Histamine H(4) receptor antagonist reduces dermal inflammation and pruritus in a hapten-induced experimental model. *Eur J Pharmacol.* (2011) 667:383–8. doi: 10.1016/j.ejphar.2011.05.037
200. Rossbach K, Schaper K, Kloth C, Gutzmer R, Werfel T, Kietzmann M, et al. Histamine H4 receptor knockout mice display reduced inflammation in a chronic model of atopic dermatitis. *Allergy.* (2016) 71:189–97. doi: 10.1111/all.12779
201. Ohsawa Y, Hirasawa N. The role of histamine H1 and H4 receptors in atopic dermatitis: from basic research to clinical study. *Allergol Int.* (2014) 63:533–42. doi: 10.2332/allergolint.13-RA-0675
202. Murata Y, Song M, Kikuchi H, Hisamichi K, Xu XL, Greenspan A, et al. Phase 2a, randomized, double-blind, placebo-controlled, multicenter, parallel-group study of a H4 R-antagonist (JNJ-39758979) in Japanese adults with moderate atopic dermatitis. *J Dermatol.* (2015) 42:129–39. doi: 10.1111/1346-8138.12726
203. Ohsawa Y, Hirasawa N. The antagonism of histamine H1 and H4 receptors ameliorates chronic allergic dermatitis via anti-pruritic and anti-inflammatory effects in NC/Nga mice. *Allergy.* (2012) 67:1014–22. doi: 10.1111/j.1398-9995.2012.02854.x
204. Liu Q, Tang Z, Surdenikova L, Kim S, Patel KN, Kim A, et al. Sensory neuron-specific GPCR Mrgprs are itch receptors mediating chloroquine-induced pruritus. *Cell.* (2009) 139:1353–65. doi: 10.1016/j.cell.2009.11.034
205. Bader M, Alenina N, Andrade-Navarro MA, Santos RA. MAS and its related G protein-coupled receptors, Mrgprs. *Pharmacol Rev.* (2014) 66:1080–105. doi: 10.1124/pr.113.008136
206. Wedi B, Gehring M, Kapp A. The pseudoallergen receptor MRGPRX2 on peripheral blood basophils and eosinophils: expression and function. *Allergy.* (2020) 75:2229–42. doi: 10.1111/all.14213
207. Steinhoff M, Buddenkotte J, Lerner EA. Role of mast cells and basophils in pruritus. *Immunol Rev.* (2018) 282:248–64. doi: 10.1111/imr.12635
208. Schmelz M. Itch processing in the skin. *Front Med.* (2019) 6:167. doi: 10.3389/fmed.2019.00167
209. Han L, Ma C, Liu Q, Weng HJ, Cui Y, Tang Z, et al. A subpopulation of nociceptors specifically linked to itch. *Nat Neurosci.* (2013) 16:174–82. doi: 10.1038/nn.3289
210. Qu L, Fan N, Ma C, Wang T, Han L, Fu K, et al. Enhanced excitability of MRGPRA3- and MRGPRD-positive nociceptors in a model of inflammatory itch and pain. *Brain.* (2014) 137:1039–50. doi: 10.1093/brain/awu007
211. Lee WJ, Kim YS, Shim WS. Korean Red Ginseng extract and ginsenoside Rg3 have anti-pruritic effects on chloroquine-induced itch by inhibition of MrgprA3/TRPA1-mediated pathway. *J Ginseng Res.* (2018) 42:470–5. doi: 10.1016/j.jgr.2017.05.004
212. Jang Y, Lee WJ, Hong GS, Shim WS. Red ginseng extract blocks histamine-dependent itch by inhibition of H1R/TRPV1 pathway in sensory neurons. *J Ginseng Res.* (2015) 39:257–64. doi: 10.1016/j.jgr.2015.01.004
213. Zhu Y, Hanson CE, Liu Q, Han L. Mrgprs activation is required for chronic itch conditions in mice. *Itch.* (2017) 2:e9. doi: 10.1097/itx.0000000000000009
214. Sikand P, Dong X, LaMotte RH. BAM8-22 peptide produces itch and nociceptive sensations in humans independent of histamine release. *J Neurosci.* (2011) 31:7563–7. doi: 10.1523/JNEUROSCI.1192-11.2011
215. Liu Q, Weng HJ, Patel KN, Tang Z, Bai H, Steinhoff M, et al. The distinct roles of two GPCRs, MrgprC11 and PAR2, in itch and hyperalgesia. *Sci Signal.* (2011) 4:ra45. doi: 10.1126/scisignal.2001925
216. Liu Q, Dong X. The role of the Mrgpr receptor family in itch. *Handb Exp Pharmacol.* (2015) 226:71–88. doi: 10.1007/978-3-662-44605-8_5

217. Kühn H, Kolkhir P, Babina M, Dull M, Frischbutter S, Fok JS, et al. Mas-related G protein-coupled receptor X2 and its activators in dermatologic allergies. *J Allergy Clin Immunol.* (2020). doi: 10.1016/j.jaci.2020.08.027. [Epub ahead of print].
218. Corbiere A, Loste A, Gaudenzio N. MRGPRX2 sensing of cationic compounds - a bridge between nociception and skin diseases? *Exp Dermatol.* (2020) 1–8. doi: 10.1111/exd.14222
219. Wu H, Zeng M, Cho EY, Jiang W, Sha O. The origin, expression, function and future research focus of a G protein-coupled receptor, mas-related gene X2 (MrgX2). *Prog Histochem Cytochem.* (2015) 50:11–7. doi: 10.1016/j.proghi.2015.06.001
220. Subramanian H, Gupta K, Ali H. Roles of Mas-related G protein-coupled receptor X2 on mast cell-mediated host defense, pseudoallergic drug reactions, and chronic inflammatory diseases. *J Allergy Clin Immunol.* (2016) 138:700–10. doi: 10.1016/j.jaci.2016.04.051
221. Fujisawa D, Kashiwakura J, Kita H, Kikukawa Y, Fujitani Y, Sasaki-Sakamoto T, et al. Expression of Mas-related gene X2 on mast cells is upregulated in the skin of patients with severe chronic urticaria. *J Allergy Clin Immunol.* (2014) 134:622–33.e9. doi: 10.1016/j.jaci.2014.05.004
222. Green DP, Limjunyawong N, Gour N, Pundir P, Dong X. A mast-cell-specific receptor mediates neurogenic inflammation and pain. *Neuron.* (2019) 101:412–20.e3. doi: 10.1016/j.neuron.2019.01.012
223. Martin-Zanca D, Hughes SH, Barbacid M. A human oncogene formed by the fusion of truncated tropomyosin and protein tyrosine kinase sequences. *Nature.* (1986) 319:743–8. doi: 10.1038/319743a0
224. Martin-Zanca D, Oskam R, Mitra G, Copeland T, Barbacid M. Molecular and biochemical characterization of the human trk proto-oncogene. *Mol Cell Biol.* (1989) 9:24–33. doi: 10.1128/MCB.9.1.24
225. Barbacid M. Structural and functional properties of the TRK family of neurotrophin receptors. *Ann N Y Acad Sci.* (1995) 766:442–58. doi: 10.1111/j.1749-6632.1995.tb26693.x
226. Skaper SD. The neurotrophin family of neurotrophic factors: an overview. *Methods Mol Biol.* (2012) 846:1–12. doi: 10.1007/978-1-61779-536-7_1
227. Nockher WA, Renz H. Neurotrophins in allergic diseases: from neuronal growth factors to intercellular signaling molecules. *J Allergy Clin Immunol.* (2006) 117:583–9. doi: 10.1016/j.jaci.2005.11.049
228. Matsumura S, Terao M, Murota H, Katayama I. Th2 cytokines enhance TrkA expression, upregulate proliferation, and downregulate differentiation of keratinocytes. *J Dermatol Sci.* (2015) 78:215–23. doi: 10.1016/j.jdermsci.2015.02.021
229. Sin AZ, Roche EM, Togias A, Lichtenstein LM, Schroeder JT. Nerve growth factor or IL-3 induces more IL-13 production from basophils of allergic subjects than from basophils of nonallergic subjects. *J Allergy Clin Immunol.* (2001) 108:387–93. doi: 10.1067/mai.2001.117459
230. Caroleo MC, Costa N, Bracci-Laudiero L, Aloe L. Human monocyte/macrophages activate by exposure to LPS overexpress NGF and NGF receptors. *J Neuroimmunol.* (2001) 113:193–201. doi: 10.1016/S0165-5728(00)00441-0
231. Nilsson G, Forsberg-Nilsson K, Xiang Z, Hallbook F, Nilsson K, Metcalfe DD. Human mast cells express functional TrkA and are a source of nerve growth factor. *Eur J Immunol.* (1997) 27:2295–301. doi: 10.1002/eji.18302 70925
232. Groneberg DA, Serowka F, Peckenschneider N, Artuc M, Grutzkau A, Fischer A, et al. Gene expression and regulation of nerve growth factor in atopic dermatitis mast cells and the human mast cell line-1. *J Neuroimmunol.* (2005) 161:87–92. doi: 10.1016/j.jneuroim.2004.12.019
233. Noga O, Englmann C, Hanf G, Grutzkau A, Guhl S, Kunkel G. Activation of the specific neurotrophin receptors TrkA, TrkB and TrkC influences the function of eosinophils. *Clin Exp Allergy.* (2002) 32:1348–54. doi: 10.1046/j.1365-2745.2002.01442.x
234. Lindsay RM, Shooter EM, Radeke MJ, Misko TP, Dechant G, Thoenen H, et al. Nerve growth factor regulates expression of the nerve growth factor receptor gene in adult sensory neurons. *Eur J Neurosci.* (1990) 2:389–96. doi: 10.1111/j.1460-9568.1990.tb00431.x
235. Ma L, Merenmies J, Parada LF. Molecular characterization of the TrkA/NGF receptor minimal enhancer reveals regulation by multiple cis elements to drive embryonic neuron expression. *Development.* (2000) 127:3777–88.
236. Freund-Michel V, Frossard N. The nerve growth factor and its receptors in airway inflammatory diseases. *Pharmacol Ther.* (2008) 117:52–76. doi: 10.1016/j.pharmthera.2007.07.003
237. Manti S, Brown P, Perez MK, Piedimonte G. The role of neurotrophins in inflammation and allergy. *Vitam Horm.* (2017) 104:313–41. doi: 10.1016/bs.vh.2016.10.010
238. Bürgi B, Otten UH, Ochensberger B, Rihs S, Heese K, Ehrhard PB, et al. Basophil priming by neurotrophic factors. Activation through the trk receptor. *J Immunol.* (1996) 157:5582–8.
239. Ehrhard PB, Ganter U, Stalder A, Bauer J, Otten U. Expression of functional trk protooncogene in human monocytes. *Proc Natl Acad Sci USA.* (1993) 90:5423–7. doi: 10.1073/pnas.90.12.5423
240. Ehrhard PB, Erb P, Graumann U, Otten U. Expression of nerve growth factor and nerve growth factor receptor tyrosine kinase Trk in activated CD4-positive T-cell clones. *Proc Natl Acad Sci USA.* (1993) 90:10984–8. doi: 10.1073/pnas.90.23.10984
241. Torcia M, Bracci-Laudiero L, Lucibello M, Nencioni L, Labardi D, Rubartelli A, et al. Nerve growth factor is an autocrine survival factor for memory B lymphocytes. *Cell.* (1996) 85:345–56. doi: 10.1016/S0092-8674(00) 81113-7
242. Dou YC, Hagstromer L, Emtestam L, Johansson O. Increased nerve growth factor and its receptors in atopic dermatitis: an immunohistochemical study. *Arch Dermatol Res.* (2006) 298:31–7. doi: 10.1007/s00403-006-0657-1
243. Bonini S, Lambiase A, Bonini S, Angelucci F, Magrini L, Manni L, et al. Circulating nerve growth factor levels are increased in humans with allergic diseases and asthma. *Proc Natl Acad Sci USA.* (1996) 93:10955–60. doi: 10.1073/pnas.93.20.10955
244. Hodeib A, El-Samad ZA, Hanafy H, El-Latief AA, El-Bendary A, Abu-Raya A. Nerve growth factor, neuropeptides and cutaneous nerves in atopic dermatitis. *Indian J Dermatol.* (2010) 55:135–9. doi: 10.4103/0019-5154.62735
245. Kubanov AA, Katunina OR, Chikin VV. Expression of neuropeptides, neurotrophins, and neurotransmitters in the skin of patients with atopic dermatitis and psoriasis. *Bull Exp Biol Med.* (2015) 159:318–22. doi: 10.1007/s10517-015-2951-4
246. Folster-Holst R, Papakonstantinou E, Rudrich U, Buchner M, Pite H, Gehring M, et al. Childhood atopic dermatitis-brain-derived neurotrophic factor correlates with serum eosinophil cationic protein and disease severity. *Allergy.* (2016) 71:1062–5. doi: 10.1111/all.12916
247. Guseva D, Rudrich U, Kotnik N, Gehring M, Patsinakidis N, Agelopoulos K, et al. Neuronal branching of sensory neurons is associated with BDNF-positive eosinophils in atopic dermatitis. *Clin Exp Allergy.* (2020) 50:577–84. doi: 10.1111/cea.13560
248. Hon KL, Lam MC, Leung TF, Kam WY, Lee KC, Li MC, et al. Nocturnal wrist movements are correlated with objective clinical scores and plasma chemokine levels in children with atopic dermatitis. *Br J Dermatol.* (2006) 154:629–35. doi: 10.1111/j.1365-2133.2006.07213.x
249. Di Marco E, Mathor M, Bondanza S, Cutuli N, Marchisio PC, Cancedda R, et al. Nerve growth factor binds to normal human keratinocytes through high and low affinity receptors and stimulates their growth by a novel autocrine loop. *J Biol Chem.* (1993) 268:22838–46. doi: 10.1016/S0021-9258(18)41604-3
250. Horiuchi Y, Bae S, Katayama I. Nerve growth factor (NGF) and epidermal nerve fibers in atopic dermatitis model NC/Nga mice. *J Dermatol Sci.* (2005) 39:56–8. doi: 10.1016/j.jdermsci.2005.03.012
251. Tominaga M, Ozawa S, Ogawa H, Takamori K. A hypothetical mechanism of intraepidermal neurite formation in NC/Nga mice with atopic dermatitis. *J Dermatol Sci.* (2007) 46:199–210. doi: 10.1016/j.jdermsci.2007.02.002
252. Takano N, Sakurai T, Kurachi M. Effects of anti-nerve growth factor antibody on symptoms in the NC/Nga mouse, an atopic dermatitis model. *J Pharmacol Sci.* (2005) 99:277–86. doi: 10.1254/jphs.FP00 50564
253. Stein AT, Ufret-Vincenty CA, Hua L, Santana LF, Gordon SE. Phosphoinositide 3-kinase binds to TRPV1 and mediates NGF-stimulated TRPV1 trafficking to the plasma membrane. *J Gen Physiol.* (2006) 128:509–22. doi: 10.1085/jgp.200 609576

254. Anand U, Otto WR, Casula MA, Day NC, Davis JB, Bountra C, et al. The effect of neurotrophic factors on morphology, TRPV1 expression and capsaicin responses of cultured human DRG sensory neurons. *Neurosci Lett.* (2006) 399:51–6. doi: 10.1016/j.neulet.2006.01.046

255. Roblin D, Yosipovitch G, Boyce B, Robinson J, Sandy J, Mainero V, et al. Topical TrkA kinase inhibitor CT327 is an effective, novel therapy for the treatment of pruritus due to psoriasis: results from experimental studies, and efficacy and safety of CT327 in a phase 2b Clinical trial in patients with psoriasis. *Acta Derm Venereol.* (2015) 95:542–8. doi: 10.2340/00015555-2047

10

Endogenous Opioid Levels do not Correlate with Itch Intensity and Therapeutic Interventions in Hepatic Pruritus

Miriam M. Düll[1], Katharina Wolf[1], Marcel Vetter[1], Peter Dietrich[1,2], Markus F. Neurath[1,3] and Andreas E. Kremer[1]*

[1] Department of Medicine 1, University Hospital Erlangen and Translational Research Center, Friedrich-Alexander-University Erlangen-Nürnberg, Erlangen, Germany, [2] Emil-Fischer-Zentrum, Institute of Biochemistry, Friedrich-Alexander-University Erlangen-Nürnberg, Erlangen, Germany, [3] Deutsches Zentrum Immuntherapie DZI, Erlangen, Germany

***Correspondence:**
Andreas E. Kremer
andreas.kremer@uk-erlangen.de

Background: Chronic pruritus affects up to 70% of patients with immune-mediated hepatobiliary disorders. Antagonists of the μ-opioid receptor (MOR) and agonists of the κ-opioid receptor (KOR) are used to treat hepatic itch, albeit with limited success. An imbalance between ligands of MOR and KOR receptors has recently been suggested as a potential mechanism of hepatic pruritus. In this study, we therefore investigated systemic levels of important endogenous opioids such as β-endorphin, dynorphin A, Leu- and Met-enkephalin in plasma of a large cohort of well-characterized patients with immune-mediated cholestatic disorders, including patients with liver cirrhosis, and during effective anti-pruritic therapy.

Methods: Plasma samples and clinical data were prospectively collected from well-characterized patients with primary/secondary sclerosing cholangitis (PSC/SSC), primary biliary cholangitis (PBC) and overlap syndromes suffering from pruritus (n = 29) and age-, gender- and disease-matched controls without pruritus (n = 27) as well as healthy controls (n = 20). General laboratory testing for hepatobiliary and renal function was performed. Levels of β-endorphin, dynorphin A, Leu- and Met-enkephalin were quantified in plasma by ELISA. Intensity of pruritus over the last week was evaluated using a visual analog scale (VAS, 0–10).

Results: PBC and PSC patients with or without pruritus did neither differ in disease entity, disease stage, nor in the presence of cirrhosis. While both dynorphin A and β-endorphin concentrations were lower in pruritic patients compared to those without pruritus and healthy controls, the MOR/KOR ligand ratio was unaltered. No significant differences were observed for Leu- and Met-enkephalin concentrations. Opioid levels correlated with neither itch intensity nor stage of disease. Cirrhotic patients displayed higher concentrations of MOR agonist Leu-enkephalin and KOR agonist dynorphin A. Endogenous opioid levels remained largely unchanged after successful treatment with the potent anti-pruritic drugs rifampicin and bezafibrate.

Conclusions: Endogenous opioid levels and the MOR/KOR ligand ratio neither correlate with itch intensity nor differentiate pruritic from non-pruritic patients with immune-mediated liver diseases. Thus, endogenous opioids may modulate signaling pathways involved in hepatic pruritus, but are unlikely to represent the major pruritogens in liver disease.

Keywords: endorphin, dynorphin, enkephalin, rifampicin, bezafibrate, cholestasis, liver, therapy

INTRODUCTION

Chronic pruritus, defined as itch lasting for 6 weeks or more, represents a serious and challenging symptom in several systemic diseases, including chronic kidney disease (CKD), hematological disorders, and hepatobiliary diseases (1, 2). Up to one fifth of patients with generalized pruritus suffers from a systemic disease (3). Hepatobiliary disorders are associated with various extrahepatic manifestations such as abdominal pain, jaundice, fatigue, but also pruritus.

Itch is more frequently prevalent in cholestatic liver diseases, which can result from reduced bile secretion and/or flow on the level of hepato- and/or cholangiocytes (4).

Chronic immune-mediated cholestatic liver diseases such as primary biliary cholangitis (PBC) and primary sclerosing cholangitis (PSC) are commonly associated with pruritus. Up to 70% of patients are affected during their course of disease (4). A significant proportion of these patients suffers from moderate to severe pruritus, which can dramatically diminish quality of life and in extreme cases, even evoke suicidal intentions (5).

Several substances, including bile salts, endogenous opioids, histamine, serotonin, progesterone metabolites and lysophosphatidic acid have been suggested as potential pruritogens. Still, the causal receptors and signaling pathways remain elusive (6).

The endogenous opioid system represents one potential factor in hepatic pruritus (7). This hypothesis is supported by the fact that itch is commonly reported as adverse effect by patients receiving opioids, in particular if administered spinally (8). Concentrations of endogenous opioids were elevated in rats after surgically-induced cholestasis (9, 10) and in a few cholestatic PBC patients (11, 12). The mRNA expression of the opioid precursor molecule preproenkephalin was found in liver tissue of cholestatic rats (13). Increased Met-enkephalin immunoreactivity was observed in liver tissue of patients with PBC or chronic hepatitis C virus infection (14, 15). Antagonists of the μ-opioid receptor (MOR) such as naloxone or naltrexone and agonists of the κ-opioid receptor (KOR) such as nalfurafine are used to treat hepatic itch, albeit with limited anti-pruritic effect (16, 17). Amongst other findings, this data led to the hypothesis that substances activating μ-opioid receptors (MOR) might induce itch while agonists of κ-opioid receptor (KOR) rather activate anti-pruritogenic pathways.

However, no correlation between systemic endogenous opioid levels and intensity of pruritus could be established so far (18).

A recent study explained this lack of correlation with the finding of an imbalance in human plasma between ligands of μ-opioid receptors (β-endorphin) and κ-opioid receptors (dynorphin A) in patients with liver diseases and pruritus. It was concluded that a disproportion between MOR and KOR binding endogenous opioids (MOR/KOR ligand ratio) might contribute to hepatic pruritus (19).

In this study, we quantified levels of important endogenous opioids including β-endorphin, dynorphin A, Leu- and Met-enkephalin in plasma of a large cohort of well-characterized patients with immune-mediated cholestatic disorders. In addition, we analyzed the change of endogenous opioid levels during effective anti-pruritic therapy.

MATERIALS AND METHODS

Patient Characteristics and Sampling

Plasma samples (in blood-sampling tubes containing ethylene-diamine-tetra-acetic acid, EDTA; Sarstedt, Nümbrecht, Germany) and clinical data were prospectively collected at the University Hospital Erlangen, Germany between 2014 to 2020. Plasma samples were centrifuged at 800 g for 10 min followed by immediate storage of plasma at −80°C until further testing.

The investigated cohort consisted of patients with primary or secondary sclerosing cholangitis (PSC/SSC), primary biliary cholangitis (PBC) and overlap syndromes. We included patients suffering from pruritus (n = 29) and age-, gender- and disease-matched controls without pruritus (n = 27) as well as age- and gender-matched healthy controls (n = 20). General laboratory testing for the hepatobiliary and renal function was performed, including assessing the values of AST (aspartate aminotransferase), ALT (alanine aminotransferase), AP (alkaline phosphatase), γGT (gamma-glutamyltransferase), total bilirubin, albumin, INR (International Normalized Ratio) and creatinine. None of the tested patients received an oral opioid antagonist (e.g., naloxone and naltrexone) or opioid-containing pain medication prior to blood sampling collection. Prevalence of cirrhosis was determined non-invasively by elastography or liver biopsy results. To evaluate the change in endogenous opioid levels during antipruritic treatment, we additionally included 22 patients who either received rifampicin (150–300 mg qd) or bezafibrate (400 mg qd) for 2–6 weeks. Except for the separately evaluated patient group treated with either rifampicin or bezafibrate, pruritic patients included in this study did not receive any oral or topical anti-pruritic drugs except for emollient or hydrating topical agents.

Clinical data and laboratory work-up of all patients are summarized in **Tables 1, 2**. Upon their visit or admission to the

TABLE 1 | Clinical and laboratory characteristics of pruritic and non-pruritic patients as well as healthy controls.

	Pruritus	No pruritus	Controls
Number of subjects	29	27	20
Male[a]	9	8	6
Female[a]	20	19	14
Age[b]	52 (42–59)	50 (34–60)	52 (44–58)
Disease entity[a]			
PBC	13	7	–
PSC/SSC	12	14	–
Overlap syndromes	4	6	–
Cirrhosis[a]	7	6	–
Laboratory values[b,c]			*p*-value
ALT (GPT, [<50 U/L])[d]	63 (37–93)	48 (25–76)	0.17
AST (GOT, [<50 U/L])[d]	62 (39–84)	41 (31–79)	0.11
γGT (<40 U/L)[e]	152 (63–286)	121 (28–224)	0.17
AP [40–130 U/L][f]	282 (144–384)	204 (120–323)	0.17
Total bilirubin (<1.1 mg/dl)	1.4 (0.8–2.5)	0.9 (0.7–1.7)	0.19
Albumin (35–55 g/L)	38.1 (36.3–42.9)	41.6 (38.8–42.9)	0.17
INR (0.85–1.15)	0.95 (0.92–1.03)	1.00 (0.95–1.05)	0.12
Creatinine (0.67–1.17 mg/dl)	0.73 (0.64–0.83)	0.71 (0.63–0.82)	0.61

Data were statistically analyzed by Mann-Whitney-U-test.
[a]Data represent the respective number of subjects.
[b]Data are shown as median (interquartile range).
[c]Reference values are shown in square brackets.
[d]Reference values according to gender, male: <50 U/L, female: <35 U/L.
[e]Reference values according to gender, male: <60 U/L, female: <40 U/L.
[f]Reference values according to gender, male: 40–130 U/L, female: 35–105 U/L.
PBC, primary biliary cholangitis; PSC/SSC, primary/secondary sclerosing cholangitis; AST, aspartate aminotransferase; ALT, alanine aminotransferase, AP, alkaline phosphatase, γGT, gamma-glutamyltransferase; INR, international normalized ratio.

hospital, patients were asked to state mean pruritus intensity over the last week on a visual analog scale (VAS, 0–10) as part of a questionnaire. Patients handed in a written informed consent according to the Declaration of Helsinki and this study was approved by the local ethics committee (approval number 238_13B).

Enzyme-Linked Immunosorbent Assays

Levels of β-endorphin, dynorphin A, Leu- and Met-enkephalin in plasma samples were quantified using commercial fluorescent EIA and ELISA kits (β-endorphin, dynorphin A, Leu-Enkephalin: Phoenix Pharmaceuticals, Burlingham, USA; Met-Enkephalin: MyBioSource, San Diego, USA) according to the respective manufacturer's guidelines. All ELISA kits had <15% intra-assay and <15% inter-assay variation. The cross-reactivity for peptides in % for the ELISA kits was as following: β-endorphin kit: 100% for β-endorphin (human), 100% for Ac-β-endorphin (human); dynorphin A kit: 100% for dynorphin A (human, rat, mouse, porcine), <0.1% for dynorphin A (1–13, porcine), and 0% for dynorphin A (1–8, porcine); Leu-enkephalin kit: 100% for Leu-Enkephalin (human), 0% for Met-enkephalin, Met-Enkephalin-Arg-Gly-Leu, Leu-Enkephalin-Arg; Met-Enkephalin kit: 100% for Met-Enkephalin (human), 0% for Leu-enkephalin.

TABLE 2 | Laboratory parameters in 22 patients before and after receiving anti-pruritic treatment with either rifampicin (150–300 mg qd) or bezafibrate (400 mg qd).

	Pre-treatment	Post-treatment	*P*-value
Laboratory values[a]			
ALT (GPT, [<50 U/L])[b,c]	62 (40–100)	52 (38–62)	0.48
AST (GOT, [<50 U/L])[c]	93 (61–139)	84 (34–116)	0.55
γGT (<40 U/L)[d]	133 (62–250)	81(52–250)	0.18
AP (40–130 U/L)[e]	196 (161–323)	165 (150–282)	0.07
Total bilirubin (<1.1 mg/dl)	4.4 (1.3–8.3)	3.8 (2.3–5.5)	0.08
Albumin (35–55 g/L)	40.3 (32.6–41.3)	40.7 (30.5–42.3)	0.89
INR (0.85–1.15)	0.98 (0.96–1.27)	1.00 (0.93–1.09)	0.34
Creatinine (0.67–1.17 mg/dl)	0.86 (0.80–0.91)	0.72 (0.64–0.87)	0.11

Data were statistically analyzed by Wilcoxon-test.
[a]Data are shown as median (interquartile range).
[b]Reference values are shown in square brackets.
[c]Reference values according to gender, male: <50 U/L, female: <35 U/L.
[d]Reference values according to gender, male: <60 U/L, female: <40 U/L.
[e]Reference values according to gender, male: 40–130 U/L, female: 35–105 U/L.
AST, aspartate aminotransferase; ALT, alanine aminotransferase, AP, alkaline phosphatase, γGT, gamma-glutamyltransferase; INR, international normalized ratio.

Data and Statistical Analyses

Statistical analyses were conducted with STATISTICA 7.0 software (StatSoft Inc., Tulsa, USA). Normality was evaluated by Shapiro-Wilk W-test. Non-parametric Mann-Whitney-U-test or Wilcoxon test was applied if data were not normally distributed and data were given as median with 25 and 75% quartiles. In case of normal distribution, values were depicted as mean ± standard error of means (SEM) and analyzed by multi-way analysis of variance (ANOVA) with least significant difference (LSD) *post hoc* testing. Spearman rank was applied to calculate correlations. Graphs and figures were generated with Origin 2020®, Corel Draw X7®, and Microsoft Excel®.

RESULTS

Patients with immune-mediated cholestatic liver diseases with ($n = 29$) and without pruritus ($n = 27$) did neither differ in disease entity, nor disease severity including the presence of liver cirrhosis (**Table 1**). Seventy percent of patients reporting on pruritus were female, in accordance with prior data indicating that women with cholestatic conditions are more often affected by pruritus than male patients (13–15). Laboratory values revealed no significant differences in transaminases levels, cholestasis parameters, surrogate markers for liver function (albumin, INR) or serum creatinine levels between pruritic and

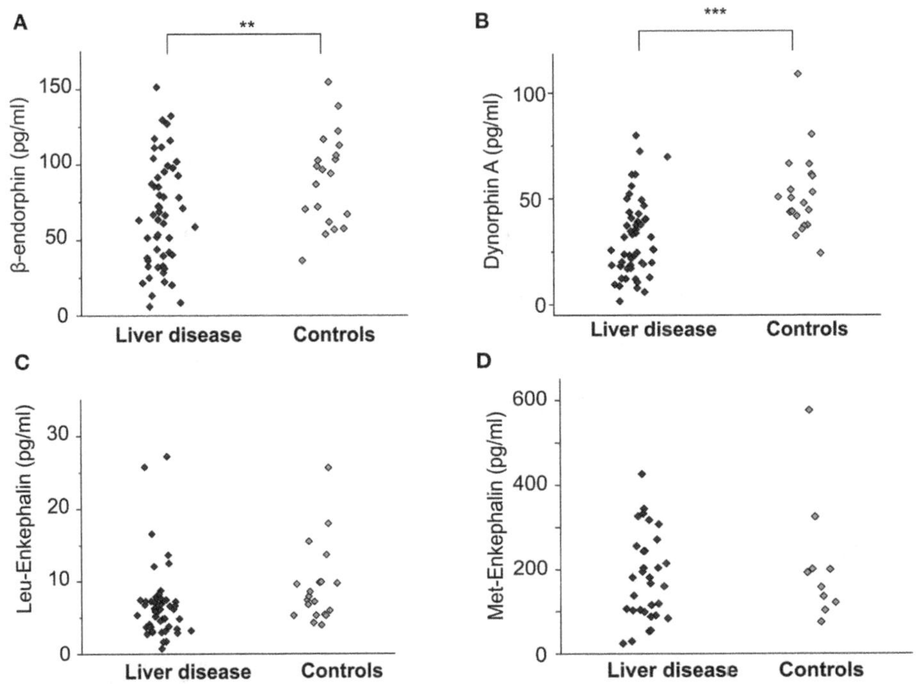

FIGURE 1 | Endogenous opioid plasma levels in patients with cholestatic liver diseases and healthy controls. Concentrations [pg/ml] of β-endorphin, dynorphin A, Leu-enkephalin and Met-enkephalin of patients with cholestatic liver diseases ($n = 56$, dark gray diamonds) and age- and gender matched controls ($n = 20$, light gray diamonds) are shown as individual values in **(A–D)**. Significantly lower levels of both β-endorphin **(A)** and dynorphin A **(B)** were observed in the patient group. The difference for Leu-enkephalin was not significant **(C)**. Data were statistically analyzed by multi-way analysis of variance (ANOVA) with least significant difference (LSD) *post hoc* testing. Significant differences are indicated by asterisks: $^{**}p < 0.01$, $^{***}p < 0.001$.

non-pruritic patients (**Table 1**). The mean pruritus VAS score over the last week was 6.2 ± 0.5 in the pruritus group. We additionally evaluated endogenous opioid levels in 22 patients pre-/post anti-pruritic treatment with either rifampicin (150–300 mg qd) or bezafibrate (400 mg qd). Transaminases and cholestasis parameters did not significantly differ before and after treatment (**Table 2**).

β-Endorphin and Dynorphin A Levels Are Lower in Pruritic Patients Without a Change to the MOR/KOR Ligand Ratio

Concentrations of β-endorphin (67.3 ± 4.9 pg/ml vs. 90.5 ± 6.9 pg/ml, $p < 0.01$, ANOVA) and dynorphin A (30.3 ± 2.5 pg/ml vs. 52.1 ± 4.3 pg/ml, $p < 0.001$, ANOVA) were significantly lower in patients with cholestatic liver diseases in general compared to healthy controls (**Figures 1A,B**). The difference in Leu-enkephalin values between patients and controls did not reach significance (6.7 ± 0.7 pg/ml vs. 9.3 ± 1.2 pg/mlL, $p = 0.053$, **Figure 1C**). Met-enkephalin levels did not differ between patients and healthy controls (**Figure 1D**). Patients suffering from pruritus had significantly lower levels of β-endorphin (49.5 ± 5.9 pg/ml, **Figure 2A**) and dynorphin A (21.8 ± 2.6 pg/ml, **Figure 2B**) compared to patients without pruritus and healthy subjects, whereas the MOR/KOR-ratio was unaltered (**Figure 2C**). No significant differences were found here for Leu- and Met-enkephalin concentrations between all groups (**Figures 2D,E**).

Leu-Enkephalin and Dynorphin A Levels Are Elevated in Patients With Cirrhosis

Cirrhotic patients ($n = 13$) had compared to non-cirrhotic patients ($n = 43$) significantly higher levels of MOR agonist Leu-enkephalin (10.6 ± 2.8 pg/ml vs. 5.8 ± 0.6 pg/ml, $p < 0.01$, ANOVA, **Figure 3A**) and KOR agonist dynorphin A (39.5 ± 4.6 ng/ml vs. 27.7 ± 2.9 ng/ml, $p < 0.05$, ANOVA, **Figure 3B**), but no significant differences were observed for β-endorphin and Met-enkephalin concentrations between those groups (**Figures 3C,D**).

Endogenous Opioid Plasma Levels and Cholestasis Parameters do Not Correlate With Pruritus Intensity in Patients With Hepatic Pruritus

None of the analyzed endogenous opioids levels correlated with the reported itch intensity, assessed as the mean itch VAS score over the last week (**Figure 4**). We obtained comparable results when the numeric rating scale (NRS) score or Worst Itch (WI)-VAS score over the last week were chosen as itch intensity outcome measures.

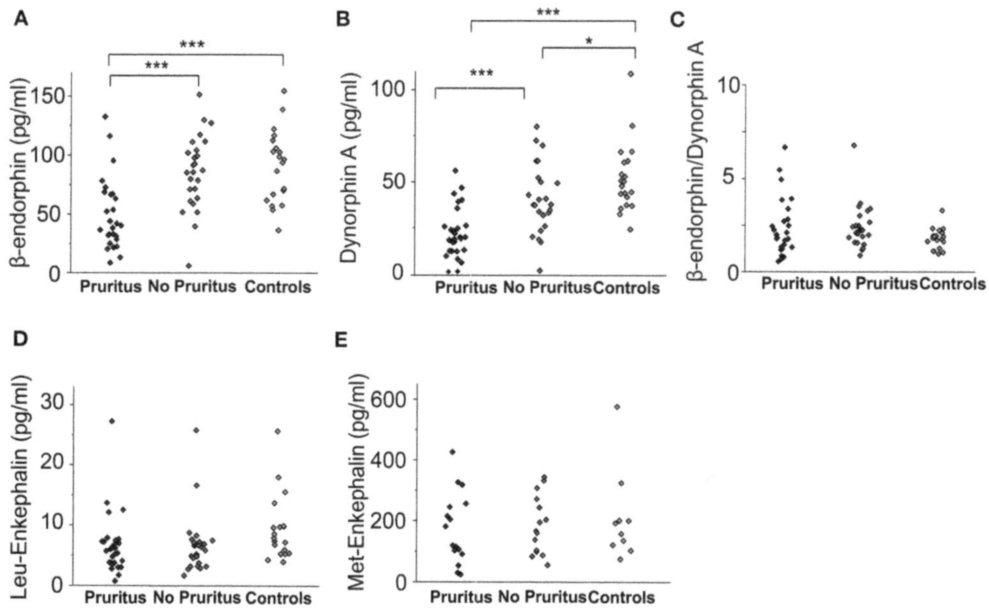

FIGURE 2 | Endogenous opioid plasma levels in patients with cholestatic liver diseases with and without associated pruritus and healthy controls. Concentrations [pg/ml] of β-endorphin **(A)** and dynorphin A **(B)** in pruritic patients ($n = 29$), non-pruritic patients ($n = 27$) and healthy controls ($n = 20$) are presented in the respective subfigures. **(C)** presents the ratio of β-endorphin to dynorphin A levels for all groups **(C)**. Met-enkephalin and Leu-enkephalin levels in patients with and without pruritus as well as healthy controls are shown in subfigures **(D)** and **(E)**. Data were statistically analyzed by multi-way analysis of variance (ANOVA) with least significant difference (LSD) *post hoc* testing. Significant differences are indicated by asterisks: $^{*}p < 0.05$, $^{***}p < 0.001$.

We also did not observe correlations between the cholestasis markers γGT, AP, or total serum bilirubin and itch intensity (**Supplementary Figure 1**).

Levels of tested endogenous opioids were additionally evaluated for correlation with the parameters of γGT, AP, and total serum bilirubin. We could not detect a correlation between any cholestasis parameter and opioid subtype (**Supplementary Figure 2**).

Effective Antipruritic Treatment Does Not Affect Endogenous Opioid Levels

Twenty two patients were treated with rifampicin (150–300 mg qd) or bezafibrate (400 mg qd) for 2–6 weeks. We assessed the endogenous opioid levels before and after treatment. Itch intensity descreased on a VAS scale by 3.8 ± 0.9 and 3.5 ± 0.9 after treatment with rifampicin and bezafibrate, respectively (**Figures 5A,B**). Although patients experienced a clinically meaningful decrease in pruritus, opioid levels remained largely unaltered (**Figures 5C–J** and **Table 3**).

DISCUSSION

In our study, dynorphin A and β-endorphin levels were both lower in pruritic patients with immune-mediated cholestatic liver diseases, whereas the MOR/KOR ligand ratio did not significantly differ from the control group.

Endogenous opioid peptides including endorphins, dynorphins and enkephalins are processed from three precursor molecules: proopiomelanocortin, prodynorphin, and proenkephalin, respectively (20). After proteolytic cleavage, they act upon binding different established opioid receptors. While dynorphins are generally described as endogenous agonists of κ-opioid receptors (KOR), endorphins and enkephalins show more affinity for μ-opioid receptors (MOR) (21).

The main location of endogenous opioid peptides and receptors is of course the central nervous system, but they are present as an established part of the enteric nervous system and other cell types (22). mRNA encoding the three endogenous opioid precursor molecules was found in several peripheral tissues, including the reproductive system, pancreas and immune cells (20). Expression and elevation of endogenous opioids in liver tissue and systemically in patients with cholestatic liver disease is limited to Met-enkephalin and enkephalin precursor molecules (23).

Opioid peptides are degraded enzymatically by various peptidases such as aminopeptidases, serine peptidases and angiotensin-converting enzyme (ACE) (24), of which some are present at the blood-brain-barrier (BBB). β-endorphin, Leu-enkephalin and Met-enkephalin cross the BBB via carrier systems such as P-glycoprotein (25, 26), which has not been reported for dynorphin A so far. It is conceivable that cholestasis alters expression or enzymatic activity of these peptidases resulting in reduced systemic levels of opioids.

There is convincing evidence for a role of the endogenous opioid system in itch transmission, for example, on the spinal level, with the μ-opioid system involved in pro-pruritic and the κ-opioid system in anti-pruritic pathways (27). It is well-known that especially epidural and spinal application of medical

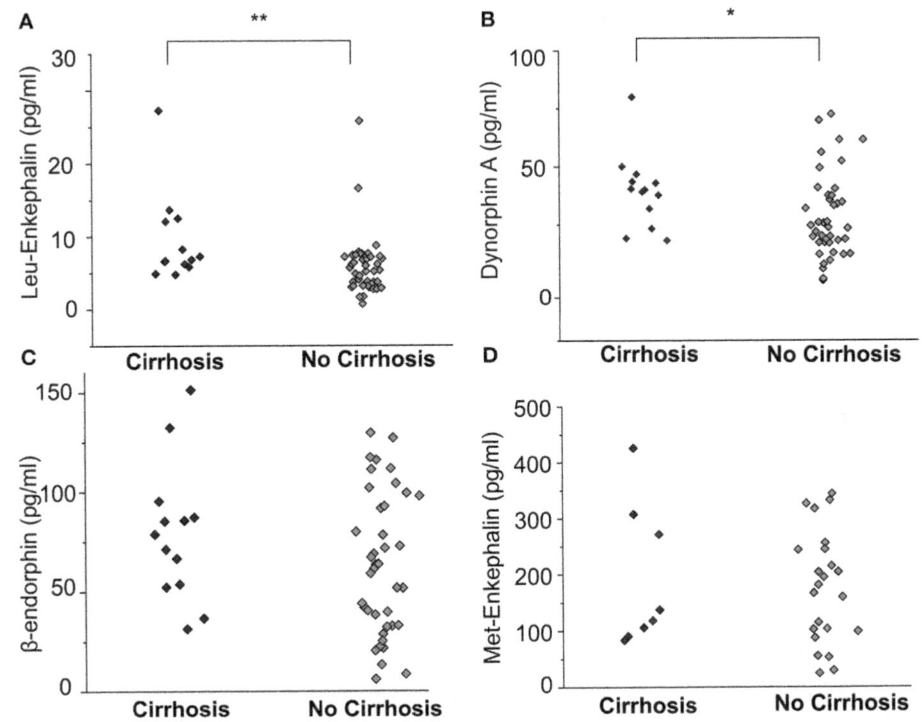

FIGURE 3 | Endogenous opioid plasma levels in patients with cholestatic liver diseases with and without cirrhosis. Leu-enkephalin and dynorphin A concentrations [pg/ml] were significantly higher in patients with liver cirrhosis (**A, B**, $n = 13$) compared to non-cirrhotic patients ($n = 43$), but no significant differences were observed for β-endorphin and Met-enkephalin concentrations between those groups **(C,D)**. Data were statistically analyzed by multi-way analysis of variance (ANOVA) with least significant difference (LSD) *post hoc* testing. Significant differences are indicated by asterisks: $^{*}p < 0.05$, $^{**}p < 0.01$.

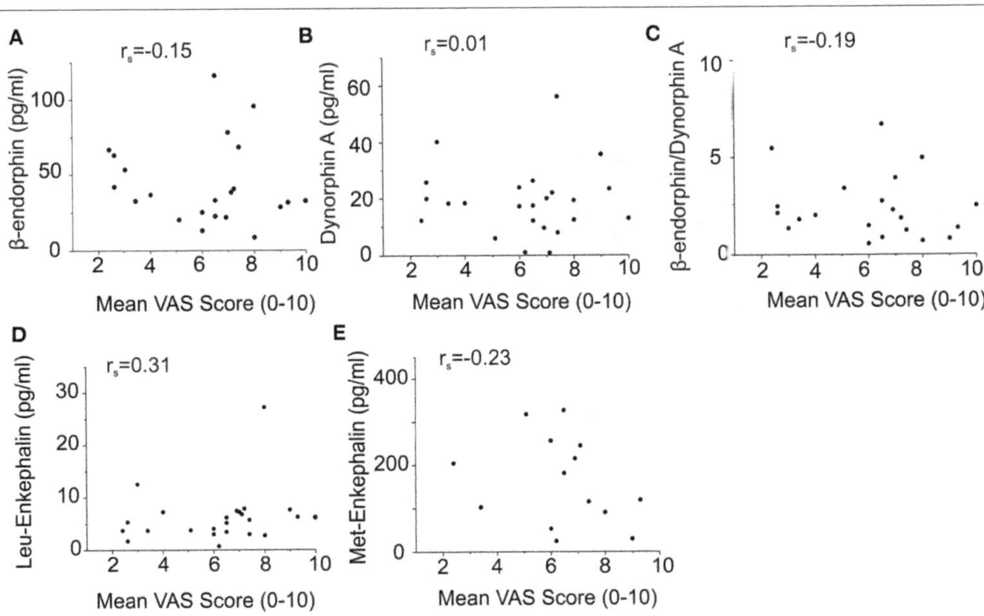

FIGURE 4 | No correlation of endogenous opioid plasma levels with mean pruritus VAS scores of patients with hepatic pruritus. Symbols (circles) represent the opioid concentration and VAS score of the individual patients, respectively. Correlations were statistically calculated using Spearman's rank. Endogenous opioid levels did not correlate with the reported itch intensity assessed as the mean itch VAS score over the last week [**(A)** β-endorphin: $r_s = -0.15$; **(B)** dynorphin A: $r_s = 0.01$; **(C)** β-endorphin/dynorphin A ratio: $r_s = -0.19$; **(D)** Leu-enkephalin: $r_s = 0.31$; **(E)** Met-enkephalin: $r_s = -0.23$].

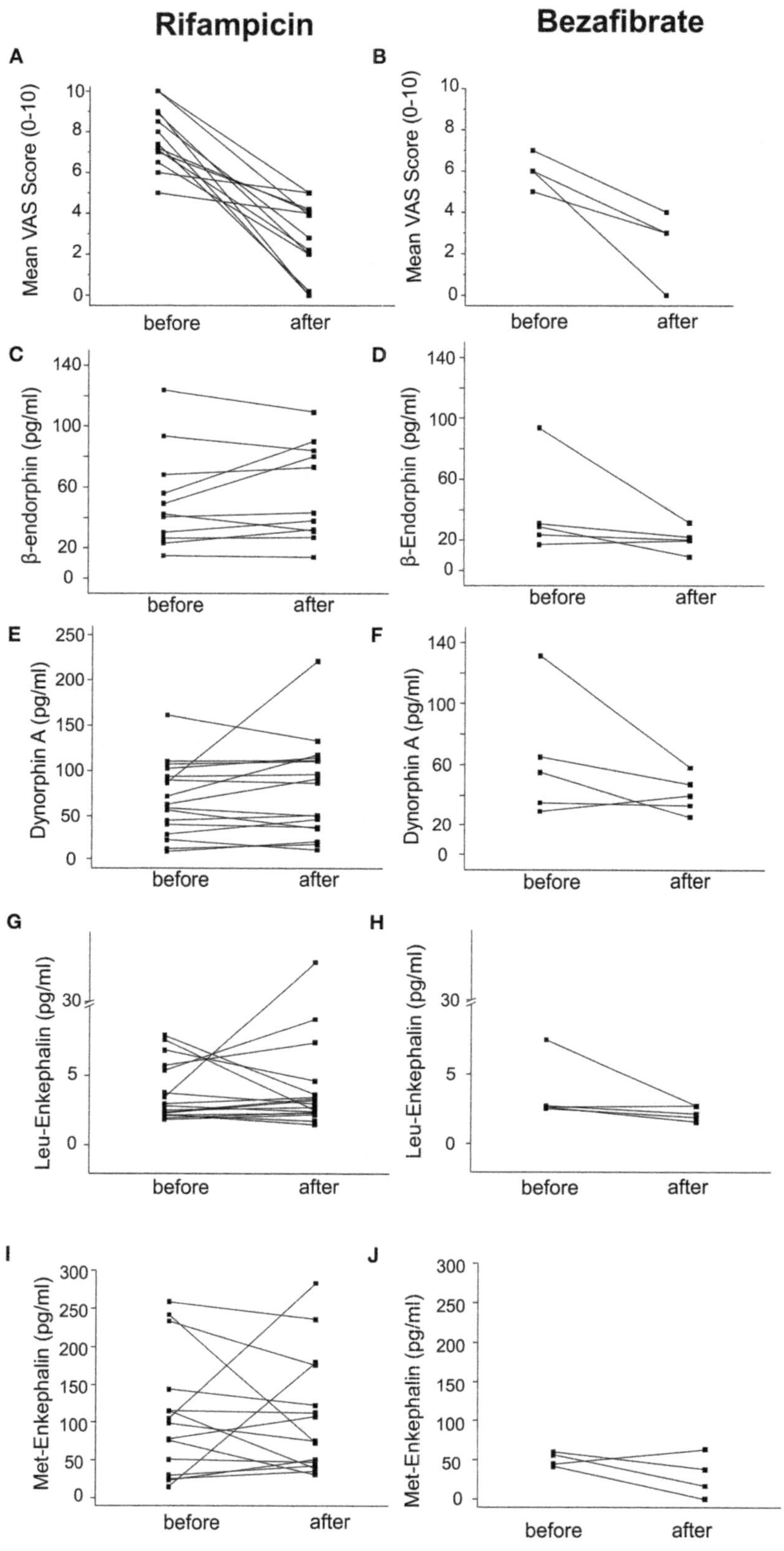

FIGURE 5 | Endogenous opioid plasma levels in patients with cholestatic liver diseases before and after anti-pruritic treatment. Endogenous opioid levels were assessed in 22 patients treated with the anti-pruritic drugs rifampicin (150–300 mg qd) or bezafibrate (400 mg qd). Black squares represent individual patient values before and after treatment. **(A)** and **(B)** indicate the mean change of VAS over the last week before and after treatment with the respective drugs. Levels of β-endorphin, dynorphin A, Leu- and Met-enkephalin did not significantly change during treatment with both drugs **(C–J)**. Data were statistically analyzed by Wilcoxon test.

TABLE 3 | Endogenous opioid concentrations in 22 patients before and after receiving anti-pruritic treatment with rifampicin (150–300 mg qd) or bezafibrate (400 mg qd).

Opioid concentrations[a]			*P*-value
	before rifampicin $n = 17$	**after rifampicin** $n = 17$	
β-endorphin (pg/ml)	49.02 (38.3–68.2)	44.4 (32.2–80.8)	0.29
Dynorphin A (pg/ml)	62.5 (39.9–93.1)	86.1 (36.4–111.1)	0.65
Leu-enkephalin (pg/ml)	2.8 (2.2–5.4)	3.0 (2.3–3.7)	0.78
Met-enkephalin (pg/ml)	98.4 (40.4–129.5)	75.6 (45.3–148.8)	0.68
	before bezafibrate $n = 5$	**after bezafibrate** $n = 5$	
β-endorphin (pg/ml)	29.0 (23.5–30.9)	20.3 (19.8–22.0)	0.14
Dynorphin A (pg/ml)	54.9 (35.0–65.30)	39.6 (33.1–47.1)	0.08
Leu-enkephalin (pg/ml)	2.6 (2.6–2.7)	2.1 (1.9–2.7)	0.08
Met-enkephalin (pg/ml)	50.7 (44.1–57.4)	27.4 (12.9–44.2)	0.25

Data were statistically analyzed by Wilcoxon-test.
[a]Data are shown as median (interquartile range).

opioids induces itch as a side effect (8). Recent data suggest that cross-activation of the human spinal cord μ-opioid receptor 1Y isoform and Gastrin-releasing Peptide Receptor (GRPR) might contribute to opioid-induced itching (28). It was also shown that different stimuli, including painful stimuli and menthol, can activate BHLHB5+ inhibitory interneurons in the spinal cord with dynorphin representing one of their released neurotransmitters. Dynorphin might subsequently inhibit GRPR+ or other downstream neurons in the itch pathway (27, 29).

For hepatic pruritus, data on the pathophysiological involvement of endogenous opioids is limited and includes findings of elevated plasma opioid levels in rats with surgically induced cholestasis (10) and Met-enkephalin immunoreactivity in liver tissue of a few patients with PBC and chronic hepatitis C virus infection (30). Other reports, however, indicated an inverse correlation with higher endogenous opioid levels at advanced histological stages of PBC, when pruritus may be alleviated despite worsening of cholestasis (18, 31).

Drugs influencing the opioid system are applied for the treatment of pruritus in systemic diseases such as chronic kidney disease-associated pruritus (CKDaP) and hepatic pruritus (1). The oral μ-opioid antagonist naltrexone induced a mild antipruritic effect in two smaller randomized placebo-controlled trials (32, 33) in cholestatic patients. A meta-analysis, comparing the itch-reducing effect of several drugs, clearly indicated inferiority of naloxone and naltrexone compared to rifampicin (17). Nalfurafine, a κ-opioid agonist, is licensed in Japan, but not in Europe or USA, for treatment of CKDaP and hepatic pruritus (1). In a randomized, placebo-controlled trial including a rather inhomogeneous group of 318 patients with different liver diseases, treatment with nalfurafine resulted in a statistically significant but clinically questionable reduction of pruritus (16). This trial and other studies on hepatic pruritus (19, 34) included patients suffering from very diverse underlying liver diseases, ranging from chronic viral hepatitis, immune-mediated cholestatic disorders including overlap syndromes, to liver cirrhosis of various causes. The selection and examination of these inhomogeneous patient collectives might have resulted in divergent laboratory findings and reactions to treatment, which we hoped to minimize here by choosing well-defined patient and control groups.

Recently, the KALM-study showed a clear benefit using intravenously applied difelikefalin, a peripherally acting κ-opioid agonist, in CKDaP (35). A current phase II trial is investigating the effects of an oral galenic of difelikefalin on pruritus in PBC patients. While influencing peripheral opioid receptors represents an interesting mechanism, especially in CKDaP, clinical data have to be awaited on its efficiency in pruritus in liver disease.

Rifampicin is a potent anti-pruritic drug in hepatic pruritus (17, 36), although its mode of action, potentially via a pregnane X receptor (PXR)-dependent mechanism, remains to be resolved. Bezafibrate, an agonist of peroxisome proliferator-activated receptors (PPAR), used to treat dyslipidemia, was shown to also exert anti-inflammatory and anti-cholestatic properties and to improve pruritus in PBC patients (37). While both drugs convincingly reduced mean and individual itch intensity in pruritic patients in our study, we could clearly show that this effective treatment did not affect systemic endogenous opioid levels.

Thornten and colleagues reported on elevelated concentrations of Leu-enkephalin in plasma of patients with liver cirrhosis due to several causes (38). Our data supports this finding with mildly increased levels of Leu-enkephalin in cirrhotic patients. However, this is likely attributed to impaired liver function rather than involvement in hepatic itch transmission as we observed no correlation between itch intensity and Leu-enkephalin concentrations in our cohort.

Our study is limited to analyses of endogenous opioid levels in plasma of patients with chronic liver diseases. It raises the question for the underlying cause of reduced levels of β-endorphin and dynorphin A in pruritic patients.

As we observed lower levels in patients with liver diseases in general compared to healthy controls, opioid concentrations might be influenced by the pathological cholestatic conditions. The lower concentrations of KOR and MOR agonists in cholestatic patients may result from increased hepatic metabolism or increased renal clearance, which warrants further investigations in animal models of intrahepatic cholestasis. Additionally, we can neither rule out that the blood brain barrier is significantly altered during cholestasis nor that a central upregulation in opioid signaling might be present in patients with chronic pruritus, which could result in decreased peripheral endogenous opioid concentrations in terms of a negative feedback loop. While other data suggest increased production and distribution of endogenous opioids in liver (39) and skin (40) in cholestatic conditions, it might be helpful to further investigate skin or liver biopsies, for example, for opioid immune reactivity and opioid receptor expression. These samples are unfortunately not available for this set of patients. With a similar plasma MOR/KOR ligand ratio in pruritic and control groups in this study, an imbalance between pro- and anti-pruritogenic subtypes of endogenous opioids is unlikely to substantially contribute to the pathophysiology of hepatic pruritus. Although an imbalance on the level of the central nervous system cannot be excluded, our data do not support a major role of peripheral endogenous opioids in the pathogenesis of hepatic pruritus.

ETHICS STATEMENT

The studies involving human participants were reviewed and approved by Ethikkommission Friedrich-Alexander-Universität Erlangen-Nürnberg. The patients/participants provided their written informed consent to participate in this study.

AUTHOR CONTRIBUTIONS

AK conceived the study. MD, KW, MV, PD, and AK collected blood specimen, clinical and laboratory patient data. MD performed ELISA analyses and wrote the manuscript. MN, AK, and PD supervised data analyses and preparation of the manuscript. All authors discussed and critically revised the manuscript.

ACKNOWLEDGMENTS

The authors thank Alina Bauer for excellent technical assistance.

SUPPLEMENTARY MATERIAL

Supplementary Figure 1 | No correlation of cholestatic parameters with itch intensity of patients with cholestatic liver diseases. The cholestatic parameters γGT **(A)**, AP **(B)**, and total serum bilirubin **(C)** did not correlate with the reported itch intensity assessed as the mean itch VAS score over the last week. Correlations were statistically calculated using Spearman's rank.

Supplementary Figure 2 | No correlation of cholestatic parameters with endogenous opioid levels in patients with cholestatic liver diseases. Levels of all tested endogenous opioids were correlated with laboratory cholestasis markers γGT, AP, and total serum bilirubin of all included patients with cholestatic liver diseases ($n = 56$). No correlation between any opioid concentration and and cholestasis parameter was observed. Correlations were statistically calculated using Spearman's rank.

REFERENCES

1. Kremer AE. What are new treatment concepts in systemic itch? *Experimental Dermatol.* (2019) 28:1485–92. doi: 10.1111/exd.14024
2. Yosipovitch G, Bernhard JD. Clinical practice. Chronic pruritus. *N Engl J Med.* (2013) 368:1625–34. doi: 10.1056/NEJMcp1208814
3. Kremer AE, Feramisco J, Reeh PW, Beuers U, Oude Elferink RP. Receptors, cells and circuits involved in pruritus of systemic disorders. *Biochim Biophys Acta.* (2014) 1842:869–92. doi: 10.1016/j.bbadis.2014.02.007
4. Dull MM, Kremer AE. Treatment of pruritus secondary to liver disease. *Curr Gastroenterol Rep.* (2019) 21:48. doi: 10.1007/s11894-019-0713-6
5. Mells GF, Pells G, Newton JL, Bathgate AJ, Burroughs AK, Heneghan MA, et al. Impact of primary biliary cirrhosis on perceived quality of life: the UK-PBC national study. *Hepatology.* (2013) 58:273–83. doi: 10.1002/hep.26365
6. Beuers U, Kremer AE, Bolier R, Elferink RP. Pruritus in cholestasis: facts and fiction. *Hepatology.* (2014) 60:399–407. doi: 10.1002/hep.26909
7. Bergasa NV. The pruritus of cholestasis: from bile acids to opiate agonists: relevant after all these years. *Med Hypotheses.* (2018) 110:86–9. doi: 10.1016/j.mehy.2017.11.002
8. Ballantyne JC, Loach AB, Carr DB. Itching after epidural and spinal opiates. *Pain.* (1988) 33:149–60. doi: 10.1016/0304-3959(88)90085-1
9. Bergasa NV, Vergalla J, Swain MG, Jones EA. Hepatic concentrations of proenkephalin-derived opioids are increased in a rat model of cholestasis. *Liver.* (1996) 16:298–302.
10. Swain MG, Rothman RB, Xu H, Vergalla J, Bergasa NV, Jones EA. Endogenous opioids accumulate in plasma in a rat model of acute cholestasis. *Gastroenterology.* (1992) 103:630–5.
11. Spivey JR, Jorgensen RA, Gores GJ, Lindor KD. Methionine-enkephalin concentrations correlate with stage of disease but not pruritus in patients with primary biliary cirrhosis. *Am J Gastroenterol.* (1994) 89:2028–32.
12. Thornton JR, Losowsky MS. Opioid peptides and primary biliary cirrhosis. *BMJ.* (1988) 297:1501–4.
13. Bergasa NV. The pruritus of cholestasis. *J Hepatol.* (2005) 43:1078–88. doi: 10.1016/j.jhep.2005.09.004
14. Kremer AE, Beuers U, Oude-Elferink RP, Pusl T. Pathogenesis and treatment of pruritus in cholestasis. *Drugs.* (2008) 68:2163–82. doi: 10.2165/00003495-200868150-00006
15. Lucey MR, Neuberger JM, Williams R. Primary biliary cirrhosis in men. *Gut.* (1986) 27:1373–6. doi: 10.1136/gut.27.11.1373
16. Kumada H, Miyakawa H, Muramatsu T, Ando N, Oh T, Takamori K, et al. Efficacy of nalfurafine hydrochloride in patients with chronic liver disease with refractory pruritus: a randomized, double-blind trial. *Hepatology Res.* (2017) 47:972–82. doi: 10.1111/hepr.12830
17. Tandon P, Rowe BH, Vandermeer B, Bain VG. The efficacy and safety of bile Acid binding agents, opioid antagonists, or rifampin in the treatment of cholestasis-associated pruritus. *Am J Gastroenterol.* (2007) 102:1528–36. doi: 10.1111/j.1572-0241.2007.01200.x
18. Kremer AE, Martens JJ, Kulik W, Rueff F, Kuiper EM, van Buuren HR, et al. Lysophosphatidic acid is a potential mediator of cholestatic pruritus. *Gastroenterology.* (2010) 139:1008–18, 18 e1. doi: 10.1053/j.gastro.2010.05.009

19. Moniaga CS, Iwamoto S, Kitamura T, Fujishiro M, Takahashi N, Kina K, et al. Plasma dynorphin A concentration reflects the degree of pruritus in chronic liver disease: a preliminary report. *Acta Derm Venereol.* (2019) 99:442–3. doi: 10.2340/00015555-3139
20. Fricker LD, Margolis EB, Gomes I, Devi LA. Five decades of research on opioid peptides: current knowledge and unanswered questions. *Mol Pharmacol.* (2020) 98:96–108. doi: 10.1124/mol.120.119388
21. Gomes I, Sierra S, Lueptow L, Gupta A, Gouty S, Margolis EB, et al. Biased signaling by endogenous opioid peptides. *Proc Natl Acad Sci U S A.* (2020) 117:11820–8. doi: 10.1073/pnas.2000712117
22. Holzer P. Opioid receptors in the gastrointestinal tract. *Regul Pept.* (2009) 155:11–7. doi: 10.1016/j.regpep.2009.03.012
23. Davis M. Cholestasis and endogenous opioids: liver disease and exogenous opioid pharmacokinetics. *Clin Pharmacokinet.* (2007) 46:825–50. doi: 10.2165/00003088-200746100-00002
24. Asvadi NH, Morgan M, Hewavitharana AK, Shaw PN, Cabot PJ. Biotransformation of beta-endorphin and possible therapeutic implications. *Front Pharmacol.* (2014) 5:18. doi: 10.3389/fphar.2014.00018
25. Banks WA, Kastin AJ, Michals EA. Tyr-MIF-1 and Met-enkephalin share a saturable blood-brain barrier transport system. *Peptides.* (1987) 8:899–903. doi: 10.1016/0196-9781(87)90078-7
26. Egleton RD, Davis TP. Development of neuropeptide drugs that cross the blood-brain barrier. *NeuroRX.* (2005) 2:44–53. doi: 10.1602/neurorx.2.1.44
27. Dong X, Dong X. Peripheral and central mechanisms of itch. *Neuron.* (2018) 98:482–94. doi: 10.1016/j.neuron.2018.03.023
28. Liu XY, Ginosar Y, Yazdi J, Hincker A, Chen ZF. Cross-talk between human spinal cord mu-opioid receptor 1Y isoform and gastrin-releasing peptide receptor mediates opioid-induced scratching behavior. *Anesthesiology.* (2019) 131:381–91. doi: 10.1097/aln.0000000000002776
29. Kardon AP, Polgár E, Hachisuka J, Snyder LM, Cameron D, Savage S, et al. Dynorphin acts as a neuromodulator to inhibit itch in the dorsal horn of the spinal cord. *Neuron.* (2014) 82:573–86. doi: 10.1016/j.neuron.2014.02.046
30. Boyella VD, Nicastri AD, Bergasa NV. Human hepatic met-enkephalin and delta opioid receptor-1 immunoreactivities in viral and autoimmune hepatitis. *Ann Hepatol.* (2008) 7:221–6. doi: 10.1016/S1665-2681(19)31851-4
31. Spivey JR, Jorgensen RA, Gores GJ, Lindor KD. Methionine-enkephalin concentrations correlate with stage of disease but not pruritus in patients with primary biliary cirrhosis. *Am J Gastroenterol.* (1994) 89:2028–32.
32. Terg R, Coronel E, Sorda J, Munoz AE, Findor J. Efficacy and safety of oral naltrexone treatment for pruritus of cholestasis, a crossover, double blind, placebo-controlled study. *J Hepatol.* (2002) 37:717–22.
33. Wolfhagen FH, Sternieri E, Hop WC, Vitale G, Bertolotti M, Van Buuren HR. Oral naltrexone treatment for cholestatic pruritus: a double-blind, placebo-controlled study. *Gastroenterology.* (1997) 113:1264–9.
34. Yoshikawa S, Asano T, Morino M, Matsumoto K, Kashima H, Koito Y, et al. Pruritus is common in patients with chronic liver disease and is improved by nalfurafine hydrochloride. *Sci Rep.* (2021) 11:3015. doi: 10.1038/s41598-021-82566-w
35. Fishbane S, Jamal A, Munera C, Wen W, Menzaghi F, Investigators K-T. A phase 3 trial of difelikefalin in hemodialysis patients with pruritus. *N Engl J Med.* (2020) 382:222–32. doi: 10.1056/NEJMoa1912770
36. Bachs L, Pares A, Elena M, Piera C, Rodes J. Effects of long-term rifampicin administration in primary biliary cirrhosis. *Gastroenterology.* (1992) 102:2077–80.
37. Corpechot C, Chazouilleres O, Rousseau A, Le Gruyer A, Habersetzer F, Mathurin P, et al. A placebo-controlled trial of bezafibrate in primary biliary cholangitis. *N Engl J Med.* (2018) 378:2171–81. doi: 10.1056/NEJMoa1714519
38. Thornton JR, Losowsky MS. Plasma leucine enkephalin is increased in liver disease. *Gut.* (1989) 30:1392–5. doi: 10.1136/gut.30.10.1392
39. Mani AR, Rasool R, Montagnese S, Dehpour AR. Endogenous opioids and liver disease. *Scand J Gastroenterol.* (2006) 41:1–11. doi: 10.1080/00365520500287533
40. Li X, Zhu J, Tao Y, Tao K. Elevated endogenous opioids in obstructive jaundice: the possible skin mechanisms. *Med Hypotheses.* (2018) 116:119–21. doi: 10.1016/j.mehy.2018.05.013

11

Causes of Pruritus in Patients Treated with Immune Checkpoint Inhibitors for Melanomas or Skin Carcinomas

*Nadia Salinas[1,2], Emmanuel Nowak[3], Maxime Etienne[1,2], Delphine Legoupil[1,2], Maxime Fouchard[1,2], Emilie Brenaut[1,2] and Laurent Misery[1,2]**

[1] Department of Dermatology, University Hospital of Brest, Brest, France, [2] Université de Brest, LIEN, Brest, France, [3] INSERM CIC 1412, University Hospital of Brest, Brest, France

***Correspondence:**
Laurent Misery
laurent.misery@chu-brest.fr

Background: Pruritus is a frequent adverse event during the use of immune checkpoint inhibitors (ICIs), with a frequency estimated to be between 11 and 47%. The underlying causes remain poorly understood.

Objectives: The main goal was to search for putative causes of pruritus occurring in patients treated with ICIs for melanomas and cutaneous carcinomas. Other objectives were to assess the association between the occurrence of pruritus and survival and between the occurrence of pruritus and other adverse events.

Methods: A monocentric retrospective descriptive study was performed using data for patients treated with ICIs (nivolumab, pembrolizumab, ipilimumab, and cemiplimab) between August 2010 and November 2019.

Results: A total of 181 patients were included (mean age: 69 years). Pruritus was reported by 25 patients (13.8%). We were able to determine three subgroups of pruritus causes under ICI use: pruritus directly related to immunotherapy, pruritus indirectly related through other pruritus-inducing side effects and pruritus unrelated to ICIs. In 6/25 patients, no more specific cause of pruritus was found at the onset of pruritus or in their backgrounds, other than ICI use.

Limitations: The study has some limitations due to unicentric and retrospective design.

Conclusion: Pruritus was found in 25/181 patients in this series; only in 6/25 patients no potential cause other than ICI could be found, and pruritus was not associated with differences in survival.

Keywords: prurit, itch, survival, melanoma, squamous cell carcinoma, immune checkpoint inhibitors

INTRODUCTION

Immune checkpoint inhibitors (ICIs) are commonly used in the therapeutic arsenal of metastatic melanoma, Merkel cell carcinoma and cutaneous squamous cell carcinoma due to their inhibitory effects on cytotoxic T-lymphocyte-associated protein 4 (anti-CTLA4) or anti-programmed death-1 (anti-PD1). Ipilimumab (anti-CTLA4), pembrolizumab and nivolumab (PD1 inhibitors) are the available ICIs used in melanoma for ipilimumab since 2014, for pembrolizumab and nivolumab since 2015. Advanced cutaneous squamous cell carcinoma has also been treated with ICIs since 2018, including cemiplimab (anti-PD1) (1–4). These treatments can induce numerous cutaneous and non-cutaneous adverse effects that are mainly due to their immunological effects (5–9). The most frequent adverse events are dysthyroidism, autoimmune hepatitis, colitis, and skin disorders (10–13). Among those, pruritus is frequently reported as a side effect of these treatments (14, 15), with an estimated incidence between 11 and 47% (16, 17). Pruritus can deeply affect the patient's quality of life and may lead to treatment discontinuation. However, ICI-related pruritus has been poorly studied to date and is not well-understood. In the literature, data on the presence and characteristics of pruritus in patients treated with ICIs have been provided, but without analyzing the causes of the pruritus (18). Indeed, it is not known whether the occurrence of pruritus is related to direct or indirect effects of ICIs. Moreover, some authors report a correlation between the occurrence of some cutaneous adverse events (but not pruritus) while taking ICIs and survival (19–23). The principal aim of our study was to analyse the putative causes of pruritus occurring without any skin lesions in patients treated with ICIs for melanomas and cutaneous carcinomas. Other objectives were to assess the association between the occurrence of pruritus and survival and between other adverse events and pruritus.

METHODS

A monocentric, retrospective and descriptive study was performed on patients treated with ICIs (nivolumab, pembrolizumab, ipilimumab, or cemiplimab) in the Department of Dermatology of the University Hospital of Brest and in the associated Department in the Hospital of Landerneau. The study was approved by the ethics committee of Brest (B2019CE.19) and was registered at clinicaltrials.gov (NCT04365244).

The inclusion criteria were as follows: age 18 years and older, treated with ICIs (nivolumab, pembrolizumab, ipilimumab, and cemiplimab) for melanoma, squamous cell carcinoma or Merkel cell carcinoma and not having formulated any opposition. The exclusion criteria were as follows: age under 18 years, adults not legally competent, presence of pruritus at inclusion, and participation refusal.

After assessing the inclusion and non-inclusion criteria, an information letter with a non-opposition form was sent to the patients. The information collected from clinical records included demographic data, history of the cancer and treatment, date of onset of pruritus and localization, pruritus characteristics, treatments, putative etiologies of pruritus, date and type of other adverse events, date of treatment discontinuation, date of illness progression, date of death, and date of loss to follow up.

The main objective was to determine the putative causes of pruritus.

The secondary objectives were to determine the presence of other side effects, to analyse survival according to the presence of pruritus and to determine whether the occurrence of pruritus is linked to other adverse events.

We conducted a descriptive analysis of the data. Quantitative data are described by their size, mean, standard deviation, median, extreme values (minimum and maximum), and number

TABLE 1 | Characteristics of patients and tumors.

	All patients (n = 181)	Patients with pruritus (n = 25)	Patients without pruritus (n = 156)	p
SEX, n (%)				
Men	92 (50.8)	12 (48.0)	80 (51.2)	0.83
Women	89 (49.2)	13 (52.0)	76 (48.7)	0.83
AGE				
Mean	69	73	69	
Median	72	76	72	
Range	27–97	41–96	27–97	
MEDICAL HISTORY, n (%)				
Cholestasis	2 (1.1)	1 (4.0)	1 (0.6)	0.25
Diabetes	16 (8.7)	4 (16.0)	12 (7.7)	0.24
Dysthyroidism	20 (11.1)	7 (28.0)	13 (8.3)	0.009*
Renal failure	8 (4.4)	3 (12.0)	5 (3.2)	0.08
Anxiety	7 (3.8)	1 (4.0)	6 (3.8)	1
Depression	16 (8.8)	4 (16.0)	12 (7.7)	0.24
Haemopathy	6 (3.3)	0	6 (3.8)	1
Skin diseases	16 (8.8)	4 (16.0)	12 (7.7)	0.24
Vitiligo	6 (3.3)	4 (16.0)	2 (1.3)	0.003*
Psoriasis	4 (2.2)	0	4 (2.6)	1
Eczema	2 (1.1)	0	2 (1.3)	1
Lichen	1 (0.5)	0	1 (0.6)	1
Rosacea	1 (0.5)	0	1 (0.6)	1
Caustic dermatitis	1 (0.5)	0	1 (0.6)	1
Pityriasis rubra pilaris	1 (0.5)	0	1 (0.6)	1
HISTOLOGICAL TYPE, n (%)				
Melanoma	175 (96.7)	23 (92.0)	152 (97.4)	0.19
SSM	53 (30.3)	11 (44.0)	42 (26.9)	0.67
MLM	13 (7.4)	0	13 (8.3)	0.21
Nodular	31 (17.7)	6 (24.0)	25 (16.0)	0.38
ALM	5 (2.8)	0	5 (3.2)	1
LM	7 (4.0)	1 (4.0)	6 (3.8)	1
Choroidal	5 (2.8)	0	5 (3.2)	1
Desmoplastic	2 (1.1)	0	2 (1.3)	1
Spitzoid	1 (0.5)	1 (4.0)	0	0.13
MD	60 (37.2)	4 (16.0)	56 (35.9)	0.04
Squamous cell carcinoma	6 (3.3)	2 (8.0)	4 (2.6)	0.20
TUMOR CHARACTERISTICS, n (%)				
Presence of ulceration	52 (28.7)	6 (24)	46 (29.5)	0.64
Breslow Mean	4.9	4.2	5.0	
Median	3.6	4.0	3.5	
Range	0–40	0.15–12	0–40	
Sentinel node Positive	8 (4.4)	1 (4.0)	7 (4.5)	1
Negative	5 (2.7)	1 (4.0)	4 (2.6)	0.52
Unmade	170 (93.9)	23 (92.0)	147 (94.2)	0.65
LOCATION, n (%)				
Head	35 (19.3)	3 (12.0)	32 (20.5)	0.41
Trunk	35 (19.3)	7 (28.0)	28 (17.9)	0.27

(Continued)

TABLE 1 | Continued

	All patients (n = 181)	Patients with pruritus (n = 25)	Patients without pruritus (n = 156)	p
Lower limbs	47 (25.9)	7 (28.0)	40 (25.6)	0.80
Upper limbs	25 (14.3)	5 (20.0)	20 (12.8)	0.33
Unknown	24 (13.2)	2 (8.0)	22 (14.1)	0.54
Neck	4 (2.2)	1 (4.0)	3 (1.9)	0.45
MD	11 (6.1)	0	11 (7.1)	0.36
METASTASIS, *n* (%)				
Site number ≥3	110 (60.7)	13 (52.0)	97 (62.2)	0.26
<3	63 (35.3)	12 (48.0)	51 (32.7)	
Brain metastasis	35 (19.3)	5 (20.0)	30 (19.2)	1
Hepatic metastasis	46 (25.4)	1 (4.0)	45 (28.8)	0.06
MUTATION STATUS (FOR MELANOMA), *n* (%)				
BRAF	44 (25.1)	6 (26.0)	38 (24.3)	1
NRAS	38 (21.7)	7 (26.1)	31 (19.9)	0.43
CKIT	6 (3.4)	0	6 (3.8)	1
MD and lack of mutation	87 (49.7)	10 (43.0)	77 (49.3)	0.39

MD, missing data.
$^*p \leq 0.05$.

of missing data. Qualitative data are described by their distributions in terms of numbers and percentages and the number of missing data. We used Excel for descriptive analyses.

Overall survival (OS) was analyzed using a multivariable Cox model with a time-dependent covariate to examine the association between pruritus onset and survival. Pruritus onset was considered a dichotomous (present/absent) time-dependent covariate without transition back from a state of present to a state of absent. Pruritus exposure also declined according to its origin: immunotherapy-induced or systemic, leading to two dichotomous time-dependent covariates without transition back from a state of present to a state of absent. Hazard ratios (HRs) were calculated with their 95% confidence intervals (95% CIs) using the PHREG procedure (SAS software, version 9.4).

RESULTS

Characteristics of the Population

One hundred and eighty-one patients were included (175 melanoma and six squamous cell carcinoma cases). Demographic data are presented in **Table 1**. In spite of our small numbers of patients when we compared patients without any pruritus to those who experienced pruritus and found significant differences in patient characteristics with regard to vitiligo and dysthyroidism (**Table 1**).

Pembrolizumab (44.7%), nivolumab (35.9%), ipilimumab (17.1%), and cemiplimab (2.3%) were prescribed as first-line treatments. The average number of infusions was 13.6; the median was 7, and the extreme values were 1–86 infusions. Thirty-six patients (19.8%) received a second line of ICIs: ipilimumab for 19, nivolumab for 10, pembrolizumab for 7, and cemiplimab for 1. The average number of second-line infusions was 5.1, with a median of 4 and extreme values of 1–36. Only six patients were treated with third-line ICIs.

Eighty-one patients (44.7%) received treatment prior to treatment with immunotherapy, including radiotherapy (38.3% of patients), chemotherapy (33.3%), targeted therapy (27.2%), and interferon alpha (18.5%). Other therapies were previously used in eight patients: cetuximab in 3, ipilimumab in 1, imiquimod in 1, masitinib in 1, and nilotinib in 1. One patient was under a research protocol and received either nivolumab or ipilimumab.

ICIs Associated With Pruritus

After the introduction of ICIs, pruritus not related to any skin disease was reported by 25 patients (13.8%); there were cases of 23 melanoma and two of squamous cell carcinoma. According to data presented in **Table 2**, pruritus occurred in 15 patients (60.0%) treated with pembrolizumab (in one of them, as a 2nd-line treatment after ipilimumab), in six patients (24.0%) treated with nivolumab, in two patients (8.0%) treated with ipilimumab (in one of them, as a 2nd-line treatment after pembrolizumab) and in two patients (8.0%) treated with cemiplimab. The average number of infusions was 25.4, the median was 21, and the extreme values were 3–81 infusions. Pruritus appeared after a mean of 8.1 months after ICIs were prescribed (median 6 months, range 0–25, 7.5 of standard deviation). On average, pruritus appeared after 12.2 infusions (median 6 and range 1–48).

Characteristics and Evolution of Pruritus

Among the 25 patients, pruritus was localized in 13 (52.0%) and was diffuse in the others. When localized, the involved areas were the trunk (nine cases, 36.0%), the upper limbs (seven cases, 28.0%), the lower limbs (six cases, 24.0%) and the neck (one case, 4.0%) (some patients had pruritus in several areas). No data on localization in seven patients were provided.

The treatment prescribed for pruritus was available in 14 cases: emollients for seven patients, antihistamines for seven patients and topical steroids for four patients. Twenty-two patients (88.0%) experienced regression of pruritus, among whom four experienced regression after treatment interruption and one experienced regression in a mean time of 79.4 days (from 10 to 280 days).

Pruritus and Other Adverse Events

Patients presented with a large variety of adverse events.

Skin disease was described in 39 (21.5%) cases: vitiligo (20 patients, 11.0%), eczema (16 patients, 8.8%), maculopapular exanthema (eight patients, 4.4%), psoriasis (six patients, 3.3%), lichen (five patients, 2.7%), folliculitis (two patients, 1.1%), and urticaria (one patient, 0.5%). For patients with pruritus we found the following associated skin adverse events (**Table 3**): vitiligo (six patients, 24%), eczema (four patients, 16%), 0 maculopapular exanthema, psoriasis (one patient, 4.0%), lichen (one patient, 4.0%), folliculitis (one patient, 0.4%), and urticaria (one patient, 4.0%). We find a significant difference in the occurrence of vitiligo when comparing the two groups. The extra-cutaneous side effects observed are reported in **Table 4**.

TABLE 2 | Treatment at the onset of pruritus.

N° patient	First line ICI's	Starting date (MM/YY)	Closing date	2nd line	Starting	Closing	Occurrence of pruritus	Occurrence in months	Regression	In days	Pruritus at last news
1	Nivolumab	09.17	10.19				07.19	22	Yes	21	No
2	Ipilimumab	03.13	06.14	Pembrolizumab	10.14	04.15	04.15	25	Yes	10	No
3	Prembrolizumab	11.15	01.17				04.16	5	Yes	252	No
4	Pembrolizumab	11.16	08.17				02.17	8	Yes	MD	No
5	Pembrolizumab	09.17	02.18	Ipilimumab	02.18	05.18	03.18	6	Yes	56	No
6	Nivolumab	01.17	10.17	Pembrolizumab	11.17	03.18	04.17	3	Yes	28	No
7	Pembrolizumab	01.19	09.19				08.19	7	No		Yes
8	Pembrolizumab	11.15	11.17				09.17	22	Yes	MD	No
9	Nivolumab	01.18	10.18				01.18	0	Yes	280	No
10	Pembrolizumab	07.17	11.17	Ipilimumab	12.17	02.18	10.17	3	Yes	21	No
11	Pembrolizumab	07.15	09.16				02.16	7	Yes	56	No
12	Pembrolizumab	03.17	09.19				12.17	9	Yes	14	No
13	Pembrolizumab	07.17	01.19				03.18	8	Yes	280	No
14	Pembrolizumab	11.15	08.16				02.16	3	Yes	42	No
15	Nivolumab	06.17	11.17	Nivolumab	01.19	05.19	08.17	2	Yes	84	No
16	Cemiplimab	08.18	09.19				10.18	2	Yes	MD	No
17	Pembrolizumab	02.18	10.19				06.18	4	No		Yes
18	Nivolumab	02.16	09.19				05.17	3	Yes	28	No
19	Pembrolizumab	09.17	07.19				05.19	20	Yes	15	No
20	Cemiplimab	08.18	09.19				03.19	7	No		Yes
21	Pembrolizumab	04.18	09.19				05.18	1	Yes	15	No
22	Pembrolizumab	02.18	10.19				04.19	14	Yes	112	No
23	Pembrolizumab	01.19	10.19				04.19	3	Yes	140	No
24	Ipilimumab	09.14	11.14	Pembrolizumab	01.18	06.18	10.14	1	Yes	28	No
25	Nivolumab	06.16	08.18				12.17	18	Yes	28	No

MD, missing data; dates are expressed in months/years. Occurrence in months: the number of months after the onset of pruritus after the start of immunotherapy. Regression: regression of pruritus in days and the persistence of the pruritus at the last follow-up.

TABLE 3 | Cutaneous adverse events.

	All patients, *n* (%) (*n* = 181)	Patients with pruritus, *n* (%) (*n* = 25)	Patients without pruritus (*n* = 156)	*p*
Vitiligo	20 (11.1)	6 (24.0)	14 (8.9)	0.03
Eczema	16 (8.3)	4 (16.0)	12 (7.7)	0.24
Maculopapular exanthema	8 (4.4)	0	8 (5.1)	0.60
Psoriasis	6 (3.3)	1 (4.0)	5 (3.2)	0.59
Lichen/lichenoid	5 (2.7)	1 (4.0)	4 (2.7)	0.52
Folliculitis	2 (1.1)	1 (4.0)	1 (0.6)	0.25
Severe toxidermia	1 (0.5)	0	1 (0.6)	1
Urticaria	1 (0.5)	1 (4.0)	0	0.13

Among these adverse events are those known to be pruritus inducers. Among the 25 patients who developed pruritus under immunotherapy, many were diagnosed with putative causes of pruritus (**Table 4**). In spite of our small numbers of patients we found, for immuno-induced effects, statistically significant differences for renal failure and hypereosinophilia.

In 6/25 patients, no more specific cause of pruritus was found at the onset of pruritus or in their backgrounds, other than ICI use. In 19/25 patients, other putative causes of pruritus were found. ICI-related adverse events that are known to be putative causes of pruritus were diagnosed before the onset of pruritus or concomitantly with the onset of pruritus: four cases of xerosis, two cases of chronic renal failure [one grade I and one grade II of the CTCAEv4 (Common Terminology Criteria for Adverse Events) classification], three cases of dysthyroidism, and two cases of cholestasis (two grade III of the CTCAEv4 classification) but no diabetes. For 10 cases, drugs (other than ICIs) that could also induce pruritus were noted. For drug causes we have selected two classes known to be responsible for pruritus. The two classes selected were antihypertensive, the class of enzyme conversion inhibitors and opiates. Last, five patients had a history of conditions that may induce pruritus: two cases of dysthyroidism, two of depression, one of diabetes, and one of vitiligo. However, these patients did not have pruritus before the introduction of ICIs and developed pruritus only after using these drugs.

TABLE 4 | Extra-cutaneous adverse events.

	All patients, *n* (%) (*n* = 181)	Patients with pruritus, *n* (%) (*n* = 25)	Patients without pruritus (*n* = 156)	*p*
ENDOCRINE				
Hypothyroidism	28 (15.5)	6 (24.0)	22 (14.1)	0.23
Hyperthyroidism	15 (8.3)	3 (12.0)	12 (7.7)	0.44
Hypophysitis	4 (2.2)	0	4 (2.6)	1
Diabetes	2 (1.1)	0	2 (1.3)	1
Adrenal insufficiency	1 (0.5)	0	1 (0.6)	1
PULMONARY				
Pneumopathy	1 (0.5)	0	1 (0.6)	1
Sarcoidosis	1 (0.5)	0	1 (0.6)	1
DIGESTIVE				
Cholestasis	52 (28.7)	8 (32.0)	44 (28.2)	0.81
Cytolysis	43 (23.7)	10 (40.0)	33 (21.1)	0.07
Colitis	10 (5.5)	2 (8.0)	8 (5.1)	0.63
Gastritis	2 (1.1)	0	2 (1.3)	1
Pancreatitis	1 (0.5)	0	1 (0.6)	1
RENAL				
Renal failure	10 (5.5)	4 (16.0)	6 (3.8)	0.03*
Nephropathy	2 (1.1)	0	2 (1.3)	1
MUSCULOSKELETAL				
Arthralgia	17 (9.4)	3 (12.0)	14 (8.9)	0.71
Myalgia	4 (2.2)	0	4 (2.6)	1
Neuropathy	3 (1.7)	0	3 (1.9)	1
OTHERS				
Hypereosinophilia	20 (11.05)	9 (36.0)	11 (7.0)	0.0002*
Dry syndrome	8 (4.4)	3 (12.0)	5 (3.2)	0.08
Uveitis	2 (0.5)	0	2 (1.3)	1

*$p \leq 0.05$.

TABLE 5 | Survival analysis based on the appearance of pruritus after adjustment with covariates (sex, cerebral, and hepatic metastases).

Variable		Hazard Ratio (95%CI)	*p*-Value
Sex	Male	1.06 (0.70, 1.59)	0.79
	Female	1	
Brain metastases	Yes	1.74 (1.07, 2.83)	0.025
	No	1	
Hepatic metastases	Yes	2.34 (1.53, 3.57)	<0.0001
	No	1	
Pruritus appearance	Yes	0.47 (0.19, 1.18)	0.11
	No	1	

The HR for each variable corresponds to adjusted analysis for the other variables.

TABLE 6 | Survival analysis according to the appearance of different pruritus subtypes after adjustment with covariates (sex, cerebral, and hepatic metastases).

Variable		Hazard Ratio (95%CI)	*p*-Value
Sex	Male	1.07 (0.71, 1.60)	0.76
	Female	1	
Brain metastases	Yes	1.76 (1.08, 2.86)	0.023
	No	1	
Hepatic metastases	Yes	2.35 (1.54, 3.60)	<0.0001
	No	1	
Pruritus appearance	Induced	0.70 (0.17, 2.89)	0.62
	Systemic	0.38 (0.12, 1.23)	0.11
	None	1	

The HR for each variable corresponds to adjusted analysis for the other variables.

Survival Analysis

Tables 5, 6 show the results of survival analyses. Adjustment with the following covariates was performed: sex, presence or absence of cerebral metastases, and presence or absence of hepatic metastases. There was a statistically significant association between the presence of cerebral or hepatic metastases and the occurrence of pruritus. There was a non-significant risk ratio for survival based on the occurrence of pruritus (HR = 0.47, 95%CI: 0.19–1.18, *p*-value = 0.11). We did not find significant risk ratios in the specific cases of pruritus directly related to ICIs (HR = 0.70, 95% CI: 0.17–2.89 and HR = 0.38, 95% CI: 0.12–1.23, respectively).

DISCUSSION

In our population, we found that 13.8% of patients developed pruritus, which corresponds to data in the literature. For example, Sibaud et al. (24) reported an incidence of 13–20%, sometimes more frequent with ipilimumab or in combination, up to 47% (25). A higher frequency of pruritus was previously reported with ipilimumab than anti-PD1. In addition, Sibaud reported a global frequency of 24.5–35.5% with ipilimumab vs. 14–21 and 17–19% with pembrolizumab and nivolumab (24), and Phillips et al. found that the trunk and limbs were more often affected than the neck. Finally, a meta-analysis evaluating the frequency of pruritus reported 26.8% in patients receiving ipilimumab, 22.4% in those receiving nivolumab, and 21.4% in those receiving pembrolizumab. When these treatments were associated, the frequency was more than 40% (26).

The main finding of our study is that causes of pruritus other than ICIs may be detected in the majority of patients. Consequently, there is a need to be cautious before considering that pruritus is a side effect of ICIs and, furthermore, to stop use of ICIs because of its development. Nonetheless, no other putative cause of pruritus was found in a quarter of patients, which is a strong argument for considering that ICIs may be the direct cause of pruritus in these patients. Finally, ICIs might also induce pruritus through side effects, such as dermatological diseases, xerosis, renal failure, cholestasis, and dysthyroidism.

There is no known role of CTLA-4 nor PD-1 in pruritus and the mechanisms of these side effects need to be elucidated.

Pruritus associated with ipilimumab is believed to be a direct result of inhibiting CTLA4 and the resulting enhanced immune system activation in the skin through amplified T cell recognition of self-antigens (14, 18). In a previous study, 14% of patients with stage IV melanoma who received ipilimumab developed pruritic skin eruptions, with CTLA4 blockade believed to be the primary cause in eight of these patients (27). Notably, these patients presented superficial, perivascular $CD4^+$-predominant T cell infiltrates with eosinophils in the dermis upon histological examination. Thus, the same pathways responsible for pruritus may also represent those involved in slowing tumor growth and increasing patient survival (18). Presumably, similar mechanisms should occur for anti-PD1 (28).

In our study, pruritus was not a rapidly occurring adverse event, appearing on average after 8.1 months and 12.2 infusions. According to Phillips, an average of 11 therapy cycles occurred before presentation in patients with pruritus only (17). Wang explained that a delayed onset of cutaneous side effects (more than 3 months) is common and that they can also occur after treatment discontinuation (29). This delay may be consistent with the presumed physiopathology of pruritus in immunotherapy.

The majority of patients experienced a regression of pruritus in our study (88%) but after cessation of treatment in only four. Most studies unfortunately do not detail the exact evolution of pruritus; nonetheless, management and therapeutic care are often described. However, this is not the case in our study because data on the management, in particular the duration of the treatments, were not necessarily available.

In our study, we found adverse events secondary to ICIs other than pruritus. Our findings involve higher numbers than in the study of Baxi, who found, for example, an incidence of 5.6% for hypothyroidism, 2.2% for pneumonitis, 0.7% for colitis, 0.2% for hepatitis, and 0.3% for hypophysitis in a total of 3,803 patients treated with anti-PD1 drugs, with any grade of severity combined (9). Indeed, our data showed 15.5% hypothyroidism, 5.5% colitis, 28.7 and 23.7% for cholestasis and cytolysis, 0.5% pneumonitis, and 2.2% hypophysitis. For cholestasis and cytolysis we took into account any increase from the high standard of ALAT, ASAT, GGT, PAL, and we did not use the CTCAE4 grade because it was not always indicated. Dermatologic IRAEs are the most frequent IRAEs. The safety profile of 10 mg/kg ipilimumab across phase II trials was associated with 47% skin IRAEs vs. 39% gastrointestinal IRAEs, 3% hepatitis, and 4% hypophysitis (10).

Skin toxicities of ICIs are variable: rash, pruritus, lichenoid dermatitis, psoriasis, vitiligo, auto-immune dermatoses, alopecia, and nail involvement, to list only the main ones (24). We also found a variety of cutaneous immune-related adverse events. The most frequent were vitiligo (11%), followed by eczema (8.3%), maculopapular exanthema (4.4%), and lichenoid dermatitis (only 2.7%). Some data in the literature show a higher rate of lichenoid dermatosis compared to our study, e.g., 17% for Boada (8). This difference can be explained by a difficulty sometimes in clinically classifying patients in the absence of histological confirmation. Different authors seem to agree that these toxicities are rarer and less severe with anti-PD1 than with ipilimumab (7).

Several authors report an association between survival and the occurrence of side effects. Eggermont evaluated the association between these factors and survival for patients with stage III melanoma treated with pembrolizumab in a double-blind randomized clinical trial comparing pembrolizumab and placebo. In the pembrolizumab arm, he found a reduction in the risk of recurrence of death after the onset of side effects (19). Chan et al. explained that dermatitis may be a sign of increased immune activation and therefore a better anti-tumor response in relation to lymphocyte infiltration. Patients who had one or more cutaneous reactions (eczema, lichenoid reactions or vitiligo-like depigmentation) were approximately half as likely to experience disease progression than patients who did not develop those IRAEs (23). In a prospective observational study, Hua reported a better tumor response in patients with vitiligo than in patients who did not develop vitiligo while on pembrolizumab (22). This suggests that the onset of vitiligo is an IRAE associated with a clinical benefit. Freeman-Keller rash and vitiligo were associated with a statistically significant overall survival difference for patients with resected and unresectable metastatic melanoma treated with nivolumab (20).

Our survival analysis did not find an association between pruritus and better survival. This might be related to the heterogeneity of tumor characteristics. Moreover, we were not able to demonstrate better survival in the population who developed pruritus without any other detected putative cause of pruritus than ICIs. Our results, although not significant, are consistent with those previously reported for other undesirable skin effects (23).

Our study had some limitations. The main limitation is that it is a monocentric and retrospective study; when files are analyzed retrospectively, data are inevitably missing, or the information is incomplete. Our results warrant further investigation in a prospective study, procuring more information on the characteristics of pruritus (notably on its severity and consequences on quality of life) and the treatment of patients. Skin biopsies could also permit analysis of histological changes in the skin as well as small-fiber neuropathies. Another limitation is the relatively small size of our sample.

In conclusion, our results indicate that pruritus can be a direct side effect of ICIs but may also be an indirect side effect or due to a concomitant disorder or treatment without any relationship to ICIs. Further studies would allow a better understanding of these three pathophysiological pathways. The occurrence of pruritus might be associated with better survival, and studies with larger sample sizes should be able to confirm this trend.

ETHICS STATEMENT

The studies involving human participants were reviewed and approved by ethics committee of Brest (B2019CE.19). The patients/participants provided their written informed consent to participate in this study.

AUTHOR CONTRIBUTIONS

NS: research work and writing article. EN: participation in the preparation of statistical analyses. DL, ME, and MF: supervision and coaching. EB and LM: supervision and coaching, and proofreading work. All authors contributed to the article and approved the submitted version.

REFERENCES

1. Feld E, Mitchell TC. Immunotherapy in melanoma. *Immunotherapy.* (2018) 10:987–98. doi: 10.2217/imt-2017-0143
2. Ahmed SR, Petersen E, Patel R, Migden MR. Cemiplimab-rwlc as first and only treatment for advanced cutaneous squamous cell carcinoma. *Expert Rev Clin Pharmacol.* (2019) 12:947–51. doi: 10.1080/17512433.2019.1665026
3. Faghfuri E, Faramarzi MA, Nikfar S, Abdollahi M. Nivolumab and pembrolizumab as immune-modulating monoclonal antibodies targeting the PD-1 receptor to treat melanoma. *Expert Rev Anticancer Ther.* (2015) 15:981–93. doi: 10.1586/14737140.2015.1074862
4. Leven C, Padelli M, Carré JL, Bellissant E, Misery L. Immune checkpoint inhibitors in melanoma: a review of pharmacokinetics and exposure-response relationships. *Clin Pharmacokinet.* (2019) 58:1393–405. doi: 10.1007/s40262-019-00789-7
5. Hwang SJE, Fernández-Peñas P. Adverse reactions to biologics: melanoma (Ipilimumab, Nivolumab, Pembrolizumab). *Curr Probl Dermatol.* (2018) 53:82–92. doi: 10.1159/000478081
6. Sibaud V, Delord JP, Chevreau C, Gangloff D, Garrido-Stowhas I. Dermatologic adverse events of the new targeted anticancer therapies used in oncodermatology. *Ann Chir Plast Esthet.* (2012) 57:106–13. doi: 10.1016/j.anplas.2012.02.002
7. de Golian E, Kwong BY, Swetter SM, Pugliese SB. Cutaneous complications of targeted melanoma therapy. *Curr Treat Options Oncol.* (2016) 17:57. doi: 10.1007/s11864-016-0434-0
8. Boada A, Carrera C, Segura S, Collgros H, Pasquali P, Bodet D, et al. Cutaneous toxicities of new treatments for melanoma. *Clin Transl Oncol.* (2018) 20:1373–84. doi: 10.1007/s12094-018-1891-7
9. Baxi S, Yang A, Gennarelli RL, Khan N, Wang Z, Boyce L, et al. Immune-related adverse events for anti-PD-1 and anti-PD-L1 drugs: systematic review and meta-analysis. *BMJ.* (2018) 360:k793. doi: 10.1136/bmj.k793
10. Di Giacomo AM, Biagioli M, Maio M. The emerging toxicity profiles of anti-CTLA-4 antibodies across clinical indications. *Semin Oncol.* (2010) 37:499–507. doi: 10.1053/j.seminoncol.2010.09.007
11. Boutros C, Tarhini A, Routier E, Lambotte O, Ladurie FL, Carbonnel F, et al. Safety profiles of anti-CTLA-4 and anti-PD-1 antibodies alone and in combination. *Nat Rev Clin Oncol.* (2016) 13:473–86. doi: 10.1038/nrclinonc.2016.58
12. Brahmer JR, Lacchetti C, Schneider BJ, Atkins MB, Brassil KJ, Caterino JM, et al. Management of immune-related adverse events in patients treated with immune checkpoint inhibitor therapy: American Society of Clinical Oncology clinical practice guideline. *J Clin Oncol.* (2018) 36:1714–68. doi: 10.1200/JCO.2017.77.6385
13. Tison A, Quéré G, Misery L, Funck-Brentano E, Danlos FX, Routier E, et al. Safety and efficacy of immune checkpoint inhibitors in patients with cancer and preexisting autoimmune disease: a nationwide, multicenter cohort study. *Arthritis Rheumatol.* (2019) 71:2100–11. doi: 10.1002/art.41068
14. Ensslin CJ, Rosen AC, Wu S, Lacouture ME. Pruritus in patients treated with targeted cancer therapies: systematic review and meta-analysis. *J Am Acad Dermatol.* (2013) 69:708–20. doi: 10.1016/j.jaad.2013.06.038
15. Wu J, Lacouture ME. Pruritus associated with targeted anticancer therapies and their management. *Dermatol Clin.* (2018) 36:315–24. doi: 10.1016/j.det.2018.02.010
16. Sibaud V, Meyer N, Lamant L, Vigarios E, Mazieres J, Delord JP. Dermatologic complications of anti-PD-1/PD-L1 immune checkpoint antibodies. *Curr Opin Oncol.* (2016) 28:254–63. doi: 10.1097/CCO.0000000000000290
17. Phillips GS, Freites-Martinez A, Wu J, Chan D, Fabbrocini G, Hellmann MD, et al. Clinical characterization of immunotherapy-related pruritus among patients seen in 2 oncodermatology clinics. *JAMA Dermatol.* (2018) 155:249–51. doi: 10.1001/jamadermatol.2018.4560
18. Fischer A, Rosen AC, Ensslin CJ, Wu S, Lacouture ME. Pruritus to anticancer agents targeting the EGFR, BRAF, and CTLA-4. *Dermatol Ther.* (2013) 26:135–48. doi: 10.1111/dth.12027
19. Eggermont AMM, Kicinski M, Blank CU, Mandala M, Long GV, Atkinson V, et al. Association between immune-related adverse events and recurrence-free survival among patients with stage III melanoma randomized to receive pembrolizumab or placebo: a secondary analysis of a randomized clinical trial. *JAMA Oncol.* (2020) 6:519–27. doi: 10.1001/jamaoncol.2019.5570
20. Freeman-Keller M, Kim Y, Cronin H, Richards A, Gibney G, Weber JS. Nivolumab in resected and unresectable metastatic melanoma: characteristics of immune-related adverse events and association with outcomes. *Clin Cancer Res.* (2016) 22:886–94. doi: 10.1158/1078-0432.CCR-15-1136
21. Simeone E, Gentilcore G, Giannarelli D, Grimaldi AM, Caracò C, Curvietto M, et al. Immunological and biological changes during ipilimumab treatment and their potential correlation with clinical response and survival in patients with advanced melanoma. *Cancer Immunol Immunother.* (2014) 63:675–83. doi: 10.1007/s00262-014-1545-8
22. Hua C, Boussemart L, Mateus C, Routier E, Boutros C, Cazenave H, et al. Association of vitiligo with tumor response in patients with metastatic melanoma treated with pembrolizumab. *JAMA Dermatol.* (2016) 152:45–51. doi: 10.1001/jamadermatol.2015.2707
23. Chan L, Hwang SJE, Byth K, Kyaw M, Carlino MS, Chou S, et al. Survival and prognosis of individuals receiving programmed cell death 1 inhibitor with and without immunologic cutaneous adverse events. *J Am Acad Dermatol.* (2020) 82:311–6. doi: 10.1016/j.jaad.2019.06.035
24. Sibaud V, Boulinguez S, Pagès C, Riffaud L, Lamant L, Chira C, et al. Dermatologic toxicities of immune checkpoint inhibitors. *Ann Dermatol Venereol.* (2018) 145:313–30. doi: 10.1016/j.annder.2018.01.047
25. Sibaud V. Dermatologic reactions to immune checkpoint inhibitors: skin toxicities and immunotherapy. *Am J Clin Dermatol.* (2018) 19:345–61. doi: 10.1007/s40257-017-0336-3
26. Almutairi AR, McBride A, Slack M, Erstad BL, Abraham I. Potential immune-related adverse events associated with monotherapy and combination therapy of Ipilimumab, Nivolumab, and Pembrolizumab for advanced melanoma: a systematic review and meta-analysis. *Front Oncol.* (2020) 10:91. doi: 10.3389/fonc.2020.00091
27. Jaber SH, Cowen EW, Haworth LR, Booher SL, Berman DM, Rosenberg SA, et al. Skin reactions in a subset of patients with stage IV melanoma treated with anti-cytotoxic T-lymphocyte antigen 4 monoclonal antibody as a single agent. *Arch Dermatol.* (2006) 142:166–72. doi: 10.1001/archderm.142.2.166
28. Perret RE, Josselin N, Knol AC, Khammari A, Cassecuel J, Peuvrel L, et al. Histopathological aspects of cutaneous erythematous-papular eruptions induced by immune checkpoint inhibitors for the treatment of metastatic melanoma. *Int J Dermatol.* (2017) 56:527–33. doi: 10.1111/ijd.13540
29. Wang LL, Patel G, Chiesa-Fuxench ZC, McGettigan S, Schuchter L, Mitchell TC, et al. Timing of onset of adverse cutaneous reactions associated with programmed cell death protein 1 inhibitor therapy. *JAMA Dermatol.* (2018) 154:1057–61. doi: 10.1001/jamadermatol.2018.1912

12

Sensitive Scalp: A Possible Association with the Use of Hair Conditioners

Emilie Brenaut[1,2], Laurent Misery[1,2], Cécile Legeas[1], Alain-Claude Roudot[2] and Anne-Sophie Ficheux[2]*

[1] Department of Dermatology, CHU Brest, Brest, France, [2] University of Brest, LIEN, Brest, France

***Correspondence:**
Emilie Brenaut
emilie.brenaut@chu-brest.fr*

A sensitive scalp is defined by the occurrence of unpleasant sensations (tingling, burning, pain, pruritus) triggered by stimuli that should not cause such sensations. Environmental factors, particularly cosmetics, can be triggering factors. The aims of this study were to assess hair cosmetic product consumption in subjects with sensitive scalp and to perform a clinical evaluation of sensitive scalp. After a dermatological examination, women between the ages of 18 and 65 years with or without a sensitive scalp completed different questionnaires. Their use of hair cosmetics (frequency, amount per application) was recorded. A total of 160 women with a mean age of 41 years were included. Twenty-seven subjects presented with seborrheic dermatitis or psoriasis, so only 133 were included in the analysis. Five percent of the subjects declared they had a very sensitive scalp, 25% had a sensitive scalp, 38% had a slightly sensitive scalp, and 32% had a scalp that was not sensitive. The mean sensitive scalp score (3S) score was 3.7 $\pm$ 1.6 in the very sensitive scalp group, 3.6 $\pm$ 2.1 in the sensitive group, 1.2 $\pm$ 1.2 in the slightly sensitive group and 0.1 $\pm$ 0.4 in the non-sensitive group. Two groups were analyzed: the 56 subjects with a sensitive scalp (3S $\geq$ 2 score) and the 56 subjects with a null 3S score. In the sensitive scalp group, 89% suffered from itch, and 45% suffered from tingling. No parameter (hormonal status, smoking, age, phototype, BMI) was associated with the 3S score. No differences in the exposure to shampoos and masks between the two groups were noted. The exposure to hair conditioners was significantly higher in the sensitive scalp group than in the group without sensitive scalp. Itch is the main symptom of a sensitive scalp. The frequency of a sensitive scalp was lower than that previously described when the subjects with scalp dermatosis were excluded. The amount of hair conditioners used was significantly higher in subjects with sensitive scalp than in those without sensitive scalp, suggesting a possible link.

Keywords: sensitive scalp, sensitive skin, cosmetic products, hair products, 3S questionnaire, BoSS questionnaire, sensitive scale

INTRODUCTION

Sensitive skin has been defined by the sensitive-skin special interest group in the International Forum for the Study of Itch (IFSI) as the occurrence of unpleasant sensations (stinging, burning, pain, pruritus, and tingling sensations) in response to stimuli that normally should not provoke such sensations (1). These symptoms are not explained by any other skin disease. Sensitive skin affects approximately half of the population and is more frequent in women than in men (2, 3). The pathophysiological mechanisms have been debated, and several hypotheses exist (4). Sensitive skin can be considered a result of a decrease in the skin tolerance threshold, which thereby impairs barrier function and leads to abnormalities in the cutaneous nervous system, making the skin hyperreactive (4–6). Sensitive skin can therefore be the clinical expression of neurogenic inflammation and can be modulated by many factors (7). Triggering factors of sensitive skin can be physical (ultraviolet, heat, cold, and wind), chemical (cosmetics, water, and pollutants), and occasionally psychological (stress) (8). A recent meta-analysis showed that the most frequent triggering factors were cosmetics, with an odds ratio of >7 (8). However, no specific information on the actual consumption of cosmetic products among people with sensitive skin is available. Thus, the SENSICOS study was designed to assess the relationship between cosmetic use and sensitive skin.

A sensitive scalp is one of the most frequent complaints related to sensitive skin. Sensitive skin can be located on different areas of the body, and sensitive scalp is a specific condition because of the presence of hairs on the head, it is associated with different symptoms (9) and nerves innervate the scalp in a specific pattern (10, 11). The first study on this condition showed that 44% of French people, more commonly women, suffer from sensitive scalp (9). Environmental factors, particularly cosmetics, probably trigger sensitive scalp (12). The aim of this study was to evaluate hair cosmetic product consumption in subjects with sensitive scalp and to clinically evaluate the factors associated with, the symptoms of, and the correlations among scores related to sensitive scalp.

MATERIALS AND METHODS

This monocentric prospective study took place in the dermatology department of the University Hospital of Brest. The aim of the SENSICOS study was to compare the cosmetic product consumption of subjects presenting with sensitive skin in a group of adult women. Recruitment was carried out in three ways: with an e-mail sent to the employees of the hospital, with an announcement in a free local newspaper and by contacting our acquaintances. In the announcement, it was written that women between 18 and 65 years old with or without sensitive skin and with any level of cosmetic product consumption were eligible.

The aim of this study was to evaluate hair cosmetic product consumption in subjects with sensitive scalp and to clinically evaluate parameters associated with sensitive scalp (associated factors, symptoms, correlations with different scores).

The inclusion criteria were women between 18 and 65 years old without any skin diseases on the face. The exclusion criteria were as follows: males, women younger than 18 years or older than 65 years, individuals with a skin facial disease (such as eczema, rosacea, acne, psoriasis, etc.), and individuals who refuse to participate. A total of 160 subjects needed to be included in this study.

The subjects were invited to visit our dermatology department for an appointment with a dermatologist. An information letter was given to all patients. The subjects did not receive any compensation. A clinical examination was performed to verify the absence of a skin disease to ensure the subject met the inclusion and exclusion criteria.

Then, all subjects completed questionnaires concerning the following factors:

- Sociodemographic and clinical data, including age, weight, hormonal status, smoking status, and socioprofessional category
- Sensitive skin factors, which were evaluated by the following question about sensitive skin, "Is your skin very sensitive, sensitive, slightly sensitive, or not sensitive at all?" Moreover, the volunteers were asked about the frequency at which they experience sensitive skin. Then, the sensitive scale, which includes items on 10 signs felt on the face in the last 3 days (skin irritability, tingling, burning and warmth, tightness, itching, pain, general discomfort and flushes) was used. The scores ranged from 0 (no intensity) to 10 (unbearable intensity). The final score (SS-10) varied between 0 and 100 (13).
- Sensitive scalp factors, which were assessed by the following question about sensitive scalp, "Is your scalp very sensitive, sensitive, slightly sensitive, not sensitive at all?" Moreover, the volunteers were asked about the frequency at which they experience sensitive scalp. The sensitive scalp score (3S) was used: it includes items (which symptoms have you experienced on your scalp?) on five sensations (itching, tingling, tightness, pain and burning sensations), with scores ranging from 0 (absent) to 4 (unbearable), so the total score ranged between 0 and 20 (14).
- The burden of sensitive skin, which was assessed with the BoSS questionnaire (15). It consists of 14 questions, which are scored from 0 (never) to 4 (always) and concern three dimensions: personal care, daily life and appearance. The total score ranges from 0 to 56.
- Cosmetic product consumption for scalp, which was assessed by the frequency of use of shampoos, hair conditioners, masks, hair dyes, and hair bleach. The subjects brought all the cosmetic products they were using at least once a week for the scalp. Then, they dispensed their shampoos, hair conditioners and masks in their hand and applied them to their scalp, and the weight of their bottles before and after application were noted to determine the amount of product used per application. The composition of each product was noted. The exposure to each product (mg/kg bw/day) was calculated with the following formula: [frequency (day^{-1}) x amount (mg/use)]/body weight (kg bw).

Statistical analysis was performed using XLSTAT 2019.1 (Addinsoft, Paris, France). Descriptive statistics are presented as the means and standard deviations (SDs) for the quantitative variables and as percentages for the qualitative variables. For group comparisons, we used the Mann-Whitney test, the Kruskal-Wallis test or Chi^2 test, as appropriate. A correlation analysis (Pearson's correlation coefficient) was used to assess the link between the 5 items involved in the calculation of the 3S score and the final score and the correlations between the following 3 scores: 3S, SS-10 and BoSS. $p < 0.05$ indicated statistical significance.

The study was registered on ClinicalTrials.gov with the title "Impact of Exposure to Cosmetics on Sensitive Skin (SENSICOS)," and the identifier was NCT03958968. The study protocol was approved by the ethics committee of Brest (29BRC18.0078).

RESULTS

Recruitment and Subjects

One hundred and sixty women volunteers were included between July and October 2019. Concerning recruitment, 38% of the subjects were acquaintances, 36% responded to the announcement in the local newspaper, and 26% responded to the e-mail sent to the hospital employees. The average age of the participants was 41 ±13 years (19–65). Among the 160 subjects included in the SENSICOS study, 27 presented with a skin disease of the scalp (24 had seborrheic dermatitis, and 3 had psoriasis). The 133 subjects analyzed had a normal skin on the scalp, without redness. The mean 3S score was 1.6 ± 1.9 in subjects without scalp dermatosis ($n = 133$) and 3.3 ± 3.2 in subjects with seborrheic dermatitis ($n = 24$), and this difference was significant ($p = 0.017$). Among the 160 subjects, 11% of the participants reported having a "very sensitive scalp," 48% reported having a "sensitive scalp," 30% reported having a "slightly sensitive scalp," and 11% reported having a scalp that was "not sensitive at all." Participants with psoriasis or seborrheic dermatitis of the scalp were excluded from the rest of the analysis because the definition of sensitive skin excluded the presence of a skin disease. Consequently, the data from only 133 subjects were analyzed.

Presence of Sensitive Scalp

Five percent of the participants reported having a "very sensitive scalp," 25% reported having a "sensitive scalp," 38% reported having a "slightly sensitive scalp," and 32% reported having a scalp that was "not sensitive at all." The mean 3S score was 1.6 ± 1.9 (range 0–9). The maximum 3S score possible is 20. The distribution of the 3S scores is presented in **Figure 1** (range 0 to 9). The intensity of each item of the 3S questionnaire is presented in **Figure 2**. The mean 3S score was 0.1 ± 0.4 in the "not sensitive at all" group, 1.2 ± 1.2 in the "slightly sensitive scalp" group, 3.6 ± 2.1 in the "sensitive scalp" group and 3.7 ± 1.6 in the "very sensitive scalp" group (**Figure 3**). The Kruskal-Wallis statistical test was used to compare the 4 groups. Statistically significant differences were observed among the 4 groups ($p < 0.0001$).

Items of the 3S Questionnaire

A positive and statistically significant correlation was found between each of the 5 items involved in the calculation of the 3S score and the final score. The strongest correlation was with itching (0.832), followed by tingling (0.666), tightness (0.555), burning (0.532), and pain (0.264). The distribution of subjects according to the intensity of the itch scalp and the 3S score is presented in **Figure 4**.

Factors Associated With a Sensitive Scalp

None of the general medical or dermatological parameters (menopause, smoking, phototype, type of skin, erythema, age, weight, height) were correlated with the 3S score (Pearson's correlation).

Correlation Between the Three Scores: The 3S, SS-10, and BoSS Scores

A positive (0.329) and statistically significant correlation ($p < 0.01$) was observed between the SS-10 score and the 3S score (**Figure 5**). A positive (0.328) and statistically significant correlation ($p < 0.01$) was observed between the BoSS score and the 3S score (**Figure 6**).

Comparisons of the Groups With and Without a Sensitive Scalp

Two groups were formed according to the 3S score: the non-sensitive scalp group included the 55 subjects with a 3S score equal to 0, and the sensitive scalp group included the 55 subjects with a 3S score higher than or equal to 2. In the sensitive scalp group, 90.9% of the subjects presented with itching, 45.5% presented with tingling, 27.3% presented with tightness, 14.5% presented with burning, and 7.3% presented with pain.

Cosmetic Product Consumption

Shampoos were used by 100% of the subjects in the two groups. Hair conditioners were used by 40% of the women in the non-sensitive scalp group vs. 53.6% in the sensitive scalp group ($p = 0.15$). Masks were used by 40% of the women in the non-sensitive scalp group vs. 48.2% in the sensitive scalp group ($p = 0.38$). Hair dyes were used by 41% of the women in the non-sensitive scalp group vs. 52.7% in the sensitive scalp group ($p = 0.18$). Hair bleach was used by 23.6% of the women in the non-sensitive scalp group vs. 20% of the persons in the sensitive scalp group ($p = 0.64$). The frequency, amount and exposure to shampoos, hair conditioners and masks in the 2 groups are presented in **Table 1**. There were no data concerning the amount or exposure to hair dyes and hair bleach because the subjects brought all the cosmetic products that they used at least once a week for the scalp. A statistically significant difference was observed in the amount of hair conditioner applied per use: this amount was lower in the non-sensitive scalp group than in the sensitive scalp group ($p = 0.03$). No statistically significant difference was observed between these two groups in the other parameters that were studied.

Types of Cosmetic Products

Shampoos for sensitive scalp were used by 20% of the women in the sensitive scalp group and 12.7% of the women in the non-sensitive scalp group ($p = 0.3$). Organic shampoos were used by 25.4% of the women in the sensitive scalp group and 20% of the women in the non-sensitive scalp group ($p = 0.49$). Shampoos for children were used by 12.7% of the women in the sensitive scalp group and 5.4% of the women in the non-sensitive scalp group ($p = 0.18$).

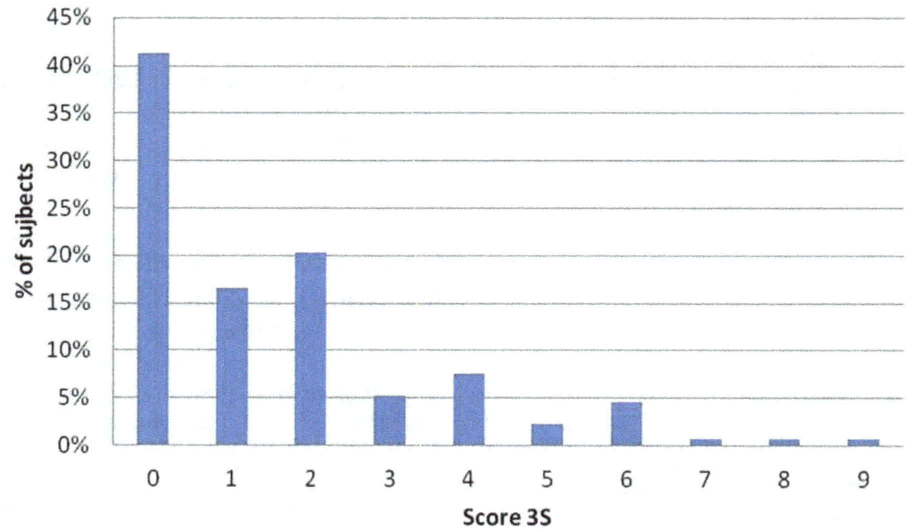

FIGURE 1 | Distribution of the 3S scores in the group of 133 subjects without scalp dermatosis.

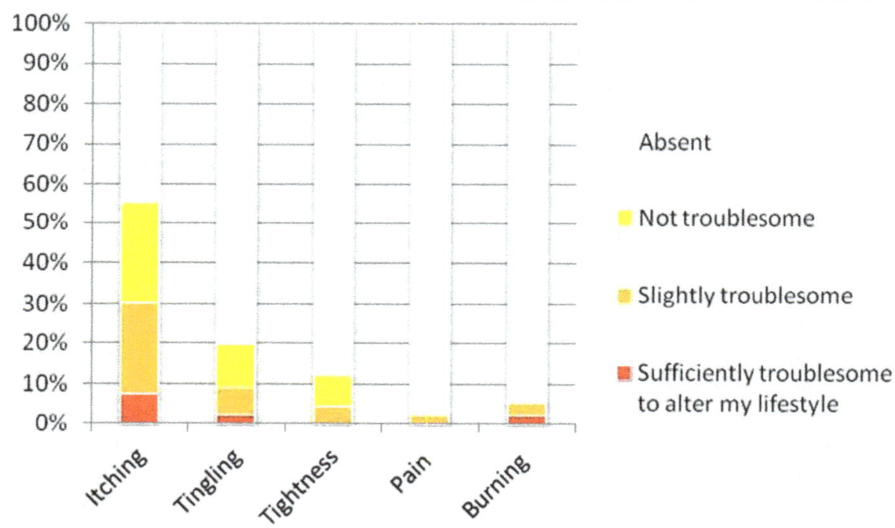

FIGURE 2 | Intensity of each item of the 3S questionnaire.

Hair care products for sensitive scalp were used by 12.7% of the women in the sensitive scalp group and 7.2% of the women in the non-sensitive scalp group ($p = 0.3$). Organic hair care products were used by 20% of the women in the sensitive scalp group and 7.2% of the women in the non-sensitive scalp group ($p = 0.05$).

Point of Purchase

Concerning the point of purchase for shampoos, 63.6, 29.1, 10.9, 9.1, 9.1, and 5.8% of the subjects with sensitive scalp and 63.1, 20, 14.5, 9.1, 5.8, and 3.8% of the subjects with non-sensitive scalp said they buy their products from supermarkets, pharmacies, beauty brands, the internet, hair salons, and organic supermarkets, respectively ($p = 0.2$, $p = 0.2$, $p = 0.6$, $p = 1$, $p = 0.4$, and $p = 0.6$).

DISCUSSION

Few studies related to sensitive scalp have been published in the literature, but sensitive skin is frequently located on the scalp. The frequency of sensitive scalp without skin dermatosis was 30% in our study, as measured by the response "very sensitive" or "sensitive," and 41.3% of the subjects had a 3S score ≥ 2. In the 27 patients with scalp dermatosis, 59% of the subjects had a "very sensitive" or "sensitive" scalp. In a recent study in which subjects were asked, "Do you have sensitive

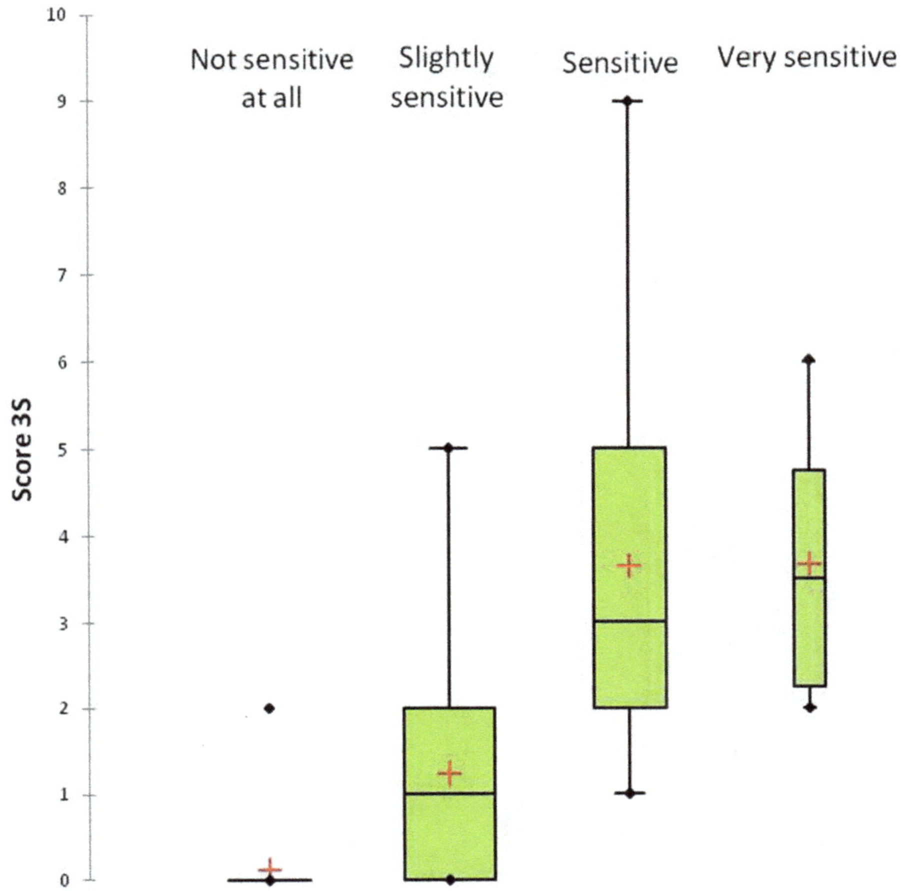

FIGURE 3 | 3S scores stratified by the severity of sensitive scalp.

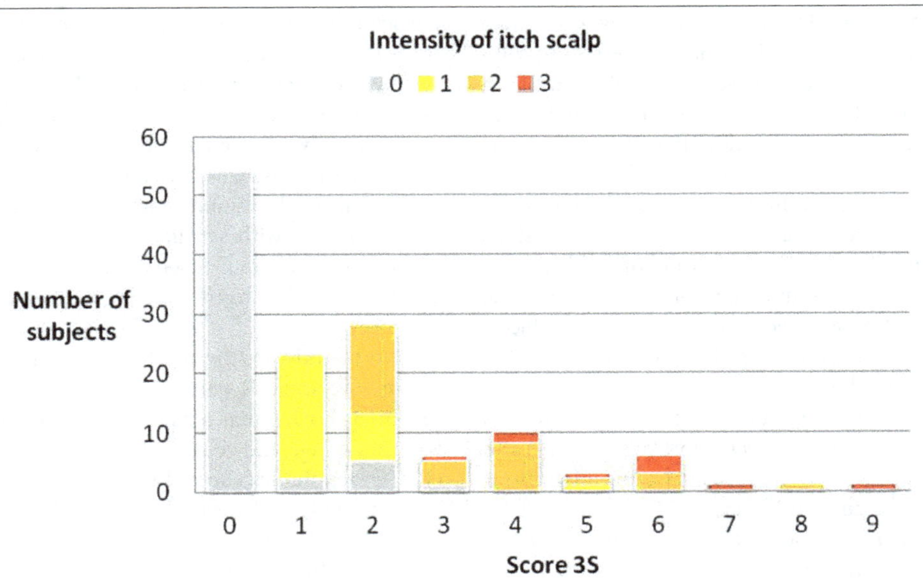

FIGURE 4 | Distribution of subjects according to the intensity of the itch scalp and the 3S score.

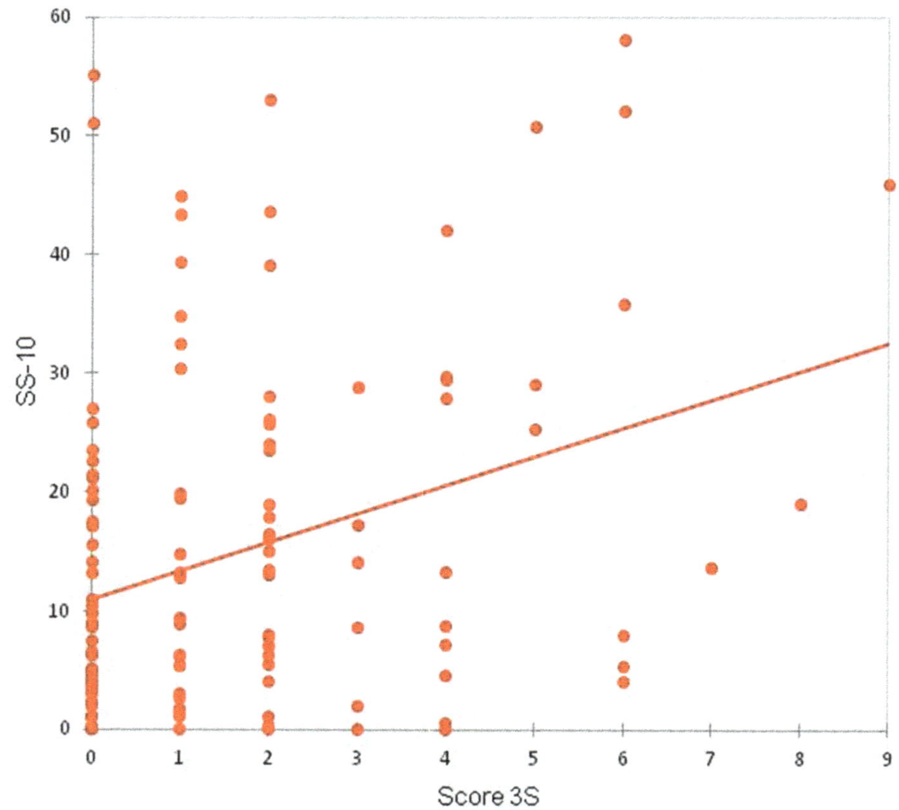

FIGURE 5 | Correlation between the SS-10 and 3S scores.

scalp?," 56% had a positive answer (12). Other studies reported frequencies of 32% (11), 36% (12), or 44.2% (6), with a higher frequency in women. These frequencies were overestimated because the authors did not exclude subjects presenting with scalp dermatosis, such as psoriasis or seborrheic dermatitis. In the majority of studies, the subjects were not examined. In the study that was designed to develop the 3S score, some subjects suffered from hair loss, dandruff, seborrheic dermatitis or psoriasis. Later, a consensual definition of sensitive skin stated that "these unpleasant sensations cannot be explained by lesions attributable to any skin disease." This definition of sensitive skin is applicable to all locations, including the scalp. In our study, the dermatological examination allowed us to include only subjects without any skin diseases on the scalp, in accordance with the new definition of sensitive skin.

We chose to include only women to focus on a homogenous population because sensitive scalp affects mostly women (9) and because they use twice as many hair cosmetic products (four products in mean) as men do (two in mean) (16).

Sensitive skin is mainly a subjective syndrome, and the diagnosis is commonly made by interviewing subjects and asking them whether they have sensitive skin. Objective tests with lactic acid or capsaicin are difficult in the presence of hairs. The sensitive scalp score (3S) was developed in 2011 as a tool to diagnose sensitive scalp, and more than 2,100 subjects were included. In the majority of studies on sensitive skin, particularly those conducted by phone or web survey, the subjects were asked whether they had very sensitive, sensitive, slightly sensitive or not sensitive scalp. The 3S has the advantage of being more precise. In our study, itching was the factor that most strongly correlated with the 3S score and was present in 90.9% of subjects, which is more frequent than on the face or other glabrous locations. Our study also showed that the scores of the subjects with sensitive scalp and those without sensitive scalp were similar. Consequently, it is not possible to define a cut-off for the diagnosis of sensitive scalp according to the 3S scores.

In our study, we did not find any risk factor for the presence of sensitive scalp. Regarding age, a study including 369 subjects in China showed that sensitive scalp were more frequent at 30–39 years of age and that the prevalence decreased after this age (17). Other studies showed that the frequency of sensitive scalp increased (14) or decreased with age (18).

We found a positive correlation between SS10 and 3S scores, suggesting that sensitive skin and a sensitive scalp are linked. The presence of sensitive scalp was positively correlated with the BoSS score, suggesting that sensitive scalp reduce quality of life. However, these results should be interpreted with caution

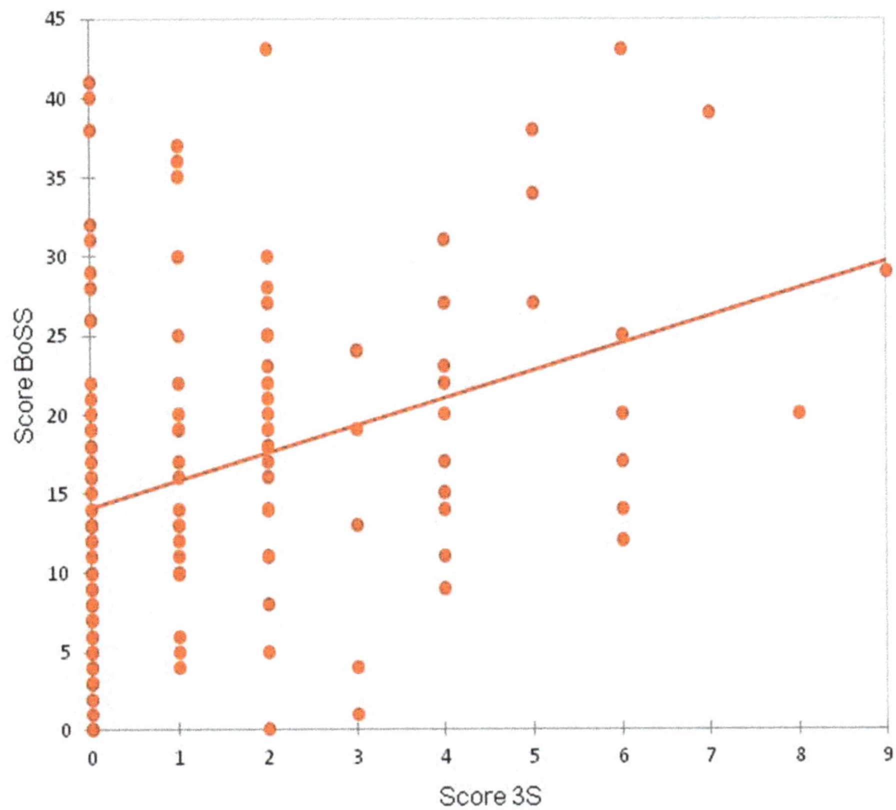

FIGURE 6 | Correlation between the 3S and BoSS scores.

because there are many low 3S scores and very few high 3S scores, which may impact the correlation.

In a study including 125 Korean adult women, the major triggering factor cited was hair care products, as it was cited as a triggering factor in 65.6% of subjects in the group with sensitive scalp (12). There are several types of cosmetics care products for the hair: the hair conditioners, the masks, the oils, the lotions, the serums. We have chosen to analyze the hair conditioners and masks because they are applied right down to the roots of the hair to the skin whereas the other are applied only on the hair. Because of the presence of surfactants and other potentially irritant substances, shampoos are supposed to be highly involved in the development of sensitive scalp, but this hypothesis was not supported in a previous study (14), and our exposure study did not show that shampoos are involved. However, we found a significant difference regarding amount used of hair conditioners, higher in the sensitive scalp group. These cosmetic products are used after the shampoo and are rinsed. We did not confirm the involvement of hair dyes, which we previously showed (18). An analysis of the composition of the various ingredients contained in products used for the scalp may provide more complete information on the link between sensitive scalp and cosmetics. It is not possible to conclude that there is a causal link between a cosmetic product and sensitive scalp. It is possible that hair conditioners cause the sensitive scalp, but it is also possible that subjects with a sensitive scalp use products to relieve their symptoms as hair conditioners.

Concerning consumption habits, the subjects with sensitive scalp seemed to buy organic products or those designed for children more often than those without sensitive scalp, but the difference was not significant, perhaps because of the limited sample size. There was no significant difference concerning the use of products labeled for sensitive scalp between the two groups, but there are quite a few products labeled for the sensitive scalp, contrary to sensitive skin. There was no significant difference concerning the point of purchase, whereas the subjects with non-sensitive scalp seemed to buy products more often in supermarkets. Among the limitations, there is a risk of recruitment bias. We cannot exclude the possibility that more people with sensitive skin responded to the announcement than those without sensitive skin, but we specified that all persons, with or without sensitive scalp, were invited to participate.

In conclusion, itching is the main symptom of sensitive scalp. The frequency of sensitive scalp was lower than that previously described when the subjects with scalp dermatosis were excluded. The exposure to hair conditioners is significantly higher in

TABLE 1 | The frequency of use, amount used and exposure to hair cosmetic products in the two groups.

		Sensitive scalp group (n = 56)	Non sensitive scalp group (n = 56)	
Shampoos	Percentage of users	100%	100%	$p = 1$
	Frequency (day^{-1})	0.56 ± 0.37 (n = 52)	0.55 ± 0.38 (n = 52)	$p = 0.81$
	Amount (g/use)	6.40 ± 5.39 (n = 53)	4.90 ± 2.91 (n = 48)	$p = 0.45$
	Exposition (mg/kg bw/day)	60.54 ± 68.91 (n = 50)	45.35 ± 36.33 (n = 47)	$p = 0.71$
Hair conditioners	Percentage of users	53.6%	40%	$p = 0.15$
	Frequency (day^{-1})	0.32 ± 0.27 (n = 28)	0.37 ± 0.30 (n = 20)	$p = 0.48$
	Amount (g/use)	5.48 ± 5.87 (n = 19)	2.88 ± 3.75 (n = 11)	$p = 0.03$
	Exposition (mg/kg bw/day)	28.52 ± 25.20 (n = 18)	18.16 ± 25.12 (n = 11)	$p = 0.07$
Masks	Percentage of users	48.2%	40%	$p = 0.38$
	Frequency (day^{-1})	0.11 ± 0.09 (n = 27)	0.13 ± 00.9 (n = 21)	$p = 0.73$
	Amount (g/use)	6.19 ± 4.03 (n = 15)	5.38 ± 4.28 (n = 10)	$p = 0.68$
	Exposition (mg/kg bw/day)	0.014 ± 0.0155 (n = 15)	0.014 ± 0.014 (n = 10)	p =0.93
Hair dyes	Percentage of users	52.7%	41%	$p = 0.18$
	Frequency (year^{-1})	6.43 ± 2.62 (n = 23)	6.66 ± 3.10 (n = 12)	$P = 0.92$
Hair bleach	Percentage of users	20%	23.6%	$p = 0.64$
	Frequency (year^{-1})	5.71 ± 3.14 (n = 7)	5.71 ± 2.14 (n = 7)	Not evaluated

subjects with sensitive scalp, suggesting that sensitive scalp might be specifically related to products that are in contact with scalp for a long time.

ETHICS STATEMENT

The studies involving human participants were reviewed and approved by ethics committee of Brest, France (29BRC18.0078). Written informed consent for participation was not required for this study in accordance with the national legislation and the institutional requirements.

AUTHOR CONTRIBUTIONS

A-SF, EB, LM, and A-CR contributed to the design of the research. EB and CL contributed to include subjects. EB and A-SF wrote the manuscript. All authors validated the final version of the manuscript.

ACKNOWLEDGMENTS

We thank Paul Fassier-Frisque for recruiting volunteers.

REFERENCES

1. Misery L, Ständer S, Szepietowski JC, Reich A, Wallengren J, Evers AWM, et al. Definition of sensitive skin: an expert position paper from the special interest group on sensitive skin of the international forum for the study of itch. *Acta Derm Venereol.* (2017) 97:4–6. doi: 10.2340/00015555-2397
2. Misery L, Jourdan E, Huet F, Brenaut E, Cadars B, Virassamynaïk S, et al. Sensitive skin in France: a study on prevalence, relationship with age and skin type and impact on quality of life. *J Eur Acad Dermatol Venereol JEADV.* (2018) 32:791–5. doi: 10.1111/jdv.14837
3. Farage MA. The prevalence of sensitive skin. *Front Med.* (2019) 6:98. doi: 10.3389/fmed.2019.00098

4. Misery L, Weisshaar E, Brenaut E, Evers AWM, Huet F, Ständer S, et al. Pathophysiology and management of sensitive skin: position paper from the special interest group on sensitive skin of the International Forum for the Study of Itch (IFSI). *J Eur Acad Dermatol Venereol JEADV.* (2020) 34:222–9. doi: 10.1111/jdv.16000
5. Richters R, Falcone D, Uzunbajakava N, Verkruysse W, van Erp P, van de Kerkhof P. What is sensitive skin? A systematic literature review of objective measurements. *Skin Pharmacol Physiol.* (2015) 28:75–83. doi: 10.1159/000363149
6. Huet F, Misery L. Sensitive skin is a neuropathic disorder. *Exp Dermatol.* (2019) 28:1470–3. doi: 10.1111/exd.13991
7. Talagas M, Misery L. Role of keratinocytes in sensitive skin. *Front Med.* (2019) 6:108. doi: 10.3389/fmed.2019.00108
8. Brenaut E, Barnetche T, Le Gall-Ianotto C, Roudot A-C, Misery L, Ficheux A-S. Triggering factors in sensitive skin from the worldwide patients' point of view: a systematic literature review and meta-analysis. *J Eur Acad Dermatol Venereol JEADV.* (2020) 34:230–8. doi: 10.1111/jdv.15985
9. Misery L, Sibaud V, Ambronati M, Macy G, Boussetta S, Taieb C. Sensitive scalp: does this condition exist? An epidemiological study. *Contact Dermatitis.* (2008) 58:234–8. doi: 10.1111/j.1600-0536.2007.01288.x
10. Saif GAB, Ericson ME, Yosipovitch G. The itchy scalp – scratching for an explanation. *Exp Dermatol.* (2011) 20:959–68. doi: 10.1111/j.1600-0625.2011.01389.x
11. Saif GAB, Alajroush A, McMichael A, Kwatra SG, Chan Y-H, McGlone F, et al. Aberrant C nerve fibre function of the healthy scalp. *Br J Dermatol.* (2012) 167:485–9. doi: 10.1111/j.1365-2133.2012.11070.x
12. Park KH, Kim J, Oh B, Lee E, Hwang-Bo J, Ha J. Evaluation of factors triggering sensitive scalp in Korean adult women. *Skin Res Technol Off J Int Soc Bioeng Skin ISBS Int Soc Digit Imaging Skin ISDIS Int Soc Skin Imaging ISSI.* (2019) 25:862–6. doi: 10.1111/srt.12747
13. Misery L, Jean-Decoster C, Mery S, Georgescu V, Sibaud V. A new ten-item questionnaire for assessing sensitive skin: the Sensitive Scale-10. *Acta Derm Venereol.* (2014) 94:635–9. doi: 10.2340/00015555-1870
14. Misery L, Rahhali N, Ambonati M, Black D, Saint-Martory C, Schmitt A-M, et al. Evaluation of sensitive scalp severity and symptomatology by using a new score. *J Eur Acad Dermatol Venereol JEADV.* (2011) 25:1295–8. doi: 10.1111/j.1468-3083.2010.03968.x
15. Misery L, Jourdan E, Abadie S, Ezzedine K, Brenaut E, Huet F, et al. Development and validation of a new tool to assess the Burden of Sensitive Skin (BoSS). *J Eur Acad Dermatol Venereol JEADV.* (2018) 32:2217–23. doi: 10.1111/jdv.15186
16. Ficheux AS, Wesolek N, Chevillotte G, Roudot AC. Consumption of cosmetic products by the French population. First part: frequency data. *Food Chem Toxicol Int J Publ Br Ind Biol Res Assoc.* (2015) 78:159–69. doi: 10.1016/j.fct.2015.01.016
17. Ma L, Guichard A, Humbert P, Zheng S, Tan Y, Yu L, et al. Evaluation of the severity and triggering factors of sensitive scalp in Chinese females. *J Cosmet Dermatol.* (2016) 15:219–25. doi: 10.1111/jocd.12203
18. Bernard A, Ficheux AS, Nedelec AS, Bourgeois P, Hornez N, Batardière A, et al. Induction of sensitive skin and sensitive scalp by hair dyeing. (2016). 4:227–39.

13

Comparative Study on Different Skin Pruritus Mouse Models

Guan Donglang†, Liu Tongtong†, Chen Dan, Zhu Chan, Wang Changming, Yu Guang, Yang Yan and Tang Zongxiang**

School of Medicine & Holistic Integrative Medicine, Nanjing University of Chinese Medicine, Nanjing, China

***Correspondence:**
Yang Yan
yangyan3727@njucm.edu.cn
Tang Zongxiang
zongxiangtang1@163.com

†These authors have contributed equally to this work

The animal model is an important tool to study the mechanism of disease formation. Different animal models of pruritus have been adopted based on the purpose of researchers in the study of the itching mechanism. Although the symptoms of various models are quite different, scratching behavior is a key indicator. Therefore, it is necessary to find an animal model that can quickly induce animal scratching and maintain the stability of scratching behavior. In this study, we compared animal models of pruritus induced by four substances and found that the scratching behavior of mice induced by urushiol not only reached the plateau stage quickly but also showed more stability in the plateau phase than that induced by 2,4-dinitrofluorobenzene, oxazolone, and imiquimod. Meanwhile, in the animal model induced by urushiol, the changes of epidermal thickening and inflammatory cell aggregation were also more obvious. In addition, pruritus induced by urushiol is prevalent all over the world, especially in the United States and Europe, involving outdoor groups such as firefighters, forest loggers, and farmers. Therefore, we believe that the urushiol-induced animal model is an ideal choice for the study of the itch formation mechanism and the development of antipruritic drugs.

Keywords: urushiol, pruritus, animal model, psoriasis, atopic dermatitis, allergic contact dermatitis

INTRODUCTION

Chronic pruritus is an obvious symptom of patients with xeroderma, psoriasis, allergic dermatitis, etc. Pruritus severely influences the quality of life of patients (1). In addition, many systemic diseases are also accompanied by pruritus, including diabetes, chronic kidney disease, and psychiatric disorders (2, 3). Itching-related skin diseases often have different symptoms, including xerosis, eczema, dermatitis, urticarial, and cutaneous pruritus (4, 5). To investigate the mechanism of this chronic itch, multiple animal models are used to simulate pruritic symptoms of clinical patients (6). Different animal models of pruritus have been adopted based on the purpose of the researchers in the study of the itching mechanism. Different mouse models of atopic dermatitis (AD), allergic contact dermatitis (ACD), acetone–ether–water (AEW), and psoriasis are widely used to simulate the symptoms of clinical patients. In the process of establishing different animal models, many chemical compounds are used to induce pruritus, including DNFB, oxazolone, imiquimod, and a mixture of acetone and ether (7, 8). Although the symptoms of various models are quite different, scratching behavior is a key indicator.

AD is a chronic eczematous skin disorder characterized by dry and itchy skin. It is a manifestation of immediate hypersensitivity mediated by immunoglobulin E (IgE); delayed-type hypersensitivity is also involved in the skin reaction of patients (9). Oxazolone and DNFB are usually used to induce AD. Oxazolone is a potent contact allergen in humans, which is usually used to induce an AD model (10, 11). It has been reported that the mechanism responsible for producing the scratching in mice after repeated application with oxazolone resembles that of the itching in patients with AD (12). Oxazolone is also used to induce colitis and respiratory allergy (13, 14). DNFB is an decoupling agent, first used to induce typical skin sensitization of the contact type in guinea pigs (15). AD is recognized as a T helper 2 (Th2)–mediated allergic disease, accompanied by increases in cytokines such as tumor necrosis factor α (TNFα), interleukin 4 (IL-4), and IL-17.

Psoriasis is defined as a chronic inflammatory skin disorder characterized by scaly skin plaques, hyperproliferative keratinocytes, and immune cell infiltration into the skin, often accompanied by itching (16). An imiquimod-induced psoriasis model is used to imitate the symptoms of patients with psoriasis in the clinic (17, 18). It has been reported that disturbances in the innate and adaptive cutaneous immune responses are responsible for the development and sustainment of psoriatic inflammation (19, 20).

Contact dermatitis is defined as an inflammation of the skin induced by direct contact of a substance with the surface of the skin. Skin exposure to irritating substances, including solvents, some chemicals, and cosmetics, often results in red, painful rather than itchy, patches on the involved skin areas (21–23). Urushiol-induced ACD is the most common environmental allergic condition in the world. Urushiol as an pruritogen wildly exists in the *Toxicodendron* (formerly *Rhus*) species—poison ivy, poi-oak, and poison sumac (24). It is mainly distributed in Eastern and Central Asia, Vietnam, Korea, Japan, North America, Africa, Australia, New Zealand, and other countries. Urushiol dermatitis patients often develop an extensive, very itchy vesiculo-bullous rash on an infiltrated base or intermittent rashes, with some lesions resembling erythema multiforme (25, 26). Early urushiol-induced ACD model experiments were done on guinea pigs (27).

Due to the complex mechanism, the research on associated with urushiol dermatitis has remained largely unexplored, and no particularly effective drug has been found. Immune cells including $CD8^+$ lymphocytes play a central role in urushiol dermatitis, regulated by $CD4^+$ T lymphocyte subpopulations (28). Cytokines including thymic stromal lymphopoietin (TSLP), serotonin (5-HT), IL-33, and endothelin (ET-1) also mediate this allergic reaction (29, 30). It was reported that the most common treatment received was oral steroids. The cost of diagnosis in the emergency department is, on average, five times that in the outpatient setting (24). Therefore, the urushiol-induced model is optimal to study the mechanism of ACD, which can be expected to magnify the prevalence of urushiol dermatitis.

Although the cause of the itch was complicated, there were still some common factors that existed. Multiple immune cells participate in pruritus of the irritated itch model mice, including mast cells and $CD4^+$ and $CD8^+$ T lymphocytes (31, 32). Like keratinocytes, mast cells are a major source of cutaneous proinflammatory mediators thought to underlie the pathology of pruritus, most importantly IL-33, IL-4, and IL-13 (29, 33, 34). So, these pruritus models have some common features to some extent. Multiple pharmaceuticals could reduce cytokines and chemokines including histamine, TSLP, IL-5, IL-6, IL-8, and IL-13 to relieve the pruritus of the AD induced by DNFB (35, 36). The levels of serum IgE, IL-4, and AD-involved cytokines, such as TNFα, interferon-γ (IFN-γ), IL-1β, TSLP, IL-33, and IL-25, also mediate inflammation in an oxazolone-induced mouse model (19, 37). Different cytokines and chemokines, such as interleukin, TNFα, INFγ, and monocyte chemotactic protein 1 (MCP-1), also increased in imiquimod-induced psoriasis (38, 39).

The aim of this research was to evaluate the skin lesions and behavior of different animal models induced by different irritants. Therefore, the number of inflammatory cytokine immune cells was measured, and the phenotype of the skin was observed.

MATERIALS AND METHODS

Animals

Male C57bl/6J mice 6–8 weeks old were used in the behavioral experiments. All animals were habituated in a room with a 12 h light–dark cycle. The temperature was sustained at 26°C, with humidity at 35%. All mice were kept in the SPF animal center at the Nanjing University of Chinese Medicine. All animal experiments were approved by the animal ethics committee of the Nanjing University of Chinese Medicine.

Pruritic Models

All mice were divided into five groups, exposed to acetone, urushiol, 2,4-dinitrofluorobenzene (DNFB), oxazolone, and imiquimod. Mice were shaved 5 or 2 days prior. Mice were sensitized with 2.0% (wt/vol) urushiol, DNFB, or oxazolone on the abdominal skin, followed by challenges on the nape of neck 5 days later with 0.5% urushiol, DNFB, or oxazolone. The imiquimod-induced pruritic model was established through painting 5% imiquimod on the neck of mice every day. Urushiol, DNFB, and oxazolone were dissolved in acetone, while imiquimod cream was painted directly. Acetone was used in control mice.

Materials

DNFB and oxazolone were purchased from Sigma. Imiquimod cream was purchased as a prescription drug (produced by Sichuan Med-shine Pharmaceutical, Co., LTD.). Urushiol was extracted from Chinese lacquer trees (HPLC≥95%) (40). Hematoxylin and eosin (H&E) staining reagent and Giemsa staining reagent were obtained from Solarbio Life Sciences.

Behavioral Experiments

Mice were habituated in a box with dimensions of 15 × 15 × 15 cm for 15 min every day before experiments. Then, urushiol, DNFB, oxazolone, and imiquimod were painted on the necks of the mice, respectively, shaved 2 days prior. Behaviors of the mice were recorded by video for at least 1 h. We recorded scratching bouts of the mice at 9:00 p.m. every day for 10 days. Scratching numbers were defined as the number of times the hind limbs scratched the neck.

Histological Analysis

Mice were decapitated quickly on the 10th day. The neck skin of the control and model mice was collected, with an area of 8 × 8 mm. Skin was posterior fixed for 24 h in 4% paraformaldehyde and then placed in 30% sugar for 3–5 days. Skin tissue slices were prepared using a frozen section with a thickness of 15 μm, for histochemical experimentation. H&E staining and toluidine blue staining were used to observe the skin lesions and mast cell. Giemsa staining was used to determine the number of inflammatory cells.

Statistical Analysis

The results are expressed as mean ± SEM. The significance of the differences between groups was calculated using Student's *t*-test and ANOVA analysis. In all analyses, a $p < 0.05$ is considered to be statistically significant.

RESULTS

Four Established Pruritic Mouse Models

To compare the different pruritic compounds that induced itch, we established four chronic pruritic models, using urushiol, DNFB, oxazolone, and imiquimod on the neck of mice. Mice were sensitized with 2.0% (wt/vol) urushiol, DNFB, or oxazolone on the abdominal skin, followed by challenges on the nape of the neck 5 days later with 0.5% urushiol, DNFB, or oxazolone (**Figure 1A**). The imiquimod-induced pruritic model was established by painting 5% imiquimod on the neck of mice every day (**Figure 1B**). Control mice were treated with acetone. Our results showed that all the model mice displayed skin lesions to different degrees compared with control mice ($p < 0.001$) (**Figure 1C**). Tissue hyperplasia was the typical characteristic of the skin lesions. The thickness of the skin hyperplasia indicated that all the model mice showed skin lesions to different degrees (**Figure 1D**). Urushiol-induced model mice showed more severe skin damage than the other three mouse models. The epidermis thickness was more obvious compared with other models (uru, 89.8 ± 3.12 μm; oxa, 43.2 ± 1.60 μm; DNFB, 80.8 ± 2.53 μm; IMQ, 75.2 ± 2.24 μm vs. con, 10.1 ± 0.34 μm, $n = 4$ or 5, $p < 0.001$) (**Figure 1E**). The results indicated that the urushiol-induced model showed the most serious skin lesions.

The Difference in Scratching Behavior in the Four Mouse Models

Different animal models were used to imitate the pruritus of patients in clinic, including psoriasis (imiquimod model), xeroderma (AEW model), AD (oxazolone model, DNFB model), and ACD (urushiol model). Pruritus was the obvious symptom of these models. To observe consecutive pruritic behavior, we recorded scratching behavior every day, rather than only at 1 h or 24 h. We found that the four mouse models could show obvious scratching behavior consistent with reported results (8, 17, 29). Except the skin lesions, we found that the scratching bouts of the four mouse models also showed a significant difference. Compared with control mice, all model mice could experience pruritus to different degrees ($p < 0.01$). Urushiol, DNFB, and oxazolone were used to induce ACD. Imiquimod often was used to establish psoriasis, which also showed skin pruritus. Our results showed that urushiol-induced model mice exhibited pruritic behavior earlier than the DNFB, oxazolone, and imiquimod groups ($n = 4$) (**Figures 2A,B**). Compared with the oxazolone group, urushiol-induced model mice showed more obvious pruritic behavior on the zeroth to third days. The pruritic

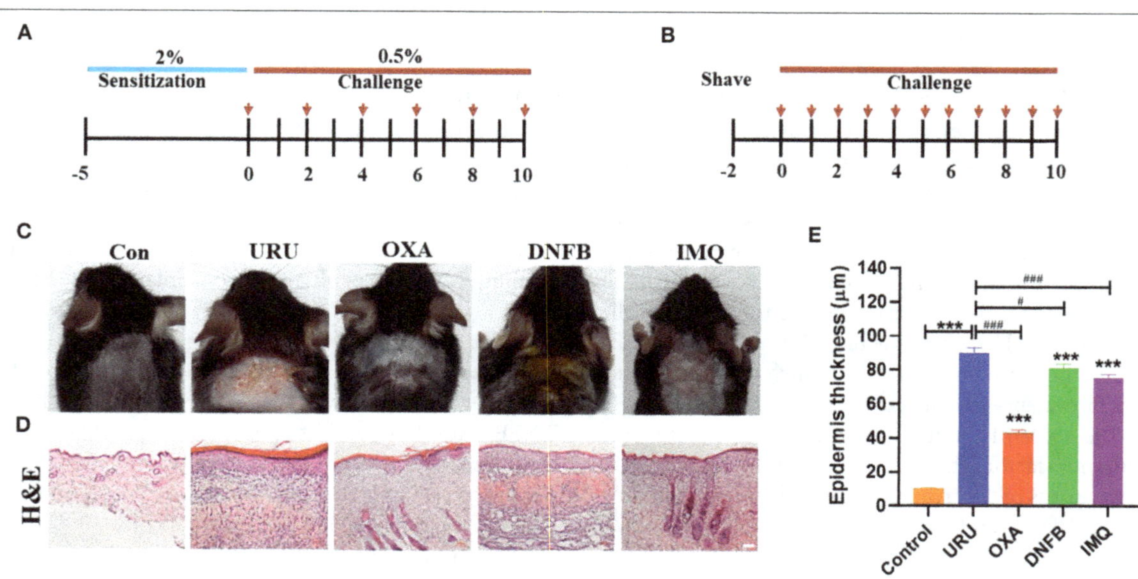

FIGURE 1 | Itchy animals induced by pruritic irritant showed severe skin lesions. **(A)** The itch model was induced by different irritants [urushiol, 2,4-dinitrofluorobenzene (DNFB), and oxazolone]. The red arrow shows the treatment day with the pruritic irritant. **(B)** The psoriasis model was induced by imiquimod. **(C)** Different itch model mice showed obvious skin lesions on the neck compared with control mice. **(D)** Hematoxylin and eosin (H&E) painting of the skin slice on the 10th day. Model mice showed thickening to different degrees. Scale bar 20 μm. **(E)** Statistics of the epidermis thickness of the model mice and control mice. Significant difference is indicated by *p*-value (*compared with control mice; #compared with urushiol-induced model mice). ***$p < 0.001$, **$p < 0.01$, *$p < 0.05$; ###$p < 0.01$.

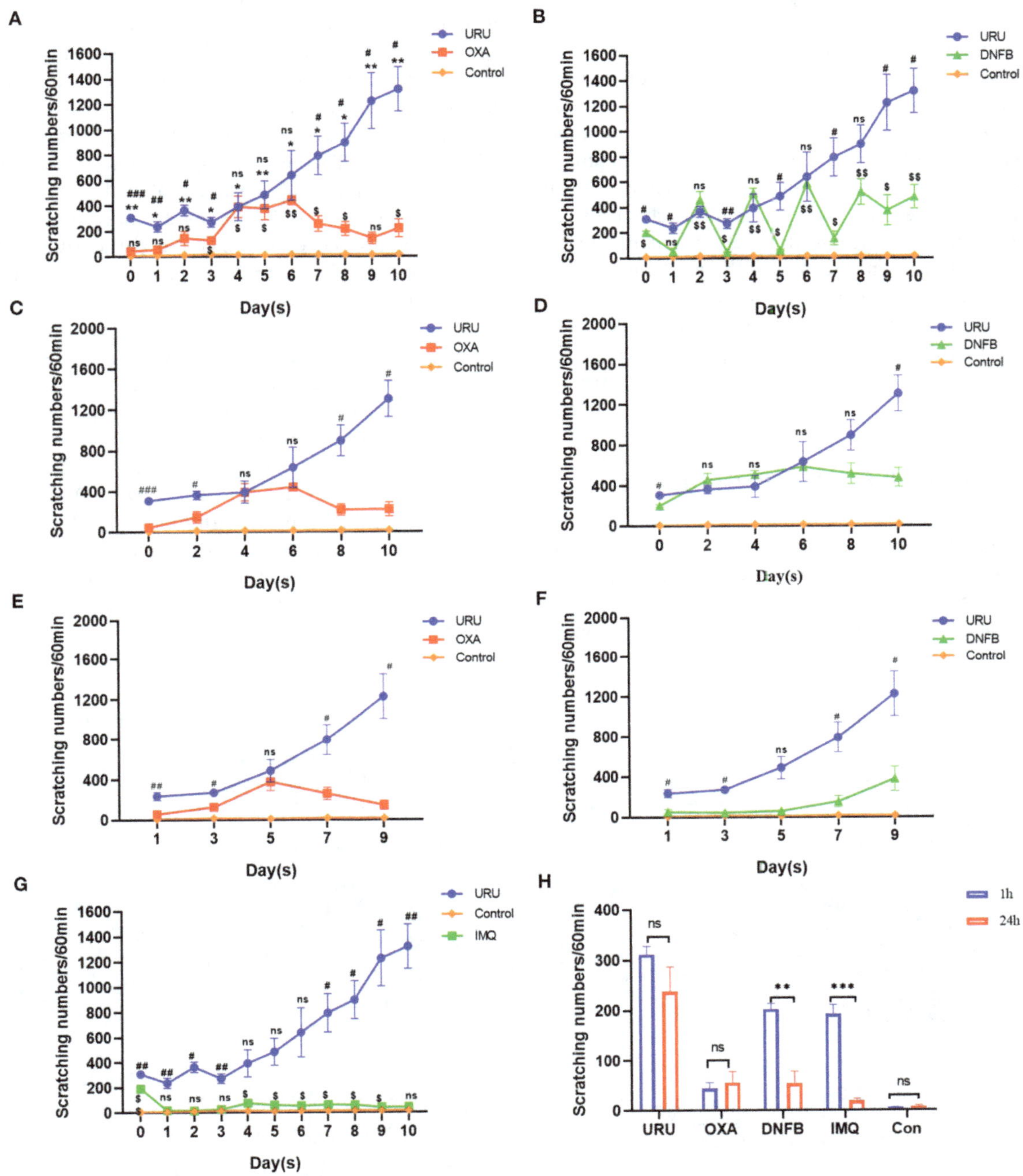

FIGURE 2 | Comparison of scratching bouts between different itch models. **(A)** Scratching bouts of the urushiol-induced mice were higher than those of oxazolone-induced mice and control mice. Significant difference is indicated by *p*-value (*shows urushiol-induced model mice compared with control mice; #shows urushiol-induced model mice compared with oxazolone group; $shows oxazolone group compared with control mice). **(B)** Pruritic behavior of the urushiol-induced mice was more obvious than that of DNFB-induced mice (#shows urushiol-induced model mice compared with DNFB group; $shows DNFB group compared with control mice). **(C)** Compared with oxazolone, urushiol induced more obvious pruritus in 1 h (evoked scratching). **(D)** Compared with DNFB, there was no obvious difference in scratching bouts induced by urushiol in 1 h (evoked scratching). **(E)** Compared with oxazolone, urushiol induced more obvious pruritus in 24 h (spontaneous scratching). **(F)** There was an obvious difference in pruritus between DNFB and urushiol model mice. **(G)** Scratching bouts of the urushiol-induced mice were higher than those of IMQ-induced mice (#shows urushiol-induced model mice compared with IMQ group; $shows IMQ group compared with control mice). **(H)** Scratching behavior of the different mice shown in 1 and 24 h on the first day. ***$p < 0.001$, **$p < 0.01$, *$p < 0.05$; ##$p < 0.01$, ###$p < 0.001$; $^{\$}p < 0.05$.

behavior of the oxazolone-induced model mice reached a plateau on the fourth day (**Figures 2A,C,E**). DNFB-induced model mice showed serious pruritus in 1 h after application of DNFB. The itchy behavior of the mice in 24 h was reduced until the eighth day (**Figures 2B,D,F**). Our results showed that imiquimod-induced psoriasis exhibited less severe pruritic behavior in mice than the urushiol group (**Figure 2G**). Especially, we found that there was no difference in scratching bouts between 1 and 24 h in the urushiol and oxazolone groups on the first day (urushiol, 307 ± 14.3 vs. 235 ± 40.5, $p = 0.20$; oxazolone, 44 ± 11.6 vs. 55 ± 22.4, $p = 0.67$) (**Figure 2H**). However, there was a significant difference between 1 and 24 h in the DNFB and imiquimod groups (DNFB, 202 ± 11.3 vs. 53 ± 24.7, $p < 0.01$; imiquimod, 192 ± 18.8 vs. 18 ± 4.4, $p < 0.001$). The different irritants inducing pruritus have different pathogenic mechanisms. We speculated that after treatment with different irritants for 1 h, there was direct stimulus to the skin of the model mice. After 24 h, pruritus tends to be stable. DNFB, as a strong sensitizer, also had multiple side effects, such as apoptotic death of skin dendritic cells occurring after exposure and promotion of tumors (41, 42). We concluded that compared with other irritants, urushiol was a relatively stable, safe, and effective irritant for itching.

Inflammatory Cells of the Irritant Itch Models

Despite the diversity of the mechanisms in different itch models of mice, inflammatory cells and cytokines have been reported to be involved in the formation of pruritus in mice (43–45). A mast cell is a kind of inflammatory cell, which we have paid close attention to recently. To speculate on whether mast cells participate in the pruritus behavior of these mouse models, we calculated the statistic degranulation percentage of mast cells, using toluidine blue painting. Our results showed that the degranulation percentage of the four mouse models was higher than that of control mice ($p < 0.001$) (**Figures 3A,B**). Therefore, we speculate that the cytokines and chemokines released by mast cells after degranulation may be the cause of pruritus in the model mice. Other than mast cells, basophils and eosinophils also participate in the itch of these mouse models. Our results showed that both basophils and eosinophils increase obviously compared with control mice ($p < 0.01$) (**Figure 3C**). To observe the inflammatory cell aggregation induced by different irritants, we compared urushiol-, oxazolone-, DNFB-, and imiquimod-induced itch models. Statistical data revealed that basophil and eosinophil aggregation induced by urushiol was more obvious compared to oxazolone and DNFB (113.6 ± 4.7; oxazolone, 82.14 ± 2.0, $p < 0.001$; DNFB, 42.5 ± 2.2, $p < 0.001$). There was no difference between the urushiol-induced model and the imiquimod-induced model (106.9 ± 2.9, $p = 0.2037$). We believe that different inflammatory cells, including mast cells, basophils and eosinophils, and cytokines, mediated the pruritus of the irritant itch.

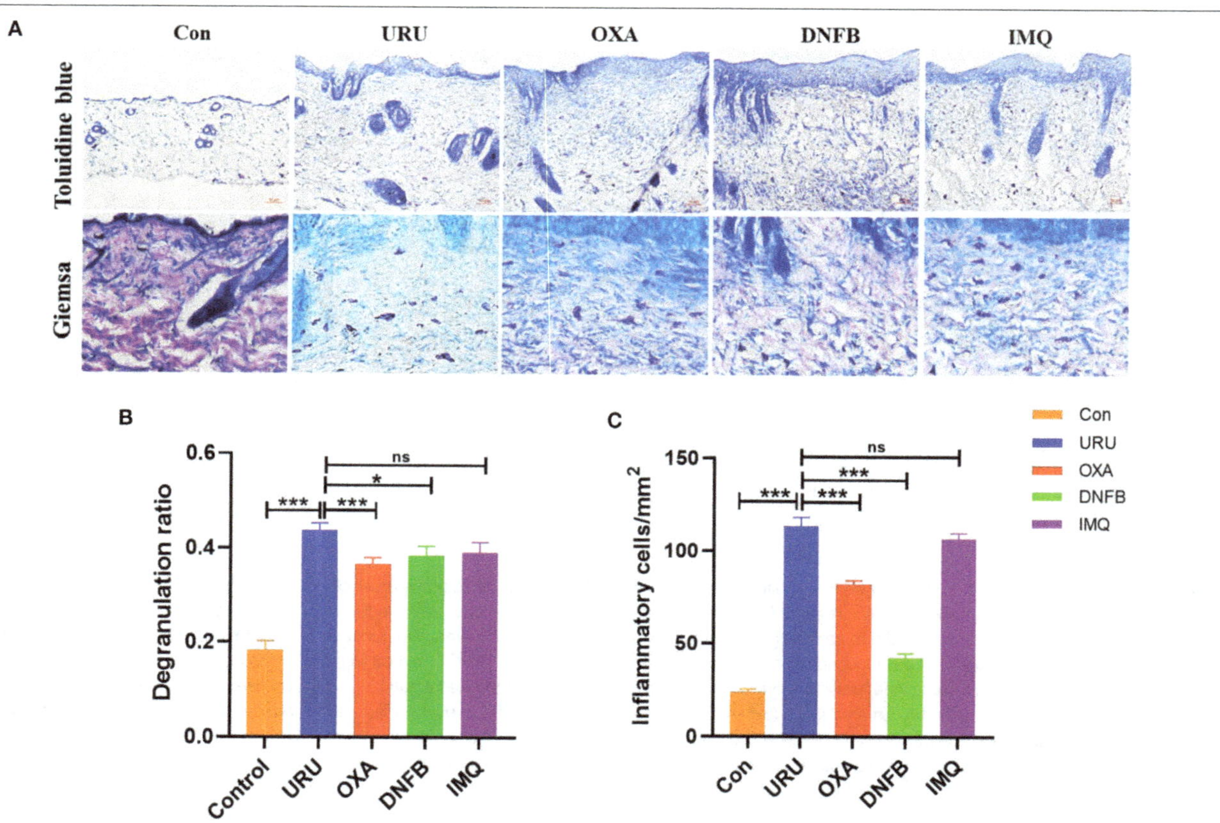

FIGURE 3 | Inflammatory cells mediated itch of the model mice. **(A)** Immunohistochemistry staining of the skin tissue. Toluidine blue staining of the model mice and control mice (upper figure), scale bar, 50 μm. Giemsa staining of the basophils and eosinophils, scale bar 25 μm (bottom of **A**). **(B)** Degranulation ratio of the model mice increased compared to control mice. **(C)** Inflammatory cells in skin tissue of the mice. $^{***}p < 0.001$, $^{**}p < 0.01$, $^{*}p < 0.05$.

DISCUSSION

Animal models of human disease refer to animals with human disease simulation performance established in various medical science research studies. The use of animal models is a very important experimental method and means in modern biomedical research, which is conducive to more convenient and effective understanding of the occurrence and development of human diseases and research on prevention and control measures. We observed four animal models simulating human pruritus and compared their pruritus characteristics and pathogenesis. It is hoped that these results can provide some references for researchers who are studying different diseases with pruritus.

Pruritus is a disease and a symptom of different diseases. For itch researchers, it is necessary and important to establish an animal model with obvious, stable, and persistent itching behavior. Scratching bouts were usually considered to be an indicator for evaluating itching in mice. Our consecutive record of the behavior showed that the scratching bouts of the urushiol-induced model were more obvious, sustained, and stable than those of DNFB-induced mice. In addition, the pruritus symptom of the urushiol-induced model mice was more severe than oxazolone- and imiquimod-induced model mice. At the same time, urushiol is more likely to induce pruritus than other irritants. Compared with other models, the urushiol-induced model is easier to establish. The characteristics of these animal models can indeed provide a choice for researchers with different directions and who are interested in itching.

The purpose of basic research is to seek effective treatment methods and approaches. The mechanisms of pruritus caused by different diseases are different, but there may be some of the same itching molecules, itch-related receptors, and immune cells in human and animal bodies, which play an important role. For example, IL-22, IL-23, IL-31, and IL-33 were increased in the skin of patients and model animals with allergic dermatitis, AD, and psoriasis (30, 46). In the skin of AD and psoriasis patients, the expression of these receptors such as phospholipase A2, substance P, Nav1.7, and TRPV1 was positively correlated with the degree of skin lesions. In addition, cytokines such as IL-17A, IL-23A, and IL-31 had elevated gene transcript levels in both itchy atopic and psoriatic skin (47). So far, although we are still unable to determine whether the pruritus in different animal models has the same material basis, we can compare and analyze the data obtained in different animal models of pruritus and find out whether there is a certain rule. In any case, the determination of itch targets will effectively promote the development of antipruritic drugs.

ETHICS STATEMENT

The animal study was reviewed and approved by Animal Ethics Committee of Nanjing University of Chinese Medicine.

AUTHOR CONTRIBUTIONS

GD and LT are mainly responsible for data collection and data analysis. CD, ZC, WC, and YG are responsible for review. YY are responsible for data analysis and writing. TZ are responsible for the writing and review. All authors contributed to the article and approved the submitted version.

REFERENCES

1. Stander S, Stander HF, Steinke S, Bruland P, Dugas M, Augustin M. Chronic pruritus care in daily practice. *Hautarzt.* (2016) 67:640–7. doi: 10.1007/s00105-016-3829-8
2. Twycross R, Greaves MW, Handwerker H, Jones EA, Libretto SE, Szepietowski JC, et al. Itch: scratching more than the surface. *Qjm-Int J Med.* (2003) 96:7–26. doi: 10.1093/qjmed/hcg002
3. Welz-Kubiak K, Reszke R, Szepietowski JC. Pruritus as a sign of systemic disease. *Clinics Dermatol.* (2019) 37:644–56. doi: 10.1016/j.clindermatol.2019.07.031
4. Barrett M, Luu M. Differential diagnosis of atopic dermatitis. *Immunol Allergy Clin.* (2017) 37:11–34. doi: 10.1016/j.iac.2016.08.009
5. Zhong CS, Elmariah SB. Phototherapy for Itch. *Dermatol Clin.* (2020) 38:145–55. doi: 10.1016/j.det.2019.08.008
6. Lorz LR, Kim MY, Cho JY. Medicinal potential of Panax ginseng and its ginsenosides in atopic dermatitis treatment. *J Ginseng Res.* (2020) 44:8–13. doi: 10.1016/j.jgr.2018.12.012
7. Chen X, Zhu C, Zhang Y, Yang N, Shi H, Yang W, et al. Antipruritic effect of ethyl acetate extract from fructus cnidii in mice with 2,4-dinitrofluorobenzene-induced atopic dermatitis. *Evid Based Complement Alternat Med.* (2020) 2020:1–14. doi: 10.1155/2020/6981386
8. Kiguchi N, Saika F, Fukazawa Y, Matsuzaki S, Kishioka S. Critical role of GRP receptor-expressing neurons in the spinal transmission of imiquimod-induced psoriatic itch. *Neuropsychopharmacol Rep.* (2020) 3:1–4. doi: 10.1002/npr2.12120
9. Tomimori Y, Muto T, Fukami H, Saito K, Horikawa C, Tsuruoka N, et al. Chymase participates in chronic dermatitis by inducing eosinophil infiltration. *Lab Invest.* (2002) 82:789–94. doi: 10.1097/01.LAB.0000018827.78602.F4
10. Asherson GL, Ptak W. Contact and delayed hypersensitivity in the mouse. I. Active sensitization and passive transfer. *Immunology.* (1968) 15:405–16.
11. Tsukumo Y, Harada D, Manabe H. Pharmacological characterization of itch-associated response induced by repeated application of oxazolone in mice. *J Pharmacol Sci.* (2010) 113:255–62. doi: 10.1254/jphs.10050FP
12. Tsukumo Y, Matsumoto Y, Miura H, Yano H, Manabe H. Gabapentin and pregabalin inhibit the itch-associated response induced by the repeated application of oxazolone in mice. *J Pharmacol Sci.* (2011) 115:27–35. doi: 10.1254/jphs.10173FP
13. Yi R, Tan F, Suo H, Li W, Zhou X, Mu J, et al. Prophylactic Effect of Lactobacillus plantarum YS4 on Oxazolone-Induced Colitis in

BALB/c Mice. *Evid Based Complement Alternat Med.* (2020) 2020:1–11. doi: 10.1155/2020/9048971

14. Kuper C F, Radonjic M, Van Triel J, Stierum R, De Groot R J, Arts J H. Oxazolone (OXA) is a respiratory allergen in Brown Norway rats. *Toxicology.* (2011) 290:59–68. doi: 10.1016/j.tox.2011.08.017
15. Landsteiner K, Chase MW. Studies on the sensitization of animals with simple chemical compounds : Ix. Skin sensitization Induced by Injection of Conjugates. *J Exp Med.* (1941) 73:431–8. doi: 10.1084/jem.73.3.431
16. Boehncke WH, Schon MP. Psoriasis. *Lancet.* (2015) 386:983–94. doi: 10.1016/S0140-6736(14)61909-7
17. Sakai K, Sanders KM, Youssef MR, Yanushefski KM, Jensen L, Yosipovitch G, et al. Mouse model of imiquimod-induced psoriatic itch. *Pain.* (2016) 157:2536–43. doi: 10.1097/j.pain.0000000000000674
18. Van Der Fits L, Mourits S, Voerman JS, Kant M, Boon L, Laman JD, et al. Imiquimod-induced psoriasis-like skin inflammation in mice is mediated via the IL-23/IL-17 axis. *J Immunol.* (2009) 182:5836–45. doi: 10.4049/jimmunol.0802999
19. Oh MS, Hong JY, Kim MN, Kwak EJ, Kim SY, Kim EG, et al. Activated leukocyte cell adhesion molecule modulates Th2 immune response in atopic dermatitis. *Allergy Asthma Immunol Res.* (2019) 11:677–90. doi: 10.4168/aair.2019.11.5.677
20. Rendon A, Schakel K. Psoriasis pathogenesis and treatment. *Int J Mol Sci.* (2019) 20:1–28. doi: 10.3390/ijms20061475
21. Bras S, Mendes-Bastos P, Amaro C, Cardoso J. Allergic contact dermatitis caused by laurel leaf oil. *Contact Dermatitis.* (2015) 72:417–9. doi: 10.1111/cod.12377
22. Fonacier LS, Sher JM. Allergic contact dermatitis. *Ann Allerg Asthma Im.* (2014) 113:9–12. doi: 10.1016/j.anai.2014.03.018
23. Park ME, Zippin JH. Allergic contact dermatitis to cosmetics. *Dermatol Clin.* (2014) 32:1–11. doi: 10.1016/j.det.2013.09.006
24. Kim Y, Flamm A, Elsohly MA, Kaplan DH, Hage RJ Jr, et al. Poison ivy, oak, and sumac dermatitis: what is known and what is new? *Dermatitis.* (2019) 30:183–90. doi: 10.1097/DER.0000000000000472
25. Raison-Peyron N, Bourrain JL, Girard C, Rance C, Dereure O. An unusual clinical presentation of allergic contact dermatitis to common ivy. *Contact Dermatitis.* (2020) 82:235–7. doi: 10.1111/cod.13442
26. White JML, Pink AE. English sunday lunch dermatitis: allergic contact dermatitis to parsnip, carrot, fennel (and ivy). *Contact Dermatitis.* (2020) 83:317–8. doi: 10.1111/cod.13593
27. Lepoittevin JP, Benezra C, Asakawa Y. Allergic contact dermatitis to Ginkgo biloba L.: relationship with urushiol. *Arch Dermatol Res.* (1989) 281:227–30. doi: 10.1007/BF00431055
28. Lopez CB, Kalergis AM, Becker MI, Garbarino JA, De Ioannes AE. CD8+ T cells are the effectors of the contact dermatitis induced by urushiol in mice and are regulated by CD4+ T cells. *Int Arch Allergy Immunol.* (1998) 117:194–201. doi: 10.1159/000024010
29. Liu B, Tai Y, Achanta S, Kaelberer MM, Caceres AI, Shao X, et al. IL-33/ST2 signaling excites sensory neurons and mediates itch response in a mouse model of poison ivy contact allergy. *Proc Natl Acad Sci USA.* (2016) 113:E7572–9. doi: 10.1073/pnas.1606608113
30. Liu B, Tai Y, Liu B, Caceres AI, Yin C, Jordt SE. Transcriptome profiling reveals Th2 bias and identifies endogenous itch mediators in poison ivy contact dermatitis. *JCI Insight.* (2019) 5:1–13. doi: 10.1172/jci.insight.124497
31. Turner CT, Zeglinski MR, Richardson KC, Santacruz S, Hiroyasu S, Wang C, et al. Granzyme B contributes to barrier dysfunction in oxazolone-induced skin inflammation through E-cadherin and FLG cleavage. *J Invest Dermatol.* (2020) 141:36–47. doi: 10.1016/j.jid.2020.05.095
32. Fang Z, Li L, Zhao J, Zhang H, Lee YK, Lu W, et al. Bifidobacteria adolescentis regulated immune responses and gut microbial composition to alleviate DNFB-induced atopic dermatitis in mice. *Eur J Nutr.* (2020) 59:3069–81. doi: 10.1007/s00394-019-02145-8
33. Du L, Hu X, Yang W, Yasheng H, Liu S, Zhang W, et al. Spinal IL-33/ST2 signaling mediates chronic itch in mice through the astrocytic JAK2-STAT3 cascade. *Glia.* (2019) 67:1680–93. doi: 10.1002/glia.23639
34. Barr T P, Garzia C, Guha S, Fletcher E K, Nguyen N, Wieschhaus A J, et al. PAR2 pepducin-based suppression of inflammation and itch in atopic dermatitis models. *J Invest Dermatol.* (2019) 139:412–21. doi: 10.1016/j.jid.2018.08.019
35. Aye A, Song YJ, Jeon YD, Jin JS. Xanthone suppresses allergic contact dermatitis *in vitro* and *in vivo*. *Int Immunopharmacol.* (2020) 78:1–10. doi: 10.1016/j.intimp.2019.106061
36. Yoou MS, Nam SY, Wan Yoon K, Jeong HJ, Kim HM. Bamboo salt suppresses skin inflammation in mice with 2, 4-dinitrofluorobenzene-induced atopic dermatitis. *Chin J Nat Med.* (2018) 16:97–104. doi: 10.1016/S1875-5364(18)30035-9
37. Jung Y, Kim JC, Park NJ, Bong SK, Lee S, Jegal H, et al. Eupatilin, an activator of PPARalpha, inhibits the development of oxazolone-induced atopic dermatitis symptoms in Balb/c mice. *Biochem Biophys Res Commun.* (2018) 496:508–14. doi: 10.1016/j.bbrc.2018.01.098
38. Yang BY, Cheng YG, Liu Y, Liu Y, Tan JY, Guan W, et al. Datura Metel L. Ameliorates imiquimod-induced psoriasis-like dermatitis and inhibits inflammatory cytokines production through TLR7/8-MyD88-NF-kappaB-NLRP3 inflammasome pathway. *Molecules.* (2019) 24:1–14. doi: 10.3390/molecules24112157
39. Hung C H, Wang C N, Cheng H H, Liao J W, Chen Y T, Chao Y W, et al. Baicalin ameliorates imiquimod-induced psoriasis-like inflammation in mice. *Planta Med.* (2018) 84:1110–7. doi: 10.1055/a-0622-8242
40. He Q, Zhang J, Tian YG, Liu YH, Wang JX, Wei H. Separation and preparation of a C15 triolefinic urushiol from raw lacquer. *J Jishou University.* (2016) 37:42–4. doi: 10.3969/j.cnki.jdxb.2016.05.010
41. Cruz MT, Duarte CB, Goncalo M, Figueiredo A, Carvalho AP, Lopes MC. The sensitizer 2,4-dinitrofluorobenzene activates caspase-3 and induces cell death in a skin dendritic cell line. *Int J Toxicol.* (2003) 22:43–8. doi: 10.1080/10915810305069
42. Maldve RE, Fischer SM. Tumor-promoting activity of 2,4-dinitrofluorobenzene. *Int J Cancer.* (1995) 60:545–53. doi: 10.1002/ijc.2910600420
43. Tian T, Chang H, He K, Ni Y, Li C, Hou M, et al. Fucoidan from seaweed Fucus vesiculosus inhibits 2,4-dinitrochlorobenzene-induced atopic dermatitis. *Int Immunopharmacol.* (2019) 75:1–9. doi: 10.1016/j.intimp.2019.105823
44. Giuffrida P, Caprioli F, Facciotti F, Di Sabatino A. The role of interleukin-13 in chronic inflammatory intestinal disorders. *Autoimmun Rev.* (2019) 18:549–55. doi: 10.1016/j.autrev.2019.03.012
45. Singh TP, Zhang HH, Hwang ST, Farber JM. IL-23- and imiquimod-induced models of experimental psoriasis in mice. *Curr Protoc Immunol.* (2019) 125:e71. doi: 10.1002/cpim.71
46. Hashimoto T, Sakai K, Sanders K M, Yosipovitch G, Akiyama T. Antipruritic effects of janus kinase inhibitor tofacitinib in a mouse model of psoriasis. *Acta Derm-Venereol.* (2019) 99:298–303. doi: 10.2340/00015555-3086
47. Nattkemper LA, Tey HL, Valdes-Rodriguez R, Lee H, Mollanazar NK, Albornoz C, et al. The genetics of chronic itch: gene expression in the skin of patients with atopic dermatitis and psoriasis with severe itch. *J Investigative Dermatol.* (2018) 138:1311–7. doi: 10.1016/j.jid.2017.12.029

14

Cholestasis-Associated Pruritus and its Pruritogens

Jacqueline A. G. M. Langedijk, Ulrich H. Beuers and Ronald P. J. Oude Elferink*

Amsterdam University Medical Centers, Tytgat Institute for Liver and Intestinal Research, Research Institute Amsterdam Gastroenterology, Endocrinology and Metabolism (AGEM), University of Amsterdam, Amsterdam, Netherlands

Correspondence:
Ronald P. J. Oude Elferink
r.p.oude-elferink@amsterdamumc.nl

Pruritus is a debilitating symptom of various cholestatic disorders, including primary biliary cholangitis (PBC), primary sclerosing cholangitis (PSC) and inherited progressive familial intrahepatic cholestasis (PFIC). The molecular mechanisms leading to cholestasis-associated pruritus are still unresolved and the involved pruritogens are indecisive. As a consequence of pruritus, patients suffer from sleep deprivation, loss of daytime concentration, auto-mutilation and sometimes even suicidal ideations. Current guideline-approved therapy of cholestasis-associated pruritus includes stepwise administration of several medications, which may alleviate complaints in some, but not all affected patients. Therefore, also experimental therapeutic approaches are required to improve patients' quality of life. This article reviews the current state of research on pruritogens and their receptors, and shortly discusses the most recent experimental therapies.

Keywords: cholestasis, bile formation, cholestasis-associated pruritus, itch, autotaxin, pruritogen

INTRODUCTION

Cholestasis is the term for diminished or impaired bile flow generated by hepatocytes and cholangiocytes. The cause of cholestasis can be intra- or extrahepatic, and can be genetic or the consequence of an inflammatory or malignant hepatobiliary disease. Next to fatigue, pruritus is the most frequent symptom in patients with chronic cholestatic disorders and may affect more than half of patients with fibrosing cholangiopathies such as primary biliary cholangitis (PBC) or primary sclerosing cholangitis (PSC) at least transiently during their disease course. Depending on the cause of cholestasis, 30–90% of patients suffer from chronic pruritus, which is unresponsive to antihistamines. Chronic pruritus can lead to loss of concentration, sleep deprivation and auto-mutilation or prurigo nodularis due to scratching (1). In most serious cases, suicidal ideations may occur and the burden of pruritus can become the primary indication for liver transplantation. Cholestasis-associated pruritus shows a diurnal rhythm with increased intensity in the late evening and early night. The itch is typically localized at the limbs and soles of the feet and at the forearms and palms of the hands, but may also be generalized.

Liver diseases over a wide range of prevalences are associated with chronic pruritus including PBC, PSC and secondary sclerosing cholangitis (SSC), cholangiocarcinoma, viral hepatitis, drug-induced cholestasis, sarcoidosis hepatis, and rare inherited forms of cholestasis. For intrahepatic cholestasis of pregnancy (ICP) pruritus is one of the mandatory diagnostic criteria and is observed in 0.5–2.0% of pregnant women, PBC is found in about 0.1% of women at an age of 50 years, whereas Alagille syndrome as an example of rare genetic diseases is found in only one of 100,000 children and adolescents. In some cases, such as PBC, pruritus can be the first symptom of the disease. Since this is a relatively rare disease, diagnosis by general practitioners or dermatologists may be difficult.

It has not been established whether environmental, geographical or life-style factors influence the prevalence or severity of cholestasis-associated itch. However, for ICP there are indications for possible environmental factors that influence the occurrence of ICP in genetically susceptible individuals. It has been postulated that the long-chain monounsaturated fatty acid erucic acid and/or selenium may play a role. Furthermore, the occurrence of ICP was exceptionally high in Chile a number of decades ago, but has drastically decreased more recently, suggesting that a change in diet or unknown lifestyle factor might play a role in ICP (2, 3).

The pathogenesis of cholestasis-associated pruritus is still poorly understood, however, based on research of the past 40 years and therapies that give relief of pruritus in a subset of patients, there is common understanding that:

- Potential pruritogens are located in the systemic circulation, as indicated by (partial) relief of pruritus after treatment with plasmapheresis, albumin dialysis or plasma separation/anion absorption.
- Direct or indirect pruritogens are excreted into bile and undergo enterohepatic circulation, as suggested by attenuation of pruritus in some patients after oral administration of anion exchange resins, and by inhibitors of the apical sodium-dependent bile acid transporter (ASBT) or effectively, but only transiently by nasobiliary drainage.
- Pruritogens are thought to be formed or biotransformed in the liver and/or the gut as indicated by effective treatment with the potent pregnane X receptor (PXR) agonist, rifampicin.
- Pruritogens affect the endogenous opioidergic and serotoninergic system, as suggested by antipruritic activity of opioid antagonists such as naltrexone and serotonin reuptake inhibitors such as sertraline.

In this review, we will discuss the current literature on cholestasis-associated pruritus, with a specific disquisition of the possible pruritogens. We will briefly deliberate the receptors involved in pruritus and current treatment options.

Abbreviations: 5-HT, serotonin; γGT, γ-glutamyltransferase; ANIT, α-naphthylisothiocyanate; AP, alkaline phosphatase; ASBT, apical sodium-dependent bile salt transporter; ATX, autotaxin; BSEP, bile salt export pump; CMH, mechano-heat-sensitive C-fiber; CMi, mechano-insensitive C-fiber; DC, deoxycholate; DRG, dorsal root ganglion; EASL, European Association for the Study of the Liver; ENPP, ectonucleotide pyrophosphatase; FXR, farnesoid X receptor; GCDC, glycochenodeoxycholate; GPCR, G-protein coupled receptor; GRP, gastrin-releasing peptide; H1R, histamine 1 receptor; H4R, histamine 4 receptor; ICP, intrahepatic cholestasis of pregnancy; IPF, idiopathic pulmonary fibrosis; LPA, lysophosphatidic acid; LPC, lysophosphatidylcholine; Mrgpra3, mas-related G-protein a3; MRGPRX1, mas-related G-protein X1; MRGPRX4, mas-related G-protein X4; NASH, non-alcoholic steatosis hepatitis; Nppb, natriuretic peptide B; NTCP, Na^+-taurocholate cotransporting polypeptide; PPAR, peroxisome proliferator-activated receptor; PAR2, protease-activated receptor 2; PAR4, protease-activated receptor 4; PBC, primary biliary cholangitis; PEBD, partial external biliary diversion; PKC, protein kinase C; PLC, phospholipase C; PM3S, progesterone metabolite 3 sulfate; PSC, primary sclerosing cholangitis; PFIC, progressive familial intrahepatic cholestasis; PXR, pregnane X receptor; SSRI, selective serotonin reuptake inhibitor; TCDC, taurochenodeoxycholate; TGR5, G-protein coupled bile salt receptor; TRPA1, transient receptor potential ankyrin 1; TRPV1, transient receptor potential vanilloid 1; UDCA, ursodeoxycholic acid.

Itch Signaling

Signaling of itch is often measured after provocation with histamine, chloroquine or cowhage, which activate the histamine 1 (H1R) or 4 (H4R) receptor (4), the Mas-related G-protein X1 in humans (MRGPRX1) or a3 in mice (mrgpra3) (5), and the protease-activated receptor 2 (PAR2) or 4 (PAR4) (6), respectively.

Histamine-induced itch signaling occurs through mechano-insensitive C-fibers (CMi) with unmyelinated nerve endings in the skin (7, 8). However, the majority of chronic itch types including cholestasis-associated pruritus cannot be relieved by anti-histamine treatment, and are therefore classified as non-histaminergic itch (9–13). Non-histaminergic itch in humans possibly signals through mechano-heat-sensitive C-fibers (CMH), as measured with cowhage provocation (14, 15).

Itch signals run from primary itch neurons in the skin through the dorsal root ganglia (DRG) to a secondary neuron in the dorsal horn of the spinal cord (16) with natriuretic peptide B (Nppb) and glutamate as the neurotransmitters (16–19). In the dorsal horn of the spinal cord, the secondary neuron crosses to the contralateral side and transmits the signal by gastrin-releasing peptide (GRP) to a tertiary neuron (16, 20, 21). This third neuron projects through the spinothalamic tract to the ventromedial nucleus of the thalamus.

In order to reduce itch, the central nervous system provokes an urge to create a local pain signal by scratching. This demonstrates that pain has an inhibitory effect on itch (22, 23). When pain is pharmacologically reduced, for example by morphine administration, itch frequently sets in at the region of reduced pain transmission (24, 25). This contra-mechanism is very likely fulfilled by inhibitory interneurons in the dorsal horn of the spinal cord, which create a constant tonus of inhibition by nociceptive to pruriceptive neurons. In genetic experiments with mice, it was shown that when these inhibitory interneurons are not formed, due to deletion of the gene for the transcription factor *Bhlhb5*, mice suffer from severe chronic itch (26).

Many receptors that are involved in pruritus are G-protein coupled receptors, which, after activation, cause an increase in intracellular calcium release and thereby activate PLC and PKC [reviewed by (27)]. PLC and PKC are often coupled to TRP-channels that amplify the intracellular cation wave and together with Na_V channels initiate an action potential, leading to itch sensation (28–31). Next to their role in coupled cation influx, these TRP-channels can also be activated directly by chemical, thermal and mechanical noxious stimuli (32–34).

Pruritogens That Are Potentially Involved in Cholestatic Itch

Bile Salts

The most abundant components of bile are bile salts, which for a long time were and still are thought by some to act as pruritogens in cholestasis. There are several subspecies of bile salts with different properties. They can bind to the intracellular farnesoid X receptor (FXR) which is a nuclear receptor that regulates a considerable transcription network, and to the transmembrane G protein-coupled receptor TGR5 that upon activation induces cAMP synthesis. A specific subset of bile salts can even cause a response through the pregnane X receptor, vitamin D receptor and constitutive androstane receptor, thereby influencing bile salt synthesis and progression of cholestasis (35).

Bile salt levels are elevated in serum of cholestatic patients (36, 37). Elimination of bile with all its substances by nasobiliary drainage, or removal of albumin-bound substances (including bile salts) by albumin dialysis, often cause a tremendous diminution in the perception of itch, although this only lasts for a few weeks to months after the intervention (38–41). The results of these therapies clearly indicate that pruritogen(s) or progenitors of pruritogens are excreted in bile, but not necessarily that bile salts are causing cholestasis-associated pruritus.

Early research aimed at binding bile salts in the gut by using anion exchange resins (and, thereby, also bile salt sequestrants) like cholestyramine, which resulted in some reduction of pruritus (42–44). However, a more recent report indicates that the later developed, more potent anion exchange resin colesevelam does not improve pruritus more than placebo, despite the fact that bile salt levels were reduced by nearly 50% (45).

The group of Bunnett intensely studied itch signaling by bile salts. They proposed that itch signaling is mediated by the bile salt receptor TGR5. TGR5 expression was detected in the soma of DRG neurons of mice (but not in nerve fibers in the skin or the dorsal horn). Activation of DRG neurons led to the release of the neuropeptide gastrin-releasing peptide (GRP) and the opioid peptide leucine-enkephalin, which are thought to be itch and analgesia transmitters (46). A year later, the same group showed that the TGR5 receptor was co-expressed with the itch channel TRPA1 and activation of this axis induced scratch activity in mice (47). Indications for the involvement of TGR5 in itch signaling seem strong, but the role for bile salts as candidate pruritogens in relation to cholestasis-associated pruritus remains inconclusive. Several clinical studies have shown that there is no correlation between bile salts in serum, urine or skin and the intensity of pruritus (48–51). Pruritus is often one of the first symptoms of cholestatic liver disease, while bile salts levels are still relatively low (52, 53). During late stages of the disease, or in obstructive cholestasis, when bile salt levels can increase to high concentrations, pruritus is sometimes reported to subside (54).

Another receptor that is postulated to be involved in bile salt-induced itch signaling is the mas-related G protein receptor X4 (MRGPRX4). Mouse Mrgpr orthologs were not activated by bile salts and therefore the human receptor was expressed in mice and scratch activity was reported to be increased upon subcutaneous injection of the pruritogen chloroquine and the bile salt deoxycholate (DC) (55). However, injection with unconjugated bile salts is not very representative for cholestasis, since conjugated primary bile salts [like taurochenodeoxycholate (TCDC) and glycochenodeoxycholate (GCDC)] are increased during cholestasis whereas the pool size of conjugates of the secondary bile salt DC is reduced in cholestasis (56). Moreover, unconjugated bile salts diffuse into cells and cause increases in cytosolic free calcium (57, 58). In the same report, mice were treated with the hepatotoxicant α-naphthylisothiocyanate (ANIT), which is a known inducer of cholestasis, serious liver damage, including hepatocellular necrosis and liver fibrosis (59–62). Scratch activity was found to be increased in mice expressing MRGPRX4 compared to control animals, but only during the first 2 days of cholestasis (56), suggesting that this signaling undergoes fairly rapid desensitization. Such a short period of scratch behavior is not representative of the human situation, in which pruritus usually lasts for months and years. Moreover, in two other reports ANIT treatment did not lead to increased scratch activity [(63) and Langedijk et al., submitted].

A second, independent, report on MRGPRX4 showed that intradermal injection of 500 μg DC induced an acute itch sensation in healthy volunteers (64). These researchers showed that MRGPRX4 mRNA is expressed in 6–8% of human DRG neurons and co-expressed with H1R, TRPV1, and $Na_V1.7$ voltage-gated sodium channel; which are all established itch-related channels. Since high concentrations of administered bile salts can lead to direct activation and degranulation of mast cells, and thereby release of histamine (65), the authors included the administration of antihistamines, which did not reduce DC-induced itch, indicating a non-histaminergic mechanism. However, DC, which showed to be the most potent ligand for MRGPRX4 among all tested bile salts, was not present in a different concentration in plasma of itchy vs. non-itchy patients with cholestasis (64). Other bile salts that showed a bigger difference were only weak agonists for MRGPRX4 (64).

Together, these results indicate that bile salts are involved in many processes, by binding to several receptors that are, among others, located on sensory neurons. However, as pruritogens for cholestatic itch, plasma bile salt concentrations do not correlate with clinical complaints of itch. The most prominent example against the theory of bile salts as pruritogens is represented by patients suffering from Na^+-taurocholate cotransporting polypeptide (NTCP)-deficiency. The plasma bile salt levels of these patients can be extremely high, but patients do not complain of pruritus (66–69).

In conclusion, human clinical observations overrule all *in vivo* and *in vitro* research and pose the strongest argument against bile salts as dominant pruritogens in cholestatic itch.

Endogenous Opioids

The role of endogenous opioids in cholestasis-associated pruritus has recently been reviewed by Bergasa (70). Here, we want to discuss the most important arguments that support or dispute the role of endogenous opioids as causative pruritogens in cholestatic liver disease.

The central mechanism of pruritus is thought to include upregulation of the μ-opioid receptor system and suppression of the κ-opioid receptor system (71). One of the first observations in relation to opioids and pruritus is the fact that the μ-receptor agonist morphine can induce pruritus in humans (24, 72), while the μ-receptor antagonist naloxone can inhibit this reaction (73, 74). Endogenous opioid levels, including methionine enkephalin, leucine enkephalin and β-endorphin (μ-receptor agonists), were increased in plasma of bile duct ligated (BDL) animals and cholestatic patients with cirrhosis (75–77). However, in a more recent study the plasma levels of these μ-receptor agonists were comparable between cholestatic patients with and without pruritus, and were not increased in women with ICP compared to regular pregnancies (48). As was shown before in PBC patients, methionine-enkephalin concentrations correlate with the stage of disease but not with the severity of pruritus (75). Most studies into the beneficial effects of opioid antagonists involved few patients (in some cases even case reports) and/or were not placebo-controlled. Although treatment with μ-receptor antagonists like naloxone and naltrexone could reduce the level of pruritus in cholestatic patients, it can also lead to an opiate withdrawal-like reaction (73, 77–81).

Next to inhibiting the μ-opioid receptor, studies have been performed on activating the κ-opioid receptor system in mice, thereby reducing scratch activity induced by substance P, histamine or morphine (82, 83). The κ-receptor agonist nalfurafine has been studied in Japan, to treat pruritus in patients with chronic kidney disease (84, 85) and chronic liver disease (71, 86, 87). Treatment showed a partial decrease in levels of pruritus without any severe adverse events. The κ-opioid receptor agonist asimadoline is being tested in a phase II clinical trial to assess its efficacy on the relief of pruritus in patients with atopic dermatitis (88). For an overview on κ-opioid receptor agonists, see (89).

LPA/ATX

We have reported in earlier studies that lysophosphatidic acid (LPA) is a potential pruritogen in cholestasis (48, 90). LPA in serum of pregnant women with ICP and in serum of PBC patients with pruritus induced an increased Ca^{2+} response when applied to neuronal cells (48). Intradermal injection of LPA in the skin of mice initiated a scratch response, which confirmed a previous independent study (48, 91). The main production of LPA comes from the phospholipase D autotaxin (ATX), which catalyzes the hydrolysis of lysophosphatidylcholine (LPC) into LPA and choline (92–94). ATX (ENPP2) belongs to the family of ectonucleotide pyrophosphatases/phosphodiesterases (ENPP1-7) and promotes multiple functions like cell migration, angiogenesis and metastasis (95). A direct causal relation between plasma ATX and production of LPA is seen in ATX heterozygous mice, which show a reduction of 50% in ATX activity and plasma LPA levels, while ATX-deficient mice die prematurely due to vascular defects (96). High ATX mRNA expression in human tissues has been described for brain, ovary, lung and kidney, while enzyme activity has been detected in blood, cerebrospinal and seminal fluid, urine and saliva [reviewed in (97)]. So far, it is still unclear which of these organs contribute to the circulating ATX levels in human plasma and cerebrospinal fluid. Recently, our group has shown that human enteroendocrine cells of the small intestine are also a source of ATX (98).

LPA can activate neuronal cells, satellite glia cells and other cell types *via* six different LPA-specific receptors (LPAR1-6) (99–101). It has been described that LPA can induce neuropathic pain *via* LPAR1, LPAR3 and LPAR5 (102). However, in a study using the cheek injection mouse model Kittaka et al. (103) showed that LPA is a mediator of only itch rather than of pain. In this study, LPA was found to activate LPAR5 which, *via* intracellular phospholipase D activation, generates intracellular LPA that can activate TRPA1 and TRPV1, and thereby induce itch sensation.

The crystal structure of ATX shows an active site containing a hydrophilic groove, a hydrophobic lipid-binding pocket and a hydrophobic channel (tunnel) (104–106). This tunnel structure is able to selectively bind steroids and bile salts that lead to inhibition of ATX activity (107). The question remains whether more compounds involved in cholestasis can bind in this tunnel, and this way influence ATX activity.

Serum ATX levels are prominently increased in cholestatic patients with pruritus compared to cholestatic patients without pruritus, and in pregnant women with ICP compared to regular pregnancy. In our study, ATX activity correlated significantly with intensity of pruritus and with the effectiveness of treatment by rifampicin, MARS and nasobiliary drainage (48, 90). Serum ATX levels also indicate a therapeutic response to treatment with bezafibrate (108), prednisolone (109) and plasmapheresis (110). Even though ATX is not excreted into bile (48), interruption of the enterohepatic circulation by nasobiliary drainage and ASBT-inhibition still led to a decrease in both circulating ATX levels and pruritus scores (48, 111–113). These findings strongly indicate a tight relation between serum ATX levels and pruritus.

On the other hand, serum ATX levels are similarly increased in (pathological) conditions without itch, including regular pregnancy, some cancer entities and chronic viral hepatitis B and C. In several liver diseases accompanied by liver fibrosis (but not itch), serum ATX levels can also act as a marker of severity of liver injury [including non-alcoholic steatosis hepatitis (NASH) (114), PBC and PSC (115, 116), hepatitis B (117) and hepatitis C (118)]. A recent study reported that ATX levels correlate with fibrosis markers but not with frequency and severity of pruritus in PBC patients (119). A paradox seems to remain in the relation of serum ATX levels to pruritus. A common factor might be involved in both pruritus and liver fibrosis and therefore share ATX as a biomarker. Together, these results suggest that research into other cholestatic factors, that play a more dominant role in the initiation and/or potentiation of pruritus in cholestasis, is warranted.

Serotonin

Serotonin (5-HT) is a neurotransmitter in the central nervous system that can directly activate sensory neurons (120–122). Serotonin can be released from mast cells in the skin and can act as a pruritogen (123–125). The serotonergic system might be deregulated in cholestatic patients (126) and in patients with atopic dermatitis (127), leading to chronic pruritus. In rats with cholestasis induced by BDL, serotonin levels in the skin and spinal cord were significantly increased compared to sham mice, and enhanced scratching behavior was noted after mechanical and heat stimulation (128). In the absence of mechanical and heat stimuli, however, these mice showed no increased spontaneous scratching activity while they were clearly cholestatic.

Seven classes of 5-HT receptors have been identified (5-HT1-7) that comprise at least fifteen subtypes, of which all but one are metabotropic GPCRs (129, 130). 5-HT2 receptors are suggested to be important for itch perception (131, 132), by signaling through $G_{q/11}$, which activates PLC (124, 129). Many pruritogens bind to metabotropic receptors on primary sensory neurons and are coupled to ionotropic channels *via* intracellular signaling pathways to allow sufficient current influx to generate action potentials (133). The cation channels TRPV1 and TRPA1 are often involved in itch transmission (134). A similar mechanism of a metabotropic receptor coupling to an ionotropic channel was found by Morita et al., where serotonin induces itch *via* activation of 5-HT7, which was shown to be coupled to TRPA1 (135). In a mouse model of atopic dermatitis, where mice were lacking 5-HT7 or TRPA1, the animals displayed reduced scratching. The authors suggest a role for 5-HT7 antagonists in the treatment of a variety of pathological itch conditions (135). By investigating the peripheral neuronal mechanisms underlying pruritus, Imamachi et al. showed that serotonin-induced pruritus in mice required the presence of PLCβ3 and TRPV1-expressing neurons, although not the TRPV1-channel itself (30). The TRPV4-channel, however, does seem to be involved as shown by reduced serotonin-evoked scratch bouts in TRPV4 knockout mice and wild type mice treated with a TRPV4 antagonist (131).

Selective serotonin reuptake inhibitors (SSRIs) have shown some effect against pruritus in cholestatic patients (136–139). They inhibit pre-synaptic reuptake of serotonin and might dull transmission of nociceptive stimuli through unmyelinated C-fibers (120, 140). When standard therapies have no effect on the reduction of pruritus, the SSRI sertraline is advised as a fourth line treatment (141). Notably, chronic pruritus is often associated with psychopathology, including anxiety and depression, where SSRIs may improve pruritus by treating underlying psychiatric comorbidities (142).

Histamine

Histamine is the best established pruritogen during acute allergic reactions, by activating histamine receptors (which are GPCRs) and TRP channels on sensory nerve endings. Antagonists of H1R are useful for the treatment of acute allergic pruritus, but are ineffective in the treatment of cholestasis-associated pruritus (141). Although plasma histamine levels have been reported to be slightly increased in cholestatic disease (143), in the study of Kremer et al., no correlation was found between plasma histamine levels and itch intensity in pruritic patients with ICP, PBC and other cholestatic disorders (48). Also skin changes consistent with histamine-mediated effects, like axon-reflex erythema (144), are not seen in cholestatic disease. Sedation with antihistamines may have a non-specific beneficial effect by improving sleep at night, but they reduce concentration during the day (145). Primary afferent neurons, responsible for histamine-induced itch in humans, belong to the group of mechano-insensitive unmyelinated C-fibers (7, 23, 146). However, a second group of C-fibers exist, that are insensitive to histamine, but sensitive to low intensity, high frequency electrical stimulation, which could explain itch without accompanying axon-reflex erythema (23, 144).

Bilirubin

Bilirubin is an essential component in bile and is the direct cause of jaundice in cholestatic diseases. It was recently hypothesized that bilirubin could act as a pruritogen by stimulating human MRGPRX4 and mouse mrgpral (147). MRGPRs are a family of GPCRs expressed in DRGs on primary sensory neurons (148, 149). In the study of Meixiong, the mouse receptor mrgpral and the human receptor MRGPRX4 were expressed in mouse DRGs that lacked expression of any other MRGPR (Mrgpr cluster KO mice). Bilirubin could activate 14 and 32% of the respective DRGs. Induction of cholestasis in mice by treatment with the hepatotoxicant ANIT led to hyperbilirubinemia and increased scratch activity, which was reduced in mrgpral KO and biliverdin reductase KO mice. From these results, the authors suggest that high serum bilirubin levels are involved in cholestasis-associated pruritus by binding to MRGPRX4 on sensory neurons (147).

Results from clinical observations, however, suggest otherwise. It has been shown multiple times that plasma bilirubin correlates poorly with pruritus intensity in cholestatic patients (50, 150). Pruritus is often observed while at the same time serum bilirubin levels are hardly elevated (141). Furthermore, many patients that suffer from pruritus are not jaundiced and vice versa, many jaundiced patients do not complain of itch. Patients with Dubin Johnson syndrome or Crigler Najjar syndrome type I have medium to very high plasma levels of bilirubin (conjugated and unconjugated, respectively) and hardly ever complain about itching (151). These results suggest that bilirubin is not a dominant pruritogen in cholestasis-associated pruritus.

Steroid Metabolites

Steroids like progesterone and estrogen might be involved in the pathogenesis of cholestasis-associated pruritus, particularly in the case of ICP. Progesterone and estrogen metabolites can be converted into steroids with a cholestatic potential (152). In women with ICP, serum concentrations of progesterone metabolites (pregnanediol sulfates) are elevated at 35–41 weeks of gestation (153, 154). These progesterone metabolites have been implicated as potential pruritogens from analyses of urine samples from ICP cases (155, 156). Progesterone metabolites can interact with the bile salt receptor FXR (153, 156), the bile salt transporter NTCP (157) and the bile salt export pump (BSEP) (158), thereby affecting bile salt homeostasis pathways and inhibiting hepatic bile salt uptake and efflux. This could possibly result in or contribute to cholestasis and hypercholanemia.

Three pregnanediol sulfates are found at increased concentrations in plasma during gestational weeks 9–15, prior to symptom onset of ICP (156). These concentrations were (weakly) associated with itch severity and were able to differentiate between women with ICP compared to those with benign pruritus gravidarum (156). One of these progesterone sulfates, 5β-pregnan-3α,-20α-diol-3-sulfate (PM3S), evoked a Tgr5-dependent scratch response in mice (156). Together, these results suggest that steroid metabolites might influence pruriception in cholestasis. Further research into steroid metabolites is needed to evaluate their mechanism in cholestasis-associated pruritus.

PAR2-Agonists

Protease-activated receptors (PARs) are implicated in somatosensory functions like itch and pain (159). They have been studied in relation to chronic itch in atopic dermatitis patients. PARs consist of four members, where PAR2 is highly expressed in keratinocytes and is thought to be involved in pruritus caused by atopic dermatitis (159–162). Activation of PAR2 in keratinocytes induces the release of pruritogenic cytokines that can induce itch through channels on sensory neurons (159). A recent study of Zhao et al. suggested that PAR2 mediates itch *via* TRPV3 signaling. Both PAR2 and TRPV1 were shown to be upregulated in the skin of patients with atopic dermatitis and in mouse models for atopic dermatitis (163).

PAR2 can be activated by the agonist SLIGRL and the proteases trypsin and tryptase. Skin application of those compounds have been shown to induce itch and scratch behavior in humans and in mice, respectively (162, 164–167). However, the shorter peptide, SLIGR, which also activates PAR2, did not induce scratching behavior but rather induced thermal hyperalgesia (168). Tryptase is a mast cell derived protease, which has been evaluated in cholestasis-associated pruritus, but a correlation with pruritus intensity could not be found (48). However, other proteases might be involved in cholestasis-associated pruritus that could signal through PAR2 and illicit itch sensation.

Gut Microbiome

Since cholestasis-associated pruritus is significantly improved by treatment with the antibiotic rifampicin (169), it seems plausible that gut microbiota are involved in cholestatic liver disease. The first link between gut microbiota and liver pathogenesis was made by Pereira et al., who hypothesized that neutrophil activators involved in inflammatory bowel disease, pass from the inflamed colon to the liver *via* the enterohepatic circulation (170). Biliary lactoferrin concentrations were increased in active ulcerative colitis and Crohn's disease, and fell with colectomy and disease remission. Patients with PSC are often also identified with inflammatory bowel disease. This suggests a potential role for gut-derived factors.

In a review of Li et al., several studies are discussed that suggest the important role of intestinal microbiota in the etiopathogenesis of cholestatic liver diseases by regulating metabolism and immune responses (171). A study in 2016 showed a reduction of several potential beneficial microbiota and enrichment of opportunistic pathogens in early-stage PBC patients compared to healthy controls (171, 172). Species richness was reduced in PBC patients, resulting in a shift in overall microbial diversity (171, 173). These results were ameliorated after ursodeoxycholic acid (UDCA) treatment. However, in both of these studies, cholestasis-associated pruritus was not measured. Probiotic studies have shown antipruritic effects in patients with atopic dermatitis (174, 175).

Recently, Hegade et al. performed a study in which they compared PBC-patients suffering from pruritus with non-symptomatic PBC patients and healthy volunteers (113). The gut microbiota showed no significant difference between those groups, suggesting that cholestasis-associated pruritus is not associated with a specific gut bacterial composition. However, after treatment with the ASBT-inhibitor linerixibat (GSK2330672), which reduces pruritus scores in PBC patients, fecal bacterial composition significantly changed from baseline. These changes might be due to the increased bile salt load in the colon resulting from ASBT inhibition (112, 113). Together, these studies do not support a major role for gut microbiota in the pathology of cholestasis-associated pruritus.

Treatment of Cholestasis-Associated Pruritus

Evidence-Based Treatments

Evidence-based and experimental treatments for cholestasis-associated pruritus have recently been reviewed (176). Here, we will provide a brief overview. In general, treatment of pruritus can be associated with a considerable placebo effect when using subjective patient-reported outcomes (177, 178). In line with European Association for the Study of the Liver (141), patients with PBC, but also various other cholestatic liver diseases are treated with ursodeoxycholic acid (UDCA). UDCA exerts potent anticholestatic effects and improves biochemical surrogate markers of prognosis such as serum bilirubin or alkaline phosphatase (ALP), histological features (179–181) and liver transplantation-free survival in PBC and, according to most recently reported preliminary data, also in PSC. A beneficial effect of UDCA on pruritus, however, was not reported in large trials.

The non-specific peroxisome proliferator-activated receptor (PPAR) agonist bezafibrate has most recently been shown to effectively improve severe to moderate pruritus in 74 patients with PSC and PBC in a prospective, randomized, double-blind, placebo-controlled trial (182, 183). Bezafibrate has first been introduced as 2nd line treatment of PBC in Japan (184) in combination with UDCA in patients incompletely responding to UDCA alone. Its anticholestatic effect and that of the PPARα agonist fenofibrate has since then been documented in various small trials (185), and finally in a prospective, randomized, placebo-controlled study in 100 patients with PBC treated over 2 years (108, 186) convincingly confirmed. In this trial, a minor antipruritic effect of bezafibrate represented one of the favorable secondary observations in PBC patients with mild pruritus. A case series describing an antipruritic effect of bezafibrate was published in 2018 (187). It remains unclear at present whether bezafibrate is superior to the selective PPARα agonist fenofibrate, which also exerts anticholestatic and antipruritic effects in PBC. With its antipruritic, anticholestatic, and anti-inflammatory effects in fibrosing cholangiopathies such as PSC or PBC and its safety profile, bezafibrate—and potentially other PPAR agonists—should become the 1st line treatment in cholestasis-associated pruritus in the future.

The antibiotic rifampicin is a potent pregnane X receptor (PXR) agonist, and, thereby, inducer of phase 1 and phase 2 biotransformation enzymes including cytochrome P450 3A4, a major drug-metabolizing enzyme. Rifampicin is widely used to reduce cholestasis-associated pruritus and is recommended as a second line antipruritic agent (81, 188). It induces biotransformation of many endogenous and exogenous compounds by phase 1 (e.g., hydroxylation) and phase 2 (e.g., glucuronidation) reactions (189–191) to more water-soluble molecules which can then be excreted *via* the renal route. The antibacterial effects of rifampicin on intestinal flora may alter metabolization and absorption of primary and secondary bile salts and pruritogens (188). Additionally, rifampicin can downregulate ATX expression *via* PXR-dependent mechanisms and, thereby, reduce formation of the pruritogen LPA (90). Currently, it is still unclear whether one or the other of these effects plays a prominent role in the anti-pruritic action of rifampicin. Adverse effects of rifampicin include discoloring of body fluids and teeth and resistance against rifampicin-sensitive bacteria. Use of rifampicin for over more than 2 weeks may enhance the risk of hepatotoxicity and therefore requires strict guidance in patients with liver disease (141).

As third-line treatment for pruritus, oral opioid antagonists like naltrexone and naloxone are used (81, 192, 193). Endogenous opioids were found to be elevated in plasma of patients with acute liver disease and cirrhosis with ascites (77) but Kremer et al. did not observe a correlation between itch and plasma opioid activity (48). Opioid antagonists are able to reduce pruritus (77, 193); however, they also can cause severe side effects similar to opioid withdrawal symptoms (79) and should be started at low daily doses.

Patients that are resistant to above-mentioned treatments can receive the selective serotonin reuptake inhibitor (SSRI) sertraline as a fourth-line treatment (137). This antidepressant can alter potential pruritic pathways involving serotonin.

In the past, cholestyramine was used as the first-line recommended treatment against pruritus. Cholestyramine is an anion-exchange resin that can bind and sequester numerous amphiphilic compounds including bile salts and (other?) potential pruritogens in the intestine (43, 194, 195). Despite the long history of use, evidence for efficacy of this treatment modality is moderate at best (141, 196). In addition, cholestyramine quite often causes gastrointestinal complaints. In a prospective, randomized, placebo-controlled trial, a more potent anion-exchange resin, colesevelam, was able to reduce bile salt levels by nearly 50%, but no effect was observed on intensity of pruritus when compared to placebo (45). Therefore, we conclude that anion-exchange resins should not anymore be ranked among evidence-based, recommended treatment options and rather should have a role as escape medication when other (above discussed) antipruritic medications fail or are not tolerated.

Invasive Treatments

Invasive treatments are indicated for patients that do not respond to abovementioned medical drug therapies. Patients can undergo extracorporeal albumin dialysis (41, 182), plasmapheresis (110, 183–185) and biliary drainage (38–40). These treatments, if effective, only last for days or a few weeks and in exceptional cases months, after which pruritus returns. Surgical partial internal/external biliary diversion can be a permanent solution in children when performed before advanced liver disease has developed (186). Liver transplantation can be performed as a last resort for severe cholestasis-associated pruritus refractory to medical and invasive therapeutic approaches.

Experimental Treatments

Pruritogens might undergo enterohepatic circulation in a similar way as bile salts do. The reuptake of bile salts and other compounds in the ileum, through the intestinal apical sodium-dependent bile acid transporter (ASBT), can be reduced by the use of ASBT-inhibitors and can give a strong reduction of itch sensation in patients. Several inhibitory pharmaceuticals have been developed, which have minimal systemic absorption, thereby only affecting absorption in the intestine. More recent ASBT inhibitors studied include linerixibat (GSK2330672) (112, 113), maralixibat (SHP625) (178) and odevixibat (A4250) (111). Clinical trials with cholestatic patients suffering from pruritus showed promising, but equivocal, results in reducing pruritus (111–113, 178). Frequent adverse events were diarrhea and abdominal discomfort possibly due to increased bile salt load in the large intestine. Notably, the majority of these adverse events resolved over time in one of the studies (178).

In a placebo-controlled trial the effect of the κ-opioid antagonist nalfurafine was found to mildly reduce cholestasis-associated itch in 318 patients with chronic cholestasis-associated itch without major side effects (86).

Since serum ATX levels correlate well with itch intensity in cholestatic patients, and the ATX product LPA can act as a pruritogen (48, 90), future therapy for cholestasis-associated pruritus might include ATX-inhibitors [reviewed in (187)]. Current research on ATX and ATX-inhibition is predominantly performed in the cancer and inflammation fields (197, 198). The ATX-LPA axis is involved in multiple functions, including cell migration, angiogenesis and metastasis (95). Future studies will have to study the safety and efficacy of ATX-inhibitors and their potential role in cholestasis-associated pruritus.

CHALLENGES AND FUTURE PERSPECTIVES OF CHOLESTASIS-ASSOCIATED PRURITUS RESEARCH

Patients with cholestatic diseases often suffer from severe, chronic pruritus, which impairs their quality of life. It is up to researchers to unravel the mechanism of cholestasis-associated pruritus, and even more importantly, to provide a treatment to reduce or resolve this burden.

This review highlights the fact that for cholestasis-associated pruritus there are many possible pruritogens, of which several are likely to play a role simultaneously. Due to different theories on the cause of cholestasis-associated pruritus, also different treatments exist of which none has yet shown to represent the final solution. Research in this field will have to continue in order to clarify the mechanism and to provide a satisfying treatment for patients with cholestasis-associated pruritus.

One of the biggest challenges in cholestasis-associated pruritus research is the possible multi-organ aspect. Besides the affected liver, multiple other organs play a potential role in cholestasis-associated pruritus, including the intestine with its enterohepatic circulation of multiple unknown compounds, the blood with all its proteins, hormones and lipids, the skin with its receptors, barriers and nerves, and the brain of which still a lot is unknown. All of these aspects can affect the production, transport, accumulation, binding, metabolism, and excretion of potential pruritogen(s).

The next questions arise; are pruritogens produced in a higher amount in patients with cholestatic disease as compared to healthy people as a consequence of cholestasis, or are they normally present and do they accumulate due to cholestatic circumstances? Is it possible that there is increased production of pruritogens as a secondary effect of accumulation of non-pruritogens? Bile formation is an important way of eliminating waste products; however, many compounds in bile are recirculated in the enterohepatic circulation, which opens the possibility of accumulation during cholestasis. We can interrupt the complete enterohepatic circulation [by anion-exchange resins, nasobiliary drainage, ASBT-inhibition or partial external biliary diversion (PEBD)], or remove hypothetical compounds from the circulation (by plasmapheresis or albumin dialysis), but we still do not know for which compounds elimination is essential. Based on the most recent studies, we would expect higher levels of pruritogens in plasma (and possibly even in bile) of patients with chronic pruritus compared to people without chronic pruritus, since elimination or filtration provides relief of pruritus. However, the possibility remains that pruritus is not caused by a change in the level of pruritogens but rather the sensitivity to them. Thus, in patients with cholestasis-associated pruritus there might be a change in sensory signaling involving receptor expression in neurons or the skin. These alternatives need to be investigated in detail still.

Another challenge in pruritus research is the way of measuring pruritus (in mice and men), which is best analyzed in a mechanic or sensory way, but mental experience is also a potent factor in human patients with pruritus. The amount or intensity of pruritus needs to be expressed in an objective value which is comparable between individuals, and not affected by side effects like emotions, mental stress or fatigue. An important challenge in pruritus research is correcting for the placebo effect of possible treatment. Several studies have shown that treatment with placebo already improves itch sensation by a great deal. Hence, a placebo group should always be included.

Detection of pruritogens involved in cholestasis might find its future in untargeted metabolomic research. All metabolites of bile, serum and possibly skin can be measured and compared between groups. The question remains whether all metabolites can yet be identified and traced back to their origin, but future research will expand the pool of identified metabolites. This approach might reveal a more specific target to unravel the mechanisms and develop a better treatment for cholestasis-associated pruritus.

AUTHOR CONTRIBUTIONS

JL wrote the review with intellectual guidance by UB and RO. All authors contributed to the article and approved the submitted version.

REFERENCES

1. Beuers U, Kremer AE, Bolier R, Elferink RP. Pruritus in cholestasis: facts and fiction. *Hepatology.* (2014) 60:399–407. doi: 10.1002/hep.26909
2. Arrese M, Macias RI, Briz O, Perez MJ, Marin JJ. Molecular pathogenesis of intrahepatic cholestasis of pregnancy. *Expert Rev Mol Med.* (2008) 10:e9. doi: 10.1017/S1462399408000628
3. Reyes H, Sulfated progesterone metabolites in the pathogenesis of intrahepatic cholestasis of pregnancy: another loop in the ascending spiral of medical knowledge. *Hepatology.* (2016) 63:1080–2. doi: 10.1002/hep.28365
4. Bell JK, McQueen DS, Rees JL. Involvement of histamine H4 and H1 receptors in scratching induced by histamine receptor agonists in Balb C mice. *Br J Pharmacol.* (2004) 142:374–80. doi: 10.1038/sj.bjp.0705754
5. Liu Q, Tang Z, Surdenikova L, Kim S, Patel KN, Kim A, et al. Sensory neuron-specific GPCR Mrgprs are itch receptors mediating chloroquine-induced pruritus. *Cell.* (2009) 139:1353–65. doi: 10.1016/j.cell.2009.11.034
6. Reddy VB, Iuga AO, Shimada SG, LaMotte RH, Lerner EA. Cowhage-evoked itch is mediated by a novel cysteine protease: a ligand of protease-activated receptors. *J Neurosci.* (2008) 28:4331–5. doi: 10.1523/JNEUROSCI.0716-08.2008
7. Schmelz M, Schmidt R, Bickel A, Handwerker HO, Torebjork HE. Specific C-receptors for itch in human skin. *J Neurosci.* (1997) 17:8003–8. doi: 10.1523/JNEUROSCI.17-20-08003.1997
8. Andrew D, Craig AD. Spinothalamic lamina I neurons selectively sensitive to histamine: a central neural pathway for itch. *Nat Neurosci.* (2001) 4:72–7. doi: 10.1038/82924
9. Yosipovitch G, Rosen JD, Hashimoto T. Itch: From mechanism to (novel) therapeutic approaches. *J Allergy Clin Immunol.* (2018) 142:1375–90. doi: 10.1016/j.jaci.2018.09.005
10. Andersen HH, Elberling J, Solvsten H, Yosipovitch G, Arendt-Nielsen L. Nonhistaminergic and mechanical itch sensitization in atopic dermatitis. *Pain.* (2017) 158:1780–91. doi: 10.1097/j.pain.0000000000000980
11. Davidson S, Zhang X, Yoon CH, Khasabov SG, Simone DA, Giesler GJ, Jr. The itch-producing agents histamine and cowhage activate separate populations of primate spinothalamic tract neurons. *J Neurosci.* (2007) 27:10007–14. doi: 10.1523/JNEUROSCI.2862-07.2007
12. Shelley WB, Arthur RP. Mucunain, the active pruritogenic proteinase of cowhage. *Science.* (1955) 122:469–70. doi: 10.1126/science.122.3167.469
13. Shelley WB, Arthur RP. Studies on cowhage (*Mucuna pruriens*) and its pruritogenic proteinase, mucunain. *AMA Arch Derm.* (1955) 72:399–406. doi: 10.1001/archderm.1955.03730350001001
14. Johanek LM, Meyer RA, Friedman RM, Greenquist KW, Shim B, Borzan J, et al. A role for polymodal C-fiber afferents in nonhistaminergic itch. *J Neurosci.* (2008) 28:7659–69. doi: 10.1523/JNEUROSCI.1760-08.2008
15. Namer B, Carr R, Johanek LM, Schmelz M, Handwerker HO, Ringkamp M. Separate peripheral pathways for pruritus in man. *J Neurophysiol.* (2008) 100:2062–9. doi: 10.1152/jn.90482.2008
16. Mishra SK, Hoon MA. The cells and circuitry for itch responses in mice. *Science.* (2013) 340:968–71. doi: 10.1126/science.1233765
17. Koga K, Chen T, Li XY, Descalzi G, Ling J, Gu J, et al. Glutamate acts as a neurotransmitter for gastrin releasing peptide-sensitive and insensitive itch-related synaptic transmission in mammalian spinal cord. *Mol Pain.* (2011) 7:47. doi: 10.1186/1744-8069-7-47
18. Lagerstrom MC, Rogoz K, Abrahamsen B, Persson E, Reinius B, Nordenankar K, et al. VGLUT2-dependent sensory neurons in the TRPV1 population regulate pain and itch. *Neuron.* (2010) 68:529–42. doi: 10.1016/j.neuron.2010.09.016

19. Liu Y, Abdel Samad O, Zhang L, Duan B, Tong Q, Lopes C, et al. VGLUT2-dependent glutamate release from nociceptors is required to sense pain and suppress itch. *Neuron.* (2010) 68:543–56. doi: 10.1016/j.neuron.2010.09.008
20. Sun YG, Chen ZF. A gastrin-releasing peptide receptor mediates the itch sensation in the spinal cord. *Nature.* (2007) 448:700–3. doi: 10.1038/nature06029
21. Sun YG, Zhao ZQ, Meng XL, Yin J, Liu XY, Chen ZF. Cellular basis of itch sensation. *Science.* (2009) 325:1531–4. doi: 10.1126/science.1174868
22. Yosipovitch G, Bernhard JD. Clinical practice. *Chronic pruritus. N Engl J Med.* (2013) 368:1625–34. doi: 10.1056/NEJMcp1208814
23. Ikoma A, Steinhoff M, Stander S, Yosipovitch G, Schmelz M. The neurobiology of itch. *Nat Rev Neurosci.* (2006) 7:535–47. doi: 10.1038/nrn1950
24. Ballantyne JC, Loach AB, Carr DB. Itching after epidural and spinal opiates. *Pain.* (1988) 33:149–60. doi: 10.1016/0304-3959(88)90085-1
25. Atanassoff PG, Brull SJ, Zhang J, Greenquist K, Silverman DG, Lamotte RH. Enhancement of experimental pruritus and mechanically evoked dysesthesiae with local anesthesia. *Somatosens Mot Res.* (1999) 16:291–8. doi: 10.1080/08990229970357
26. Ross SE, Mardinly AR, McCord AE, Zurawski J, Cohen S, Jung C, et al. Loss of inhibitory interneurons in the dorsal spinal cord and elevated itch in Bhlhb5 mutant mice. *Neuron.* (2010) 65:886–98. doi: 10.1016/j.neuron.2010.02.025
27. Dong X, Dong X. Peripheral and central mechanisms of itch. *Neuron.* (2018) 98:482–94. doi: 10.1016/j.neuron.2018.03.023
28. Wilson SR, Gerhold KA, Bifolck-Fisher A, Liu Q, Patel KN, Dong X, et al. TRPA1 is required for histamine-independent, Mas-related G protein-coupled receptor-mediated itch. *Nat Neurosci.* (2011) 14:595–602. doi: 10.1038/nn.2789
29. Amadesi S, Cottrell GS, Divino L, Chapman K, Grady EF, Bautista F, et al. Protease-activated receptor 2 sensitizes TRPV1 by protein kinase Cepsilon- and A-dependent mechanisms in rats and mice. *J Physiol.* (2006) 575:555–71. doi: 10.1113/jphysiol.2006.111534
30. Imamachi N, Park GH, Lee H, Anderson DJ, Simon MI, Basbaum AI, et al. TRPV1-expressing primary afferents generate behavioral responses to pruritogens via multiple mechanisms. *Proc Natl Acad Sci USA.* (2009) 106:11330–5. doi: 10.1073/pnas.0905605106
31. Jurcakova D, Ru F, Kollarik M, Sun H, Krajewski J, Undem BJ. Voltage-gated sodium channels regulating action potential generation in itch-, nociceptive-, and low-threshold mechanosensitive cutaneous C-fibers. *Mol Pharmacol.* (2018) 94:1047–56. doi: 10.1124/mol.118.112839
32. Kittaka H, Tominaga M. The molecular and cellular mechanisms of itch and the involvement of TRP channels in the peripheral sensory nervous system and skin. *Allergol Int.* (2017) 66:22–30. doi: 10.1016/j.alit.2016.10.003
33. Moore C, Gupta R, Jordt SE, Chen Y, Liedtke WB. Regulation of pain and itch by TRP channels. *Neurosci Bull.* (2018) 34:120–42. doi: 10.1007/s12264-017-0200-8
34. Xie Z, Hu H. TRP channels as drug targets to relieve itch. *Pharmaceuticals (Basel).* (2018) 11:100. doi: 10.3390/ph11040100
35. Schaap FG, Trauner M, Jansen PL. Bile acid receptors as targets for drug development. *Nat Rev Gastroenterol Hepatol.* (2014) 11:55–67. doi: 10.1038/nrgastro.2013.151
36. Trottier J, Bialek A, Caron P, Straka RJ, Heathcote J, Milkiewicz P, et al. Metabolomic profiling of 17 bile acids in serum from patients with primary biliary cirrhosis and primary sclerosing cholangitis: a pilot study. *Dig Liver Dis.* (2012) 44:303–10. doi: 10.1016/j.dld.2011.10.025
37. Woolbright BL, Dorko K, Antoine DJ, Clarke JI, Gholami P, Li F, et al. Bile acid-induced necrosis in primary human hepatocytes and in patients with obstructive cholestasis. *Toxicol Appl Pharmacol.* (2015) 283:168–77. doi: 10.1016/j.taap.2015.01.015
38. Hegade VS, Krawczyk M, Kremer AE, Kuczka J, Gaouar F, Kuiper EM, et al. The safety and efficacy of nasobiliary drainage in the treatment of refractory cholestatic pruritus: a multicentre European study. *Aliment Pharmacol Ther.* (2016) 43:294–302. doi: 10.1111/apt.13449
39. Beuers U, Gerken G, Pusl T. Biliary drainage transiently relieves intractable pruritus in primary biliary cirrhosis. *Hepatology.* (2006) 44:280–1. doi: 10.1002/hep.21271
40. Stapelbroek JM, van Erpecum KJ, Klomp LW, Venneman NG, Schwartz TP, van Berge Henegouwen GP, et al. Nasobiliary drainage induces long-lasting remission in benign recurrent intrahepatic cholestasis. *Hepatology.* (2006) 43:51–3. doi: 10.1002/hep.20998
41. Pares A, Herrera M, Aviles J, Sanz M, Mas A. Treatment of resistant pruritus from cholestasis with albumin dialysis: combined analysis of patients from three centers. *J Hepatol.* (2010) 53:307–12. doi: 10.1016/j.jhep.2010.02.031
42. Carey JB, Jr., Bile acids in the serum of jaundiced patients. *Gastroenterology.* (1961) 41:285–7. doi: 10.1016/S0016-5085(19)35143-1
43. Datta DV, Sherlock S. Cholestyramine for long term relief of the pruritus complicating intrahepatic cholestasis. *Gastroenterology.* (1966) 50:323–32. doi: 10.1016/S0016-5085(66)80071-9
44. Oster ZH, Rachmilewitz EA, Moran E, Stein Y. Relief of pruritus by cholestyramine in chronic liver disease. *Isr J Med Sci.* (1965) 1:599–606.
45. Kuiper EM, van Erpecum KJ, Beuers U, Hansen BE, Thio HB, de Man RA, et al. The potent bile acid sequestrant colesevelam is not effective in cholestatic pruritus: results of a double-blind, randomized, placebo-controlled trial. *Hepatology.* (2010) 52:1334–40. doi: 10.1002/hep.23821
46. Alemi F, Kwon E, Poole DP, Lieu T, Lyo V, Cattaruzza F, et al. The TGR5 receptor mediates bile acid-induced itch and analgesia. *J Clin Invest.* (2013) 123:1513–30. doi: 10.1172/JCI64551
47. Lieu T, Jayaweera G, Zhao P, Poole DP, Jensen D, Grace M, et al. The bile acid receptor TGR5 activates the TRPA1 channel to induce itch in mice. *Gastroenterology.* (2014) 147:1417–28. doi: 10.1053/j.gastro.2014.08.042
48. Kremer AE, Martens JJ, Kulik W, Rueff F, Kuiper EM, van Buuren HR, et al. Lysophosphatidic acid is a potential mediator of cholestatic pruritus. *Gastroenterology.* (2010) 139:1008–18. doi: 10.1053/j.gastro.2010.05.009
49. Bartholomew TC, Summerfield JA, Billing BH, Lawson AM, Setchell KD. Bile acid profiles of human serum and skin interstitial fluid and their relationship to pruritus studied by gas chromatography-mass spectrometry. *Clin Sci (Lond).* (1982) 63:65–73. doi: 10.1042/cs0630065
50. Freedman MR, Holzbach RT, Ferguson DR. Pruritus in cholestasis—no direct causative role for bile-acid retention. *Am J Med.* (1981) 70:1011–6. doi: 10.1016/0002-9343(81)90857-3
51. Ghent CN, Bloomer JR, Klatskin G. Elevations in skin tissue levels of bile-acids in human cholestasis—relation to serum levels and to pruritus. *Gastroenterology.* (1977) 73:1125–30. doi: 10.1016/S0016-5085(19)31870-0
52. Geenes V, Williamson C. Intrahepatic cholestasis of pregnancy. *World J Gastroenterol.* (2009) 15:2049–66. doi: 10.3748/wjg.15.2049
53. Kremer AE, Beuers U, Oude-Elferink RP, Pusl T. Pathogenesis and treatment of pruritus in cholestasis. *Drugs.* (2008) 68:2163–82. doi: 10.2165/00003495-200868150-00006
54. Murphy GM, Ross A, Billing BH. Serum bile acids in primary biliary cirrhosis. *Gut.* (1972) 13:201–6. doi: 10.1136/gut.13.3.201
55. Meixiong J, Vasavda C, Snyder SH, Dong X. MRGPRX4 is a G protein-coupled receptor activated by bile acids that may contribute to cholestatic pruritus. *Proc Natl Acad Sci USA.* (2019) 116:10525–30. doi: 10.1073/pnas.1903316116
56. Beuers U, Spengler U, Zwiebel FM, Pauletzki J, Fischer S, Paumgartner G. Effect of ursodeoxycholic acid on the kinetics of the major hydrophobic bile acids in health and in chronic cholestatic liver disease. *Hepatology.* (1992) 15:603–8. doi: 10.1002/hep.1840150409
57. Dziki AJ, Batzri S, Harmon JW, Molloy M. Cellular hypercalcemia is an early event in deoxycholate injury of rabbit gastric mucosal cells. *Am J Physiol.* (1995) 269:G287–96. doi: 10.1152/ajpgi.1995.269.2.G287
58. Lau BW, Colella M, Ruder WC, Ranieri M, Curci S, Hofer AM. Deoxycholic acid activates protein kinase C and phospholipase C *via* increased Ca2+ entry at plasma membrane. *Gastroenterology.* (2005) 128:695–707. doi: 10.1053/j.gastro.2004.12.046
59. Joshi N, Ray JL, Kopec AK, Luyendyk JP. Dose-dependent effects of alpha-naphthylisothiocyanate disconnect biliary fibrosis from hepatocellular necrosis. *J Biochem Mol Toxicol.* (2017) 31:1–7. doi: 10.1002/jbt.21834
60. Golbar HM, Izawa T, Ichikawa C, Tanaka M, Juniantito V, Sawamoto O, et al. Slowly progressive cholangiofibrosis induced in rats by alpha-naphthylisothiocyanate (ANIT), with particular references to characteristics of macrophages and myofibroblasts. *Exp Toxicol Pathol.* (2013) 65:825–35. doi: 10.1016/j.etp.2012.12.001

61. Tjandra K, Sharkey KA, Swain MG. Progressive development of a Th1-type hepatic cytokine profile in rats with experimental cholangitis. *Hepatology.* (2000) 31:280–90. doi: 10.1002/hep.510310204
62. Xu J, Lee G, Wang H, Vierling JM, Maher JJ. Limited role for CXC chemokines in the pathogenesis of alpha-naphthylisothiocyanate-induced liver injury. *Am J Physiol Gastrointest Liver Physiol.* (2004) 287:G734–41. doi: 10.1152/ajpgi.00300.2003
63. Cipriani S, Renga B, D'Amore C, Simonetti M, De Tursi AA, Carino A, et al. Impaired itching perception in murine models of cholestasis is supported by dysregulation of GPBAR1 signaling. *PLoS ONE.* (2015) 10:e0129866. doi: 10.1371/journal.pone.0129866
64. Yu H, Zhao T, Liu S, Wu Q, Johnson O, Wu Z, et al. MRGPRX4 is a bile acid receptor for human cholestatic itch. *Elife.* (2019) 8:48431. doi: 10.7554/eLife.48431
65. Quist RG, Ton-Nu HT, Lillienau J, Hofmann AF, Barrett KE. Activation of mast cells by bile acids. *Gastroenterology.* (1991) 101:446–56. doi: 10.1016/0016-5085(91)90024-F
66. Vaz FM, Paulusma CC, Huidekoper H, de Ru M, Lim C, Koster J, et al. Sodium taurocholate cotransporting polypeptide (SLC10A1) deficiency: conjugated hypercholanemia without a clear clinical phenotype. *Hepatology.* (2015) 61:260–7. doi: 10.1002/hep.27240
67. Van Herpe F, Waterham HR, Adams CJ, Mannens M, Bikker H, Vaz FM, et al. NTCP deficiency and persistently raised bile salts: an adult case. *J Inherit Metab Dis.* (2017) 40:313–5. doi: 10.1007/s10545-017-0031-9
68. Erlinger S, NTCP deficiency: a new inherited disease of bile acid transport. *Clin Res Hepatol Gastroenterol.* (2015) 39:7–8. doi: 10.1016/j.clinre.2014.07.011
69. Vaz FM, Huidekoper HH, Paulusma CC. Extended abstract: deficiency of sodium taurocholate cotransporting polypeptide (SLC10A1): a new inborn error of metabolism with an attenuated phenotype. *Dig Dis.* (2017) 35:259–60. doi: 10.1159/000450984
70. Bergasa NV. The pruritus of cholestasis: from bile acids to opiate agonists: relevant after all these years. *Med Hypotheses.* (2018) 110:86–9. doi: 10.1016/j.mehy.2017.11.002
71. Kamimura K, Yokoo T, Kamimura H, Sakamaki A, Abe S, Tsuchiya A, et al. Long-term efficacy and safety of nalfurafine hydrochloride on pruritus in chronic liver disease patients: patient-reported outcome based analyses. *PLoS ONE.* (2017) 12:e0178991. doi: 10.1371/journal.pone.0178991
72. Cousins MJ, Mather LE. Intrathecal and epidural administration of opioids. *Anesthesiology.* (1984) 61:276–310. doi: 10.1097/00000542-198409000-00008
73. Bergasa NV, Talbot TL, Alling DW, Schmitt JM, Walker EC, Baker BL, et al. A controlled trial of naloxone infusions for the pruritus of chronic cholestasis. *Gastroenterology.* (1992) 102:544–9. doi: 10.1016/0016-5085(92)90102-5
74. Bernstein JE, Swift RM, Soltani K, Lorincz AL. Antipruritic effect of an opiate antagonist, naloxone hydrochloride. *J Invest Dermatol.* (1982) 78:82–3. doi: 10.1111/1523-1747.ep12497974
75. Spivey JR, Jorgensen RA, Gores GJ, Lindor KD. Methionine-enkephalin concentrations correlate with stage of disease but not pruritus in patients with primary biliary cirrhosis. *Am J Gastroenterol.* (1994) 89:2028–32.
76. Swain MG, Rothman RB, Xu H, Vergalla J, Bergasa NV, Jones EA. Endogenous opioids accumulate in plasma in a rat model of acute cholestasis. *Gastroenterology.* (1992) 103:630–5. doi: 10.1016/0016-5085(92)90857-U
77. Thornton JR, Losowsky MS. Opioid peptides and primary biliary cirrhosis. *BMJ.* (1988) 297:1501–4. doi: 10.1136/bmj.297.6662.1501
78. Jones EA, Dekker LR. Florid opioid withdrawal-like reaction precipitated by naltrexone in a patient with chronic cholestasis. *Gastroenterology.* (2000) 118:431–2. doi: 10.1016/S0016-5085(00)70225-3
79. Mansour-Ghanaei F, Taheri A, Froutan H, Ghofrani H, Nasiri-Toosi M, Bagherzadeh AH, et al. Effect of oral naltrexone on pruritus in cholestatic patients. *World J Gastroenterol.* (2006) 12:1125–8. doi: 10.3748/wjg.v12.i7.1125
80. Shawcross DL, Jalan R. Delayed opioid withdrawal-like reaction in primary biliary cirrhosis following naloxone therapy. *Gastroenterology.* (2001) 121:743–4. doi: 10.1053/gast.2001.27714
81. Tandon P, Rowe BH, Vandermeer B, Bain VG. The efficacy and safety of bile Acid binding agents, opioid antagonists, or rifampin in the treatment of cholestasis-associated pruritus. *Am J Gastroenterol.* (2007) 102:1528–36. doi: 10.1111/j.1572-0241.2007.01200.x
82. Togashi Y, Umeuchi H, Okano K, Ando N, Yoshizawa Y, Honda T, et al. Antipruritic activity of the kappa-opioid receptor agonist, TRK-820. *Eur J Pharmacol.* (2002) 435:259–64. doi: 10.1016/S0014-2999(01)01588-6
83. Umeuchi H, Togashi Y, Honda T, Nakao K, Okano K, Tanaka T, et al. Involvement of central mu-opioid system in the scratching behavior in mice, and the suppression of it by the activation of kappa-opioid system. *Eur J Pharmacol.* (2003) 477:29–35. doi: 10.1016/j.ejphar.2003.08.007
84. Kumagai H, Ebata T, Takamori K, Muramatsu T, Nakamoto H, Suzuki H. Effect of a novel kappa-receptor agonist, nalfurafine hydrochloride, on severe itch in 337 haemodialysis patients: a Phase III, randomized, double-blind, placebo-controlled study. *Nephrol Dial Transplant.* (2010) 25:1251–7. doi: 10.1093/ndt/gfp588
85. Wikstrom B, Gellert R, Ladefoged SD, Danda Y, Akai M, Ide K, et al. Kappa-opioid system in uremic pruritus: multicenter, randomized, double-blind, placebo-controlled clinical studies. *J Am Soc Nephrol.* (2005) 16:3742–7. doi: 10.1681/ASN.2005020152
86. Kumada H, Miyakawa H, Muramatsu T, Ando N, Oh T, Takamori K, et al. Efficacy of nalfurafine hydrochloride in patients with chronic liver disease with refractory pruritus: a randomized, double-blind trial. *Hepatol Res.* (2017) 47:972–82. doi: 10.1111/hepr.12830
87. Yagi M, Tanaka A, Namisaki T, Takahashi A, Abe M, Honda A, et al. Is patient-reported outcome improved by nalfurafine hydrochloride in patients with primary biliary cholangitis and refractory pruritus? A post-marketing, single-arm, prospective study. *J Gastroenterol.* (2018) 53:1151–8. doi: 10.1007/s00535-018-1465-z
88. *clinicaltrial.gov: Safety, Pharmacokinetics and Preliminary Efficacy of Asimadoline in Pruritus Associated With Atopic Dermatitis.* Study Director: Dawn McGuire, Tioga Pharmaceuticals, Inc. (2017).
89. Cowan A, Kehner GB, Inan S. Targeting itch with ligands selective for κ opioid receptors. In: Cowan A, Yosipovitch G, editors. *Pharmacology of Itch.* Berlin, Heidelberg: Springer Berlin Heidelberg (2015). p. 291–314.
90. Kremer AE, van Dijk R, Leckie P, Schaap FG, Kuiper EM, Mettang T, et al. Serum autotaxin is increased in pruritus of cholestasis, but not of other origin, and responds to therapeutic interventions. *Hepatology.* (2012) 56:1391–400. doi: 10.1002/hep.25748
91. Hashimoto T, Ohata H, Momose K. Itch-scratch responses induced by lysophosphatidic acid in mice. *Pharmacology.* (2004) 72:51–6. doi: 10.1159/000078632
92. Tanaka M, Okudaira S, Kishi Y, Ohkawa R, Iseki S, Ota M, et al. Autotaxin stabilizes blood vessels and is required for embryonic vasculature by producing lysophosphatidic acid. *J Biol Chem.* (2006) 281:25822–30. doi: 10.1074/jbc.M605142200
93. Tokumura A, Majima E, Kariya Y, Tominaga K, Kogure K, Yasuda K, et al. Identification of human plasma lysophospholipase D, a lysophosphatidic acid-producing enzyme, as autotaxin, a multifunctional phosphodiesterase. *J Biol Chem.* (2002) 277:39436–42. doi: 10.1074/jbc.M205623200
94. Umezu-Goto M, Kishi Y, Taira A, Hama K, Dohmae N, Takio K, et al. Autotaxin has lysophospholipase D activity leading to tumor cell growth and motility by lysophosphatidic acid production. *J Cell Biol.* (2002) 158:227–33. doi: 10.1083/jcb.200204026
95. Moolenaar WH, Perrakis A. Insights into autotaxin: how to produce and present a lipid mediator. *Nat Rev Mol Cell Biol.* (2011) 12:674–9. doi: 10.1038/nrm3188
96. van Meeteren LA, Ruurs P, Stortelers C, Bouwman P, van Rooijen MA, Pradere JP, et al. Autotaxin, a secreted lysophospholipase D, is essential for blood vessel formation during development. *Mol Cell Biol.* (2006) 26:5015–22. doi: 10.1128/MCB.02419-05
97. Jankowski M, Autotaxin: its role in biology of melanoma cells and as a pharmacological target. *Enzyme Res.* (2011) 2011:194857. doi: 10.4061/2011/194857
98. Bolier R, Tolenaars D, Kremer AE, Saris J, Pares A, Verheij J, et al. Enteroendocrine cells are a potential source of serum autotaxin in men. *Biochim Biophys Acta.* (2016) 1862:696–704. doi: 10.1016/j.bbadis.2016.01.012
99. Meyer Zu Heringdorf D. Lysophospholipid receptor-dependent and -independent calcium signaling. *J Cell Biochem.* (2004) 92:937–48. doi: 10.1002/jcb.20107

100. van Meeteren LA, Moolenaar WH. Regulation and biological activities of the autotaxin-LPA axis. *Prog Lipid Res.* (2007) 46:145–60. doi: 10.1016/j.plipres.2007.02.001
101. Robering JW, Gebhardt L, Wolf K, Kuhn H, Kremer AE, Fischer MJM. Lysophosphatidic acid activates satellite glia cells and Schwann cells. *Glia.* (2019) 67:999–1012. doi: 10.1002/glia.23585
102. Choi JW, Chun J. Lysophospholipids and their receptors in the central nervous system. *Biochim Biophys Acta.* (2013) 1831:20–32. doi: 10.1016/j.bbalip.2012.07.015
103. Kittaka H, Uchida K, Fukuta N, Tominaga M. Lysophosphatidic acid-induced itch is mediated by signalling of LPA5 receptor, phospholipase D and TRPA1/TRPV1. *J Physiol.* (2017) 595:2681–98. doi: 10.1113/JP273961
104. Hausmann J, Kamtekar S, Christodoulou E, Day JE, Wu T, Fulkerson Z, et al. Structural basis of substrate discrimination and integrin binding by autotaxin. *Nat Struct Mol Biol.* (2011) 18:198–204. doi: 10.1038/nsmb.1980
105. Inoue K, Tanaka N, Haga A, Yamasaki K, Umeda T, Kusakabe Y, et al. Crystallization and preliminary X-ray crystallographic analysis of human autotaxin. *Acta Crystallogr Sect F Struct Biol Cryst Commun.* (2011) 67:450–3. doi: 10.1107/S174430911005311X
106. Nishimasu H, Okudaira S, Hama K, Mihara E, Dohmae N, Inoue A, et al. Crystal structure of autotaxin and insight into GPCR activation by lipid mediators. *Nat Struct Mol Biol.* (2011) 18:205–12. doi: 10.1038/nsmb.1998
107. Keune WJ, Hausmann J, Bolier R, Tolenaars D, Kremer A, Heidebrecht T, et al. Steroid binding to Autotaxin links bile salts and lysophosphatidic acid signalling. *Nat Commun.* (2016) 7:11248. doi: 10.1038/ncomms11248
108. Kremer AE, Le Cleac'h A, Lemoinne S, Wolf K, De Chaisemartin L, Chollet-Martin S, et al. Antipruritic effect of bezafibrate and serum autotaxin measures in patients with primary biliary cholangitis. *Gut.* (2019) 68:1902–3. doi: 10.1136/gutjnl-2018-317426
109. Sumida H, Nakamura K, Yanagida K, Ohkawa R, Asano Y, Kadono T, et al. Decrease in circulating autotaxin by oral administration of prednisolone. *Clin Chim Acta.* (2013) 415:74–80. doi: 10.1016/j.cca.2012.10.003
110. Heerkens M, Dedden S, Scheepers H, Van Paassen P, Masclee A, de Die-Smulders C, et al. Effect of plasmapheresis on cholestatic pruritus and autotaxin activity during pregnancy. *Hepatology.* (2019) 69:2707–10. doi: 10.1002/hep.30496
111. Al-Dury S, Wahlstrom A, Wahlin S, Langedijk J, Elferink RO, Stahlman M, et al. Pilot study with IBAT inhibitor A4250 for the treatment of cholestatic pruritus in primary biliary cholangitis. *Sci Rep.* (2018) 8:6658. doi: 10.1038/s41598-018-25214-0
112. Hegade VS, Kendrick SF, Dobbins RL, Miller SR, Thompson D, Richards D, et al. Effect of ileal bile acid transporter inhibitor GSK2330672 on pruritus in primary biliary cholangitis: a double-blind, randomised, placebo-controlled, crossover, phase 2a study. *Lancet.* (2017) 389:1114–23. doi: 10.1016/S0140-6736(17)30319-7
113. Hegade VS, Pechlivanis A, McDonald JAK, Rees D, Corrigan M, Hirschfield GM, et al. Autotaxin, bile acid profile and effect of ileal bile acid transporter inhibition in primary biliary cholangitis patients with pruritus. *Liver Int.* (2019) 39:967–75. doi: 10.1111/liv.14069
114. Fujimori N, Umemura T, Kimura T, Tanaka N, Sugiura A, Yamazaki T, et al. Serum autotaxin levels are correlated with hepatic fibrosis and ballooning in patients with non-alcoholic fatty liver disease. *World J Gastroenterol.* (2018) 24:1239–49. doi: 10.3748/wjg.v24.i11.1239
115. Joshita S, Umemura T, Usami Y, Yamashita Y, Norman GL, Sugiura A, et al. Serum autotaxin is a useful disease progression marker in patients with primary biliary cholangitis. *Sci Rep.* (2018) 8:8159. doi: 10.1038/s41598-018-26531-0
116. Wunsch E, Krawczyk M, Milkiewicz M, Trottier J, Barbier O, Neurath MF, et al. Serum autotaxin is a marker of the severity of liver injury and overall survival in patients with cholestatic liver diseases. *Sci Rep.* (2016) 6:30847. doi: 10.1038/srep30847
117. Joshita S, Ichikawa Y, Umemura T, Usami Y, Sugiura A, Shibata S, et al. Serum autotaxin is a useful liver fibrosis marker in patients with chronic hepatitis B virus infection. *Hepatol Res.* (2018) 48:275–85. doi: 10.1111/hepr.12997
118. Yamazaki T, Joshita S, Umemura T, Usami Y, Sugiura A, Fujimori N, et al. Association of serum autotaxin levels with liver fibrosis in patients with chronic hepatitis C. *Sci Rep.* (2017) 7:46705. doi: 10.1038/srep46705
119. Fujino H, Tanaka M, Imamura M, Morio K, Ono A, Nakahara T, et al. Pruritus in patients with chronic liver disease and serum autotaxin levels in patients with primary biliary cholangitis. *BMC Gastroenterol.* (2019) 19:169. doi: 10.1186/s12876-019-1092-z
120. Beck PW, Handwerker HO. Bradykinin and serotonin effects on various types of cutaneous nerve fibers. *Pflugers Arch.* (1974) 347:209–22. doi: 10.1007/BF00592598
121. Akiyama T, Carstens MI, Carstens E. Facial injections of pruritogens and algogens excite partly overlapping populations of primary and second-order trigeminal neurons in mice. *J Neurophysiol.* (2010) 104:2442–50. doi: 10.1152/jn.00563.2010
122. Klein A, Carstens MI, Carstens E. Facial injections of pruritogens or algogens elicit distinct behavior responses in rats and excite overlapping populations of primary sensory and trigeminal subnucleus caudalis neurons. *J Neurophysiol.* (2011) 106:1078–88. doi: 10.1152/jn.00302.2011
123. Kushnir-Sukhov NM, Brown JM, Wu Y, Kirshenbaum A, Metcalfe DD. Human mast cells are capable of serotonin synthesis and release. *J Allergy Clin Immunol.* (2007) 119:498–9. doi: 10.1016/j.jaci.2006.09.003
124. McNeil B, Dong X. Peripheral mechanisms of itch. *Neurosci Bull.* (2012) 28:100–10. doi: 10.1007/s12264-012-1202-1
125. Zhao ZQ, Liu XY, Jeffry J, Karunarathne WK, Li JL, Munanairi A, et al. Descending control of itch transmission by the serotonergic system *via* 5-HT1A-facilitated GRP-GRPR signaling. *Neuron.* (2014) 84:821–34. doi: 10.1016/j.neuron.2014.10.003
126. Schworer H, Hartmann H, Ramadori G. Relief of cholestatic pruritus by a novel class of drugs: 5-hydroxytryptamine type 3 (5-HT3) receptor antagonists: effectiveness of ondansetron. *Pain.* (1995) 61:33–7. doi: 10.1016/0304-3959(94)00145-5
127. Soga F, Katoh N, Inoue T, Kishimoto S. Serotonin activates human monocytes and prevents apoptosis. *J Invest Dermatol.* (2007) 127:1947–55. doi: 10.1038/sj.jid.5700824
128. Tian B, Wang XL, Huang Y, Chen LH, Cheng RX, Zhou FM, et al. Peripheral and spinal 5-HT receptors participate in cholestatic itch and antinociception induced by bile duct ligation in rats. *Sci Rep.* (2016) 6:36286. doi: 10.1038/srep36286
129. Bockaert J, Claeysen S, Becamel C, Dumuis A, Marin P. Neuronal 5-HT metabotropic receptors: fine-tuning of their structure, signaling, and roles in synaptic modulation. *Cell Tissue Res.* (2006) 326:553–72. doi: 10.1007/s00441-006-0286-1
130. Hoyer D, Martin G. 5-HT receptor classification and nomenclature: towards a harmonization with the human genome. *Neuropharmacology.* (1997) 36:419–28. doi: 10.1016/S0028-3908(97)00036-1
131. Akiyama T, Ivanov M, Nagamine M, Davoodi A, Carstens MI, Ikoma A, et al. Involvement of TRPV4 in serotonin-evoked scratching. *J Invest Dermatol.* (2016) 136:154–60. doi: 10.1038/JID.2015.388
132. Yamaguchi T, Nagasawa T, Satoh M, Kuraishi Y. Itch-associated response induced by intradermal serotonin through 5-HT2 receptors in mice. *Neurosci Res.* (1999) 35:77–83. doi: 10.1016/S0168-0102(99)00070-X
133. Snyder LM, Kuzirian MS, Ross SE. An unexpected role for TRPV4 in serotonin-mediated itch. *J Invest Dermatol.* (2016) 136:7–9. doi: 10.1016/j.jid.2015.11.010
134. Ross SE. Pain and itch: insights into the neural circuits of aversive somatosensation in health and disease. *Curr Opin Neurobiol.* (2011) 21:880–7. doi: 10.1016/j.conb.2011.10.012
135. Morita T, McClain SP, Batia LM, Pellegrino M, Wilson SR, Kienzler MA, et al. HTR7 Mediates serotonergic acute and chronic itch. *Neuron.* (2015) 87:124–38. doi: 10.1016/j.neuron.2015.05.044
136. Browning J, Combes B, Mayo MJ. Long-term efficacy of sertraline as a treatment for cholestatic pruritus in patients with primary biliary cirrhosis. *Am J Gastroenterol.* (2003) 98:2736–41. doi: 10.1111/j.1572-0241.2003.08662.x
137. Mayo MJ, Handem I, Saldana S, Jacobe H, Getachew Y, Rush AJ. Sertraline as a first-line treatment for cholestatic pruritus. *Hepatology.* (2007) 45:666–74. doi: 10.1002/hep.21553
138. Stander S, Bockenholt B, Schurmeyer-Horst F, Weishaupt C, Heuft G, Luger TA, et al. Treatment of chronic pruritus with the selective serotonin re-uptake inhibitors paroxetine and fluvoxamine: results of an open-labelled,

two-arm proof-of-concept study. *Acta Derm Venereol.* (2009) 89:45–51. doi: 10.2340/00015555-0553
139. Thebaut A, Habes D, Gottrand F, Rivet C, Cohen J, Debray D, et al. Sertraline as an additional treatment for cholestatic pruritus in children. *J Pediatr Gastroenterol Nutr.* (2017) 64:431–5. doi: 10.1097/MPG.0000000000001385
140. Sommer C, Serotonin in pain and analgesia: actions in the periphery. *Mol Neurobiol.* (2004) 30:117–25. doi: 10.1385/MN:30:2:117
141. European Association for the Study of the Liver. EASL clinical practice guidelines: management of cholestatic liver diseases. *J Hepatol.* (2009) 51:237–67. doi: 10.1016/j.jhep.2009.04.009
142. Gupta MA, Gupta AK. Depression modulates pruritus perception. A study of pruritus in psoriasis, atopic dermatitis and chronic idiopathic urticaria. *Ann NY Acad Sci.* (1999) 885:394–5. doi: 10.1111/j.1749-6632.1999.tb08697.x
143. Gittlen SD, Schulman ES, Maddrey WC. Raised histamine concentrations in chronic cholestatic liver disease. *Gut.* (1990) 31:96–9. doi: 10.1136/gut.31.1.96
144. Ikoma A, Handwerker H, Miyachi Y, Schmelz M. Electrically evoked itch in humans. *Pain.* (2005) 113:148–54. doi: 10.1016/j.pain.2004.10.003
145. Jones EA, Bergasa NV. Evolving concepts of the pathogenesis and treatment of the pruritus of cholestasis. *Can J Gastroenterol.* (2000) 14:33–40. doi: 10.1155/2000/747495
146. Schmelz M, Schmidt R, Weidner C, Hilliges M, Torebjork HE, Handwerker HO. Chemical response pattern of different classes of C-nociceptors to pruritogens and algogens. *J Neurophysiol.* (2003) 89:2441–8. doi: 10.1152/jn.01139.2002
147. Meixiong J, Vasavda C, Green D, Zheng Q, Qi L, Kwatra SG, et al. Identification of a bilirubin receptor that may mediate a component of cholestatic itch. *Elife.* (2019) 8:44116. doi: 10.7554/eLife.44116
148. Dong X, Han S, Zylka MJ, Simon MI, Anderson DJ. A diverse family of GPCRs expressed in specific subsets of nociceptive sensory neurons. *Cell.* (2001) 106:619–32. doi: 10.1016/S0092-8674(01)00483-4
149. Flegel C, Schobel N, Altmuller J, Becker C, Tannapfel A, Hatt H, et al. RNA-Seq analysis of human trigeminal and dorsal root ganglia with a focus on chemoreceptors. *PLoS ONE.* (2015) 10:e0128951. doi: 10.1371/journal.pone.0128951
150. Kremer AE, Gonzales E, Schaap FG, Oude Elferink RP, Jacquemin E, Beuers U. Serum autotaxin activity correlates with pruritus in pediatric cholestatic disorders. *J Pediatr Gastroenterol Nutr.* (2016) 62:530–5. doi: 10.1097/MPG.0000000000001044
151. Strassburg CP. Hyperbilirubinemia syndromes (Gilbert-Meulengracht, Crigler-Najjar, Dubin-Johnson, Rotor syndrome). *Best Pract Res Clin Gastroenterol.* (2010) 24:555–71. doi: 10.1016/j.bpg.2010.07.007
152. Reyes H, Sjovall J. Bile acids and progesterone metabolites in intrahepatic cholestasis of pregnancy. *Ann Med.* (2000) 32:94–106. doi: 10.3109/07853890009011758
153. Abu-Hayyeh S, Papacleovoulou G, Lovgren-Sandblom A, Tahir M, Oduwole O, Jamaludin NA, et al. Intrahepatic cholestasis of pregnancy levels of sulfated progesterone metabolites inhibit farnesoid X receptor resulting in a cholestatic phenotype. *Hepatology.* (2013) 57:716–26. doi: 10.1002/hep.26055
154. Meng LJ, Reyes H, Palma J, Hernandez I, Ribalta J, Sjovall J. Profiles of bile acids and progesterone metabolites in the urine and serum of women with intrahepatic cholestasis of pregnancy. *J Hepatol.* (1997) 27:346–57. doi: 10.1016/S0168-8278(97)80181-X
155. Glantz A, Reilly SJ, Benthin L, Lammert F, Mattsson LA, Marschall HU. Intrahepatic cholestasis of pregnancy: amelioration of pruritus by UDCA is associated with decreased progesterone disulphates in urine. *Hepatology.* (2008) 47:544–51. doi: 10.1002/hep.21987
156. Abu-Hayyeh S, Ovadia C, Lieu T, Jensen DD, Chambers J, Dixon PH, et al. Prognostic and mechanistic potential of progesterone sulfates in intrahepatic cholestasis of pregnancy and pruritus gravidarum. *Hepatology.* (2016) 63:1287–98. doi: 10.1002/hep.28265
157. Abu-Hayyeh S, Martinez-Becerra P, Sheikh Abdul Kadir SH, Selden C, Romero MR, Rees M, et al. Inhibition of Na+-taurocholate Co-transporting polypeptide-mediated bile acid transport by cholestatic sulfated progesterone metabolites. *J Biol Chem.* (2010) 285:16504–12. doi: 10.1074/jbc.M109.072140
158. Vallejo M, Briz O, Serrano MA, Monte MJ, Marin JJ. Potential role of trans-inhibition of the bile salt export pump by progesterone metabolites in the etiopathogenesis of intrahepatic cholestasis of pregnancy. *J Hepatol.* (2006) 44:1150–7. doi: 10.1016/j.jhep.2005.09.017
159. Akiyama T, Lerner EA, Carstens E. Protease-activated receptors and itch. *Handb Exp Pharmacol.* (2015) 226:219–35. doi: 10.1007/978-3-662-44605-8_13
160. Briot A, Deraison C, Lacroix M, Bonnart C, Robin A, Besson C, et al. Kallikrein 5 induces atopic dermatitis-like lesions through PAR2-mediated thymic stromal lymphopoietin expression in Netherton syndrome. *J Exp Med.* (2009) 206:1135–47. doi: 10.1084/jem.20082242
161. Kempkes C, Buddenkotte J, Cevikbas F, Buhl T, Steinhoff M. Role of PAR-2 in neuroimmune communication and itch. In: Carstens E, Akiyama T, editors. *Itch: Mechanisms and Treatment.* Boca Raton, FL: CRC Press/Taylor & Francis (2014).
162. Steinhoff M, Neisius U, Ikoma A, Fartasch M, Heyer G, Skov PS, et al. Proteinase-activated receptor-2 mediates itch: a novel pathway for pruritus in human skin. *J Neurosci.* (2003) 23:6176–80. doi: 10.1523/JNEUROSCI.23-15-06176.2003
163. Zhao J, Munanairi A, Liu XY, Zhang J, Hu L, Hu M, et al. PAR2 Mediates itch *via* TRPV3 signaling in keratinocytes. *J Invest Dermatol.* (2020) 140:1524–32. doi: 10.1016/j.jid.2020.01.012
164. Ui H, Andoh T, Lee JB, Nojima H, Kuraishi Y. Potent pruritogenic action of tryptase mediated by PAR-2 receptor and its involvement in anti-pruritic effect of nafamostat mesilate in mice. *Eur J Pharmacol.* (2006) 530:172–8. doi: 10.1016/j.ejphar.2005.11.021
165. Thomsen JS, Sonne M, Benfeldt E, Jensen SB, Serup J, Menne T. Experimental itch in sodium lauryl sulphate-inflamed and normal skin in humans: a randomized, double-blind, placebo-controlled study of histamine and other inducers of itch. *Br J Dermatol.* (2002) 146:792–800. doi: 10.1046/j.1365-2133.2002.04722.x
166. Shimada SG, Shimada KA, Collins JG. Scratching behavior in mice induced by the proteinase-activated receptor-2 agonist, SLIGRL-NH2. *Eur J Pharmacol.* (2006) 530:281–3. doi: 10.1016/j.ejphar.2005.11.012
167. Costa R, Marotta DM, Manjavachi MN, Fernandes ES, Lima-Garcia JF, Paszcuk AF, et al. Evidence for the role of neurogenic inflammation components in trypsin-elicited scratching behaviour in mice. *Br J Pharmacol.* (2008) 154:1094–103. doi: 10.1038/bjp.2008.172
168. Liu Q, Weng HJ, Patel KN, Tang Z, Bai H, Steinhoff M, et al. The distinct roles of two GPCRs, MrgprC11 and PAR2, in itch and hyperalgesia. *Sci Signal.* (2011) 4:ra45. doi: 10.1126/scisignal.2001925
169. Ghent CN, Carruthers SG. Treatment of pruritus in primary biliary cirrhosis with rifampin. Results of a double-blind, crossover, randomized trial. *Gastroenterology.* (1988) 94:488–93. doi: 10.1016/0016-5085(88)90442-8
170. Pereira SP, Rhodes JM, Campbell BJ, Kumar D, Bain IM, Murphy GM, et al. Biliary lactoferrin concentrations are increased in active inflammatory bowel disease: a factor in the pathogenesis of primary sclerosing cholangitis? *Clin Sci (Lond).* (1998) 95:637–44. doi: 10.1042/cs0950637
171. Li Y, Tang R, Leung PSC, Gershwin ME, Ma X. Bile acids and intestinal microbiota in autoimmune cholestatic liver diseases. *Autoimmun Rev.* (2017) 16:885–96. doi: 10.1016/j.autrev.2017.07.002
172. Lv LX, Fang DQ, Shi D, Chen DY, Yan R, Zhu YX, et al. Alterations and correlations of the gut microbiome, metabolism and immunity in patients with primary biliary cirrhosis. *Environ Microbiol.* (2016) 18:2272–86. doi: 10.1111/1462-2920.13401
173. Tang R, Wei Y, Li Y, Chen W, Chen H, Wang Q, et al. Gut microbial profile is altered in primary biliary cholangitis and partially restored after UDCA therapy. *Gut.* (2018) 67:534–41. doi: 10.1136/gutjnl-2016-313332
174. Matsumoto M, Aranami A, Ishige A, Watanabe K, Benno Y. LKM512 yogurt consumption improves the intestinal environment and induces the T-helper type 1 cytokine in adult patients with intractable atopic dermatitis. *Clin Exp Allergy.* (2007) 37:358–70. doi: 10.1111/j.1365-2222.2007.02642.x
175. Matsumoto M, Ebata T, Hirooka J, Hosoya R, Inoue N, Itami S, et al. Antipruritic effects of the probiotic strain LKM512 in adults with atopic dermatitis. *Ann Allergy Asthma Immunol.* (2014) 113:209–16.e7. doi: 10.1016/j.anai.2014.05.002
176. Patel SP, Vasavda C, Ho B, Meixiong J, Dong X, Kwatra SG. Cholestatic pruritus: emerging mechanisms and therapeutics. *J Am Acad Dermatol.* (2019) 81:1371–8. doi: 10.1016/j.jaad.2019.04.035

177. Darragh M, Chang JW, Booth RJ, Consedine NS. The placebo effect in inflammatory skin reactions: the influence of verbal suggestion on itch and weal size. *J Psychosom Res.* (2015) 78:489–94. doi: 10.1016/j.jpsychores.2015.01.011
178. Mayo MJ, Pockros PJ, Jones D, Bowlus CL, Levy C, Patanwala I, et al. A Randomized, controlled, phase 2 study of maralixibat in the treatment of itching associated with primary biliary cholangitis. *Hepatol Commun.* (2019) 3:365–81. doi: 10.1002/hep4.1305
179. Beuers U, Drug insight: mechanisms and sites of action of ursodeoxycholic acid in cholestasis. *Nat Clin Pract Gastroenterol Hepatol.* (2006) 3:318–28. doi: 10.1038/ncpgasthep0521
180. Corpechot C, Carrat F, Bonnand AM, Poupon RE, Poupon R. The effect of ursodeoxycholic acid therapy on liver fibrosis progression in primary biliary cirrhosis. *Hepatology.* (2000) 32:1196–9. doi: 10.1053/jhep.2000.20240
181. Pares A, Caballeria L, Rodes J, Bruguera M, Rodrigo L, Garcia-Plaza A, et al. Long-term effects of ursodeoxycholic acid in primary biliary cirrhosis: results of a double-blind controlled multicentric trial. UDCA-Cooperative Group from the Spanish Association for the Study of the Liver. *J Hepatol.* (2000) 32:561–6. doi: 10.1016/S0168-8278(00)80216-0
182. Pares A, Cisneros L, Salmeron JM, Caballeria L, Mas A, Torras A, et al. Extracorporeal albumin dialysis: a procedure for prolonged relief of intractable pruritus in patients with primary biliary cirrhosis. *Am J Gastroenterol.* (2004) 99:1105–10. doi: 10.1111/j.1572-0241.2004.30204.x
183. Alallam A, Barth D, Heathcote EJ. Role of plasmapheresis in the treatment of severe pruritus in pregnant patients with primary biliary cirrhosis: case reports. *Can J Gastroenterol.* (2008) 22:505–7. doi: 10.1155/2008/969826
184. Krawczyk M, Liebe R, Wasilewicz M, Wunsch E, Raszeja-Wyszomirska J, Milkiewicz P. Plasmapheresis exerts a long-lasting antipruritic effect in severe cholestatic itch. *Liver Int.* (2017) 37:743–7. doi: 10.1111/liv.13281
185. Pusl T, Denk GU, Parhofer KG, Beuers U. Plasma separation and anion adsorption transiently relieve intractable pruritus in primary biliary cirrhosis. *J Hepatol.* (2006) 45:887–91. doi: 10.1016/j.jhep.2006.08.008
186. Verkade HJ, Thompson RJ, Arnell H, Fischler B, Gillberg PG, Mattsson JP, et al. Systematic review and meta-analysis: partial external biliary diversion in progressive familial intrahepatic cholestasis. *J Pediatr Gastroenterol Nutr.* (2020) 71:176–83. doi: 10.1097/MPG.0000000000002789
187. Barbayianni E, Magrioti V, Moutevelis-Minakakis P, Kokotos G. Autotaxin inhibitors: a patent review. *Expert Opin Ther Pat.* (2013) 23:1123–32. doi: 10.1517/13543776.2013.796364
188. Khurana S, Singh P. Rifampin is safe for treatment of pruritus due to chronic cholestasis: a meta-analysis of prospective randomized-controlled trials. *Liver Int.* (2006) 26:943–8. doi: 10.1111/j.1478-3231.2006.01326.x
189. Acocella G. Pharmacokinetics and metabolism of rifampin in humans. *Rev Infect Dis.* (1983) 5(Suppl. 3):S428–32. doi: 10.1093/clinids/5.Supplement_3.S428
190. Thebaut A, Debray D, Gonzales E. An update on the physiopathology and therapeutic management of cholestatic pruritus in children. *Clin Res Hepatol Gastroenterol.* (2018) 42:103–9. doi: 10.1016/j.clinre.2017.08.007
191. Wietholtz H, Marschall H-U, Jan S, Matern S. Stimulation of bile acid 6α-hydroxylation by rifampin. *J Hepatol.* (1996) 24:713–8. doi: 10.1016/S0168-8278(96)80268-6
192. Bergasa NV, Sabol SL, Young WS, III, Kleiner DE, Jones EA. Cholestasis is associated with preproenkephalin mRNA expression in the adult rat liver. *Am J Physiol.* (1995) 268:G346–54. doi: 10.1152/ajpgi.1995.268.2.G346
193. Terg R, Coronel E, Sorda J, Munoz AE, Findor J. Efficacy and safety of oral naltrexone treatment for pruritus of cholestasis, a crossover, double blind, placebo-controlled study. *J Hepatol.* (2002) 37:717–22. doi: 10.1016/S0168-8278(02)00318-5
194. Rust C, Sauter GH, Oswald M, Buttner J, Kullak-Ublick GA, Paumgartner G, et al. Effect of cholestyramine on bile acid pattern and synthesis during administration of ursodeoxycholic acid in man. *Eur J Clin Invest.* (2000) 30:135–9. doi: 10.1046/j.1365-2362.2000.00606.x
195. Carey JB, Jr., Williams G. Relief of the pruritus of jaundice with a bile-acid sequestering resin. *JAMA.* (1961) 176:432–5. doi: 10.1001/jama.1961.03040180034008
196. European Association for the Study of the Liver. EASL clinical practice guidelines: The diagnosis and management of patients with primary biliary cholangitis. *J Hepatol.* (2017) 67:145–72. doi: 10.1016/j.jhep.2017.03.022
197. Castagna D, Budd DC, Macdonald SJ, Jamieson C, Watson AJ. Development of autotaxin inhibitors: an overview of the patent and primary literature. *J Med Chem.* (2016) 59:5604–21. doi: 10.1021/acs.jmedchem.5b01599
198. Herr DR, Chew WS, Satish RL, Ong WY. Pleotropic roles of autotaxin in the nervous system present opportunities for the development of novel therapeutics for neurological diseases. *Mol Neurobiol.* (2020) 57:372–92. doi: 10.1007/s12035-019-01719-1

15

Clinical Characteristics of Itch in Renal Transplant Recipients

Piotr K. Krajewski[1], Piotr Olczyk[2], Magdalena Krajewska[2], Wojciech Krajewski[3] and Jacek C. Szepietowski[1]*

[1] Department of Dermatology, Venereology and Allergology, Wroclaw Medical University, Wroclaw, Poland, [2] Department of Nephrology and Transplantation Medicine, Wroclaw Medical University, Wroclaw, Poland, [3] Department of Urology and Oncologic Urology, Wrocław Medical University, Wrocław, Poland

***Correspondence:**
Jacek C. Szepietowski
jacek.szepietowski@umed.wroc.pl

Background: Chronic itch is the most common symptom in dermatology. End-stage renal disease-associated chronic itch (ESRDCI) is a common burden affecting up to 35% of patients treated with hemodialysis. Kidney transplant (KTx) is believed to be the best renal replacement therapy leading to the elimination of ESRDCI. The study was undertaken to characterize and assess the prevalence of itch among patients after renal transplantation.

Methods: Between October 2019 and January 2020, we analyzed the data of 197 patients comprising 121 males (61.4%) and 76 females (38.6%) and aged 54.5 ± 13.6 years. The data collection was performed with a specially designed questionnaire. Level of itch after renal transplantation was assessed with the use of a Numeral Rating Scale, a Visual Rating Scale, and 4-Item Itch Questionnaire. Moreover, the previous 3 days of itching were evaluated.

Results: The patients suffered from chronic renal disease for 20.2 ± 12.3 years, with a mean time of pre-transplant dialysis of 2.6 ± 2.4 years and a mean time after the KTx of 8.0 ± 6.5 years. The itch was present in 38.6% of the patients during the hemodialysis, and in 73.7% of cases, the itch ceased completely after the successful transplantation. Moreover, only 2.63% of the cases had no improvement. Nevertheless, the itch was reported in 42 (21.3%) renal transplant recipients (RTR), and in 22 (52.4%) cases, the itch appeared after transplantation. The majority of patients suffering from itch were women (54.8%). Itch in the last 3 days was reported in 21 patients. The itch's severity was assessed with a numerical rating scale (NRS), with the worst severity measured at 6 ± 2.2 points indicating moderate itch. In most cases (57.1%), itch affected multiple body areas. Extremities (50%) and the back (50%) were among the most frequently affected areas. The sensation had a mostly short duration and was most frequently reported in the evening. Only eight patients suffered for the whole day. Hot water was the most frequently reported (16.7%) alleviating factor, whilst sweat was responsible for itch aggravation in 35.9% of cases.

Conclusion: Our analysis on representative patients' population indicates that itch after KTx is an important problem. Moreover, it is worth noting that more than half of the RTR did not suffer from itch during dialysis.

Keywords: renal transplant, itch, chronic kidney disease, ESRDCI, renal transplant recipients

INTRODUCTION

Chronic kidney disease (CKD) is recognized as a one of the leading public health problems, affecting up to 13.4% of the global population (1). Moreover, up to 10.6% of people suffer from advanced stages of the disease (stage 3–5) (2). CKD is defined as abnormal renal structure or function with health implications of at least a 3-month duration (1). The diagnostic criteria also include glomerular filtration rate (GFR) < 60 ml/min/1.73m^2, markers of kidney damage (albuminuria, abnormal urine sedimentation rate, tubular disorders), histologic and radiologic abnormalities, or a history of renal transplantation (3). CKD may be classified in one of the five stages using patients' GFR and one of the three stages based on the patients' albuminuria (2). The loss of kidney function leads to the development of many complications such as anemia, hyperparathyroidism and mineral bone disease, cardiovascular diseases, dyslipidemias, and cancer (4). The disease is associated with frequent and longer hospitalizations, rehospitalization, and premature morbidity (1, 5). One of the associated symptoms of CKD is end-stage renal disease-associated chronic itch (ESRDCI), also known as uremic itch. It is a burdensome symptom that may affect up to 13% of CKD patients (stages 1–5) and up to 35% (lifetime prevalence) of patients treated with hemodialysis (HD) (6). The pathophysiology is not fully understood. Due to the unknown pathomechanism, the treatment of ESRDCI is still a big challenge, and the results are often not satisfactory (7). Kidney transplant (KTx) is considered the best renal replacement therapy; however, its influence on itch was not sufficiently studied (8). The available data suggest that renal transplant recipients (RTR) may suffer from itch less frequently than patients treated with hemodialysis (9–11). Due to the insufficient reports and observations on small groups, we have decided to conduct a study and assess an actual prevalence of itch in RTR. Moreover, we have correlated itch severity with possible pathogenetic factors.

MATERIALS AND METHODS

Study Participants

The studied population consisted of 197 RTR, who are under monthly supervision of the Department of Nephrology and Transplantation Medicine of Wroclaw Medical University. The exclusion criteria included being under the age of 18 years, inability to cooperate and fill out the questionnaire, having a history of chronic dermatological disorders, and having undergone a non-functioning renal transplant. After the inclusion criteria was met by 197 individuals, a medical interview with each patient was performed. Baseline data, including age, sex, BMI, comorbidities, chronic medication, duration of CKD, time of dialysis before KTx, and time after transplantation, were collected.

Itch Assessment

Itch presence during the whole period after transplantation as well as during the last 3 days was documented. Additionally, localization, the most common aggravating and alleviating factors, specific anti-itch treatments, and usage of emollients were recorded. Moreover, the patients were asked about the presence of itch before and possible improvement after KTx. Itch intensity (worst itch during the last 3 days) was assessed with the following instruments: Numeral Rating Scale (NRS), Verbal Rating Scale (VRS), and 4-Item Itch Questionnaire (4IIQ). Moreover, the patients were asked to evaluate the worst itch intensity during the whole period after KTx. Later, the reported itch was compared to the itch caused by mosquito bites, assessed by RTR with NRS. The VRS is a four-point scale and consists of a list of adjectives describing various levels of symptom intensity: 0 = no itch, 1 = mild itch, 2 = moderate itch, and 3 = severe itch (12). The NRS is comprised of one item and represents the numbers 0 ("no itch") to 10 ("worst imaginable itch"). The cut-off points for itch NRS are as follows: mild itch (>0 to <3 points), moderate (≥3 to <7 points), severe (≥7 to <9 points), and very severe (≥9 points) (13). 4IIQ was developed and validated by our group some years ago. It assesses not only itch intensity (0–5 points), but also the frequency of itch episodes (0–5 points), areas of affected skin (0–3 points), and sleep disturbance (0–6 points) as a course of chronic itch. The maximum score for this scale is 19 points (14–16).

Lab Tests Assessments

Results of blood tests conducted periodically on all of the patients, including transplant function (eGFR, creatinine and uremia levels), liver function (ASPAT, ALAT, bilirubin level), calcium and phosphate metabolism (including parathormone levels), hemoglobin, glucose level, and medication level (cyclosporin or tacrolimus), were collected and analyzed in relationship with the presence and severity of itch.

Statistical Analysis

Statistical analysis was performed using Statistica v. 12 (StatSoft Kraków). The minimum, maximum, mean, and standard deviation numbers were calculated. Analyzed quantitative variables were compared using Mann-Whitney U test and Spearman and Pearson correlations; for qualitative data, the chi-squared test was used. A 2-sided P value ≤ 0.05 was considered to be statistically significant.

RESULTS

Patients' Characteristics

The group consisted of 197 patients—121 men (61.4%) and 76 women (38.6%). The mean age of the population was 54.5 ± 13.6 years. The group was characterized as slightly overweight with a mean BMI of 26.2 ± 4.4. The majority of patients (88.3%) was treated with three drug immunosuppressive therapies (calcineurin inhibitors, antiproliferative drugs, and glucocorticosteroids [GKS]), while almost every patient (96.4%) was taking GKS. The patients who suffered from CKD for 20.2 ± 12.3 years were treated with hemodialysis for 2.6 ± 2.4 years before RTx and were 7.9 ± 6.5 years after KTx. The majority of RNR suffered from hypertension (161 patients, 81.7%), and 36 subjects suffered from diabetes (18.3%) (**Table 1**).

TABLE 1 | Patients' characteristics.

	Whole group (n = 197)	Itch (n = 42)	No itch (n = 155)
Age in years (mean ± SD)	54.5 ± 13.6	55.7 ± 13.9	54.2 ± 13.6
Sex (Male %)	121 (61.4)	**19 (45.2)***	**102 (65.8)***
BMI in kg/m^2 (mean ± SD)	26.2 ± 4.4	26.4 ± 4.6	26.1 ± 4.3
CKD duration in years (mean ± SD)	20.2 ± 12.3	20.2 ± 11.5	20.2 ± 12.5
Time on HD before KTx in years(mean ± SD)	2.57 ± 2.4	2.2 ± 1.6	2.7 ± 2.6
Time after KTx in years (mean ± SD)	7.9 ± 6.5	8.7 ± 6.9	7.8 ± 6.4
Immunosuppression			
GKS (%)	190 (96.5)	38 (90.5)	149 (96.1)
Tacrolimus (%)	174 (88.3)	35 (83.3)	139 (89.7)
Cyclosporine A (%)	38 (19.3)	7 (16.7)	31 (20%)
Comorbidities			
Diabetes (%)	36 (18.3)	9 (21.4)	35 (22.6)
Hypertension (%)	161 (81.7)	36 (85.7)	125 (80.7)

$p = 0.005$ (in bold); CKD, chronic kidney disease; SD, standard deviation; BMI, body mass index.

Itch Assessment

Among the studied group of RTR, itch was a common symptom during the period of hemodialysis treatment (76 patients, 38.57%); however, only 42 patients (21.3%) reported itch after KTx. In 56 patients (73.7%), itch disappeared completely after the transplantation. In the majority of them (43 subjects), the relief was instant. In the rest of the subjects, relief was gradual (**Figure 1**). In the majority of RTR suffering from itch (22 patients, 52.4%), relief appeared after successful transplantation, while the rest (20 patients, 47.6%) reported residual itch from hemodialysis period with lower (18 people) or similar (two people) severity (**Figures 2, 3**). The WI-NRS itch was at 5.98 ± 2.17 points, which was similar to the itch reported after a mosquito bite (5.36 ± 2.2 points). Among 42 itchy RTR, half (21 people) reported itch in the previous 3 days, and its intensity was assessed as 4.23 ± 1.51 points on WI-NRS. Following the cut-offs for NRS, the majority of patients reported moderate itch (85.7%), two of them mild (9.5%), and only one person was suffering from severe itch (4.8%). According to VRS, 52.38% (11 patients) of RTR who suffered from itch described it as moderate, eight of them (38.1%) described it as mild, and only two (9.52%) described it as severe (**Figure 3**). Women suffered from itch significantly more than men ($p = 0.005$). Most frequently, the itch affected multiple locations (47.6%), with extremities and back being the most involved (50% of the patients for both locations). In only four patients (9.5%) the sensation was generalized; it affected only one location in the rest of patients (**Table 2**). Among alleviating factors, patients most often reported very hot and cold water; however, this strategy of relief only helped 16.67 and 14.3% of patients, respectively. The most common aggravating factor was sweat (35.7%) and warm airflow (33.3%). Most frequently, itch occurred in the evening (85.3%) and mostly for a short period of time (85.3%). In eight patients (19%), itch continuously present during the whole day. Only 17 patients (40.5%) were using emollients daily, and four had taken mediation in order to alleviate itching (**Table 3**). Among possible risk factors, we have found a significant difference ($p = 0.024$) in alkaline phosphatase (ALP) levels between itchy and non-itchy patients (76.1 ± 48.0 and 85.9 ± 33.5 U/l, respectively). There was no correlation found between prevalence (**Table 4**) or intensity of itch and graft function, the rest of laboratory tests, duration of CKD, time after KTx, time on hemodialysis, and medications administered (detailed data not shown).

DISCUSSION

Chronic itch (CI) is one of the most common symptoms in medicine. The International Forum for the Study of Itch (IFSI) defines it as a sensation that provokes the desire to scratch lasting for at least 6 weeks (17). The actual prevalence of CI is not clear. Studies show that about 8–9% of the adult population experience acute itch, while up to 16.8% experience CI (18). The incidences for both acute and chronic itch seem to increase with age. Acute itch affects up to 60% people in the elderly population every week. The incidence of CI varies among different age groups, being at 12.3% for young adults and even 20.3% for elderly persons. CI may be caused by both dermatological and systemic diseases (17). Among possible systemic causes of chronic itch, authors often mention hepatobiliary diseases, malignancies, infectious diseases, neurological disorders, metabolic diseases, endocrine diseases, and kidney diseases (16, 17, 19, 20). CI poses a high burden and is associated with decrease in quality of life of affected individuals (21).

ESRDCI or uremic itch is defined as CI associated with significant reduction in renal function in patients suffering from CKD. It usually worsens along with decreasing kidney function and may be experienced in up to 35% of individuals with stage 5 CKD treated with hemodialysis (6, 22). Lack of full understanding of pathomechanisms makes treatment difficult and often not fully effective. The frequently reported therapies include drugs such as opioid agonists and antagonists, gabapentin and pregabalin, phototherapy, and antidepressants (7).

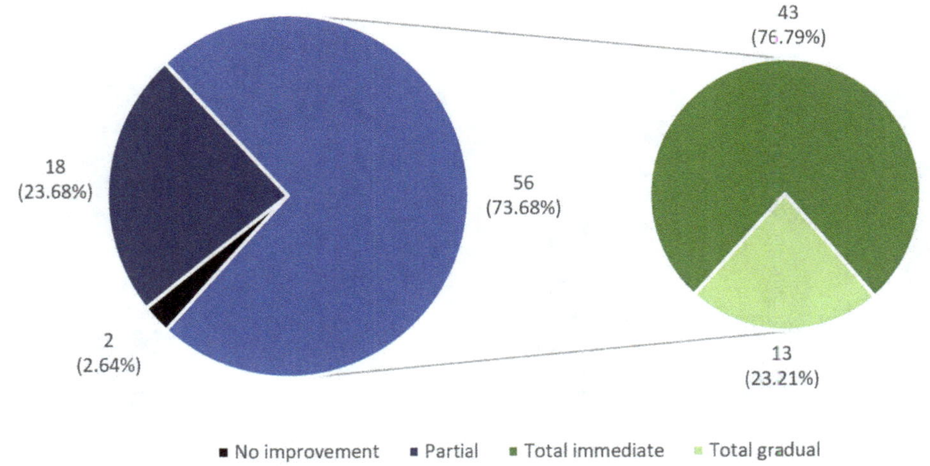

FIGURE 1 | Improvement in itch after kidney transplantation.

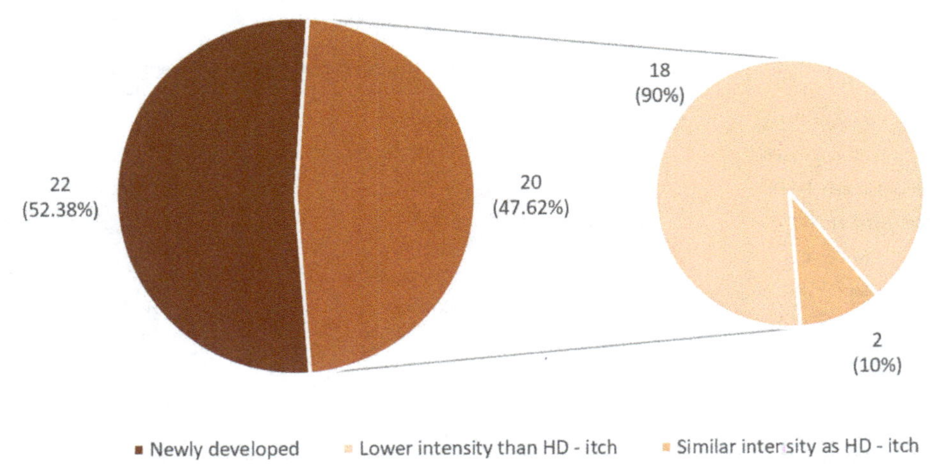

FIGURE 2 | Itch in renal transplant recipients.

The knowledge of the possible effect of KTx on uremic itch is very limited (8) and was reviewed by our group earlier this year. Our study is the first one to evaluate the prevalence of itch on a bigger sample size of RTR. The results of our work confirmed that itch is important burden in RTRs and affects 21.3% of them. The prevalence of itch in our group was different to the studies performed previously. According to the latest study by Schricker et al. (10), only 17% of the patients reported itch, while 12% were diagnosed with CI. Moreover, similarly to our study, authors have found a decrease in the itch prevalence after successful KTx. The mean intensity of recent itch was also lower than in our population (3.2 points and 4.2 points, respectively); however, those results may be different due to the time period taken into consideration (previous 24 h and 3 days, respectively). Correspondingly, Avermete et al. (23) reported only a 2% itch incidence in RTR, and Tăranu et al. (24) reported 5.3%, which was later explained as a drug-induced itch. Moreover, according to Altmeyer et al. (25), both itch and histopathological changes disappeared completely after KTx. In comparison to Panuccio et al. (9), we have reported a much lower itch prevalence (32% of RNRs). Nevertheless, it was still higher than in the healthy controls (11%). Similarly, the incidence of CI was lower than for HD patients; unfortunately, the authors did not mention itch intensity in any group. Our results were similar to those presented by Moloney et al. (26), who reported a 24.9% CI prevalence among 173 RTRs. The burden of CKD-associated itch is well documented (21). The decreased quality of life in

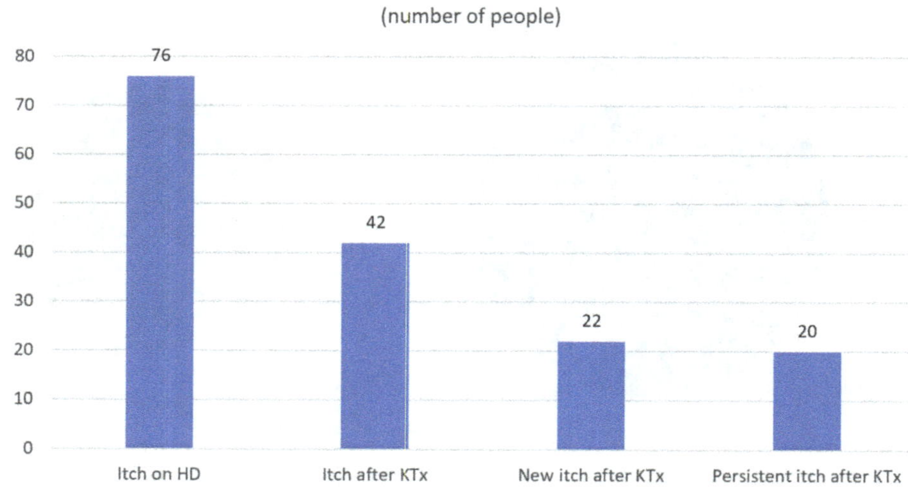

FIGURE 3 | Differences in prevalence of pre- and post-transplantation itch.

TABLE 2 | Characteristics of itch in renal transplant recipients.

		Itchy patients ($n = 42$)
Sex	Men, *n* (%)	19 (45.2)
	Women, *n* (%)	23 (54.8)
WI-NRS after renal transplantation (mean ± SD)		5.9 ± 2.2
Previous 3-day WI - NRS (mean ± SD) ($n = 21$)		4.2 ± 1.5
Previous 3-day VRS ($n = 21$)	Mild, *n* (%)	8 (38.1)
	Moderate *n* (%)	11 (52.4)
	Severe, *n* (%)	2 (9.5)
	Very severe *n* (%)	0
Itch treatment	Emollients, *n* (%)	17 (40.5)
	Antihistaminic, *n* (%)	4 (9.5)
Localization	Single, *n* (%)	18 (42.9)
	Multiple, *n* (%)	20 (47.6)
	Generalized	4 (9.5)
	Back	21 (50)
	Extremities	21 (50)
	Head	12 (28.6)
	Thorax	7 (16.7)
	Anogenital area	5 (11.9)
	Abdomen	9 (21.4)

n, number of patients; SD, standard deviation; WI-NRS, Worst Itch-Numeral Rating Scale; VRS, Verbal Rating Scale.

TABLE 3 | Factors responsible for aggravation or alleviation of itch intensity in renal transplant recipients.

Influencing factor, %	Exacerbation	Alleviation	No impact
Sleep	14.3	11.9	73.8
Physical activity	7.1	14.3	78.6
Stress	23.8	0.0	76.2
Fatigue	28.6	0.0	71.4
Diet	2.4	0.0	97.6
Very hot water	28.6	16.7	54.8
Cold water	2.4	14.3	83.3
Dry air	33.3	0.0	66.7
Sweating	35.7	2.4	61.9
Cold	2.4	9.5	88.1
Heat	21.4	9.5	69.1

RTRs was observed in many studies. Moloney et al. (26) reported that itch had large impact on lives of 57% of kidney recipients suffering from CI. Interestingly, according to Amro et al. (11) RTRs reported a statistically significant clinical decrease in the negative influence on life quality by itching in comparison to the period before transplantation.

The pathogenesis of CKD-associated itch is yet to be fully discovered. However, among possible mechanisms, authors often mention high urea and creatinine blood levels, disturbances in peripheral endogenous opioid system, hyperparathyroidism, neuropathy, xerosis, microinflammation, and neuropathy (27–31). From the most popular risk factors, which have been associated with the pathomechanisms of ESRDCI (7), none have been proven to play a role in the development of itch after successful renal transplant until today. We have correlated possible risk factors with the intensity of itch in RTRs; however, no statistically significant correlation was found. Additionally, no difference in the above-mentioned aspects was found between patients with persistent and newly developed itch. Similar results to our study were obtained by Pannucio et al. (9), who correlated itch intensity and ESRDCI

TABLE 4 | Differences in laboratory results between itchy and non-itchy patients.

	Itch ($n = 42$)	No itch ($n = 155$)	*P*
ALAT (U/l)	25.2 ± 16.3	23.8 ± 12.7	0.934
ASPAT (U/l)	26.9 ± 10.1	24.0 ± 8.8	0.127
Billirubin (mg/dl)	0.7 ± 0.3	0.8 ± 0.3	0.218
CRP (mg/l)	6.4 ± 14.2	7.6 ± 15.1	0.845
ALP (U/l)	76.1 ± 48.0	85.9 ± 33.5	**0.024**
GGTP (U/l)	36.0 ± 34.5	45.7 ± 51.3	0.217
Glucose (mg/dl)	106.4 ± 36.5	105.9 ± 33.3	0.913
eGFR (ml/min/m^2)	55.0 ± 21.0	52.2 ± 16.8	0.780
Creatinine (mg/dl)	1.4 ± 0.5	1.5 ± 0.6	0.136
Uremic acid (mg/dl)	6.6 ± 1.3	8.4 ± 9.3	0.116
Magnesium (mmol/l)	1.8 ± 0.2	1.8 ± 0.2	0.889
Potassium (mmol/l)	4.2 ± 0.3	4.3 ± 0.4	0.180
Calcium (mmol/l)	9.89 ± 0.6	9.9 ± 0.6	0.596
Hb (mg/dl)	13.8 ± 1.7	14.3 ± 1.9	0.719

*ALAT, Alanine aminotransferase; ASPAT, Aspartate aminotransferase; CRP, C -reaktive protein; ALP, Alkaline phosphatase; GGT, Gamma-glutamyltransferase; eGFR, Estimated glomerular filtration rate; Hb, Hemoglobin. *p = 0.005.*

risk factors including inflammation, bone mineral disorders, immunosuppressive therapy, and transplant function. On the other hand, a moderate positive correlation was found between CI intensity and transplant function ($r = 0.3$, $p = 0.018$) in the study by Schricker et al. (10), which was not established in our group. However, we did find a statistically significant difference in itch incidence between sexes ($p = 0.005$). We believe it is due to the different itch perception in modulation in women, as shown in the paper by Stumpf et al. (32). Interestingly, we have found significantly decreased levels of ALP in patients with itch. It is well documented that increased ALP may be a sign of hepatobiliary disorders, including cholestasis and hepatic cirrhosis (33). Those disorders are strongly correlated with high itch prevalence in those patients (34). On the other hand, low ALP levels have never been associated with incidence of itch. Although the patomechanism of itch in RNR is not clear, it is most probably multifactorial and the polypharmacy in those patients could contribute to the development and intensity of itch. Regarding the most frequent exacerbating factors, our patients reported sweat and warm airflow. These factors are similar to those present in atopic dermatitis or psoriasis (14, 35). Regarding sweat, there are multiple mechanisms that may induce or aggravate itch (e.g., abnormality in sweat components or "sweat allergy"). On the other hand, itch exacerbations due to warm air may be produced by abnormal hyperesthesia of the RNRs' skin. The sensitization of peripheral nerve may cause patients to feel thermal stimulation as itch (35).

We understand that our study has some limitations. Due to the lack of reports on severity of itch during hemodialysis in our patients, we could not assess an actual decrease in itch. However, we believe that because of the long period of time (7.9 ± 6.5 years) following KTx, the reported severity might be biased. There is no agreement on the role of the dry skin in the pathogenesis of ESRDCI (36). Therefore, in this project, we have not analyzed the relationship of itch prevalence or intensity to dryness of the skin. Moreover, there was no possibility to assess atopic predisposition. As there are almost no studies on itch in RNR, in this project we concentrated on incidence and intensity of itch in this group of subjects, and therefore we did not assess the burden of itch. We are aware that the assessment of itch's consequences, including quality of life impairment, will add value to the field. Additionally, it is important to remember that every patient in our group was taking calcineurin inhibitors, either cyclosporine A or tacrolimus. The treatment, besides its anti-rejection mechanisms, may have influenced the incidence and severity of itch. Both of the drugs were proven to be effective as anti-itch agents in animals (37), and cyclosporine A was effective in patients with prurigo nodularis and lichen planus (38, 39). Nevertheless, we have not observed a difference in prevalence and intensity of itch between different calcineurin inhibitors, and it is not possible to perform a study within RTRs without one of these two drugs involved.

In conclusion, to the best of our knowledge, this is the biggest study assessing the prevalence and intensity of itch in RTRs. It is also one of the few studies that correlated itch with common uremic itch risk factors. We have shown and confirmed that successful KTx may be of benefit in the treatment of ESRDCI. Nevertheless, it is worth noting that the majority of itch in RNR was developed after transplantation. The pathomechanism is still unknown, and future studies on representative samples are necessary to make this topic clearer.

ETHICS STATEMENT

The studies involving human participants were reviewed and approved by Bioethics committee of Wroclaw Medical University. The patients/participants provided their written informed consent to participate in this study.

AUTHOR CONTRIBUTIONS

PK: research concept and design, collection and/or assembly of data, data analysis and interpretation, writing the article, and final approval of article. PO: collection and/or assembly of data, data analysis and interpretation, and writing the article. MK and WK: research concept and design, data analysis and interpretation, writing the article, and critical revision of the article. JS: research concept and design, data analysis and interpretation, writing the article, critical revision of the article, and final approval of article. All authors contributed to the article and approved the submitted version.

REFERENCES

1. Lv JC, Zhang LX. Prevalence and disease burden of chronic kidney disease. *Adv Exp Med Biol.* (2019) 1165:3–15. doi: 10.1007/978-981-13-8871-2_1
2. Hill NR, Fatoba ST, Oke JL, Hirst JA, O'Callaghan CA, Lasserson DS, et al. Global prevalence of chronic kidney disease - a systematic review and meta-analysis. *PLoS ONE.* (2016) 11:e0158765. doi: 10.1371/journal.pone.0158765
3. Gajewski P, Szczeklik A, Wydawnictwo Medycyna P. *Interna Szczeklika 2019.* Kraków: Medycyna Praktyczna (2019).
4. Webster AC, Nagler EV, Morton RL, Masson P. Chronic kidney disease. *Lancet.* (2017) 389:1238–52. doi: 10.1016/S0140-6736(16)32064-5
5. Saunders MR, Ricardo AC, Chen J, Anderson AH, Cedillo-Couvert EA, Fischer MJ, et al. Neighborhood socioeconomic status and risk of hospitalization in patients with chronic kidney disease: a chronic renal insufficiency cohort study. *Medicine.* (2020) 99:e21028. doi: 10.1097/MD.0000000000021028
6. Hayani K, Weiss M, Weisshaar E. Clinical findings and provision of care in haemodialysis patients with chronic itch: new results from the German epidemiological haemodialysis itch study. *Acta Derm Venereol.* (2016) 96:361–6. doi: 10.2340/00015555-2280
7. Reszke R, Szepietowski JC. End-stage renal disease chronic itch and its management. *Dermatol Clin.* (2018) 36:277–92. doi: 10.1016/j.det.2018.02.007
8. Krajewski PK, Krajewska M, Szepietowski JC. Pruritus in renal transplant recipients: current state of knowledge. *Adv Clin Exp Med.* (2020) 29:769–72. doi: 10.17219/acem/122174
9. Panuccio V, Tripepi R, Bellantoni M, Saporito L, Quattrone S, Lacava V, et al. Pruritus and quality of life in renal transplant patients. *Clin Transplant.* (2017) 31:e12893. doi: 10.1111/ctr.12893
10. Schricker S, Weisshaar E, Kupfer J, Mettang T. Prevalence of pruritus in a single cohort of long-term kidney transplant recipients. *Acta Derm Venereol.* (2020) 100:adv00066. doi: 10.2340/00015555-3421
11. Amro A, Waldum-Grevbo B, von der Lippe N, Brekke FB, Miaskowski C, Os I. Symptom clusters from dialysis to renal transplantation: a five-year longitudinal study. *J Pain Symptom Manage.* (2016) 51:512–9. doi: 10.1016/j.jpainsymman.2015.10.012
12. Kido-Nakahara M, Katoh N, Saeki H, Mizutani H, Hagihara A, Takeuchi S, et al. Comparative cut-off value setting of pruritus intensity in visual analogue scale and verbal rating scale. *Acta Derm Venereol.* (2015) 95:345–6. doi: 10.2340/00015555-1972
13. Reich A, Chatzigeorkidis E, Zeidler C, Osada N, Furue M, Takamori K, et al. Tailoring the cut-off values of the visual analogue scale and numeric rating scale in itch assessment. *Acta Derm Venereol.* (2017) 97:759–60. doi: 10.2340/00015555-2642
14. Reszke R, Bialynicki-Birula R, Szepietowski JC. Itch in Psoriasis: a new look at well-known subject. *Acta Derm Venereol.* (2019) 99:429–34. doi: 10.2340/00015555-3147
15. Reszke R, Bialynicki-Birula R, Lindner K, Sobieszczanska M, Szepietowski JC. Itch in elderly people: a cross-sectional study. *Acta Derm Venereol.* (2019) 99:1016–21. doi: 10.2340/00015555-3271
16. Stefaniak AA, Zubkiewicz-Kucharska A, Matusiak L, Noczynska A, Szepietowski JC. Itch in children with type 1 diabetes: a cross-sectional study. *Dermatol Ther.* (2020) 10:745–56. doi: 10.1007/s13555-020-00403-w
17. Weisshaar E, Szepietowski JC, Dalgard FJ, Garcovich S, Gieler U, Gimenez-Arnau AM, et al. European S2k guideline on chronic pruritus. *Acta Derm Venereol.* (2019) 99:469–506. doi: 10.2340/00015555-3164
18. Stander S, Schafer I, Phan NQ, Blome C, Herberger K, Heigel H, et al. Prevalence of chronic pruritus in Germany: results of a cross-sectional study in a sample working population of 11,730. *Dermatology.* (2010) 221:229–35. doi: 10.1159/000319862
19. Welz-Kubiak K, Reszke R, Szepietowski JC. Pruritus as a sign of systemic disease. *Clin Dermatol.* (2019) 37:644–56. doi: 10.1016/j.clindermatol.2019.07.031
20. Weisshaar E, Weiss M, Mettang T, Yosipovitch G, Zylicz Z, Special Interest Group of the International Forum on the Study of I. Paraneoplastic itch: an expert position statement from the special interest group (SIG) of the international forum on the study of itch (IFSI). *Acta Derm Venereol.* (2015) 95:261–5. doi: 10.2340/00015555-1959
21. Szepietowski JC, Sikora M, Kusztal M, Salomon J, Magott M, Szepietowski T. Uremic pruritus: a clinical study of maintenance hemodialysis patients. *J Dermatol.* (2002) 29:621–7. doi: 10.1111/j.1346-8138.2002.tb00191.x
22. Murtagh FE, Addington-Hall JM, Edmonds PM, Donohoe P, Carey I, Jenkins K, et al. Symptoms in advanced renal disease: a cross-sectional survey of symptom prevalence in stage 5 chronic kidney disease managed without dialysis. *J Palliat Med.* (2007) 10:1266–76. doi: 10.1089/jpm.2007.0017
23. Avermaete A, Altmeyer P, Bacharach-Buhles M. Skin changes and tumours after renal transplantation. *Nephron.* (2002) 91:188–94. Discussion: 94–6. doi: 10.1159/000058391
24. Taranu T, Covic A, Buhaescu I, Taranu T. Drug-induced dermatological pathology in renal transplantation patients. *Rev Med Chir Soc Med Nat Iasi.* (2005) 109:36–9.
25. Altmeyer P, Kachel HG, Schafer G, Fassbinder W. Normalization of uremic skin changes following kidney transplantation. *Hautarzt.* (1986) 37:217–21.
26. Moloney FJ, Keane S, O'Kelly P, Conlon PJ, Murphy GM. The impact of skin disease following renal transplantation on quality of life. *Br J Dermatol.* (2005) 153:574–8. doi: 10.1111/j.1365-2133.2005.06699.x
27. Weisshaar E. Epidemiology of uraemic itch: new data. *Eur J Pain.* (2016) 20:32–6. doi: 10.1002/ejp.761
28. Simonsen E, Komenda P, Lerner B, Askin N, Bohm C, Shaw J, et al. Treatment of uremic pruritus: a systematic review. *Am J Kidney Dis.* (2017) 70:638–55. doi: 10.1053/j.ajkd.2017.05.018
29. Kaysen GA. The microinflammatory state in uremia: causes and potential consequences. *J Am Soc Nephrol.* (2001) 12:1549–57.
30. Chorazyczewska W, Reich A, Szepietowski JC. Lipid content and barrier function analysis in uraemic pruritus. *Acta Derm Venereol.* (2016) 96:402–3. doi: 10.2340/00015555-2266
31. Furue M, Ebata T, Ikoma A, Takeuchi S, Kataoka Y, Takamori K, et al. Verbalizing extremes of the visual analogue scale for pruritus: a consensus statement. *Acta Derm Venereol.* (2013) 93:214–5. doi: 10.2340/00015555-1446

32. Stumpf A, Burgmer M, Schneider G, Heuft G, Schmelz M, Phan NQ, et al. Sex differences in itch perception and modulation by distraction–an FMRI pilot study in healthy volunteers. *PLoS ONE.* (2013) 8:e79123. doi: 10.1371/journal.pone.0079123
33. Fernandez NJ, Kidney BA. Alkaline phosphatase: beyond the liver. *Vet Clin Pathol.* (2007) 36:223–33. doi: 10.1111/j.1939-165X.2007.tb00216.x
34. Mittal A. Cholestatic itch management. *Curr Probl Dermatol.* (2016) 50:142–8. doi: 10.1159/000446057
35. Murota H, Katayama I. Exacerbating factors of itch in atopic dermatitis. *Allergol Int.* (2017) 66:8–13. doi: 10.1016/j.alit.2016.10.005
36. Yosipovitch G, Tur E, Morduchowicz G, Boner G. Skin surface pH, moisture, and pruritus in haemodialysis patients. *Nephrol Dial Transplant.* (1993) 8:1129–32.
37. Yamashita H, Ito T, Kato H, Asai S, Tanaka H, Nagai H, et al. Comparison of the efficacy of tacrolimus and cyclosporine A in a murine model of dinitrofluorobenzene-induced atopic dermatitis. *Eur J Pharmacol.* (2010) 645:171–6. doi: 10.1016/j.ejphar.2010.07.031
38. Steinhoff M, Cevikbas F, Ikoma A, Berger TG. Pruritus: management algorithms and experimental therapies. *Semin Cutan Med Surg.* (2011) 30:127–37. doi: 10.1016/j.sder.2011.05.001
39. Siepmann D, Luger TA, Stander S. Antipruritic effect of cyclosporine microemulsion in prurigo nodularis: results of a case series. *J Dtsch Dermatol Ges.* (2008) 6:941–6. doi: 10.1111/j.1610-0387.2008.06745.x

16

Itch in Atopic Dermatitis – What is New?

*Franz J. Legat**

Department of Dermatology, Medical University of Graz, Graz, Austria

Correspondence:
Franz J. Legat
franz.legat@medunigraz.at

Atopic dermatitis (AD) is among the most frequent inflammatory skin diseases in humans, affecting up to 20% of children and 10% of adults in higher income countries. Chronic pruritus is a disease-defining symptom of AD, representing the most burdensome symptom for patients. Severe chronic pruritus causes significant sleep disturbances and impaired quality of life, as well as increased anxiety, depression and suicidal behavior. Until recently, skin care, topical corticosteroids, and calcineurin-inhibitors were primarily used to treat mild to moderate AD, while phototherapy and immunosuppressive agents such as corticosteroids, cyclosporine, and methotrexate were used to treat patients with moderate to severe AD. The potential short- and long-term adverse events associated with these treatments or their insufficient therapeutic efficacy limited their use in controlling pruritus and eczema in AD patients over longer periods of time. As our understanding of AD pathophysiology has improved and new systemic and topical treatments have appeared on the market, targeting specific cytokines, receptors, or their intracellular signaling, a new era in atopic dermatitis and pruritus therapy has begun. This review highlights new developments in AD treatment, placing a specific focus on their anti-pruritic effects.

Keywords: pruritus, itch, atopic dermatitis, biologics, JAK inhibitors

INTRODUCTION

AD is one of the most frequent inflammatory skin diseases in humans, affecting up to 20% of children living in higher-income countries. The first signs of the disease usually develop between the 3rd and 6th months of life, and about 60% of cases occur within the first two years of life; 80% of affected children experience symptoms before the 6th year of life. AD is more common in adults than previously thought, with up to nearly 10% affected. These cases result from persistent or recurrent childhood AD or the new onset of AD later in life. Up to 30% of pediatric and 50% of adult AD patients suffer from moderate to severe forms of the disease (1–3). Overall, AD incidence is increasing worldwide, indicating that an environmental factor is contributing to the development of the disease (4).

No biologic marker has yet been defined for the disease; thus, AD is still diagnosed by examining clinical signs and symptoms and using various diagnostic criteria. The most widely used criteria, described by Hanifin and Rajka, define AD with essential, common and associated symptoms (5). These diagnostic criteria use pruritus, eczematous skin lesions, and the chronic or relapsing course of the disease as essential elements to define AD. Upon clinical inspection, eczematous skin lesions observed in patients with a typical age-related distribution may initially attract our attention, but pruritus is usually the "primary symptom" experienced by the affected patients. The point prevalence of chronic pruritus in AD ranges from 87 to 100%, but, in fact, all patients who actively suffer from the disease also suffer from chronic pruritus (6). In mild and moderate forms of AD, patients experience pruritus as the most burdensome symptom overall. But even in severe cases with widespread skin involvement and extensive oozing and crusting, pruritus is still the patients' major concern and a significant burden of the disease (7, 8). In addition to pruritus, patients frequently report experiencing skin pain. For this reason, this topic requires more attention and study in AD patients (9).

Pruritus strongly and negatively impacts the quality of life of affected patients, who complain most frequently about sleep disturbances due to itch. They report that they have difficulties to fall asleep and wake up repeatedly at night, which reduces the overall sleeping time and quality (8). This lack of physical and psychological regeneration at night can considerably reduce daytime attention levels and negatively affect school and work performance levels. The negative effects on the patient's private life and relationships with family and friends are equally significant. Thus, it is not surprising that AD patients with severe pruritus are at higher risk for psychological disorders such as anxiety, depression, and suicidal behavior (8).

Until recenly, topical corticosteroids (TCS) and calcineurin inhibitors (TCI) were the only topical treatments available to treat mild to moderate AD. To treat moderate to severe AD in patients, the only systemic treatments available were phototherapy or photochemotherapy (PUVA) as well as immunosuppressant drugs, such as cyclosporine, methotrexate, azathioprine, or mycophenolate mofetil (10, 11). Acute, severe exacerbations of AD have been and are still treated with systemic corticosteroids, which are associated with a risk of rebound exacerbations after their cessation.

The recent availability of dupilumab, an IL4Ra-antibody, has signaled the beginning of a new era in AD treatment. Based on the increased knowledge of AD pathophysiology, many new substances for topical or systemic treatments of AD are currently in development and being investigated in clinical trials. This will significantly increase our treatment options against both atopic eczematous lesions and chronic pruritus in the near future (12, 13).

PATHOPHYSIOLOGY OF ITCH IN AD

Genetic predisposition (e.g., filaggrin gene mutation), immune dysfunction and environmental factors (e.g., irritants, allergens, microbiome), and their interactions with each other, play significant roles in AD (1, 2). The cutaneous neurosensory system occupies a central position within this "pathophysiological triangle" of barrier disruptions, immune dysfunction, and external impacts on the skin (**Figure 1**). Barrier dysfunction within this triangle enables the intrusion of allergens, irritants, or microbial constituents, which eventually stimulate the innate and adaptive immune systems. The immune reactions and released mediators again affect the epidermal barrier, e.g., by reducing filaggrin production (1, 2). Sensory nerves are in close contact with resident and infiltrating skin cells; they can interact intensively with these cells and the mediators released during acute and chronic disease stages (14). Cellular and soluble factors that play a role in eczema development and perpetuation are also important factors in pruritus induction in AD (1, 2, 6). Inflammatory mediators of AD can also sensitize sensory nerves, inducing the phenomena of "hyperknesis" (i.e., increased sensitivity of nerves to pruritic stimuli) and "alloknesis" (i.e., non-pruritic stimuli are perceived as itch). These aspects may contribute to the chronic nature of pruritus in AD (6, 14).

Cutaneous sensory nerves densely innervate all skin layers, including the epidermis, and extend to the stratum corneum. In the skin intercellular spaces, these sensory nerves come in close contact with resident (e.g., keratinocytes, dendritic cells), and infiltrating cells (e.g., lymphocytes, mast cells, eosinophils) and interact with these via a myriad of mediators and receptors (15). These cutaneous sensory nerves in the upper dermal layers include pruriceptive afferent sensory nerves, which convey an itch-signal upon stimulation *via* dorsal root ganglia cells and their central projections to the dorsal horn of the spinal cord. The itch signal is then transferred via interneurons to nerve fibers of the lateral spinothalamic tract, which cross to the contralateral side, and extend to the thalamus. From this point, the signal is distributed to multiple brain regions. In the brain, the signal induces an itching sensation and elicits scratching behavior (16). Researchers have measured an increased density of sensory nerve fibers in skin with AD; therefore, this skin is in a state of neural sensitization, primed to react to signals and interact with the cutaneous environment. An increased concentration of neurotrophins (e.g., the nerve growth factor (NGF) from keratinocytes or the brain-derived neurotrophic factor (BDNF) from neural projections and eosinophils), together with a decreased concentration of the epidermal axon repulsion factor semaphorin A, which is capable of antagonizing the effects of neurotrophins by enhancing nerve sprouting, resulting in hyper-innervation of the inflamed atopic skin (17, 18). This hyper-innervation may eventually lower the threshold for itch induction (i.e., hyperknesis) and favor the induction of itch by non-pruritic stimuli (i.e., alloknesis).

Studies have distinguished histamine-sensitive and histamine-insensitive pruriceptive sensory nerves in the cutaneous neuronal network (14). Antihistaminic drugs have displayed only minor or no effects against pruritus in AD, other than having a soporific effect on patients. This finding indicates that histamine plays only a minor role in AD-associated itch, at least *via* the stimulation of H1 receptors (14). However, histamine may still play a role in AD inflammation and pruritus. Blocking H4 receptors located on immune cells and sensory nerves with specific H4-antagonists had at least some anti-pruritic effects on experimental pruritus (19). Clinical trials, however, showed that no significant reductions in pruritus or eczema occurred in AD patients (20).

These findings show that pruritus in AD is primarily perceived via non-histaminergic sensory nerves. In addition, inflammatory mediators seem to play a central role in AD pathophysiology and can stimulate non-histaminergic sensory nerves, which eventually induces atopic pruritus (14).

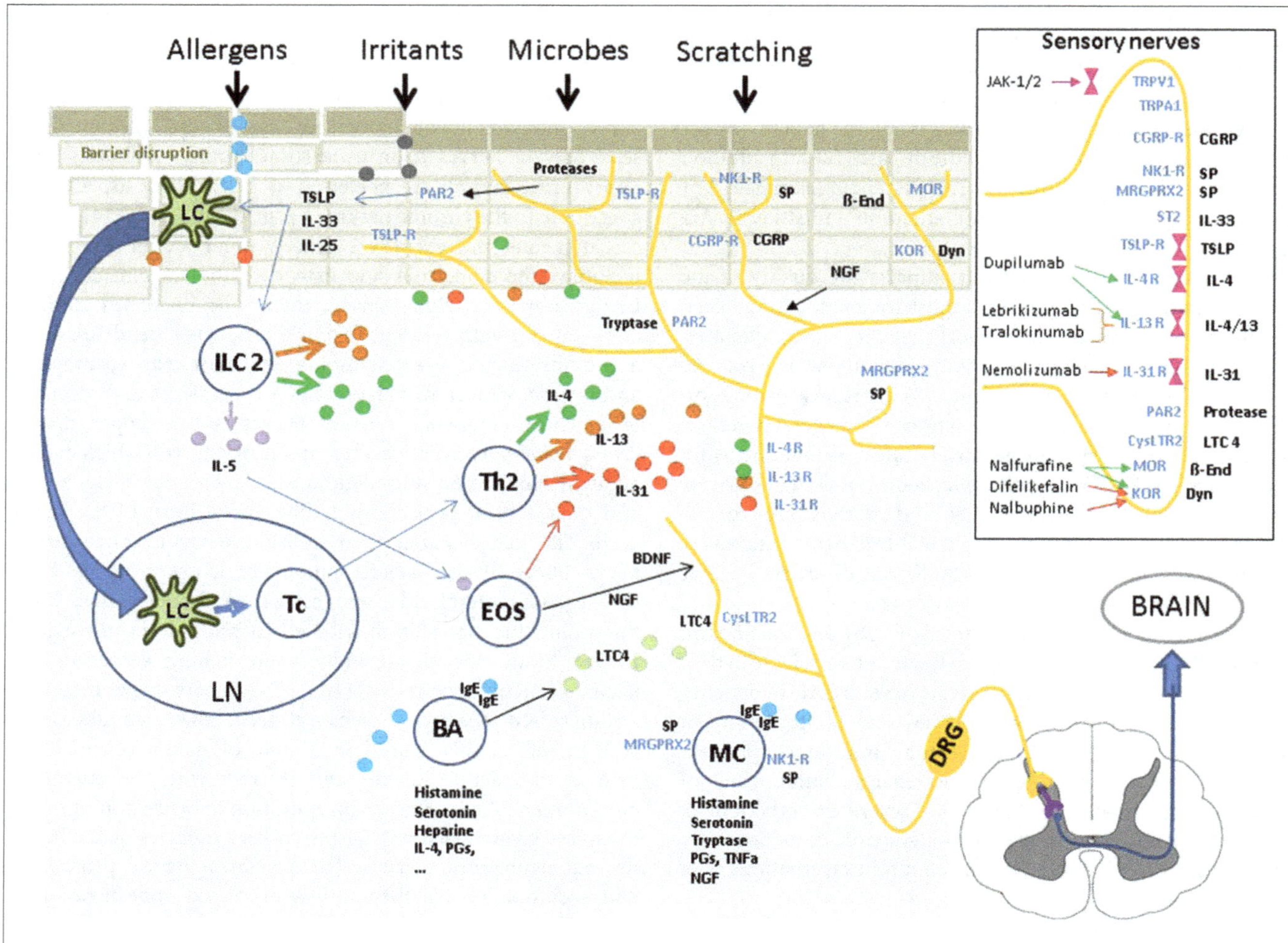

FIGURE 1 | The cutaneous neurosensory system occupies a central position within the "pathophysiological triangle" of epidermal barrier disruption, immune dysfunction, and environmental impacts due to external stimuli. The cutaneous sensory nerves are in close contact with resident and infiltrating cells and are affected by a myriad of mediators from these cells. Upon stimulation, the signal is mediated *via* pruriceptive nerve fibers and the dorsal root ganglia extending to the dorsal horn of the spinal cord. From there, the signal is transferred via interneurons to fibers of the lateral spinothalamic tract, which cross over to the contralateral side, extend up to the thalamus and, finally, reach multiple brain regions, where the nervous signal is perceived as an itching sensation, and scratching is induced. Insert: Multiple itch transmitting receptors are located on sensory nerve fibers, some of which are associated with intracellular Janus kinases. Targeting these receptors or the intracellular Janus kinases with specific inhibitors has shown to have significant antipruritic effects. IL, interleukin; TSLP, Thymic stromal lymphopoetin; NK1-R,neurokinin-1 receptor; CGRP/-R, Calcitonin gene-related peptide /-receptor; MRGPRX2, Mas-related G-protein coupled receptor X2; IgE, Immunoglobulin E; PAR2, Protease activated receptor 2; TRPV1/A1, Transient receptor potential vanilloid 1/ankyrin 1 channel; LTC4, leukotriene C4; CysLTC4, LTC4 receptor; MOR, mu-opioid receptor; KOR, kappa-opioid receptor; Dyn, Dynorphin; ß-End, ß-Endorphin; SP, substance P; ST2, IL-33-receptor.

Alarmins and Neuropeptides

These mediators include the so-called alarmins, such as thymic stromal lymphopoetin (TSLP), interleukin (IL)-33, and IL-25. They are released by keratinocytes when they come into contact with various irritants, allergens, or bacterial products (1). Alarmin induction is enhanced when the epidermal barrier is significantly disrupted. In AD, this can be due to an underlying filaggrin gene mutation, the cutaneous inflammation itself, which disturbs the production of epidermal barrier constituents, or by an altered microbiome. In addition, itch-induced scratching also damages the epidermal barrier by mechanically irritating the skin (1, 21).

Irritants, allergens and bacterial products that contact the skin often contain an array of proteolytic enzymes; these can activate protease-activated receptors (PAR) by the proteolytic cleavage of their extracellular N-termini (22). PAR-2 receptors are located on keratinocytes and sensory nerves, and researchers have argued that the stimulation of PAR-2 is a major pathway for non-histaminergic pruritus in AD and the induction of neurogenic inflammation, resulting in the release of neuropeptides such as substance P (SP) and calcitonin gene-related peptide (CGRP) (23). In AD patients, the skin is exposed to various proteolytic enzymes from exogenous (e.g., bacteria or house dust mites) or endogenous sources (e.g., tryptase, trypsin and kallikreins, mainly KLK5) that are released by epithelial or immune cells during inflammation processes, highlighting the importance of this pathway in the early disease phases (24, 25). Recent findings by Zhao et al. (26) revealed intriguingly that PAR-2 activation appears to be located upstream of TSLP and that stimulation of TRPV3 can induce TSLP release. TSLP activates other immune cells, but can also directly stimulate pruriceptive sensory nerve fibers to induce itch (27), a finding that has also been shown for the alarmin IL-33 (28). Thus, keratinocytes could boost and transform irritating stimuli from external or internal sources into itch signals via PAR-2 stimulation and the release of mediators such as TSLP. PAR-2 and TSLP could also be significant "neuro-epidermal communication" elements in AD; in a newly developed mouse model with epidermal overexpression, PAR-2 was recently shown to induce and exacerbate AD signs and symptoms, and especially pruritus (25).

PAR-2, *via* the stimulation of sensory nerves, also induces neurogenic inflammation and the release of neuropeptides such as SP and CGRP (29). SP affects sensory nerves and keratinocytes as well as inflammatory cells (e.g., lymphocytes, mast cells, eosinophils, and basophils) *via* high-affinity neurokinin (NK)-1 receptors and Mas-related G-protein coupled receptors (MrgprX2) (30). Stimulation of MrgprX2 is also involved in SP-induced mast cell degranulation, which stimulates mast cells to release of more inflammatory and pruritogenic mediators, such as histamine, leukotrienes, prostaglandins, TNF-a, proteases, and NGF (30). Interestingly, in a mouse model of acute contact dermatitis, Meixong et al. showed that Mrgprb2 (the murine form of MrgprX2) activation of mast cells differed from classical IgE-mediated stimulation in that it induced a preferential release of tryptase and the eventual induction of non-histaminergic itch, probably *via* PAR-2 activation. Whether MrgprX2 receptors are also mast cell-associated targets in pruritus of AD patients remains to be determined (31).

However, SP can also stimulate pruritus due to the effect of MRGPR-X2 on sensory nerves. This may represent an additional or even the preferred pathway by which SP stimulates pruritus in AD. In part, this may explain why a recent clinical trial in AD patients with the specific NK1R-antagonist serlopitant showed numerical but not significant reduction in pruritus (32), while tradipitant, another NK1-receptor antagonist, slightly but significantly reduced itch in these patients (33). In patients with chronic prurigo, serlopitant also significantly reduced pruritus in a phase-2 study; however, it numerically but not significantly reduced pruritus in two phase-3 studies (32). This indicates that both NK-1 and MrgprX2 receptors obviously play a role in SP-induced pruritus, but the extent to which these two receptors are involved in atopic pruritus in various disease stages requires further evaluation.

The neuropeptide CGRP also affects sensory nerves, blood vessels and immune cells (e.g., dendritic cells and T-cells), facilitates the infiltration of inflammatory cells and propagates a Th2 immune response (15). Similarly, CGRP stimulates the release of IL-13 from circulating CLA+ T-cells in AD; an increased IL-13 release from T-cells has been observed in more severely affected AD patients with more intense pruritus (34). Thus, the neurosensory system – with its antidromic axon reflex of neurogenic inflammation and local release of neuropeptides – occupies the frontline of defense against environmental impacts on the skin, even before the innate or adaptive immune systems are activated.

Interkeukins (IL)-4, IL-13, and IL-31

The release of the alarmins TSLP, IL-33, and IL-25, together with neuropeptides, not only trigger the induction and perception of itch; they also eventually stimulate the innate and adaptive immune systems. This stimulation initiates and further propagates the predominant Th2 immune response in AD. Subsequently, several pro-inflammatory mediators are released, either directly by type 2 innate lymphoid cells (ILC2) or Th2 effector lymphocytes or indirectly *via* the stimulation of mast cells, basophils, or eosinophils. Many of these mediators can either directly or indirectly stimulate pruritus in AD (1, 2).

The cytokines IL-4 and IL-13 play a central role in AD pathophysiology and also play a significant role in AD itch. These cytokines are produced and released mainly from ILC2 and Th2 cells. By activating specific receptors which share the IL-4Ra chain, they have multiple effects on epidermal and dermal cells as well as on sensory nerve fibers (1, 2). *In vitro* and *in vivo* experiments in mice have underlined the potential of IL-4 and IL-13 to sensitize sensory nerves to itch by lowering the sensitivity thresholds to other pruritogenic stimuli, such as histamine, IL-31 and TSLP (35). However, other studies have shown that both IL-4 and IL-13 also can directly stimulate pruritus in mice and that the application of combinations of these mediators even accelerated itch induction (36).

Involved sensory nerve fibers carry the transient receptor potential (TRP) V1 and TRPA1, which are unspecific cation channels (37). Once these nerves have been stimulated by IL-4, IL-13, or IL-31*via* their specific receptors, the activation of TRPV1 and/or TRPA1 induces calcium influx, which eventually induces the release of action potentials *via* the sodium channels NaV1.7, NaV1.8, or NaV1.9. TRPV1 and TRPA1 must be present for these pruritogens to induce itch or sensitize sensory nerves to other pruritogens (37, 38).

IL-4 and IL-13 also affect the skin barrier and disturb its function by downregulating essential skin barrier proteins such as filaggrin, involucrin, and loricrin (1, 2, 39). This downregulation causes the release of proteolytic enzymes, stimulating PAR-2, and the release of alarmins (IL-25, IL-33, TSLP). This series of events closes a feed-forward loop and fuels atopic inflammation as well as pruritus. IL-4 and IL-13 have also recently been shown to induce the selective expression of kallikrein (KLK)-7 in normal human epidermal keratinocytes. One recent study also implicated KLK-7 in itch induction, regardless of inflammation in AD, *via* an unknown epidermal-neural mechanism (40, 41). These cytokines, however, also affect key immunologic cells such as other lymphocytes, mast cells, eosinophils, and basophils that carry the IL-4 and/or IL-13 receptors. By triggering the release of preformed and newly produced mediators from these cells (e.g., histamine, tryptase, endothelin-1, eotaxin, IL-31), IL-4 and IL-13 further contribute to the stimulation of sensory nerves and the induction of itch in AD (42).

IL-31, the so-called "itch-cytokine" plays a major role in this respect, as it is primarily released by Th2 cells and can directly stimulate specific IL-31 receptors (IL-31R) on sensory nerves, inducing an itching sensation (35). In addition, stimulation of IL-31R, which consists of the IL-31 receptor alpha chain (IL-31Ra) and the Oncostatin M receptor-beta chain, also stimulates the sprouting and branching of these sensory nerves, increasing their sensitivity to IL-31, and other pruritogens (43). By both directly inducing itch and sensitizing nerves to further pruritic stimuli, IL-31 plays a significant role in AD pruritus. This process of neural sensitization by IL-31 may significantly contribute to the development of chronic itch. Specifically, it may play a critical role in the so-called "itch-scratch-cycle," a phenomenon which strongly promotes the development of highly pruritic nodular chronic prurigo, i.e., prurigo nodularis. Interestingly, high levels of IL-31 have been found in these pruriginous skin lesions (44). Chronic prurigo is frequently associated with atopic diathesis or a history of previous AD, and it can sometimes be found in combination with atopic eczema in AD patients with severe chronic pruritus (45).

Janus kinase/Signal Transducer and Activator of Transcription

Several of the aforementioned mediators either directly stimulate pruritus or sensitize sensory nerves to other pruritogenic stimuli. Once these mediators have bound to their specific receptors, they transmit their signals via the Janus kinase (JAK)/Signal transducer and activator of transcription (STAT) pathway.

The JAK family has four members: JAK1, JAK2, JAK3, and TYK2 (46). Cytokines that are important for pruritus in AD (e.g., IL-31, IL-4, IL-13, and TSLP) transmit their signals *via* JAK-1 and JAK-2 into the cells. The deletion or inhibition of JAK-1/2 in animal models significantly reduced itch signaling induced by these mediators (35). In humans, JAKs were shown to play a critical role in pruritus when tofacitinib, an oral JAK 1/3 inhibitor, significantly reduced pruritus in elderly patients who suffered from chronic pruritus of unknown origin (35). IL-31, IL-4, IL-13, TSLP, and IL-5, as well as other cytokines influence inflammation and pruritus in AD. The potential to inhibit JAK-1 and JAK-2 with selective JAK-inhibitors opens a new treatment avenue, indicating that it may be possible to block several important itch mediators simultaneously. This avenue should enable us to treat chronic pruritus in AD and other chronically pruritic diseases more effectively (47).

Opioid System

The central and peripheral opioid system is involved in chronic pruritus. The μ-opioid (ß-endorphin/μ-opioid receptor) and k-opioid (dynorphin A/k-opioid receptor) systems are involved in pruritus modulation (48). Stimulating μ-opioid receptors (MOR) (e.g., with morphine for pain treatment) induces itch, while inhibiting MOR with naloxone or naltrexone or stimulating k-opioid receptors (KOR) with specific agonists can reduce itch (49). Researchers have identified a relative imbalance between the KOR and MOR system with a downregulation of KOR in the epidermis of AD patients. Photochemotherapy (PUVA) could be used to rebalance the deviant KOR/MOR systems by downregulating MOR (its ligand ß-endorphin remained unchanged) and upregulating the reduced dynorphin levels to normal (KOR remained unchanged), leading to itch reduction in AD patients (48). One study found a significant decrease in KOR in patients with end-stage renal disease (ESDR) under hemodialysis, who suffered from chronic itch, as compared to patients without chronic itch, while the expression of KOR correlated significantly and negatively with itch intensity (50). The KOR agonist dynorphin can be used to modulate itch perception by, for example, interacting with KOR on interneurons in the spinal cord (51). Treating ESRD patients who suffered from chronic itch with the KOR agonist nalfurafine had significant antipruritic effects (52). The topical application of nalfurafine also had an antipruritic effect in a murine model of AD (53). Phototherapy can be used to reduce itch in both EDSR and AD patients and may also have an antipruritic effect, at least in part, because it affects the peripheral opioid system in the skin; e.g., the resulting dynorphin release can eventually act on peripheral sites as well as central KOR (54).

SYSTEMIC TREATMENTS

In recent years, scientists have gained a significant amount of knowledge about the pathophysiology and key mediators of inflammation and itch in AD (2). While several agents have been newly developed to treat AD, the results seen *in vitro* and in animal studies still need to be translated from laboratory to the bedside. In the following sub-sections, descriptions of the new treatments are provided. Future studies will provide even further information about whether these agents really be used to improve eczema and chronic pruritus under real-world conditions in daily clinical practice.

IL-4/IL-13 Blockade

When dupilumab, the first biological agent to be developed to specifically target the IL-4 receptor alpha (IL-4Ra) chain, was licensed in 2017, we entered a new era in AD treatment. Dupilumab inhibits the interactions between IL-4 and IL-13 and their receptors, which share the same IL-4Ra subunit (55).

Two monotherapy studies (SOLO 1 and SOLO 2) clearly showed that dupilumab improved atopic eczematous skin lesions. The agent significantly reached the primary endpoint, reducing the investigator global assessment (IGA) to clear or almost clear and significantly reducing the Eczema Area and Severity Index (EASI) as compared to a placebo. Dupilumab also significantly reduced the weekly average of daily peak pruritus on the numerical rating scale (NRS) from 0 (= no itch) to 10 (= worst imaginable itch) by about 50% as compared to about 20% in controls (56). The significant anti-pruritic effect of dupilumab as compared to the controls was confirmed in subsequent studies (55), and the results of a *post-hoc* analysis of data from four randomized, controlled trials showed that dupilumab could significantly reduce itch by as early as the 2nd day of treatment in adults and the 5th day of treatment in adolescents. Thus, the agent displayed not only good but also rapid itch reduction in AD (57). Similar effects on eczema and pruritus were recently shown with dupilumab treatment in children aged 6–11 years (55, 58).

In addition, dupilumab could significantly reduce pruritus in difficult to treat, highly pruritic diseases such as chronic prurigo and bullous pemphigoid. This finding indicates that IL-4 and IL-13 play important roles in chronic pruritus and that blocking these cytokines could help to relieve pruritus in diseases other than AD (59). However, with dupilumab, it has not yet been possible to determine the relative contributions of IL-4 or IL-13 to these effects. In fact, other researchers have assumed that IL-13 is the primary mediator of AD in peripheral tissues, and some have speculated that dupilumab blocks IL-13 as a primary mechanism of effect in AD (60).

Tralokinumab and lebrikizumab, two biologics that specifically target IL-13, were recently developed, enabling researchers to evaluate the importance of IL-13 in eczema and pruritus in AD. Although, no direct comparisons with dupilumab have been made, both tralokinumab and lebrikizumab significantly reduce eczema and pruritus in AD. In three phase 3 trials, tralokinumab, as monotherapy or in combination with TCS, significantly improved eczema. Tralokinumab also reduced pruritus by $\geq$ 4 points on the NRS in a significantly higher proportion of patients than in controls, regardless of their concomitant treatment with TCS (45.4 vs. 34.1% in ECZTRA3) or without TCS (20.0 vs. 10.3% in ECZTRA1 and 25.0 vs. 9.5% in ECZTRA2) (61, 62).

Likewise, lebrikizumab also significantly reduced eczema scores in a phase 2b trial. Lebrikizumab was given subcutaneously in a dose of 125 or 250 mg every 4 weeks (with a double loading dose) or in a dose of 250 mg every 2 weeks (without a double loading dose). This treatment enabled significantly more patients to reach a clinically relevant peak-pruritus reduction of $\geq$4 points NRS as compared to controls (i.e., 41.8, 47.4, and 70.0% as compared to the placebo with 27.3%). Notably, a significant difference in itch reduction was seen as early as day 2 in the high-dose group (63).

Since the study designs differed, we cannot directly compare the effects of tralokinumab and lebrikizumab on pruritus with each other or with the effects of dupilumab. However, these studies clearly show that blocking IL-13 can significantly reduce pruritus in AD. Whether the effects of IL-13 blockade can be enhanced by also blocking IL-4 remains to be determined in a future head-to-head trial with dupilumab, although, it is unlikely that these direct comparisons will be performed very soon.

IL-31 Blockade

The IL-31Ra antagonist nemolizumab had a highly significant antipruritic effect in patients with moderate to severe AD (64). This study was remarkable, because "peak pruritus" on a numerical rating scale (PP-NRS) was chosen as the primary outcome parameter. Therefore, this challenged the idea that IL-31 was the "primary itch mediator" in AD. In this study, nemolizumab was subcutaneously applied in doses of 0.1, 0.5, or 2.0 mg/kg at baseline and every 4 weeks; significant reductions of 43.7, 59.8, and 63.1%, respectively, as compared to 20.9% by placebo, were seen in peak pruritus over the 12-week trial period (64). Two other placebo-controlled phase 2 trials using fixed regimens confirmed the excellent anti-pruritic effect of nemolizumab (65, 66). In an open-label, long-term extension study of the previous 12-week study, patients were further treated with 0.5 mg/kg of nemolizumab every 4 weeks; the pruritus could be reduced by 89.6% by week 64 (67). The improvement in eczema progressed more slowly than the itch reduction. Thus, EASI was reduced by 47.8% after 12 weeks, but could also be improved by 75.8% after 64 weeks (no control group for comparison) in this long-term extension study (67).

The significant antipruritic effect of nemolizumab could also recently be demonstrated in patients with nodular chronic prurigo (i.e., prurigo nodularis (PN)) (68). PN is a treatment-resistant, distinct disease characterized by severe chronic pruritus, chronic scratching, and pruriginous nodular skin lesions (45). Four weeks after receiving one subcutaneous injection of nemolizumab (0.5 mg/kg), pruritus was reduced by 4.5 points NRS from baseline (i.e., 53.0%) as compared to only 1.7 points (i.e., 20.2%) in placebo-treated prurigo patients. At 12 weeks (i.e., 4 weeks after receiving the last of 3 monthly subcutaneous injections), the itch was even reduced by 61.9% as compared to 25.7% in controls. In addition, the extent of healed nodular skin lesions was significantly better than that seen in controls (68). Phase 3 and long-term extension studies in AD and PN with nemolizumab are currently ongoing; the outcomes of these studies should improve our knowledge about treatment possibilities for these diseases (for AD, ClinicalTrials.gov Identifier: NCT03985943 and NCT03989349 and NCT03989206; and for PN, NCT04501666, NCT04501679, NCT04204616).

These data indicate that, firstly, pruritus in AD and chronic prurigo can be significantly reduced by specifically targeting IL-31, breaking the "itch-scratch-cycle" and eventually enabling nodular prurigo to heal and eczema to improve in AD (64, 68). Secondly, blocking IL-31 with nemolizumab appears more effectively reduce atopic pruritus than eczema (65), while blocking IL-4/IL-13 appears to have a stronger inhibitory effect on eczema than on pruritus (56). To clearly understand the true relative effects of different drugs in specific diseases, these must be compared in head-to-head studies. However, pruritus and eczema in AD have traditionally been believed to be tightly connected with each other, and AD was often described as an "itch that rashes" (69). As new treatments and agents that block specific mediators appear, the regulation of pruritus and eczema in AD may turn out to be more differentiated than previously thought. This knowledge may help us to further customize AD treatments to meet the primary needs of our patients in the future.

JAK Inhibitors

The findings of Oetjen et al. (35) highlighted the importance of the mediators IL-4, IL-13, and IL-31 for the induction and maintenance of itch in AD. In their experiments, the inhibition of the JAK/STAT pathway, which mediates the intracellular signaling of these cytokines, significantly reduced atopic itch in mice. JAK-1 inhibition displayed especially significant effects on pruritus. In their study, Oetjen et al. (35) also showed that the oral JAK1/3 inhibitor tofacitinib could successfully reduce itch in patients with chronic pruritus of unknown origin.

Baricitinib is the first oral JAK inhibitor to be recently approved by the European Medicines Agency (EMA) for the treatment of patients with moderate to severe AD. This agent selectively blocks JAK-1 and JAK-2. In two phase 3 monotherapy studies (70) and one phase 3 combination study with topical TCS (71), baricitinib significantly reduced pruritus in test patients as compared to controls (who received placebo or TCS alone) throughout the whole observation period of 16 weeks. Baricitinib monotherapy (4 mg) reduced pruritus by 36.6 and 46.9% (vs. 12 and 16.6% in controls) in BREEZE-AD1 and BREEZE-AD2, respectively, by week 16 (70). In BREEZE-AD7, in which the additional use of TCS was allowed, baricitinib (4 mg) reduced pruritus by ≥4-point NRS in 52 and 44% of the patients (vs. 11 and 20% in placebo) at 4 weeks and 16 weeks, respectively (71). The rapid onset of itch reduction after baricitinib provision was recognized as a remarkable feature of this agent, with this onset occurring as early as 2 days after initiating treatment (71). The primary outcome parameters in these studies (i.e., the reduction of IGA and EASI) were also significantly met. Baricitinib (4 mg) not only reduced itch, but also significantly reduced sleep disturbance and improved quality of life, both of which are important patient-oriented outcome measures that improve the overall quality of life in AD patients. As a final bonus, baricitinib also significantly reduced skin pain (70, 71).

Other JAK inhibitors are currently in the pipeline for AD treatment. The most advanced in their developmental programs are upadacitinib and abrocitinib, both of which are considered selective JAK-1 inhibitors. In a recent phase 2b trial, upadacitinib reduced pruritus significantly and rapidly in moderate to severe AD patients, with a maximal itch reduction of 70% at the highest dose (i.e., 30 mg) as compared to a 10% reduction in the placebo group. In this study, eczema was also significantly reduced (72). The data from phase 3 trials will be published soon. Similarly, in a recent phase 3 trial, abrocitinib significantly reduced itch in moderate to severe AD patients aged ≥12 years. At the highest dose, abrocitinib (200 mg) effected a ≥4-point reduction in pruritus in 57% of patients (vs. 15% in the placebo group) within 12 weeks; it also significantly improved atopic eczematous skin lesion. Abrocitinib (200 mg) had already significantly reduced pruritus by the first day after starting treatment (73, 74). It will be interesting to see the not-yet-published results of a recent trial that directly compares abrocitinib with dupilumab.

One outstanding phenomenon observed in all these studies with JAK-1 or JAK-1/2 inhibitors is the speed of onset in itch reduction, which the patients experienced already within the first days of treatment. This rapid improvement in pruritus is probably due to the inhibition of several pruritic mediators (e.g., IL-4, IL-13, IL-31, and TSLP) by inhibiting their intracellular signal transduction. Together with a rapid improvement in sleep quality and overall quality of life, the patients' motivation to continue the oral treatment with JAK inhibitors increases. This is an important consideration, as *per-se* daily oral treatments are subject to lower treatment compliance as compared with subcutaneous injections of biologics every 2–4 weeks.

Other Systemic Treatments

Alarmins

Although, the alarmins (e.g., TSLP and IL-33) are thought to influence AD pathophysiology, a clinical phase 2 trial in which TSLP was blocked with the specific antibody tezepelumab did not result in convincing improvements in eczema or pruritus (75). In addition, phase 2 trials with monoclonal antibodies against IL-33 were prematurely terminated due to their insufficient effects on AD. Simply because significant effects have not been observed when blocking these alarmins, however, may not necessarily mean that they do not play a role in AD itch. The study design (i.e., combination treatments with TCS, patients' characteristics and stages of the disease (acute vs. chronic AD)) can significantly influence the study outcomes. Since TSLP and IL-33 are mediators in the early phases of AD, blocking these mediators could be more important in early stages or flare-ups of the disease rather than in the chronic AD patients who are included in most AD studies. A recent finding by Wang et al. also supports a differential view of itch flare-ups as compared to chronic itch in AD patients. While previous AD trials using anti-IgE therapy had yielded mixed results in AD, the authors showed that allergen exposure is capable of inducing acute itch flare-ups *via* the stimulation of basophils that carry allergen-specific IgE, eventually releasing leukotriene (LT) C4, which then activates specific CysLTR2 receptors on sensory nerves and induces itch (76).

Opioid Receptor Antagonists/Agonists

With the new treatments in AD and their promising antipruritic effects, do we need more? In fact, the significant itch reduction rates of 40–70% or ≥4-point NRS reduction in about 50% of patients will already satisfy many patients. Still, many AD patients may still suffer from pruritus, and additional antipruritic "add-on treatments" for these patients may be desirable.

This goal could be reached by targeting the central and peripheral opioid system involved in chronic pruritus of AD and in end-stage renal disease (ESRD) (48). Pruritus in AD patients has been successfully reduced with the MOR antagonists naloxone or naltrexone, but the use of these agents is associated with undesirable adverse events like dizziness, drowsiness, or vomiting, hindering their broader use (49).

Newly developed KOR agonists, such as nalfurafine, or the combined MOR antagonist/KOR agonist nalbuphine have recently shown mild but significant efficacy in reducing pruritus in ESRD patients. These appear to be associated with a lower risk for central nervous adverse events (77). Currently, nalfurafine is only licensed for uremic and cholestatic pruritus in Japan. An oral extended-release formulation of nalbuphine is currently under investigation for its antipruritic effect in PN (ClinicalTrials.gov Identifier: NCT03497975). Difelikefalin (previously CR845), a peripheral KOR agonist that is intravenously applied in a dose of 0.5 μg per kg thrice weekly for 12 weeks, demonstrated significant antipruritic effects in ESRD patients under hemodialysis without displaying any dysphoria or hallucinations as adverse events (78). Oral difelikefalin, in doses of 0.25, 0.5, or 1.0 mg twice weekly, is currently under investigation for its effect on pruritus in moderate to severe AD (ClincialTrial.gov Identifier NCT04018027).

Once these drugs have been approved for the treatment of chronic pruritus in AD or chronic prurigo, it will be very interesting to see if these drugs can be used to further reduce pruritus in patients who are been given biologics or JAK inhibitors, but who are not yet free of pruritus.

Topical Antipruritic/Anti-Inflammatory Substances

Systemic therapies for moderate to severe AD appear to have developed appreciably in recent years. However, most AD patients do not have a severe form of the disease, and many with mild to moderate forms of the disease have only circumscribed eczema but still suffer from severe pruritus. In addition, many patients do not want to be systemically treated, regardless of the severity of their disease, for various reasons. Thus, in the future topical agents will still play roles in the anti-inflammatory and antipruritic treatment of AD.

Until recently, TCS and TCI were the only "specific" topical treatments for AD. Crisaborole, a phosphodiesterase four (PDE4) inhibitor, was licensed for topical treatment of AD in 2016. Inhibition of PDE4 increases cAMP in targeted cells and reduces inflammatory mediators, eventually reducing eczema and itch associated with AD lesions. In phase 3 clinical trials, crisaborole already reduced itch significantly within the first 8 days of treatment, and the reduction remained significant throughout the 4-week study period. In addition, a significant reduction in atopic skin lesions was observed (79, 80). Although, the difference between crisaborole and placebo in reducing itch was not overwhelming, crisaborole was only associated with minor adverse events (e.g., burning or stinging), and did not cause skin atrophy.

Other new agents to treat AD are in clinical trials or already licensed. Topical JAK inhibitors are especially promising candidates as anti-inflammatory and anti-pruritic topical treatments in inflammatory skin diseases, such as AD and psoriasis. Recent studies with topical formulations of tofacitinib (a JAK1/3 inhibitor), ruxolitinib (a JAK1/2 inhibitor), and delgocitinib (a pan-JAK inhibitor that blocks all members of the JAK family) have shown promising results in reducing both eczema and especially pruritus in AD lesions (81). Delgocitinib has recently been approved for the topical treatment of AD in Japan (82). Topical JAK inhibitors are advantageous for AD patients with circumscribed pruritic AD lesions, because they can be used to control itch and the disease effectively in patients with mild to moderate AD, but also avoid the possible adverse events associated with the use of systemic JAK inhibitors (81).

Another interesting newly developed agent is tapinarof, a selective agonist for the aryl hydrocarbon receptor (AhR), also known as the dioxin receptor. Stimulation of AhR results in a decreased expression of pro-inflammatory cytokines, enhancement of the skin barrier function and a reduction in oxidative stress (83). Medicinal coal tar and soybean tar Glyteer, which have been used as anti-inflammatory agents to treat AD and psoriasis, also activate this receptor (84). In a recent phase 2b study, tapinarof 1% cream significantly reduced itch in adolescent and adult AD patients and reduced eczema (85). Significantly more patients experienced ≥ 3 points of NRS reduction at weeks 4 and 12 after starting the treatment, and a clear differentiation between the tapinarof and vehicle groups was shown, starting at week 2. In adult psoriasis patients, tapinarof cream also improved psoriasis lesions and significantly reduced itch (86).

CONCLUSION

Chronic pruritus is the most burdensome symptom experienced by patients with AD of all grades of severity. Pruritus is the primary cause of significant impairments in the quality of life of affected patients, impacting their well-being in multiple ways. The chronic itching associated with the disease can disturb the patients' sleep and reduce their performance in their private and professional lives. It can even have significant, negative psychological consequences, such as increased anxiety and depression. The high out-of-pocket and healthcare costs associated with the treatment of pruritus and eczema puts an additional economic burden on AD patients and communities. The advent of new and effective treatments for AD promises significant improvements in care options for AD patients in the near future. Every new topical or systemic agent that has proven anti-eczematous and anti-pruritic effects will help us improve our understanding of AD pathophysiology. The improved understanding and further investigations into the anti-eczematous and anti-pruritic effects of AD treatments will also enable us to customize our therapy to meet the needs of our AD patients in the present and the future.

AUTHOR CONTRIBUTIONS

The author confirms being the sole contributor of this work and has approved it for publication.

REFERENCES

1. Weidinger S, Beck LA, Bieber T, Kabashima K, Irvine AD. Atopic dermatitis. *Nat Rev Dis Primers.* (2018) 4:1. doi: 10.1038/s41572-018-0001-z
2. Langan SM, Irvine AD, Weidinger S. Atopic dermatitis. *Lancet.* (2020) 396:345-360. *Erratum in: Lancet.* (2020) 396:758. doi: 10.1016/S0140-6736(20)31286-1
3. Barbarot S, Auziere S, Gadkari A, Girolomoni G, Puig L, Simpson EL, et al. Epidemiology of atopic dermatitis in adults: results from an international survey. *Allergy.* (2018) 73:1284–93. doi: 10.1111/all.13401
4. Stefanovic N, Flohr C, Irvine AD. The exposome in atopic dermatitis. *Allergy.* (2020) 75:63–74. doi: 10.1111/all.13946
5. Hanifin JM, Rajka G. Diagnostic features of atopic dermatitis. *Acta Derm Venereol.* (1980) 92:44–7.

6. Mollanazar NK, Smith PK, Yosipovitch G. Mediators of chronic pruritus in atopic dermatitis: getting the itch out? *Clin Rev Allergy Immunol.* (2016) 51:263–92. doi: 10.1007/s12016-015-8488-5
7. Silverberg JI, Gelfand JM, Margolis DJ, Boguniewicz M, Fonacier L, Grayson MH, et al. Patient burden and quality of life in atopic dermatitis in US adults: a population-based cross-sectional study. *Ann Allergy Asthma Immunol.* (2018) 121:340–7. doi: 10.1016/j.anai.2018.07.006
8. Simpson EL, Bieber T, Eckert L, Wu R, Ardeleanu M, Graham NM, et al. Patient burden of moderate to severe atopic dermatitis (AD): insights from a phase 2b clinical trial of dupilumab in adults. *J Am Acad Dermatol.* (2016) 74:491–8. doi: 10.1016/j.jaad.2015.10.043
9. Ständer S, Simpson EL, Guttman-Yassky E, Thyssen JP, Kabashima K, Ball SG, et al. Clinical relevance of skin pain in atopic dermatitis. *J Drugs Dermatol.* (2020) 19:921–6. doi: 10.36849/JDD.2020.5498
10. Wollenberg A, Barbarot S, Bieber T, Christen-Zaech S, Deleuran M, Fink-Wagner A, et al. Consensus-based European guidelines for treatment of atopic eczema (atopic dermatitis) in adults and children: part I. *J Eur Acad Dermatol Venereol.* (2018) 32:657–82. *Erratum in: J Eur Acad Dermatol Venereol.* (2019) 33:1436. doi: 10.1111/jdv.14891
11. Wollenberg A, Barbarot S, Bieber T, Christen-Zaech S, Deleuran M, Fink-Wagner A, et al. Consensus-based European guidelines for treatment of atopic eczema (atopic dermatitis) in adults and children: part II. *J Eur Acad Dermatol Venereol.* (2018) 32:850–78. doi: 10.1111/jdv.14888
12. Paller AS, Kabashima K, Bieber T. Therapeutic pipeline for atopic dermatitis: end of the drought? *J Allergy Clin Immunol.* (2017) 140:633–43. doi: 10.1016/j.jaci.2017.07.006
13. Bieber T. Novel therapies based on the pathophysiology of atopic dermatitis. *J Dtsch Dermatol Ges.* (2019) 17:1150–62. doi: 10.1111/ddg.13965
14. Yosipovitch G, Berger T, Fassett MS. Neuroimmune interactions in chronic itch of atopic dermatitis. *J Eur Acad Dermatol Venereol.* (2020) 34:239–50. doi: 10.1111/jdv.15973
15. Choi JE, Di Nardo A. Skin neurogenic inflammation. *Semin Immunopathol.* (2018) 40:249–59. doi: 10.1007/s00281-018-0675-z
16. Yosipovitch G, Bernhard JD. Clinical practice. Chronic pruritus. *N Engl J Med.* (2013) 368:1625–34. doi: 10.1056/NEJMcp1208814
17. Tominaga M, Ogawa H, Takamori K. Decreased production of semaphorin 3A in the lesional skin of atopic dermatitis. *Br J Dermatol.* (2008) 158:842–4. doi: 10.1111/j.1365-2133.2007.08410.x
18. Guseva D, Rüdrich U, Kotnik N, Gehring M, Patsinakidis N, Agelopoulos K, et al. Neuronal branching of sensory neurons is associated with BDNF-positive eosinophils in atopic dermatitis. *Clin Exp Allergy.* (2020) 50:577–84. doi: 10.1111/cea.13560
19. Dunford PJ, Williams KN, Desai PJ, Karlsson L, McQueen D, Thurmond RL. Histamine H4 receptor antagonists are superior to traditional antihistamines in the attenuation of experimental pruritus. *J Allergy Clin Immunol.* (2007) 119:176–83. doi: 10.1016/j.jaci.2006.08.034
20. Werfel T, Layton G, Yeadon M, Whitlock L, Osterloh I, Jimenez P, et al. Efficacy and safety of the histamine H_4 receptor antagonist ZPL-3893787 in patients with atopic dermatitis. *J Allergy Clin Immunol.* (2019) 143:1830–7.e4. doi: 10.1016/j.jaci.2018.07.047
21. Chu CY. Treatments for childhood atopic dermatitis: an update on emerging therapies. *Clin Rev Allergy Immunol.* (2020). doi: 10.1007/s12016-020-08799-1
22. Gieseler F, Ungefroren H, Settmacher U, Hollenberg MD, Kaufmann R. Proteinase-activated receptors (PARs) - focus on receptor-receptor-interactions and their physiological and pathophysiological impact. *Cell Commun Signal.* (2013) 11:86. doi: 10.1186/1478-811X-11-86
23. Steinhoff M, Neisius U, Ikoma A, Fartasch M, Heyer G, Skov PS, et al. Proteinase-activated receptor-2 mediates itch: a novel pathway for pruritus in human skin. *J Neurosci.* (2003) 23:6176–80. doi: 10.1523/JNEUROSCI.23-15-06176.2003
24. Buhl T, Ikoma A, Kempkes C, Cevikbas F, Sulk M, Buddenkotte J, et al. Protease-activated receptor-2 regulates neuro-epidermal communication in atopic dermatitis. *Front Immunol.* (2020) 11:1740. doi: 10.3389/fimmu.2020.01740
25. Briot A, Deraison C, Lacroix M, Bonnart C, Robin A, Besson C, et al. Kallikrein 5 induces atopic dermatitis-like lesions through PAR2-mediated thymic stromal lymphopoietin expression in netherton syndrome. *J Exp Med.* (2009) 206:1135–47. doi: 10.1084/jem.20082242
26. Zhao J, Munanairi A, Liu XY, Zhang J, Hu L, Hu M, et al. par2 mediates itch via trpv3 signaling in keratinocytes. *J Invest Dermatol.* (2020) 140:1524–32. doi: 10.1016/j.jid.2020.01.012
27. Wilson SR, The L, Batia LM, Beattie K, Katibah GE, McClain SP, et al. The epithelial cell-derived atopic dermatitis cytokine TSLP activates neurons to induce itch. *Cell.* (2013) 155:285–95. doi: 10.1016/j.cell.2013.08.057
28. Liu B, Tai Y, Achanta S, Kaelberer MM, Caceres AI, Shao X, et al. IL-33/ST2 signaling excites sensory neurons and mediates itch response in a mouse model of poison ivy contact allergy. *Proc Natl Acad Sci U S A.* (2016) 113:E7572–9. doi: 10.1073/pnas.1606608113
29. Steinhoff M, Vergnolle N, Young SH, Tognetto M, Amadesi S, Ennes HS, et al. Agonists of proteinase-activated receptor 2 induce inflammation by a neurogenic mechanism. *Nat Med.* (2000) 6:151–8. doi: 10.1038/72247
30. Azimi E, Reddy VB, Pereira PJS, Talbot S, Woolf CJ, Lerner EA. Substance p activates mas-related G protein-coupled receptors to induce itch. *J Allergy Clin Immunol.* (2017) 140:447–53.e3. doi: 10.1016/j.jaci.2016.12.980
31. Meixiong J, Anderson M, Limjunyawong N, Sabbagh MF, Hu E, Mack MR, et al. Activation of mast-cell-expressed mas-related G-protein-coupled receptors drives non-histaminergic itch. *Immunity.* (2019) 50:1163–71.e5. doi: 10.1016/j.immuni.2019.03.013
32. Ständer S, Spellman MC, Kwon P, Yosipovitch G. The NK1 receptor antagonist serlopitant for treatment of chronic pruritus. *Expert Opin Investig Drugs.* (2019) 28:659–66. doi: 10.1080/13543784.2019.1638910
33. Welsh SE, Xiao C, Kaden AR, Brzezynski JL, Mohrman MA, Wang J, et al. Neurokinin-1 receptor antagonist tradipitant has mixed effects on itch in atopic dermatitis: results from EPIONE, a randomized clinical trial. *J Eur Acad Dermatol Venereol.* (2020) 35:e338–40. doi: 10.1101/2020.06.21.20136911
34. Antúnez C, Torres MJ, López S, Rodriguez-Pena R, Blanca M, Mayorga C, et al. Calcitonin gene-related peptide modulates interleukin-13 in circulating cutaneous lymphocyte-associated antigen-positive T cells in patients with atopic dermatitis. *Br J Dermatol.* (2009) 161:547–53. doi: 10.1111/j.1365-2133.2009.09318.x
35. Oetjen LK, Mack MR, Feng J, Whelan TM, Niu H, Guo CJ, et al. Sensory neurons co-opt classical immune signaling pathways to mediate chronic itch. *Cell.* (2017) 171:217–28.e13. doi: 10.1016/j.cell.2017.08.006
36. Campion M, Smith L, Gatault S, Métais C, Buddenkotte J, Steinhoff M. Interleukin-4 and interleukin-13 evoke scratching behaviour in mice. *Exp Dermatol.* (2019) 28:1501–4. doi: 10.1111/exd.14034
37. Cevikbas F, Wang X, Akiyama T, Kempkes C, Savinko T, Antal A, et al. A sensory neuron-expressed IL-31 receptor mediates T helper cell-dependent itch: involvement of TRPV1 and TRPA1. *J Allergy Clin Immunol.* (2014) 133:448–60. doi: 10.1016/j.jaci.2013.10.048
38. Cevikbas F, Lerner EA. Physiology and pathophysiology of itch. *Physiol Rev.* (2020) 100:945–82. doi: 10.1152/physrev.00017.2019
39. Howell MD, Kim BE, Gao P, Grant AV, Boguniewicz M, Debenedetto A, et al. Cytokine modulation of atopic dermatitis filaggrin skin expression. *J Allergy Clin Immunol.* (2007) 120:150–5. doi: 10.1016/j.jaci.2007.04.031
40. Morizane S, Yamasaki K, Kajita A, Ikeda K, Zhan M, Aoyama Y, et al. TH2 cytokines increase kallikrein 7 expression and function in patients with atopic dermatitis. *J Allergy Clin Immunol.* (2012) 130:259–61.e1. doi: 10.1016/j.jaci.2012.03.006
41. Guo CJ, Mack MR, Oetjen LK, Trier AM, Council ML, Pavel AB, et al. Kallikrein 7 promotes atopic dermatitis-associated itch independently of skin inflammation. *J Invest Dermatol.* (2020) 140:1244–52.e4. doi: 10.1016/j.jid.2019.10.022
42. Moyle M, Cevikbas F, Harden JL, Guttman-Yassky E. Understanding the immune landscape in atopic dermatitis: The era of biologics and emerging therapeutic approaches. *Exp Dermatol.* (2019) 28:756–68. doi: 10.1111/exd.13911
43. Feld M, Garcia R, Buddenkotte J, Katayama S, Lewis K, Muirhead G, et al. The pruritus- and TH2-associated cytokine IL-31 promotes growth of sensory nerves. *J Allergy Clin Immunol.* (2016) 138:500–8.e24. doi: 10.1016/j.jaci.2016.02.020

44. Sonkoly E, Muller A, Lauerma AI, Pivarcsi A, Soto H, Kemeny L, et al. IL-31: a new link between T cells and pruritus in atopic skin inflammation. *J Allergy Clin Immunol.* (2006) 117:411–7. doi: 10.1016/j.jaci.2005.10.033
45. Pereira MP, Steinke S, Zeidler C, Forner C, Riepe C, Augustin M, et al. European academy of dermatology and venereology European prurigo project: expert consensus on the definition, classification and terminology of chronic prurigo. *J Eur Acad Dermatol Venereol.* (2018) 32:1059–65. doi: 10.1111/jdv.14570
46. Villarino AV, Kanno Y, O'Shea JJ. Mechanisms and consequences of Jak-STAT signaling in the immune system. *Nat Immunol.* (2017) 18:374–84. doi: 10.1038/ni.3691
47. Rodrigues MA, Torres T. JAK/STAT inhibitors for the treatment of atopic dermatitis. *J Dermatolog Treat.* (2020) 31:33–40. doi: 10.1080/09546634.2019.1577549
48. Tominaga M, Ogawa H, Takamori K. Possible roles of epidermal opioid systems in pruritus of atopic dermatitis. *J Invest Dermatol.* (2007) 127:2228–35. doi: 10.1038/sj.jid.5700942
49. Phan NQ, Lotts T, Antal A, Bernhard JD, Ständer S. Systemic kappa opioid receptor agonists in the treatment of chronic pruritus: a literature review. *Acta Derm Venereol.* (2012) 92:555–60. doi: 10.2340/00015555-1353
50. Wieczorek A, Krajewski P, Kozioł-Gałczyńska M, Szepietowski JC. Opioid receptors expression in the skin of haemodialysis patients suffering from uraemic pruritus. *J Eur Acad Dermatol Venereol.* (2020) 34:2368–72. doi: 10.1111/jdv.16360
51. Kardon AP, Polgar E, Hachisuka J, Snyder LM, Cameron D, Savage S, et al. Dynorphin acts as a neuromodulator to inhibit itch in the dorsal horn of the spinal cord. *Neuron.* (2014) 82:573–86. doi: 10.1016/j.neuron.2014.02.046
52. Inui S. Nalfurafine hydrochloride to treat pruritus: a review. *Clin Cosmet Investig Dermatol.* (2015) 8:249–55. doi: 10.2147/CCID.S55942
53. Elliott G, Vanwersch R, Soeberdt M, Metze D, Lotts T, Ständer S, et al. Topical nalfurafine exhibits anti-inflammatory and anti-pruritic effects in a murine model of AD. *J Dermatol Sci.* (2016) 84:351–54. doi: 10.1016/j.jdermsci.2016.09.008
54. Legat FJ. The antipruritic effect of phototherapy. *Front Med.* (2018) 5:333. doi: 10.3389/fmed.2018.00333
55. Fourzali K, Golpanian RS, Yosipovitch G. Dupilumab use in atopic dermatitis and beyond in skin diseases. *Immunotherapy.* (2020) 12:1221–35. doi: 10.2217/imt-2020-0175
56. Simpson EL, Bieber T, Guttman-Yassky E, Beck LA, Blauvelt A, Cork MJ, et al. Two phase 3 trials of dupilumab versus placebo in atopic dermatitis. *N Engl J Med.* (2016) 375:2335–48. doi: 10.1056/NEJMoa1610020
57. Silverberg JI, Yosipovitch G, Simpson EL, Kim BS, Wu JJ, Eckert L, et al. Dupilumab treatment results in early and sustained improvements in itch in adolescents and adults with moderate to severe atopic dermatitis: analysis of the randomized phase 3 studies SOLO 1 and SOLO 2, AD ADOL, and CHRONOS. *J Am Acad Dermatol.* (2020) 82:1328–36. doi: 10.1016/j.jaad.2020.02.060
58. Paller AS, Siegfried EC, Thaçi D, Wollenberg A, Cork MJ, Arkwright PD, et al. Efficacy and safety of dupilumab with concomitant topical corticosteroids in children 6 to 11 years old with severe atopic dermatitis: a randomized, double-blinded, placebo-controlled phase 3 trial. *J Am Acad Dermatol.* (2020) 83:1282–93. *Erratum in: J Am Acad Dermatol.* (2020). doi: 10.1016/j.jaad.2020.06.054
59. Hendricks AJ, Yosipovitch G, Shi VY. Dupilumab use in dermatologic conditions beyond atopic dermatitis - a systematic review. *J Dermatolog Treat.* (2019) 12:1–10. doi: 10.1080/09546634.2019.1689227
60. Bieber T. Interleukin-13: Targeting an underestimated cytokine in atopic dermatitis. *Allergy.* (2020) 75:54–62. doi: 10.1111/all.13954
61. Wollenberg A, Blauvelt A, Guttman-Yassky E, Worm M, Lynde C, Lacour JP, et al. Tralokinumab for moderate-to-severe atopic dermatitis: results from two 52-week, randomized, double-blind, multicentre, placebo-controlled phase III trials (ECZTRA 1 and ECZTRA 2). *Br J Dermatol.* (2020) 184:437–49. doi: 10.1111/bjd.19574
62. Silverberg JI, Toth D, Bieber T, Alexis AF, Elewski BE, Pink AE, et al. Tralokinumab plus topical corticosteroids for the treatment of moderate-to-severe atopic dermatitis: results from the double-blind, randomized, multicentre, placebo-controlled phase III ECZTRA 3 trial. *Br J Dermatol.* (2020) 184: 450–63. doi: 10.1111/bjd.19573
63. Guttman-Yassky E, Blauvelt A, Eichenfield LF, Paller AS, Armstrong AW, Drew J, et al. Efficacy and safety of lebrikizumab, a high-affinity interleukin 13 inhibitor, in adults with moderate to severe atopic dermatitis: a phase 2b randomized clinical trial. *JAMA Dermatol.* (2020) 156:411–20. doi: 10.1001/jamadermatol.2020.0079
64. Ruzicka T, Hanifin JM, Furue M, Pulka G, Mlynarczyk I, Wollenberg A, et al. Anti-interleukin-31 receptor a antibody for atopic dermatitis. *N Engl J Med.* (2017) 376:826–35. doi: 10.1056/NEJMoa1606490
65. Silverberg JI, Pinter A, Pulka G, Poulin Y, Bouaziz JD, Wollenberg A, et al. Phase 2B randomized study of nemolizumab in adults with moderate-to-severe atopic dermatitis and severe pruritus. *J Allergy Clin Immunol.* (2020) 145:173–82. doi: 10.1016/j.jaci.2019.08.013
66. Kabashima K, Matsumura T, Komazaki H, Kawashima M, Nemolizumab-JP01 Study Group. Trial of nemolizumab and topical agents for atopic dermatitis with pruritus. *N Engl J Med.* (2020). 383:141–50. doi: 10.1056/NEJMoa1917006
67. Kabashima K, Furue M, Hanifin JM, Pulka G, Wollenberg A, Galus R, et al. Nemolizumab in patients with moderate-to-severe atopic dermatitis: randomized, phase II, long-term extension study. *J Allergy Clin Immunol.* (2018) 142:1121–30.e7. doi: 10.1016/j.jaci.2018.03.018
68. Ständer S, Yosipovitch G, Legat FJ, Lacour JP, Paul C, Narbutt J, et al. Trial of nemolizumab in moderate-to-severe prurigo nodularis. *N Engl J Med.* (2020) 382:706–16. doi: 10.1056/NEJMoa1908316
69. Romeo SP. Atopic dermatitis: the itch that rashes. *Pediatr Nurs.* (1995) 21:157–63.
70. Simpson EL, Lacour JP, Spelman L, Galimberti R, Eichenfield LF, Bissonnette R, et al. Baricitinib in patients with moderate-to-severe atopic dermatitis and inadequate response to topical corticosteroids: results from two randomized monotherapy phase III trials. *Br J Dermatol.* (2020) 183:242–55. doi: 10.1111/bjd.18898
71. Reich K, Kabashima K, Peris K, Silverberg JI, Eichenfield LF, Bieber T, et al. Efficacy and safety of baricitinib combined with topical corticosteroids for treatment of moderate to severe atopic dermatitis: a randomized clinical trial. *JAMA Dermatol.* (2020) 156:1333–43. doi: 10.1001/jamadermatol.2020.3260
72. Guttman-Yassky E, Thaçi D, Pangan AL, Hong HC, Papp KA, Reich K, et al. Upadacitinib in adults with moderate to severe atopic dermatitis: 16-week results from a randomized, placebo-controlled trial. *J Allergy Clin Immunol.* (2020) 145:877–84. doi: 10.1016/j.jaci.2019.11.025
73. Simpson EL, Sinclair R, Forman S, Wollenberg A, Aschoff R, Cork M, et al. Efficacy and safety of abrocitinib in adults and adolescents with moderate-to-severe atopic dermatitis (JADE MONO-1): a multicentre, double-blind, randomised, placebo-controlled, phase 3 trial. *Lancet.* (2020) 396:255–266. doi: 10.1016/S0140-6736(20)30732-7
74. Silverberg JI, Simpson EL, Thyssen JP, Gooderham M, Chan G, Feeney C, et al. Efficacy and safety of abrocitinib in patients with moderate-to-severe atopic dermatitis: a randomized clinical trial. *JAMA Dermatol.* (2020) 156:863–73. doi: 10.1001/jamadermatol.2020.1406
75. Simpson EL, Parnes JR, She D, Crouch S, Rees W, Mo M, et al. Tezepelumab, an anti-thymic stromal lymphopoietin monoclonal antibody, in the treatment of moderate to severe atopic dermatitis: a randomized phase 2a clinical trial. *J Am Acad Dermatol.* (2019) 80:1013–21. doi: 10.1016/j.jaad.2018.11.059
76. Wang F, Trier AM, Li F, Kim S, Chen Z, Chai JN, et al. A basophil-neuronal axis promotes itch. *Cell.* 2021 184:422-440.e17. doi: 10.1016/j.cell.2020.12.033
77. Kremer AE. What are new treatment concepts in systemic itch? *Exp Dermatol.* (2019) 28:1485–92. doi: 10.1111/exd.14024
78. Fishbane S, Jamal A, Munera C, Wen W, Menzaghi F, KALM-1 Trial Investigators. A phase 3 trial of difelikefalin in hemodialysis patients with pruritus. *N Engl J Med.* (2020). 382:222–32. doi: 10.1056/NEJMoa1912770
79. Paller AS, Tom WL, Lebwohl MG, Blumenthal RL, Boguniewicz M, Call RS, et al. Efficacy and safety of crisaborole ointment, a novel, nonsteroidal phosphodiesterase 4 (PDE4) inhibitor for the topical treatment of atopic dermatitis (AD) in children and adults. *J Am Acad Dermatol.* (2016) 75:494–503.e6. *Erratum in: J Am Acad Dermatol.* (2017). 76:777. doi: 10.1016/j.jaad.2016.05.046
80. Yosipovitch G, Gold LF, Lebwohl MG, Silverberg JI, Tallman AM, Zane LT. Early relief of pruritus in atopic dermatitis with crisaborole ointment, a non-steroidal, phosphodiesterase 4 inhibitor. *Acta Derm Venereol.* (2018) 98:484–9. doi: 10.2340/00015555-2893

81. Solimani F, Meier K, Ghoreschi K. emerging topical and systemic JAK inhibitors in dermatology. *Front Immunol.* (2019) 10:2847. doi: 10.3389/fimmu.2019.02847
82. Dhillon S. *Drugs.* (2020). 80:609–15. doi: 10.1007/s40265-020-01291-2
83. Smith SH, Jayawickreme C, Rickard DJ, Nicodeme E, Bui T, Simmons C, et al tapinarof is a natural AhR agonist that resolves skin inflammation in mice and humans. *J Invest Dermatol.* (2017) 137:2110–9. doi: 10.1016/j.jid.2017.05.004
84. Furue M, Hashimoto-Hachiya A, Tsuji G. Aryl hydrocarbon receptor in atopic dermatitis and psoriasis. *Int J Mol Sci.* (2019) 20:5424. doi: 10.3390/ijms20215424
85. Peppers J, Paller AS, Maeda-Chubachi T, Wu S, Robbins K, Gallagher K, et al. A phase 2, randomized dose-finding study of tapinarof (GSK2894512 cream) for the treatment of atopic dermatitis. *J Am Acad Dermatol.* (2019) 80:89–98.e3.doi: 10.1016/j.jaad.2018.06.047
86. Gold LS, Bhatia N, Tallman AM, Rubenstein DS. A phase IIb, randomized clinical trial of tapinarof cream for the treatment of plaque psoriasis: secondary efficacy and patient-reported outcomes. *J Am Acad Dermatol.* (2020) 84:624–31.doi: 10.1016/j.jaad.2020.04.181

ZBTB20 in Nociceptive Neurons of the Trigeminal Ganglia Regulates Pruritus

Xin Jia[1,2†], *Meng-Han Dai*[1,3†], *An-Jing Ren*[4†], *Ting-Ting Wang*[1,5], *Weiping J. Zhang*[4,6*] and *Ling Zhang*[1,2*]

[1] The First Rehabilitation Hospital of Shanghai, Tongji University School of Medicine, Shanghai, China, [2] Key Laboratory of Spine and Spinal Cord Injury Repair and Regeneration of Ministry of Education, Orthopaedic Department of Tongji Hospital, School of Medicine, Tongji University, Shanghai, China, [3] Department of Anesthesiology, Renmin Hospital, Hubei University of Medicine, Shiyan, China, [4] Department of Pathophysiology, Naval Medical University, Shanghai, China, [5] Department of Dermatology, Tongren Hospital Shanghai Jiao Tong University School of Medicine, Shanghai, China, [6] NHC Key Laboratory of Hormones and Development, Tianjin Institute of Endocrinology, Tianjin Medical University Chu Hsien-I Memorial Hospital, Tianjin, China

***Correspondence:**
Ling Zhang
lzhang0808@tongji.edu.cn
Weiping J. Zhang
wzhang@smmu.edu.cn

†These authors have contributed equally to this work

Recent studies have shown that ZBTB20, a zinc-finger protein containing transcription factor, is highly expressed in small-diameter primary sensory neurons in mice, and modulates pain through regulating TRP channels. However, whether ZBTB20 regulates itch sensation has not been demonstrated. In this study, small-diameter primary sensory neuron-specific ZBTB20 knockout (PN-ZB20KO) mice were used to investigate the role of ZBTB20 in the regulation of itch sensation. First, both histamine-dependent and non-histamine-dependent itch behaviors induced by injection of histamine and chloroquine (CQ) into the cheek were significantly diminished in PN-ZB20KO mice. Second, double immunohistochemistry showed that ZBTB20 was mainly expressed in CGRP-labeled small peptidergic neurons and was expressed at low levels in IB4-labeled small non-peptidergic and NF200-labeled large neurons in the trigeminal ganglia (TG). ZBTB20 was also expressed in most TRPV1$^+$ and TRPA1$^+$ neurons and to a lesser extent in TRPM8$^+$ neurons in the TG. Furthermore, cheek injection of histamine and CQ enhanced the mRNA expression of TRPV1 and TRPA1 but not TRPM8 in the TG. Moreover, TRPV1 and TRPA1 knockout (KO) mice exhibited attenuation of itch behavior induced by histamine and CQ, respectively. Finally, silencing endogenous ZBTB20 with recombinant lentivirus expressing a short hairpin RNA against ZBTB20 (LV-shZBTB20) in TG neurons attenuated histamine- and non-histamine-induced itch and downregulated TRP channels in the TG. Our study suggests that ZBTB20 plays an important role in mediating itch in small primary sensory neurons.

Keywords: itch, TRPA1, TRPV1, ZBTB20, trigeminal ganglia, pain, pruritus

INTRODUCTION

The zinc finger protein ZBTB20 regulates development and metabolism in multiple systems and is essential for postnatal survival in mice (1). ZBTB20 has been found to play a crucial role in the development and function of the central nervous system, such as the development of dendritic and synaptic structures (2), the maturation of CA1 neurons (3), and the generation of neuronal layers in the developing cortex (2, 4). However, the function of ZBTB20 in the peripheral nervous system has not been fully investigated.

Recently, ZBTB20 was specifically knocked out in nociceptive neurons in mice, alerting the expression of transient potential (TRP) channels, including TRPV1, TRPA1, and TRPM8, and thus resulting in abnormal mechanical pain, heat pain and inflammatory pain (5). TRP channels are a large family composed of 28 members in mammals that can be divided into seven subfamilies, including TRPA, TRPC, TRPM, TRPN, TRPML, TRPP, and TRPV, based on their amino acid sequence homology (6, 7). Many TRP channels have been found to participate in the transduction of thermal, chemical, and mechanical sensations (8, 9). TRPV1, TRPA1, and TRPM8, which have long been reported to play important roles in the transduction of a variety of noxious stimuli (10, 11), have recently been implicated in the processing of itch sensation (12, 13).

Itch, an unpleasant sensation that provokes the scratch reflex (14), can be classified as histamine-dependent and non-histamine-dependent according to the sensitivity of the sensation to antihistamine treatment (15). Histamine and non-histamine itch have been reported to be mediated by distinct TRP signaling pathways (16–18). Although itch and pain are both mediated by primary sensory neurons, the cell bodies of which are located in the dorsal root ganglia (DRG) or trigeminal ganglia (TG) (14), they are distinguished by unique behavioral responses (19). While pain evokes acute withdrawal behaviors to escape from nociceptive stimuli, itch leads to a scratch reflex and brings attention to the affected area to remove pruritogens and provides temporary relief. Itch was previously thought to be a kind of minor pain and not an independent sensory modality. Recently, progress has been made toward elucidating the molecular mechanism underlying itch. Itch and pain are now clearly understood to be distinct sensory modalities involving distinct neural and molecular pathways in primary sensory neurons and the spinal cord (20–25). Given the similarities and differences between pain and itch sensation, it is worth investigating whether ZBTB20 in primary sensory neurons regulates itch.

In the present study, we used PN-ZB20KO mice and gene silencing of ZBTB20 in the TG to specifically detect whether ZBTB20 in primary sensory neurons mediates itch sensation. We found that ZBTB20 was involved in both histamine- and non-histamine-dependent itch, and the effect was likely mediated by TRPA1 and TRPV1 channels in TG neurons.

MATERIALS AND METHODS

Animals

ZBTB20 mutant (ZBTB20$^{flox/flox}$; Nav1.8-Cre) mice, named PN-ZB20KO mice, were described previously (5). Floxed/Cre-negative, non-floxed Cre-positive, or wild-type (WT) mice were used as littermate controls. C57BL/6 mice were purchased from SLAC Laboratory Animal Company (Shanghai, China). All mice, including TRPV1 knockout (KO) and TRPA1 KO mice and their littermates, were provided food and water *ad libitum* and housed under a 12-h/12-h light/dark cycle. The temperature in the animal facility was maintained at 22 ± 1°C, and the relative humidity was 40–60%. The mice were allowed to adapt to the environment for 1 week before the experiment was initiated. Animal care procedures and experimental protocols were reviewed and approved by the Animal Study Committee of Tongji University School of Medicine (Shanghai, China).

Drug and Administration

Pruritogens and algogen (histamine, H7125; chloroquine (CQ), C6628; capsaicin, M2028) were purchased from Sigma-Aldrich (St. Louis, MO, USA). To induce itch responses in the facial region, histamine (50 μg) and chloroquine (40 μg) were dissolved in 10 μL of PBS, and capsaicin (10 μg) dissolved in 10 μL of solution (7% Tween 80:20% ethanol:73% PBS) was intradermally injected into the cheek region as reported previously (26–28).

Behavioral Test

The mouse cheek model was established to distinguish pain and itch behaviors (19). Itch and pain responses were evaluated as described previously (26, 27). The right cheek of each mouse was shaved 2 days before the behavioral experiment, and histamine, CQ and capsaicin were intradermally injected into the right cheek. A video camera (SONY HDR-Cx240) was positioned above the mice to record their behavior, and the numbers of ipsilateral forelimb wipes and hindlimb scratch bouts in the injection site in 5-min intervals over a 30-min period were determined in a blinded manner.

Real-Time Quantitative RT-PCR

The mRNA levels of ZBTB20, TRPA1, TRPV1, and TRPM8 were analyzed by RT-PCR. The mice were decapitated, and the bilateral TGs were collected with sterilized instruments 30 min after histamine and CQ administration into bilateral cheeks. Total RNA was extracted with an RNA Extraction Kit (Takara). Isolated RNA was reverse-transcribed to synthesize first strand cDNA using a cDNA synthesis kit (Tiangen). The ABI 7500 Real-Time PCR System and SYBR Green I (Tiangen) were used for PCR. Real-time PCR mixtures were prepared, and the reaction conditions were set following the kit instructions. GAPDH was served as an internal control. The melting curve was used to evaluate the reliability of the PCR results. The threshold cycle (CT) value (the inflection point of the amplification curve) was determined, and the relative expression of target genes was calculated using the $2^{-\Delta\Delta Ct}$ method. The primer sequences for ZBTB20, TRPV1, TRPA1, TRPM8, and GAPDH are shown in **Table 1**.

Immunohistochemistry

Mice were anesthetized with 10% chloral hydrate and perfused through the ascending aorta with PBS followed by 4%

TABLE 1 | Primers sequence for RT-PCR.

Primer	Forward	Reverse
ZBTB20	CGGCGAGCGCTCCCTCTACAGTG	GCTTGCGGCAGTGCGTGGTCT
TRPV1	GGGAGGCCTGGCTTCTACTTTG	TGCCGGCACTCTGGTTCGT
TRPA1	GGCAATGTGGAGCAATAGCG	CAATAAGCTGCCCAAAGGTC
TRPM8	ACATCCCCTTCCCCTTCGTT	TCGCCAGCCTTACTTGATGTTATT
GAPDH	CCAATGTGTCCGTCGTGGATC	GTTGAAGTCGCAGGAGACAAC

paraformaldehyde in 0.1 M phosphate buffer (pH 7.4). After perfusion, the TGs were removed and post-fixed with 4% paraformaldehyde for 4 h. The samples were cut into 14-μm-thick frozen sections on a cryostat. The sections were incubated with primary antibodies (mouse anti-TRPV1, 1:1,000, Abcam; rabbit anti-TRPA1, 1:500, Abcam; rabbit anti-TRPM8, 1:500, Abcam; mouse anti-CGRP, 1:1,000, Abcam; mouse anti-NF200, 1:1,000, Abcam; mouse anti-IB4-FITC, 1:1,000, Sigma; rabbit anti-ZBTB20, 1:1,000, Atlas Antibodies AB; rat anti-ZBTB20, 1:2,000, Abcam) overnight at 4°C, followed by secondary antibodies (Alexa Fluor 555 donkey anti-rabbit IgG, 1:1,000 and Alexa Fluor 488-conjugated donkey anti-mouse IgG 1:1,000, Invitrogen) at room temperature for 2 h. The sections were then observed under an epifluorescence microscope. All images were made into figures using Adobe Photoshop (Adobe Systems Incorporated, San Jose, CA), with only minor adjustments to the contrast and brightness settings if necessary.

RNA Inference and TG Stereotaxic Injection

The recombinant lentivirus that expressed a short hairpin RNA (LV-shRNA) against ZBTB20 (shZBTB20) was used to silence endogenous ZBTB20 (29). Mice were anesthetized with 1% sodium pentobarbital (100 mg/kg, i.p.) and then placed in a stereotaxic apparatus. The skull of mice was exposed through the midline incision of scalp, and the microinjection glass pipette was inserted into TG through bilateral craniotomy with a hand-held drill (relative to bregma: anteroposterior (AP), −0.5 mm; mediolateral (ML), ±2.2 mm; dorsoventral (DV), −5.8 mm according to the mouse atlas of Paxinos and Watson). LV-shZBTB20 or scrambled shRNA (2.0×10^8 TU/mL, 300 nL in volume) was microinjected into the bilateral TG at a rate of 25 nL per min with glass micropipettes. After a week of recovery, the mice were injected with histamine, CQ and capsaicin intradermally into the cheek for the behavior test. The bilateral TGs were collected for the measurement of the expression of ZBTB20 and TRP channels and immunohistochemistry study.

Statistical Analyses

All data are expressed as the mean ± SEM. Statistical analyses were performed with GraphPad 7.0. Differences between groups were compared using 2-tailed Student's *t*-test. The time course data were analyzed by two-way ANOVA followed by a test of

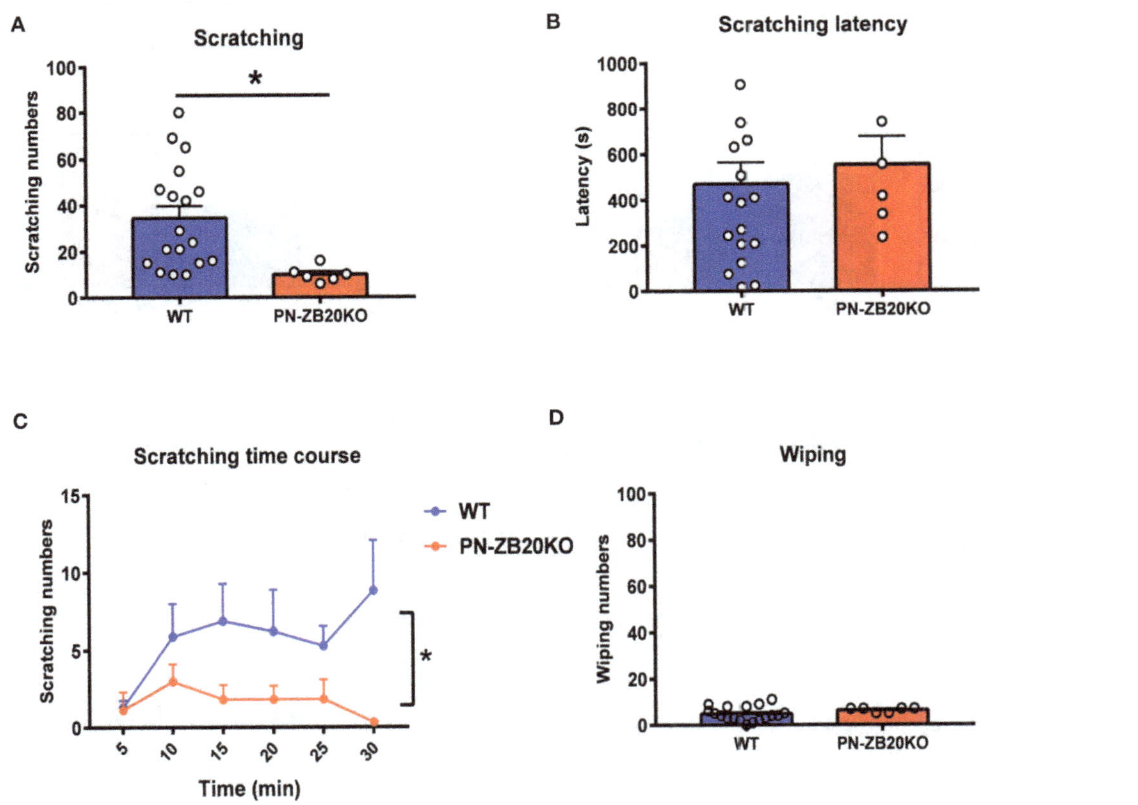

FIGURE 1 | Histamine-induced itch was dramatically attenuated in PN-ZB20KO mice. **(A)** The scratching behavior induced by injection of histamine (50 μg in 10 μL PBS) into the mouse cheek was decreased significantly in PN-ZB20KO mice compared to control mice (*t*-test, $^*p < 0.05$). **(B)** The latency to scratch following histamine injection did not change in PN-ZB20KO mice compared to control mice (*t*-test, $p > 0.05$). **(C)** The time course of scratching behavior induced by histamine administration. Two-way ANOVA, [$F_{(1, 22)} = 6.989$; $p = 0.0148$, $^*p < 0.05$]. **(D)** The wiping induced by histamine was maintained at a low level and did not change after histamine administration (*t*-test, $p > 0.05$). N = 6–18 for each group.

homogeneity of variance. The criterion for statistical significance was $p < 0.05$.

RESULTS

ZBTB20 in Primary Sensory Neurons Is Involved in the Modulation of Histamine-Dependent and Non-histamine-Dependent Itch

To examine whether ZBTB20 in primary neurons is involved in itch transmission, we first established a mouse cheek model to measure histamine- or CQ-induced itch behavior, which represent histamine- and non-histamine-dependent itch, respectively. After the pruritogens were injected into the cheek of each mouse, the total number of scratches and wipes every 5 min for 30 min was calculated. The latency to scratching or wiping behavior following chemical injection was also recorded. The results showed that scratching behaviors induced by histamine (5 μg/μL, 10 μL) (**Figures 1A,C**) and CQ (4 μg/μL, 10 μL) (**Figures 2A,C**) were robustly inhibited in PN-ZB20KO mice compared with WT mice. However, little forelimb wiping was observed in PN-ZB20KO mice, and there were no differences in this behavior between the two groups (**Figures 1D, 2D**). Furthermore, the latency to scratch following CQ injection was increased significantly in PN-ZB20KO mice compared with WT mice (**Figure 2B**), further indicating the attenuation of CQ-induced itch. The results above suggest that ZBTB20 in primary sensory neurons plays an important role in mediating histamine- and non-histamine-induced itch. In addition, the number of forelimb wipes induced by capsaicin was significantly reduced in PN-ZB20KO mice compared to WT mice (**Figure 3**), which is in line with a previous report (5) and further verifies the function of ZBTB20 in modulating inflammatory pain.

ZBTB20 Is Expressed in Small Peptidergic Neurons and Colocalizes With TRP Channels in the TG

Previous studies have shown that ZBTB20 is colocalized with peripherin and exists in 80% of nav1.8-positive neurons, indicating that ZBTB20 mainly exists in small neurons in the DRG (5). However, the cellular distribution of ZBTB20 in primary sensory neurons, especially the percentage of ZBTB20

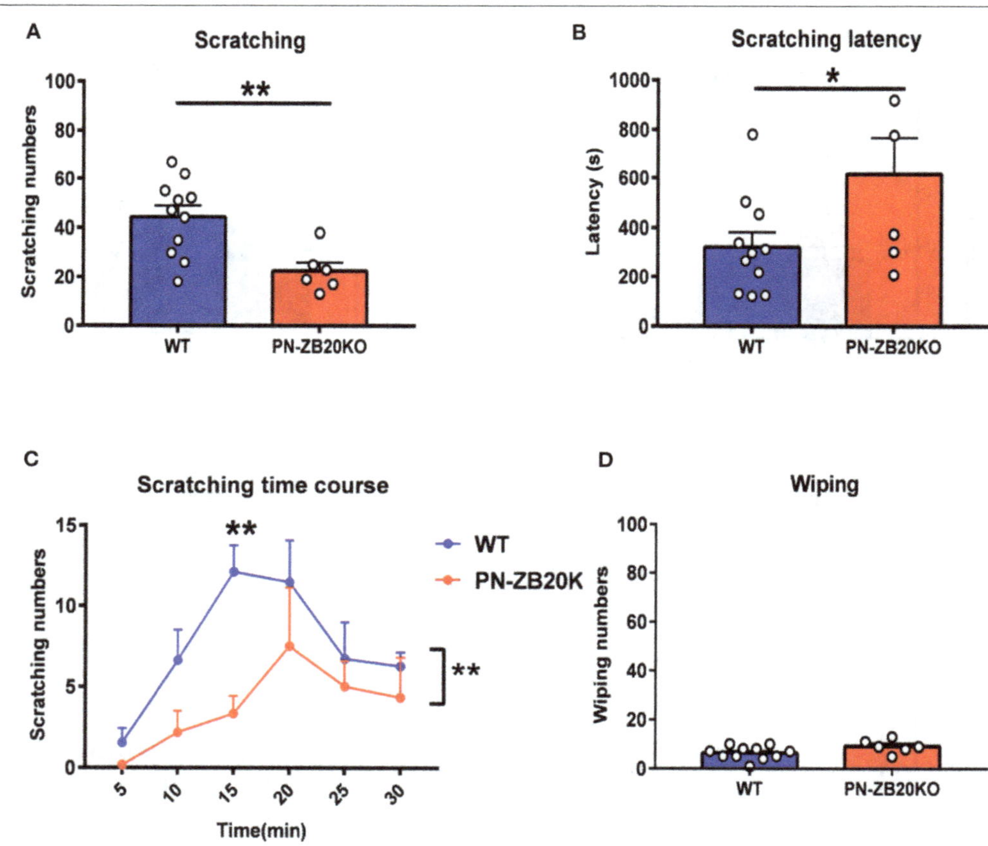

FIGURE 2 | CQ-induced itch was dramatically attenuated in PN-ZB20KO mice. **(A)** The scratching behavior induced by injection of CQ (40 μg in 10 μL PBS) into the mouse cheek was decreased significantly in PN-ZB20KO mice compared to control mice (*t*-test, $^{**}p < 0.01$). **(B)** The latency to scratch following CQ injection significantly increased in PN-ZB20KO mice compared to control mice (*t*-test, $^{*}p < 0.05$). **(C)** The time course of scratching behavior induced by CQ administration. Two-way ANOVA [$F_{(1, 15)} = 10.27$; $p = 0.0059$, $^{**}p < 0.01$]. **(D)** The wiping induced by CQ was maintained at a low level and did not change after histamine administration (*t*-test, $p > 0.05$). $N = 6$–11 for each group.

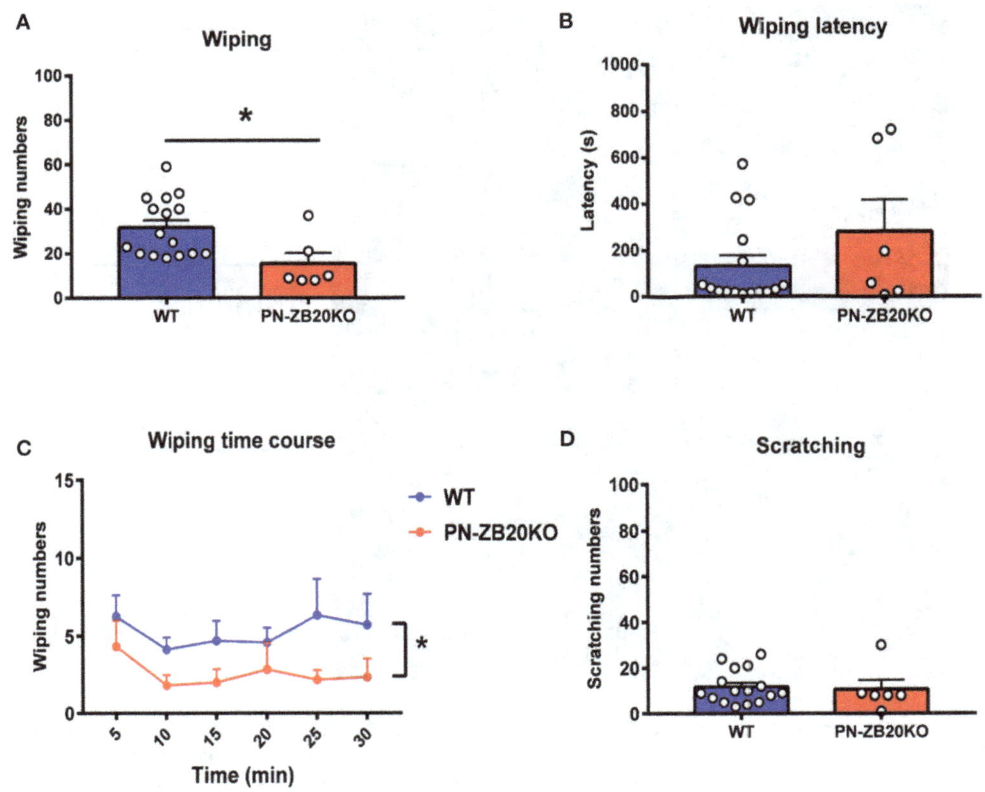

FIGURE 3 | Capsaicin-induced wiping was dramatically attenuated in PN-ZB20KO mice. **(A)** The wiping behavior induced by injection of capsaicin (10 μg in 10 μL of solution) into the mouse cheek was decreased dramatically in PN-ZB20KO mice compared to control mice (*t*-test *$p < 0.05$). **(B)** The latency to wiping following capsaicin injection did not change in PN-ZB20KO mice compared to control mice (*t*-test, $p > 0.05$). **(C)** The time course of wiping induced by capsaicin administration. Two-way ANOVA [$F_{(1, 20)} = 6.958$; $p = 0.0158$, *$p < 0.05$]. **(D)** The scratching induced by capsaicin was maintained at a low level and did not change after capsaicin administration. $N = 6$–16 for each group.

expressed in different TG neurons, has not been demonstrated. We detected the expression of ZBTB20 in the TG by double immunofluorescence, and the results showed that ZBTB20 was expressed in 78.9% of CGRP$^+$ neurons (**Figures 4A,B**), 27.6% of IB4 $^+$ (**Figures 4C,D**) and 13.4% of NF200$^+$ neurons (**Figures 4E,F**). We further investigated the colocalization of ZBTB20 with TRP channels and found that ZBTB20 was expressed in 80.9% of TRPV1$^+$, 51.7% of TRPA1$^+$ and 36.2% of TRPM8$^+$ neurons in the TG (**Figures 5A–F**). These results suggested that ZBTB20 is mainly distributed in small peptidergic neurons and coexists with the majority of TRPV1 and TRPA1, implicating ZBTB20 in the modulation of both pain and itch.

Pruritogens Increase the mRNA Expression of TRPV1 and TRPA1 in the TG

Because TRP channels are very important for itch transduction in primary neurons, we next measured the TRP channel mRNA expression induced by histamine and CQ. The results showed that the mRNA expression of TRPV1 and TRPA1 but not TRPM8 in the TG was upregulated significantly by cheek injection of histamine and CQ (**Figures 6B–D**). Moreover, the mRNA expression of ZBTB20 was also upregulated by cheek injection of the two types of pruritogens (**Figure 6A**). Our results indicated that ZBTB20 may mediate pruritus by regulating TRPV1 and TRPA1.

TRPV1 and TRPA1 KO Mice Exhibit Attenuation of Itch Induced by Histamine and CQ

To further verify the role of TRPV1 and TRPA1 in itch sensation, TRPV1 and TRPA1 KO mice were used. We found that scratching induced by histamine was inhibited in TRPV1 KO mice compared to WT mice (**Figure 7A**), while scratching induced by CQ was attenuated in TRPA1 KO mice compared with WT mice (**Figure 7B**). The data are in line with a previous study (11, 18, 30, 31) and further suggest that TRPV1 and TRPA1 modulate histamine- and non-histamine-dependent acute itch.

Silencing ZBTB20 in TG Suppressed Histamine-Dependent and Non-histamine-Dependent Itch

To further verify the effect of ZBTB20 on itch behavior, we silenced endogenous ZBTB20 expression in primary mouse TG neurons using recombinant lentivirus expressing a short hairpin

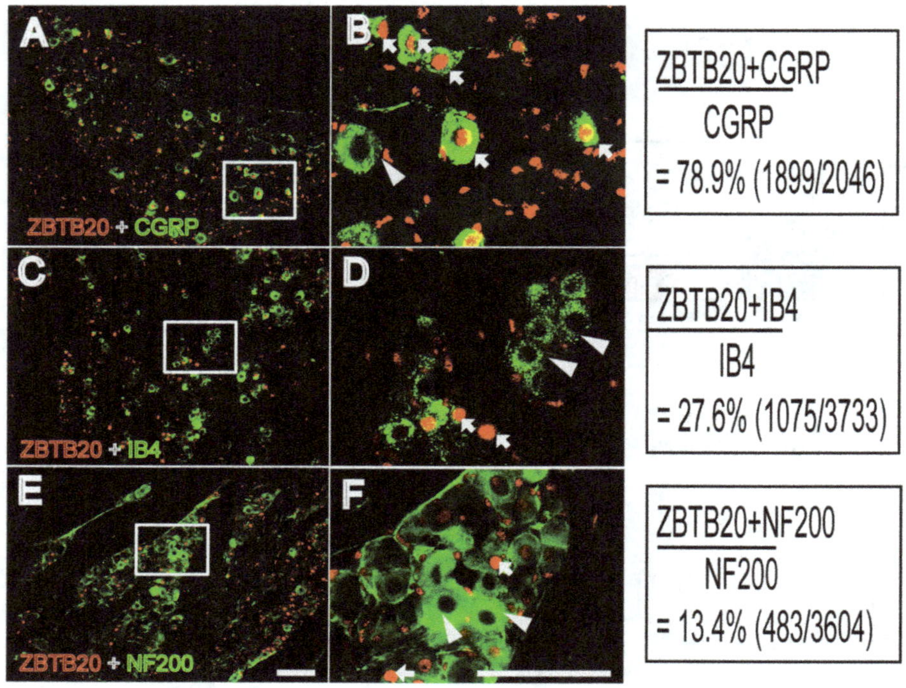

FIGURE 4 | Colocalization of ZBTB20 with CGRP, IB4, and NF200 in the trigeminal ganglia. **(A,B)** Colocalization of ZBTB20 with CGPR. **(C,D)** Colocalization of ZBTB20 with IB4. **(E,F)** Colocalization of ZBTB20 with NF200. **Figures B,D,F** are high magnifications of the boxes in **Figures A,C,E**. The arrowhead indicates the colocalization of ZBTB20 with CGRP, IB4, and NF200 in **Figures B,D,F**. The arrow indicates the expression of CGRP, IB4, and NF200 without colocalization with ZBTB20 in **Figures B,D,F**. $N = 3$; bar =50 μm.

RNA against ZBTB20 (LV-shZBTB20) or a scramble shRNA as a mock control (29). The scratching numbers induced by histamine and CQ were dramatically attenuated by knocking down ZBTB20 in the TG (**Figures 8A–F**). In addition, the wiping numbers induced by capsaicin were also significantly attenuated after ZBTB20 RNA interference in the TG (**Figure 8**). The mRNA levels of ZBTB20, TRPV1, TRPA1, and TRPM8 were significantly decreased in the LV-shZBTB20 group compared with the scrambled shRNA control group (**Figure 8J**). After the behavior test, we also verified the knockdown effect of LV-shZBTB20 on ZBTB20 expression in the TG by immunofluorescence (**Figures 8K,L**).

DISCUSSION

In the present study, we used PN-ZB20KO mice and RNA interference to assess the function of ZBTB20 in the progression of itch. Our results showed that ZBTB20 in primary sensory neurons was involved in both histamine- and non-histamine-dependent itch and that the effect was likely mediated by TRPA1 and TRPV1 channels.

ZBTB20 is highly expressed in the nervous system and is essential for postnatal survival in mice (1). As previously described, the ZBTB20 gene is deleted specifically in nociceptors at E14 using Nav1.8-Cre, but deletion of this gene does not affect the formation, survival or diversification of nociceptors (5). It is well-known that pain and itch are transmitted by nociceptive primary sensory neurons. Hence, these PN-ZB20KO mice are suitable for the study of pain as well as itch. Given that ZBTB20 affects pain by regulating TRP channels in primary sensory neurons, it is worth investigating whether ZBTB20 regulates itch.

Pain and itch are distinguished by unique behavioral responses. While pain leads to withdrawal reflexes and other types of avoidance behavior, itch induces the urge to scratch. In the standard rodent model of itch, pruritogens are applied to the nape of the neck, and scratches with the hindpaw are evaluated and considered itch-responsive behavior (32, 33). However, mice also scratch with the hindpaw when capsaicin, which induces pain sensation, is injected into the nape of the neck. It was discovered that when the agents are injected into the cheek, mice scratch the injection site with their hind limbs in response to histamine (itch) and wipe with their forelimbs in response to capsaicin (pain) (19). Therefore, since 2008, the mouse cheek model reported by Shimada and LaMotte has been widely used to differentiate itch and pain behaviors. In our study, scratch behavior was largely attenuated in PN-ZB20KO mice compared to WT mice when histamine and CQ were administered to the cheek, indicating that ZBTB20 in primary sensory neurons modulates both histamine- and non-histamine-dependent itch sensation. In addition, we found that wiping behavior induced by capsaicin was dramatically decreased in PN-ZB20KO mice compared to WT mice, which is in line with our previous report (5), showing that ZBTB20 is involved in inflammatory pain; these

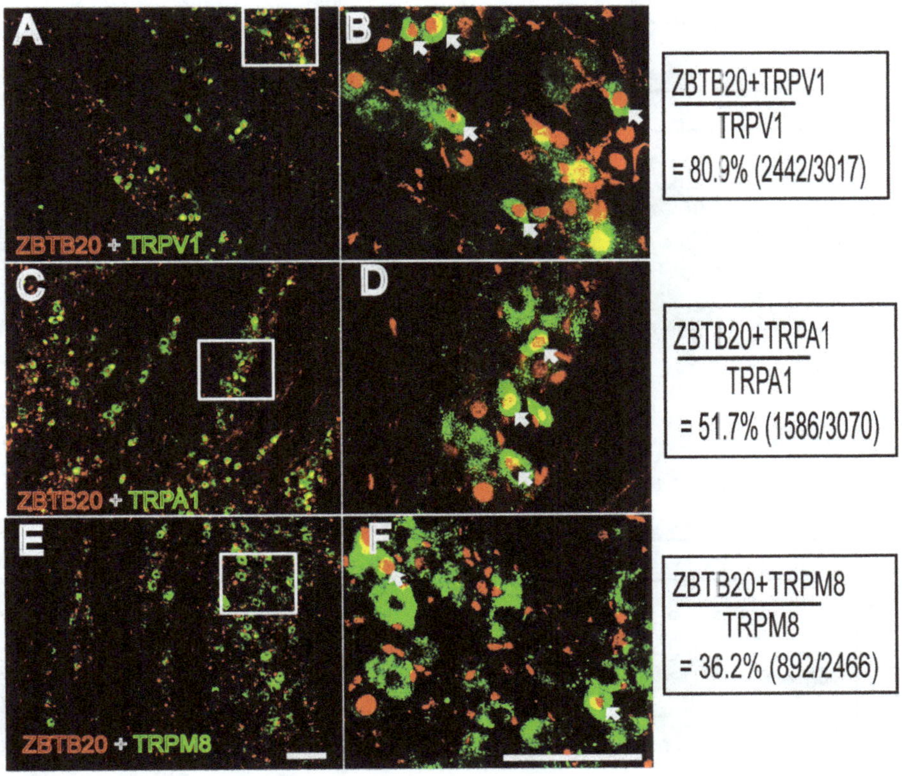

FIGURE 5 | Colocalization of ZBTB20 with TRPV1, TPRA1, and TRPM8 in the trigeminal ganglia **(A,B)** Colocalization of ZBTB20 with TRPV1. **(C,D)** Colocalization of ZBTB20 with TRPA1. **(E,F)** Colocalization of ZBTB20 with TRPM8. **Figures B,D,F** are high magnifications of the boxes in **Figures A,C,E**. The arrowhead indicates the colocalization of ZBTB20 with TRPV1, TRPA1, and TRPM8 in **Figures B,D,F**. $N = 3$; bar =50 μm.

data further confirm the function of ZBTB20 in modulating both pain and itch.

Nociceptive primary sensory neurons are located in the DRG and TG, which are homologs of each other and transmit nociception from the body and craniofacial neurons, respectively. The nociceptive neurons in the DRG and TG can be chemically divided into two subsets: peptidergic and non-peptidergic neurons. Peptidergic neurons synthesize neuropeptides such as calcitonin gene-related peptide (CGRP) and substance P (SP) and respond to nerve growth factor. Non-peptidergic neurons, which express the c-Ret neurotrophin receptor, are capable of binding isolectin IB4 and responding to glial-derived neurotrophic factors (34, 35). Because we administered chemicals to the cheek in this study, ZBTB20 expression in the TG was measured. We therefore used CGRP and IB4 to label these two subsets of neurons in the TG and found that ZBTB20 was expressed in most CGRP $^+$ small peptidergic neurons and a few IB4$^+$ small non-peptidergic neurons and NF200$^+$ large neurons. This result further suggests that ZBTB20 is involved in regulating TRP channels, since TRPV1 is expressed in a population of unmyelinated neurons that express the neuropeptide CGRP within rodent sensory ganglia (7). Although ZBTB20 is expressed by precursor cells for all neuronal types (36), it becomes more restricted in the majority of neurons expressing TRPV1, TRPA1, and TPRM8 in the DRG (5). To further investigate the colocalization of ZBTB20 with TRP channels in TG neurons, we performed double immunostaining for ZBTB20 and TRP channels and found that ZBTB20 was expressed in most TRPV1$^+$ (80.9%) and TRPA1$^+$ (51.7%) neurons and to a lesser extent in TRPM8$^+$ (36.2%) neurons in the TG, suggesting that there may be differences in neuron mechanisms in the DRG and TG where primary sensory neurons are located. Nevertheless, our results confirmed a previous report and provided detailed information regarding the expression of ZBTB20 in the TG.

TRP channels are molecular sensors for mechanical, chemical, and thermal changes. Recently, growing evidence has indicated that TRP channels also play an important role in itch signaling (13), and different TRP channels are required for different types of itch. For example, TRPV1 mediates histamine-induced itch by coupling with histamine H1R and H4R (32, 37). TRPA1 is involved in non-histamine-dependent itch induced by CQ and BAM8-22. TRPV1 or TRPA1 KO mice exhibit less histamime- or CQ-evoked scratching behavior (18). In addition, some pruritogens, such as lysophosphatidic acid (LPA), squaric acid dibutylester (SADBE) and IL31, induce itch that is mediated by both TRPV1 and TRPA1 (38–40). It has been demonstrated that mice with TRPV1 exclusively expressed in MrgprA3$^+$ neurons exhibit only itch and not pain behavior in response to capsaicin (22), indicating that there are two subpopulations of TRPV1

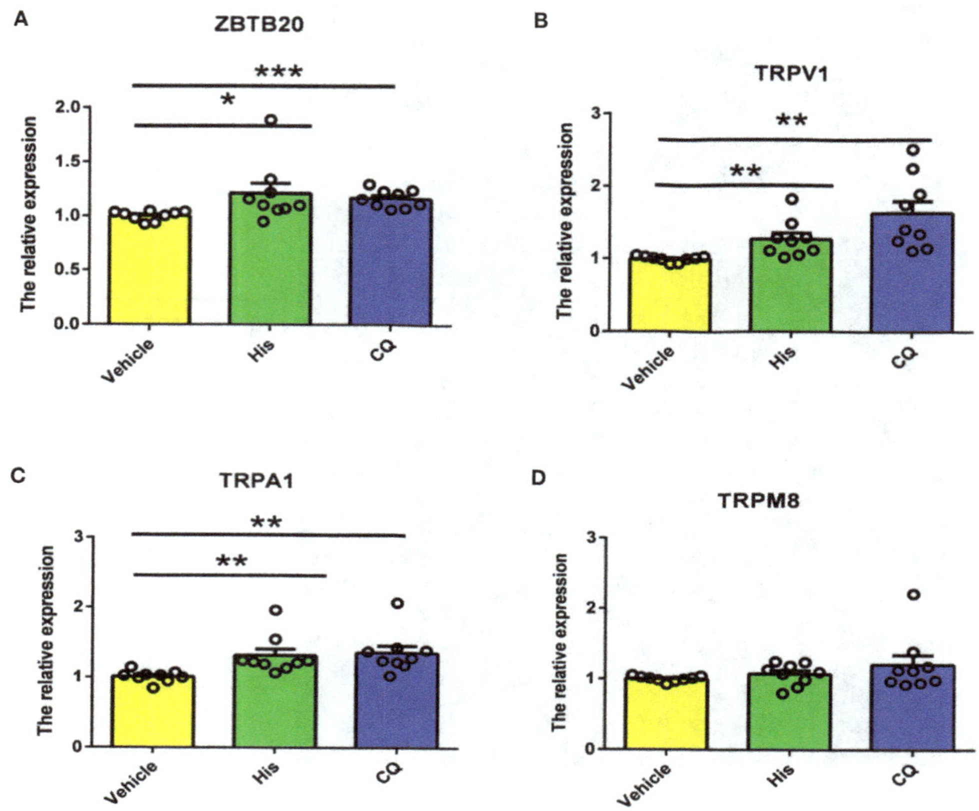

FIGURE 6 | Histamine and CQ increased the mRNA expression of ZBTB20, TRPV1, and TRPA1 but not TRPM8 in the trigeminal ganglia. **(A)** The mRNA expression of ZBTB20 in the TG was increased after histamine and CQ injection into the cheek (*t*-test, $^{*}p < 0.05$, $^{***}p < 0.001$ vs. the vehicle group). **(B)** The mRNA expression of TRPV1 in the TG was increased after histamine and CQ injection into the cheek (*t*-test, $^{**}p < 0.01$ vs. the vehicle group). **(C)** The mRNA expression of TRPA1 in the TG was increased after histamine and CQ injection into the cheek (*t*-test, $^{**}p < 0.01$ vs. the vehicle group). **(D)** The mRNA expression of TRPM8 in the TG was not increased after histamine and CQ injection into the cheek (*t*-test, $p > 0.05$ vs. the vehicle group). $N = 9$ for each group.

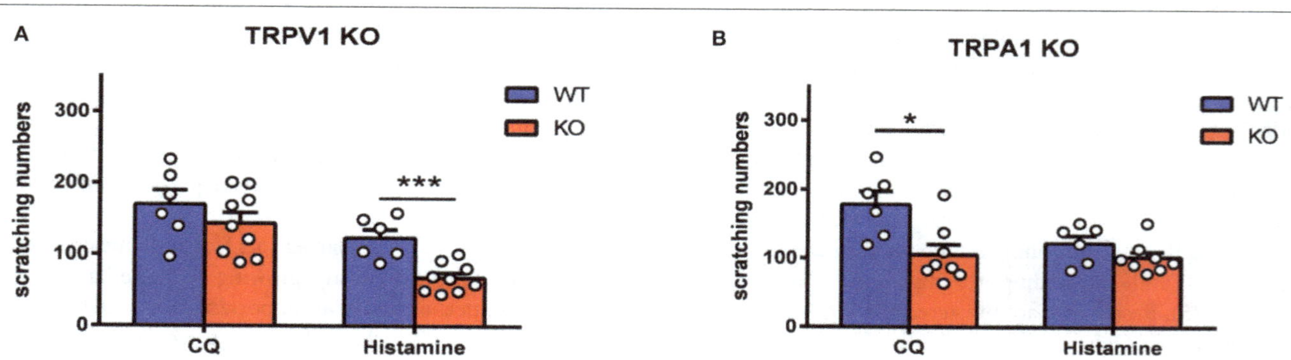

FIGURE 7 | Itch behavior was attenuated in TRPV1 KO and TRPA1 KO mice. **(A)** Histamine-induced scratching was reduced dramatically in TRPV1 KO mice (*t*-test, $^{***}p < 0.001$ vs. the WT group). **(B)** CQ-induced scratching was reduced dramatically in TRPA1 KO mice (*t*-test, $^{*}p < 0.05$ vs. the WT group). $N = 6$-9 for each group.

neurons in the primary sensory ganglia that distinctly mediate itch and pain. However, whether ZBTB20 regulates itch-related TRP channels has not been reported. Our data demonstrated that both histamine and CQ increase the mRNA expression of ZBTB20, TRPV1, and TRPA1 in the TG, providing evidence that ZBTB20 probably modulates TRP channels in itch-specific neurons. In contrast to TRPV1 and TRPA1, TRPM8 inhibits itch and is required for cooling and menthol-mediated itch inhibition (41). Although previous results have shown that ZBTB20 affects pain behavior by regulating TRPA1, TRPV1, and TRPM8, in our study, TRPM8 expression was not altered after pruritogen administration, further indicating that pain and

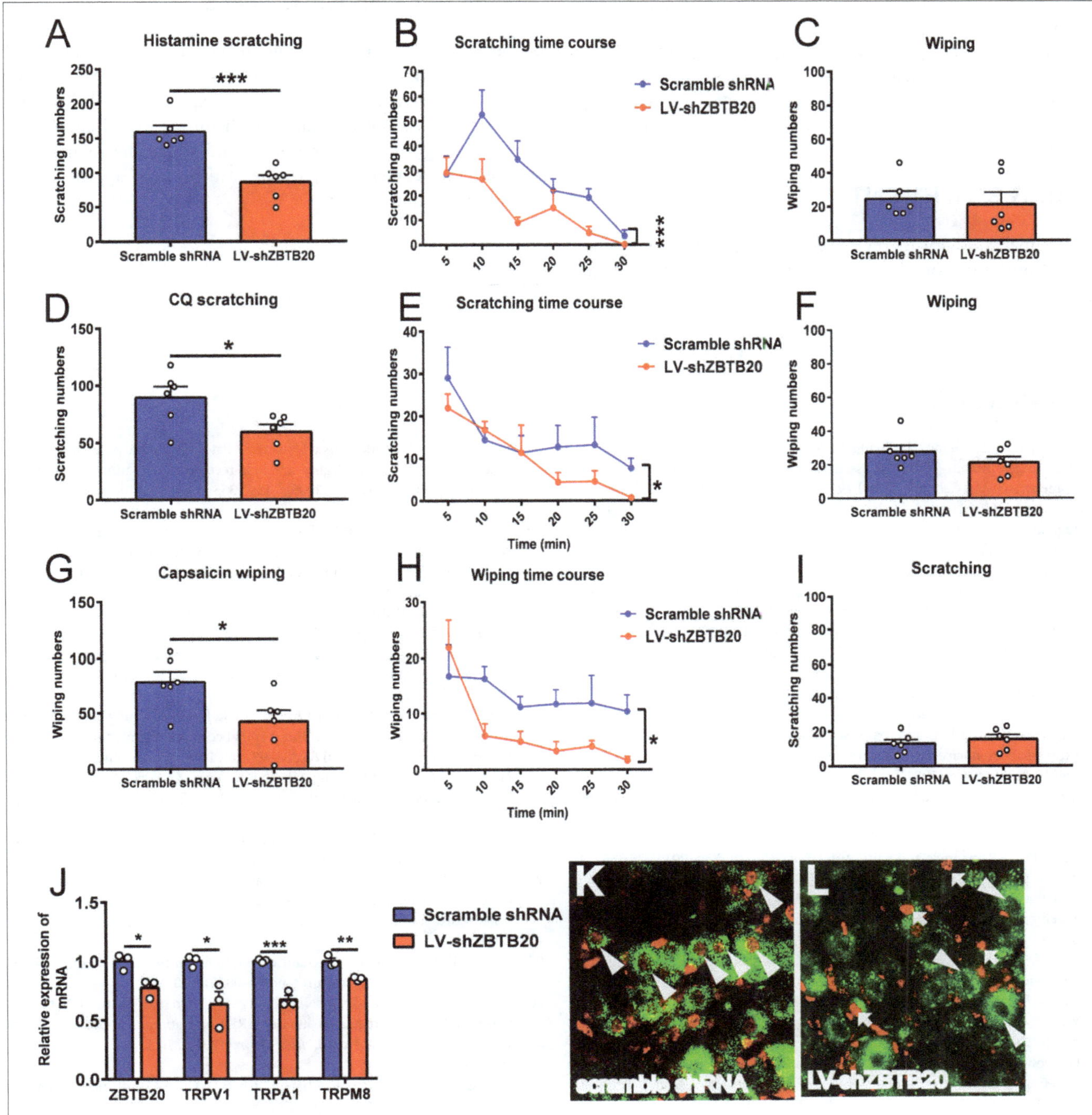

FIGURE 8 | The itch and pain behavior induced by histamine, CQ or capsaicin after silencing endogenous ZBTB20 in the TG. **(A)** The scratching induced by histamine (50 μg in 10 μL PBS) was decreased dramatically in LV-shZBTB20 mice compared to scramble shRNA mice (*t*-test, $^{***}p < 0.001$). **(B)** The time course of scratching induced by histamine in LV-shZBTB20 and scramble shRNA mice [$F_{(1,\ 10)} = 29.06$; $p = 0.0003$, $^{***}p < 0.001$]. **(C)** The wiping induced by histamine was maintained at a low level and did not change after histamine injection (*t*-test, $p > 0.05$). **(D)** The scratching induced by CQ (4 μg in 10 μL PBS) was decreased dramatically in LV-shZBTB20 mice compared to scramble shRNA mice (*t*-test, $^{*}p < 0.05$). **(E)** The time course of scratching induced by CQ LV-shZBTB20 and scramble shRNA mice [$F_{(1,\ 15)} = 10.27$; $p = 0.0059$, $^{*}p < 0.05$]. **(F)** The wiping induced by CQ was maintained at a low level and did not change after CQ treatment (*t*-test, $p > 0.05$). **(G)** The wiping induced by capsaicin (10 μg in 10 μL of solution) was decreased dramatically in LV-shZBTB20 mice compared to scramble shRNA mice (*t*-test, $^{*}p < 0.05$). **(H)** The time course of wiping induced by capsaicin in LV-shZBTB20 and scramble shRNA mice [$F_{(1,\ 10)} = 6.548$; $p = 0.0284$, $^{*}p < 0.05$]. **(I)** The scratching induced by capsaicin was maintained at a low level and did not change after capsaicin treatment. $N = 6$ for each group. **(J)** The mRNA expression of ZBTB20, TRPV1, TRPA1, and TRPM8 in the TG was decreased significantly in LV-shZBTB20 mice compared to scramble shRNA mice (*t*-test, $^{*}p < 0.05$, $^{**}p < 0.01$, $^{***}p < 0.001$). $N = 3$ for each group. **(K,L)** Example showing immunofluorescent staining of ZBTB20 with scramble shRNA and LV-shZBTB20 in TG neurons. The arrowhead indicates colocalization of ZBTB20 (red) with scramble shRNA (green) **(K)**. The arrow indicates ZBTB20 (red), and the arrowhead indicates LV-shZBTB20 (green) **(L)**. $N = 3$; bar =50 μm.

itch are two different modalities that have distinct molecular signaling pathways.

In summary, our results demonstrated that ZBTB20 acts as a critical regulator of pruritus in primary sensory neurons, which could through TRPA1 and TRPV1 channels. Our study will help to unravel the cellular and molecular bases of itch sensation.

ETHICS STATEMENT

The animal study was reviewed and approved by Animal Study Committee of Tongji University School of Medicine Shanghai, China.

AUTHOR CONTRIBUTIONS

XJ and M-HD performed the behavioral experiments and RT-PCR. XJ and A-JR performed RNA interference experiments. T-TW participated in the behavior experiments. T-TW and A-JR performed the immunohistochemistry experiments. WZ and LZ designed the experiments and wrote the manuscript. All authors contributed to the article and approved the submitted version.

REFERENCES

1. Sutherland AP, Zhang H, Zhang Y, Michaud M, Xie Z, Patti ME, et al. Zinc finger protein Zbtb20 is essential for postnatal survival and glucose homeostasis. *Mol Cell Biol.* (2009) 29:2804–15. doi: 10.1128/MCB.01667-08
2. Doeppner TR, Herz J, Bahr M, Tonchev AB, Stoykova A. Zbtb20 regulates developmental neurogenesis in the olfactory bulb and gliogenesis after adult brain injury. *Mol Neurobiol.* (2019) 56:567–82. doi: 10.1007/s12035-018-1104-y
3. Ren A, Zhang H, Xie Z, Ma X, Ji W, He DZ, et al. Regulation of hippocampus-dependent memory by the zinc finger protein Zbtb20 in mature CA1 neurons. *J Physiol.* (2012) 590:4917–32. doi: 10.1113/jphysiol.2012.234187
4. Tonchev AB, Tuoc TC, Rosenthal EH, Studer M, Stoykova A. Zbtb20 modulates the sequential generation of neuronal layers in developing cortex. *Mol Brain.* (2016) 9:65. doi: 10.1186/s13041-016-0242-2
5. Ren AJ, Wang K, Zhang H, Liu A, Ma X, Liang Q, et al. ZBTB20 regulates nociception and pain sensation by modulating TRP channel expression in nociceptive sensory neurons. *Nat Commun.* (2014) 5:4984. doi: 10.1038/ncomms5984
6. Montell C, Birnbaumer L, Flockerzi V. The TRP channels, a remarkably functional family. *Cell.* (2002) 108:595–8. doi: 10.1016/s0092-8674(02)00670-0
7. Julius D. TRP channels and pain. *Annu Rev Cell Dev Biol.* (2013) 29:355–84. doi: 10.1146/annurev-cellbio-101011-155833
8. Chatzigeorgiou M, Yoo S, Watson JD, Lee WH, Spencer WC, Kindt KS, et al. Specific roles for DEG/ENaC and TRP channels in touch and thermosensation in *C. elegans nociceptors Nat Neurosci.* (2010) 13:861–8. doi: 10.1038/nn.2581
9. Wu LJ, Sweet TB, Clapham DE. International union of basic and clinical pharmacology. LXXVI Current progress in the mammalian TRP ion channel family. *Pharmacol Rev.* (2010) 62:381–404. doi: 10.1124/pr.110.002725
10. Wang H, Woolf CJ. Pain TRPs. *Neuron.* (2005) 46:9–12. doi: 10.1016/j.neuron.2005.03.011
11. Patapoutian A, Tate S, Woolf CJ. Transient receptor potential channels: targeting pain at the source. *Nat Rev Drug Discov.* (2009) 8:55–68. doi: 10.1038/nrd2757
12. Wilson SR, The L, Batia LM, Beattie K, Katibah GE, McClain SP, et al. The epithelial cell-derived atopic dermatitis cytokine TSLP activates neurons to induce itch. *Cell.* (2013) 155:285–95. doi: 10.1016/j.cell.2013.08.057
13. Moore C, Gupta R, Jordt SE, Chen Y, Liedtke WB. Regulation of pain and itch by TRP channels. *Neurosci Bull.* (2018) 34:120–42. doi: 10.1007/s12264-017-0200-8
14. Ikoma A, Steinhoff M, Stander S, Yosipovitch G, Schmelz M. The neurobiology of itch. *Nat Rev Neurosci.* (2006) 7:535–47. doi: 10.1038/nrn1950
15. Han L, Dong X. Itch mechanisms and circuits. *Annu Rev Biophys.* (2014) 43:331–55. doi: 10.1146/annurev-biophys-051013-022826
16. Ward L, Wright E, McMahon SB. A comparison of the effects of noxious and innocuous counterstimuli on experimentally induced itch and pain. *Pain.* (1996) 64:129–38. doi: 10.1016/0304-3959(95)00080-1
17. Liu Q, Tang Z, Surdenikova L, Kim S, Patel KN, Kim A, et al. Sensory neuron-specific GPCR Mrgprs are itch receptors mediating chloroquine-induced pruritus. *Cell.* (2009) 139:1353–65. doi: 10.1016/j.cell.2009.11.034
18. Wilson SR, Gerhold KA, Bifolck-Fisher A, Liu Q, Patel KN, Dong X, et al. TRPA1 is required for histamine-independent, Mas-related G protein-coupled receptor-mediated itch. *Nat Neurosci.* (2011) 14:595–602. doi: 10.1038/nn.2789
19. Shimada SG, LaMotte RH. Behavioral differentiation between itch and pain in mouse. *Pain.* (2008) 139:681–7. doi: 10.1016/j.pain.2008.08.002
20. Sun YG, Chen ZF. A gastrin-releasing peptide receptor mediates the itch sensation in the spinal cord. *Nature.* (2007) 448:700–3. doi: 10.1038/nature06029
21. Ross SE, Mardinly AR, McCord AE, Zurawski J, Cohen S, Jung C, et al. Loss of inhibitory interneurons in the dorsal spinal cord and elevated itch in Bhlhb5 mutant mice. *Neuron.* (2010) 65:886–98. doi: 10.1016/j.neuron.2010.02.025
22. Han L, Ma C, Liu Q, Weng HJ, Cui Y, Tang Z, et al. A subpopulation of nociceptors specifically linked to itch. *Nat Neurosci.* (2013) 16:174–82. doi: 10.1038/nn.3289
23. Mishra SK, Hoon MA. The cells and circuitry for itch responses in mice. *Science.* (2013) 340:968–71. doi: 10.1126/science.1233765
24. Bourane S, Duan B, Koch SC, Dalet A, Britz O, Garcia-Campmany L, et al. Gate control of mechanical itch by a subpopulation of spinal cord interneurons. *Science.* (2015) 350:550–4. doi: 10.1126/science.aac8653
25. Lay M, Dong X. Neural Mechanisms of Itch. *Annu Rev Neurosci.* (2020) 43:187–205. doi: 10.1146/annurev-neuro-083019-024537
26. Zhang L, Jiang GY, Song NJ, Huang Y, Chen JY, Wang QX, et al. Extracellular signal-regulated kinase (ERK) activation is required for itch sensation in the spinal cord. *Mol Brain.* (2014) 7:25. doi: 10.1186/1756-6606-7-25
27. Jiang GY, Dai MH, Huang K, Chai GD, Chen JY, Chen L, et al. Neurochemical characterization of pERK-expressing spinal neurons in histamine-induced itch. *Sci Rep.* (2015) 5:12787. doi: 10.1038/srep12787
28. Huang K, Hu DD, Bai D, Wu ZY, Chen YY, Zhang YJ, et al. Persistent extracellular signal-regulated kinase activation by the histamine H4 receptor in spinal neurons underlies chronic itch. *J Invest Dermatol.* (2018) 138:1843–50. doi: 10.1016/j.jid.2018.02.019
29. Ren AJ, Chen C, Zhang S, Liu M, Wei C, Wang K, et al. Zbtb20 deficiency causes cardiac contractile dysfunction in mice. *FASEB J.* (2020) 34:13862–76. doi: 10.1096/fj.202000160RR
30. Shim WS, Tak MH, Lee MH, Kim M, Kim M, Koo JY, et al. TRPV1 mediates histamine-induced itching *via* the activation of phospholipase A2 and 12-lipoxygenase. *J Neurosci.* (2007) 27:2331–7. doi: 10.1523/JNEUROSCI.4643-06.2007

31. Tsagareli MG, Nozadze I, Tsiklauri N, Carstens MI, Gurtskaia G, Carstens E. Thermal hyperalgesia and mechanical allodynia elicited by histamine and non-histaminergic itch mediators: respective involvement of TRPV1 and TRPA1. *Neuroscience.* (2020) 449:35–45. doi: 10.1016/j.neuroscience.2020.09.048
32. Green AD, Young KK, Lehto SG, Smith SB, Mogil JS. Influence of genotype, dose and sex on pruritogen-induced scratching behavior in the mouse. *Pain.* (2006) 124:50–8. doi: 10.1016/j.pain.2006.03.023
33. Shimada SG, Shimada KA, Collins JG. Scratching behavior in mice induced by the proteinase-activated receptor-2 agonist, SLIGRL-NH2. *Eur J Pharmacol.* (2006) 530:281–3. doi: 10.1016/j.ejphar.2005.11.012
34. Dong X, Han S, Zylka MJ, Simon MI, Anderson DJ. A diverse family of GPCRs expressed in specific subsets of nociceptive sensory neurons. *Cell.* (2001) 106:619–32. doi: 10.1016/s0092-8674(01)00483-4
35. Pinto LG, Souza GR, Kusuda R, Lopes AH, Sant'Anna MB, Cunha FQ, et al. Non-peptidergic nociceptive neurons are essential for mechanical inflammatory hypersensitivity in mice. *Mol Neurobiol.* (2019) 56:5715–28. doi: 10.1007/s12035-019-1494-5
36. Sharma N, Flaherty K, Lezgiyeva K, Wagner DE, Klein AM, Ginty DD. The emergence of transcriptional identity in somatosensory neurons. *Nature.* (2020) 577:392–8. doi: 10.1038/s41586-019-1900-1
37. Imamachi N, Park GH, Lee H, Anderson DJ, Simon MI, Basbaum AI, et al. TRPV1-expressing primary afferents generate behavioral responses to pruritogens *via* multiple mechanisms. *Proc Natl Acad Sci USA.* (2009) 106:11330–5. doi: 10.1073/pnas.0905605106
38. Cevikbas F, Kempkes C, Buhl T, Mess C, Buddenkotte J, Steinhoff M. *Itch: Mechanisms and Treatment.* Boca Raton, FL: CRC Press (2014).
39. Feng J, Yang P, Mack MR, Dryn D, Luo J, Gong X, et al. Sensory TRP channels contribute differentially to skin inflammation and persistent itch. *Nat Commun.* (2017) 8:980. doi: 10.1038/s41467-017-01056-8
40. Kittaka H, Uchida K, Fukuta N, Tominaga M. Lysophosphatidic acid-induced itch is mediated by signalling of LPA5 receptor, phospholipase D and TRPA1/TRPV1. *J Physiol.* (2017) 595:2681–98. doi: 10.1113/JP273961
41. Xie Z, Hu H. TRP Channels as Drug Targets to Relieve Itch. *Pharmaceuticals (Basel).* (2018) 11:100. doi: 10.3390/ph11040100

18

Interleukin-31 Signaling Bridges the Gap Between Immune Cells, the Nervous System and Epithelial Tissues

Jana Maria Nemmer [1†], Marcus Kuchner [1†], Angeliki Datsi [1,2†], Péter Oláh [1,3], Valérie Julia [4], Ulrike Raap [5] and Bernhard Homey [1]*

[1] Department of Dermatology, Medical Faculty, University Hospital Düsseldorf, Heinrich-Heine-University Düsseldorf, Düsseldorf, Germany, [2] Medical Faculty, Institute for Transplantation Diagnostics and Cell Therapy, University Hospital Düsseldorf, Heinrich-Heine-University Düsseldorf, Düsseldorf, Germany, [3] Department of Dermatology, Venereology and Oncodermatology, Medical Faculty, University of Pécs, Pécs, Hungary, [4] Galderma Pharmaceuticals, Vevey, Switzerland, [5] Division of Experimental Allergy and Immunodermatology, Department of Dermatology, University of Oldenburg, Oldenburg, Germany

***Correspondence:**
Bernhard Homey
bernhard.homey@Med.Uni-Duesseldorf.De

† These authors have contributed equally to this work and share first authorship

Pruritus represents one of the most common symptoms in dermatology and general medicine. Chronic pruritus severely impairs the quality of life of affected patients. During the last two decades a number of modulators and mediator of pruritus have been identified. Recently, Interleukin (IL)-31 and its receptor complex attracted significant interest, as clinical phase two studies demonstrated therapeutic efficacy of the neutralizing IL-31 receptor A (IL-31RA) antibody nemolizumab in patients suffering from atopic dermatitis or prurigo nodularis. IL-31 has also been shown to play relevant roles in allergic contact dermatitis, urticaria, mastocytosis, allergic rhinitis and asthma. Here, we summarize the current knowledge of the novel cytokine IL-31 and its receptor regarding cellular origin, regulation, signaling pathways and their involvement in biological processes such as pruritus, neuronal growth, inflammation, barrier dysfunction and tissue remodeling.

Keywords: atopic dematitis, interleukin-31, interleukin-31 receptor, neuroinflammation, pruritus

INTRODUCTION

Pruritus represents an important archaic sensation, and its evolutionary role is to sensitize the host to a distinct body site in order to remove invading parasites or plant matter. Chronic pruritus severely impairs the quality of life of affected patients and represents a significant unmet medical need. In 2004, Dillon et al. first demonstrated the involvement of IL-31 signaling in the development of pruritus and atopic dermatitis-like skin lesions (1). Subsequently an emerging body of evidence supported a central role of IL-31 and its receptor in bridging the immune system with neurons, epithelial surfaces and connective tissue. Recently, phase two clinical trials demonstrated therapeutic efficacy of the neutralizing IL-31RA antibody nemolizumab in patients suffering from atopic dermatitis or prurigo nodularis (2, 3). In addition, IL-31 also plays a role in T_H2-driven and autoimmune diseases such as contact dermatitis, urticaria, mastocytosis, allergic rhinitis; but also systemic sclerosis, dermatomyositis, and lupus erythematosus (4–12). Here, we summarize the current knowledge on the novel cytokine IL-31 and its receptor regarding cellular origin, regulation, signaling pathways and their involvement in biological processes such as pruritus, neuronal growth, inflammation, barrier dysfunction and tissue remodeling.

INTERLEUKIN-31

IL-31 represents a member of the IL-6 family of cytokines, which share a four-helical structure and the majority signals through receptor complexes containing glycoprotein 130 (gp130). This family consists of nine members including IL-6, IL-11, ciliary neurotrophic factor (CNTF), leukemia inhibitory factor (LIF), oncostatin M (OSM), cardiotrophin 1 (CT-1), cardiotrophin-like cytokine (CLC), IL-27 and IL-31. Members of the IL-6 family are predominantly expressed under proinflammatory conditions and realize pleiotropic functions in immune-related processes (13). The *IL31* gene is located on chromosome 12q24.31 (1). Recent studies support the production of IL-31 in a variety of leukocyte subsets including T cells, eosinophils, basophils, mast cells, monocytes and dendritic cells. However, it is widely accepted that effector memory T cells with a T_H2 phenotype represent the major source of IL-31 (4, 14–18). Interestingly, findings linking IL-31 expression with patients suffering from *Dedicator of cytokinesis protein 8* (*DOCK8*) deficiency-related hyper IgE syndrome pointed to an important upstream regulation pathway. *DOCK8* loss-of-function mutations lead to a combined immunodeficiency with elevated serum levels of IgE, eosinophilia, decreased number of B and T cells as well as severe atopic dermatitis with increased IL-31 expression (19). Subsequent *in vitro*- as well as *in vivo*-studies demonstrated that DOCK8 is a negative regulator of the nuclear translocation of Endothelial PAS domain-containing protein 1 (EPAS1). This function is dependent of STK4 (MST1), a serine threonine kinase involved in apoptosis (20, 21). Knockdown of the *MST1* gene led to an increased translocation of EPAS1 to the nucleus in alignment with *DOCK8* knockout models showing elevated IL-31 expression (21). Consequently, clinical symptoms of patients with STK4 (*MST1*) mutations leading to deficiency at the protein level are resembling those with DOCK8 deficiency (22). EPAS1 is regulated by IL-4-mediated signal transducer and activator of transcription 6 (STAT6) signaling in $CD4^+$ T cells (23). Jabara et al. reported that DOCK8 is constitutively associated with myeloid differentiation primary response protein (MyD88), an adaptor protein of Toll-like receptors (TLR) (24). Hence it is interesting to speculate whether microbes such as *S. aureus* may influence IL-31 production through TLR engagement.

Interleukin-31 Receptor

Within the IL-6 family IL-31 is special, since it shares the four helical structure but does not signal through a receptor complex containing gp130. Instead, it binds to a heterodimeric receptor composed of the IL-31RA chain and the oncostatin M receptor (OSMR) β chain. The *IL31RA* gene is located on chromosome 5q11.2, 24 kb downstream of *IL6ST* (25, 26). From a phylogenetical view, IL-31RA is paralogous to gp130, although they share only 28% amino acid identity. It has five fibronectin type III (FNIII)-like domains and shares the WSxWS motif and the conserved cysteines with other type I cytokine receptors within the cytokine binding domain [as reviewed in (27)]. Horejs-Hoeck et al. showed that STAT1 is a relevant transcription factor to activate the promoter region of the *IL31RA* gene following IFN-γ stimulation and this regulation pathway was confirmed in several studies and cell types (28). Cytokine effects are based on their capacity to assemble receptor complexes to bring the associated kinases in spatial proximity for phosphorylation. Therefore, the expression pattern of relevant receptor chains in target cells determines their ability to respond to specific cytokine signals. The OSMRβ chain is considered to be widely expressed (29). Hence the limiting factor for IL-31 signal transduction appears to be the expression of the IL-31RA chain. Recent studies demonstrate that multiple leukocyte subsets, as well as epithelial and stromal cells express IL-31RA in steady state or more importantly under activated conditions (14, 17, 28, 30, 31). At first, the expression of IL-31RA on itch-conducting dorsal root ganglia (DRG) neurons attracted significant attention (4). Non-immune cells such as keratinocytes, fibroblasts and a distinct subset of DRG neurons also express and signal via IL-31RA (18, 31, 32). Binding of IL-31 to the receptor complex leads to phosphorylation of STAT1, STAT3 and STAT5 via the associated Janus kinase (JAK) 1 and JAK2 (33, 34). Besides JAK/STAT signaling the IL-31 receptor complex activates MEK/ERK and PI3K/Akt pathways as well as the JNK pathway (33, 35–37). Negative feedback mechanisms of IL-31RA signaling include suppressor of cytokine signaling (SOCS)1- and SOCS3-dependent inhibition of STAT3 activation (34). Interestingly, OSMR is a shared subunit of the receptor complexes of IL-31 and OSM, although their biological functions differ. While IL-31 is involved in many T_H2-driven diseases as mentioned above, OSM plays an important role in hematopoiesis and cancer development (38). It will be of interest to elucidate the distinct roles of IL-31 and OSM. Taken together, the diverse distribution of its receptor enables IL-31 to target the nervous system, immune functions, epithelial surfaces and stromal cells.

Nervous System

Within the cytokine superfamily IL-31 has a unique position, because it bridges the gap between the immune and the peripheral nervous systems (see **Figure 1**). During recent years, several independent studies confirmed the expression and signaling of IL-31RA and OSMRβ in a subset of murine as well as human DRG neurons (4, 18, 39–41). These findings stimulated further research on IL-31 targeting sensory neurons. Cevikbas et al. demonstrated in murine behavioral studies that IL-31 induces itch but not pain and mediates its effects independent of mast cells by activating the ion channels TRPV1 and TRPA1. In DRG neurons IL-31 induces intracellular Ca^{2+} mobilization as well as STAT3 and ERK phosphorylation (18). Following the activation of afferent DRG neurons, neurotransmitters such as natriuretic polypeptide b (Nppb) forward the signal further to the dorsal horn of the spinal cord, where the gastrin-releasing peptide receptor (Grpr) system is subsequently activated transmitting the signal further to projection neurons that transport the information to the brain (42–45). Recently, Meng et al. showed that IL-31 stimulation increased *Nppb* in DRG neurons *in vitro* and *in vivo* and induced soluble *N*-ethylmaleimide-sensitive-factor attachment receptor (SNARE)-dependent brain natriuretic peptide (BNP) release (46). In pharmacological studies, Ma et al. demonstrated that activation of the spinal neuropeptide Y system dampens IL-31-induced scratching behavior through activation of neuropeptide Y_2 receptor on DRG neurons (47). Notably, noxious signals activate neuropeptide Y interneurons, and this may explain, how the infliction of pain, e.g., through scratching, heat, cold, etc., may reduce itch perception in atopic dermatitis patients. Next to the initiation of pruritus signals, Feld et al. recently demonstrated that IL-31 also induces a distinct transcriptional program in sensory neurons, leading to nerve elongation and branching both *in vitro* and *in vivo*. Hence the increased density of neuronal networks in the skin may help us understand why atopic dermatitis patients experience increased sensitivity to minimal stimuli inducing sustained itch (48).

Immune Functions

Since the IL-31 receptor heterodimer is expressed on a variety of different leukocyte subsets including monocytes, macrophages, dendritic cells, eosinophils, mast cells and basophils, it is interesting to have a closer look at immune functions that are targeted by IL-31. Recently, Raap et al. demonstrated that basophils upon IL-31 stimulation do not release histamine but secrete large amounts of IL-4 and IL-13 (14). This is of particular importance since IL-4 is a critical factor for the differentiation of T cells into a T_H2 phenotype and the source of IL-4 in this dendritic cell-driven process is still debated (49, 50). Thus, IL-31 secretion may serve as an early upstream signal during the development of type 2 skin inflammation. In eosinophils and dendritic cells IL-31 induced a set of proinflammatory cytokines and chemokines including TNF-α, IL-1β, IL-6, CXCL1, CXCL8, CCL2 and CCL5 and CCL22 (16, 51). Through these molecules, IL-31 may recruit neutrophils (CXCL1, CXCL8), dendritic cells (CCL2), T_H1 (CCL5) and T_H2 (CCL22) cells to sites of inflammation or promote angiogenesis (CXCL1, CXCL8) and tissue remodeling (CCL2, IL-6) (52, 53). On the other

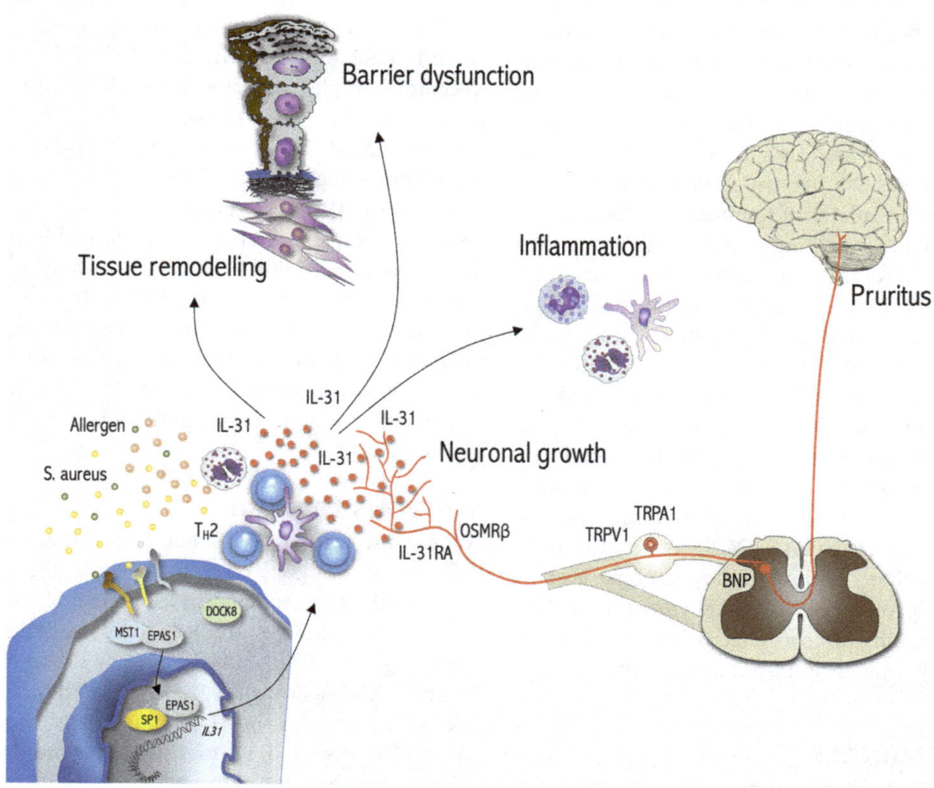

FIGURE 1 | IL-31 signaling bridges the gap between the immune system, neurons and epithelial surfaces. During T cell activation DOCK8 dissociates from EPAS1 enabling EPAS1 to translocate to the nucleus. Within the nucleus EPAS1 forms a complex with SP1 initiating *IL31* transcription. T_H2 cells are a major source of IL-31 production. In IL-31RA/OSMRß-expressing sensory neurons IL-31 induces the activation of ion channels (TRPV1, TRPA1) and transmits pruritus signals via BNP to the CNS. Moreover, IL-31 stimulates neuronal growth and the branching of sensory nerves. Furthermore, IL-31 targets immune cells such as mast cells, eosinophils, basophils and monocytes/dendritic cells to induce inflammation. Within the skin, IL-31 impairs keratinocyte differentiation as well as barrier function and in turn activates keratinocytes to produce cytokines, chemokines and pruritus mediators amplifying skin inflammation and itch. Interestingly, IL-31 also interacts with dermal fibroblasts initiating tissue remodeling by inducing collagen production and cytokine as well as chemokine expression. Hence, IL-31 signaling exerts pleiotropic effects beyond pruritus.

hand, cytokines such as TNF-α, IL-1β, and IL-6 may directly affect T cell, B cell and dendritic cell functions as well as activate surrounding stromal or epithelial cells (54). Hence, IL-31 signaling is able to amplify inflammation via different self-reinforcing loops.

Epithelial Surfaces

In 2004, Dillon et al. demonstrated for the first time the expression of IL-31RA and OSMRß in epidermal keratinocytes and IL-31 stimulation resulted in chemokine (CXCL1, CCL1, CCL4, CCL17, CCL19, CCL22, and CCL23) expression (1). Subsequently, a number of studies confirmed IL-31 receptor expression on keratinocytes and showed downstream signaling leading to STAT3 and ERK phosphorylation. Recent findings in 2D and 3D keratinocyte culture systems unravel, that IL-31 stimulation also modulates keratinocyte differentiation and disrupts epithelial barrier function (55–57). Cornelissen et al. demonstrated that IL-31 induced cell cycle arrest in keratinocytes and inhibited proliferation (55). Moreover, IL-31 elicited a differentiation defect with decreased filaggrin expression and impaired barrier functions facilitating transepidermal allergen penetration in organotypic keratinocyte cultures (55–57). Next to the production of chemokines, IL-31-stimulated keratinocytes contribute to skin inflammation through the expression of key proinflammatory mediators including IL-1α, IL-1β, IL-6, S100A7, S100A8, S100A9, β-defensin-2, β-defensin-3 (57). Moreover, IL-31-induced BNP release from sensory neurons may activate keratinocytes to produce proinflammatory cytokines and chemokines (46). Hence, inflammation circuits between epithelial surfaces, nerves and immune cells are connected and amplified via IL-31 signaling.

More recently, another keratinocyte-driven circuit potentially amplifying pruritus has been proposed. Andoh et al. demonstrated that intradermal injection of IL-31 induced thromboxane synthase in epidermal keratinocytes and significantly increased the concentration of thromboxane B_2, a metabolite of the pruritus mediator thromboxane A_2 (58). Moreover, keratinocytes produced the pruritus mediator leukotriene B_4 (LTB4) following IL-31 treatment and the LTB4 receptor antagonist CMHVA as well as the 5-lipoxygenase inhibitor, zileuton, suppressed the scratching behavior of mice intradermally injected with IL-31 (59).

Thus, next to the direct engagement of peripheral sensory neurons, IL-31 may sustain pruritus via keratinocyte activation and the release of other pruritus mediators (58–60). Notably, besides epidermal keratinocytes, bronchial and gut epithelial cells have been shown to be a target of IL-31 (61, 62).

Tissue Remodeling

Given the pleiotropic functions of IL-6 family members it has been reasonable to also investigate the role of IL-31 in tissue remodeling. Several studies report a direct effect of IL-31 on fibroblasts (17, 63). IL-31 signaling resulted in STAT3 phosphorylation and the activation of ERK, JNK and AKT (17). It is important to note that pro-fibrotic processes often follow STAT3 signaling pathways representing a considerable checkpoint for tissue fibrosis (64). Indeed, high levels of IL-31 were reported in plasma, fibrotic skin and lung lesions of systemic sclerosis (SSc) patients (10). Moreover, IL-31RA was upregulated in fibrotic skin and lung fibroblasts. Gene expression analysis of IL-31-treated dermal fibroblasts revealed a total of 561 differentially expressed genes with 200 genes involved in

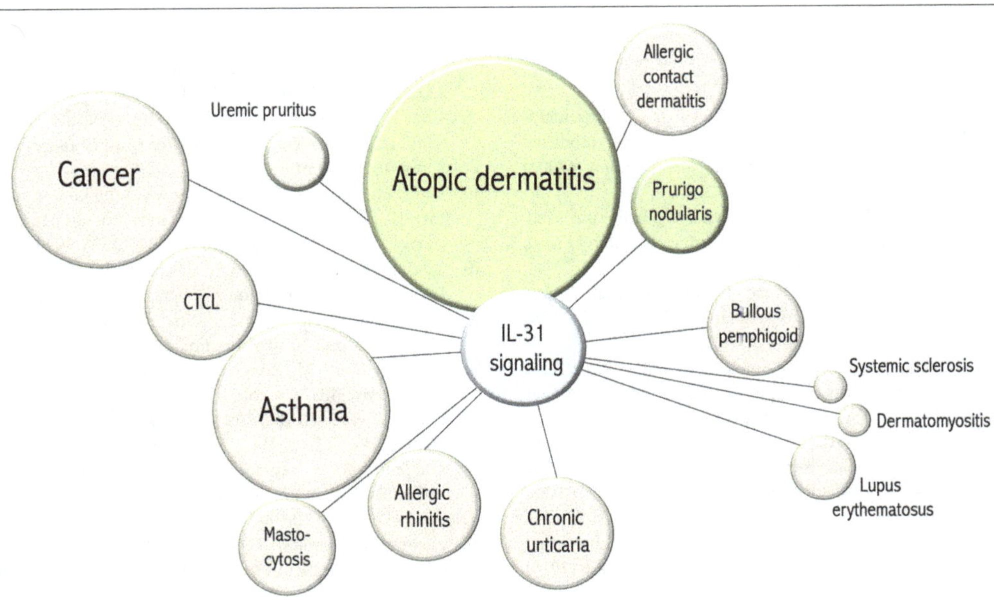

FIGURE 2 | Disease associations of IL-31 signaling. The circle diameter of each item correlates to the number of disease-associated publications listed in PubMed (pubmed.ncbi.nlm.nih.gov). The green color of an item corresponds to the therapeutic efficacy in clinical trials of targeting IL-31 signaling. The distance of an item from the center indicates whether IL-31 signaling hypothetically could serve as a therapeutic target.

processes such as cell proliferation and growth. Furthermore, the authors showed that IL-31 stimulated dermal fibroblast activated STAT3 and PI3K/Akt pathways and induced collagen I production (10). Several expression studies in fibroblasts also support that IL-31 stimulation promotes inflammation and tissue remodeling through the induction of IL-6, IL-16, IL-32, CCL2, CCL13, CCL15, CXCL1, CXCL3, CXCL8, and CXCL10 and matrix metalloproteinases (MMP-1, MMP-3, MMP-7 and MMP-25) (63).

Taken together, IL-31 represents a master regulator of neuroimmune inflammation and bridges the gap between immune cells, the nervous system and epithelial tissues.

DISCUSSION

During recent years a variety of diseases have been associated with IL-31 signaling (see **Figure 2**). An initial focus was directed on processes accompanied with pruritus and following, at least partly, concepts of type 2 inflammation. These included atopic dermatitis, allergic contact dermatitis, urticaria, mastocytosis, allergic rhinitis and asthma (4–9). Given the role of IL-31 signaling in the development of itch it is interesting to speculate whether IL-31 may also be involved in the stimulation of sneezing, coughing or bronchial hyperreactivity. In this context, other epithelial surfaces such as the gut and conditions such as irritable bowel syndrome also come to mind. STAT1 related regulation of IL-31RA may link this pathway also with autoimmune diseases such as systemic sclerosis, dermatomyositis and lupus erythematosus (10–12). A subset of affected patients experience severe pruritus but IL-31 signaling in autoimmune inflammation may also facilitate fibrosis and amplify inflammatory circuits. These are interesting aspects that need to be further explored in the future. Among autoimmune skin diseases, bullous pemphigoid has a unique position since patients develop autoantibodies against hemidesmosomes (BP180, BP230), eosinophilia, urticarial skin lesions, blisters and suffer from severe pruritus. A number of studies demonstrated the expression of IL-31 and its receptor in this condition and bullous pemphigoid appears to be a very interesting candidate for clinical studies targeting IL-31 signaling (65–68). Early on IL-31 expression and serum levels have been investigated in patients suffering from cutaneous T cell lymphoma (69–71). Notably, an increasing body of literature links IL-31 with malignant diseases such as endometrial carcinoma, lung cancer, myeloproliferative disorders, mastocytosis, cutaneous T cell lymphoma and follicular B cell lymphoma (7, 69, 71–76). The role of IL-31 in malignant diseases remains largely obscure but this aspect is worth to closely follow in the future. Taken together, IL-31 is a neuroimmune cytokine and IL-31RA signaling represents a master regulator of inflammation that bridges the gap between immune cells, the nervous system and epithelial tissues.

AUTHOR CONTRIBUTIONS

JN, MK, AD, BH, and VJ conceptualization and writing. UR and BH critical revision of manuscript. BH and PO editing. All authors contributed to the article and approved the submitted version.

REFERENCES

1. Dillon SR, Sprecher C, Hammond A, Bilsborough J, Rosenfeld-Franklin M, Presnell SR, et al. Interleukin 31, a cytokine produced by activated T cells, induces dermatitis in mice. *Nat Immunol.* (2004) 5:752–60. doi: 10.1038/ni1084
2. Ruzicka T, Hanifin JM, Furue M, Pulka G, Mlynarczyk I, Wollenberg A, et al. Anti-interleukin-31 receptor A antibody for atopic dermatitis. *N Engl J Med.* (2017) 376:826–35. doi: 10.1056/NEJMoa1606490
3. Ständer S, Yosipovitch G, Legat FJ, Lacour JP, Paul C, Narbutt J, et al. Trial of nemolizumab in moderate-to-severe prurigo nodularis. *N Engl J Med.* (2020) 382:706–16. doi: 10.1056/NEJMoa1908316
4. Sonkoly E, Muller A, Lauerma AI, Pivarcsi A, Soto H, Kemeny L, et al. IL-31: a new link between T cells and pruritus in atopic skin inflammation. *J Allergy Clin Immunol.* (2006) 117:411–7. doi: 10.1016/j.jaci.2005.10.033
5. Neis MM, Peters B, Dreuw A, Wenzel J, Bieber T, Mauch C, et al. Enhanced expression levels of IL-31 correlate with IL-4 and IL-13 in atopic and allergic contact dermatitis. *J Allergy Clin Immunol.* (2006) 118:930–7. doi: 10.1016/j.jaci.2006.07.015
6. Raap U, Wieczorek D, Gehring M, Pauls I, Ständer S, Kapp A, et al. Increased levels of serum IL-31 in chronic spontaneous urticaria. *Exp Dermatol.* (2010) 19:464–6. doi: 10.1111/j.1600-0625.2010.01067.x
7. Hartmann K, Wagner N, Rabenhorst A, Pflanz L, Leja S, Förster A, et al. Serum IL-31 levels are increased in a subset of patients with mastocytosis and correlate with disease severity in adult patients. *J Allergy Clin Immunol.* (2013) 132:232–5. doi: 10.1016/j.jaci.2012.11.008
8. Chai R, Liu B, Qi F. The significance of the levels of IL-4, IL-31 and TLSP in patients with asthma and/or rhinitis. *Immunotherapy.* (2017) 9:331–7. doi: 10.2217/imt-2016-0131
9. Lei Z, Liu G, Huang Q, Lv M, Zu R, Zhang GM, et al. SCF and IL-31 rather than IL-17 and BAFF are potential indicators in patients with allergic asthma. *Allergy.* (2008) 63:327–32. doi: 10.1111/j.1398-9995.2007.01566.x
10. Yaseen B, Lopez H, Taki Z, Zafar S, Rosario H, Abdi BA, et al. Interleukin-31 promotes pathogenic mechanisms underlying skin and lung fibrosis in scleroderma. *Rheumatology.* (2020) 59:2625–36. doi: 10.1093/rheumatology/keaa195
11. Kim HJ, Zeidi M, Bonciani D, Pena SM, Tiao J, Sahu S, et al. Itch in dermatomyositis: the role of increased skin interleukin-31. *Br J Dermatol.* (2018) 179:669–78. doi: 10.1111/bjd.16498
12. Huang HT, Chen JM, Guo J, Lan Y, Wei YS. The association of interleukin-31 polymorphisms with interleukin-31 serum levels and risk of systemic lupus erythematosus. *Rheumatol Int.* (2016) 36:799–805. doi: 10.1007/s00296-016-3422-6
13. Garbers C, Hermanns HM, Schaper F, Müller-Newen G, Grötzinger J, Rose-John S, et al. Plasticity and cross-talk of interleukin 6-type cytokines. *Cytokine Growth Factor Rev.* (2012) 23:85–97. doi: 10.1016/j.cytogfr.2012.04.001
14. Raap U, Gehring M, Kleiner S, Rüdrich U, Eiz-Vesper B, Haas H, et al. Human basophils are a source of - and are differentially activated

by - IL-31. *Clin Exp Allergy.* (2017) 47:499–508. doi: 10.1111/cea.12875

15. Niyonsaba F, Ushio H, Hara M, Yokoi H, Tominaga M, Takamori K, et al. Antimicrobial peptides human beta-defensins and cathelicidin LL-37 induce the secretion of a pruritogenic cytokine IL-31 by human mast cells. *J Immunol.* (2010) 184:3526–34. doi: 10.4049/jimmunol.0900712
16. Cheung PF, Wong CK, Ho AW, Hu S, Chen DP, Lam CW. Activation of human eosinophils and epidermal keratinocytes by Th2 cytokine IL-31: implication for the immunopathogenesis of atopic dermatitis. *Int Immunol.* (2010) 22:453–67. doi: 10.1093/intimm/dxq027
17. Wong CK, Leung KM, Qiu HN, Chow JY, Choi AO, Lam CW. Activation of eosinophils interacting with dermal fibroblasts by pruritogenic cytokine IL-31 and alarmin IL-33: implications in atopic dermatitis. *PLoS ONE.* (2012) 7:e29815. doi: 10.1371/journal.pone.0029815
18. Cevikbas F, Wang X, Akiyama T, Kempkes C, Savinko T, Antal A, et al. A sensory neuron-expressed IL-31 receptor mediates T helper cell-dependent itch: Involvement of TRPV1 and TRPA1. *J Allergy Clin Immunol.* (2014) 133:448–60. doi: 10.1016/j.jaci.2013.10.048
19. Zhang Q, Davis JC, Lamborn IT, Freeman AF, Jing H, Favreau AJ, et al. Combined immunodeficiency associated with DOCK8 mutations. *N Engl J Med.* (2009) 361:2046–55. doi: 10.1056/NEJMoa0905506
20. Graves JD, Draves KE, Gotoh Y, Krebs EG, Clark EA. Both phosphorylation and caspase-mediated cleavage contribute to regulation of the Ste20-like protein kinase Mst1 during CD95/Fas-induced apoptosis. *J Biol Chem.* (2001) 276:14909–15. doi: 10.1074/jbc.M010905200
21. Yamamura K, Uruno T, Shiraishi A, Tanaka Y, Ushijima M, Nakahara T, et al. The transcription factor EPAS1 links DOCK8 deficiency to atopic skin inflammation via IL-31 induction. *Nat Commun.* (2017) 8:13946. doi: 10.1038/ncomms13946
22. Halacli SO, Ayvaz DC, Sun-Tan C, Erman B, Uz E, Yilmaz DY, et al. STK4 (MST1) deficiency in two siblings with autoimmune cytopenias: a novel mutation. *Clin Immunol.* (2015) 161:316–23. doi: 10.1016/j.clim.2015.06.010
23. Elo LL, Järvenpää H, Tuomela S, Raghav S, Ahlfors H, Laurila K, et al. Genome-wide profiling of interleukin-4 and STAT6 transcription factor regulation of human Th2 cell programming. *Immunity.* (2010) 32:852–62. doi: 10.1016/j.immuni.2010.06.011
24. Jabara HH, McDonald DR, Janssen E, Massaad MJ, Ramesh N, Borzutzky A, et al. DOCK8 functions as an adaptor that links TLR-MyD88 signaling to B cell activation. *Nat Immunol.* (2012) 13:612–20. doi: 10.1038/ni.2305
25. Diveu C, Lelièvre E, Perret D, Lak-Hal AH, Froger J, Guillet C, et al. GPL, a novel cytokine receptor related to GP130 and leukemia inhibitory factor receptor. *J Biol Chem.* (2003) 278:49850–9. doi: 10.1074/jbc.M307286200
26. Ghilardi N, Li J, Hongo JA, Yi S, Gurney A, de Sauvage FJ. A novel type I cytokine receptor is expressed on monocytes, signals proliferation, and activates STAT-3 and STAT-5. *J Biol Chem.* (2002) 277:16831–6. doi: 10.1074/jbc.M201140200
27. Zhang Q, Putheti P, Zhou Q, Liu Q, Gao W. Structures and biological functions of IL-31 and IL-31 receptors. *Cytokine Growth Factor Rev.* (2008) 19:347–56. doi: 10.1016/j.cytogfr.2008.08.003
28. Horejs-Hoeck J, Schwarz H, Lamprecht S, Maier E, Hainzl S, Schmittner M, et al. Dendritic cells activated by IFN-γ/STAT1 express IL-31 receptor and release proinflammatory mediators upon IL-31 treatment. *J Immunol.* (2012) 188:5319–26. doi: 10.4049/jimmunol.1101044
29. *GTEx Portal - OSMR.* (2020). Available online at: https://www.gtexportal.org/home/gene/OSMR (accessed december 6, 2020).
30. Bilsborough J, Leung DY, Maurer M, Howell M, Boguniewicz M, Yao L, et al. IL-31 is associated with cutaneous lymphocyte antigen-positive skin homing T cells in patients with atopic dermatitis. *J Allergy Clin Immunol.* (2006) 117:418–25. doi: 10.1016/j.jaci.2005.10.046
31. Jawa RS, Chattopadhyay S, Tracy E, Wang Y, Huntoon K, Dayton MT, et al. Regulated expression of the IL-31 receptor in bronchial and alveolar epithelial cells, pulmonary fibroblasts, and pulmonary macrophages. *J Interferon Cytokine Res.* (2008) 28:207–19. doi: 10.1089/jir.2007.0057
32. Kasraie S, Niebuhr M, Baumert K, Werfel T. Functional effects of interleukin 31 in human primary keratinocytes. *Allergy.* (2011) 66:845–52. doi: 10.1111/j.1398-9995.2011.02545.x
33. Kasraie S, Niebuhr M, Werfel T. Interleukin (IL)-31 activates signal transducer and activator of transcription (STAT)-1, STAT-5 and extracellular signal-regulated kinase 1/2 and down-regulates IL-12p40 production in activated human macrophages. *Allergy.* (2013) 68:739–47. doi: 10.1111/all.12152
34. Maier E, Mittermeir M, Ess S, Neuper T, Schmiedlechner A, Duschl A, et al. Prerequisites for functional interleukin 31 signaling and its feedback regulation by suppressor of cytokine signaling 3 (SOCS3). *J Biol Chem.* (2015) 290:24747–59. doi: 10.1074/jbc.M115.661306
35. Dambacher J, Beigel F, Seiderer J, Haller D, Göke B, Auernhammer CJ, et al. Interleukin 31 mediates MAP kinase and STAT1/3 activation in intestinal epithelial cells and its expression is upregulated in inflammatory bowel disease. *Gut.* (2007) 56:1257–65. doi: 10.1136/gut.2006.118679
36. Diveu C, Lak-Hal AH, Froger J, Ravon E, Grimaud L, Barbier F, et al. Predominant expression of the long isoform of GP130-like (GPL) receptor is required for interleukin-31 signaling. *Eur Cytokine Netw.* (2004) 15:291–302.
37. Chattopadhyay S, Tracy E, Liang P, Robledo O, Rose-John S, Baumann H. Interleukin-31 and oncostatin-M mediate distinct signaling reactions and response patterns in lung epithelial cells. *J Biol Chem.* (2007) 282:3014–26. doi: 10.1074/jbc.M609655200
38. Stephens JM, Elks CM. Oncostatin M: potential implications for malignancy and metabolism. *Curr Pharm Des.* (2017) 23:3645–57. doi: 10.2174/1381612823666170704122559
39. Bando T, Morikawa Y, Komori T, Senba E. Complete overlap of interleukin-31 receptor A and oncostatin M receptor beta in the adult dorsal root ganglia with distinct developmental expression patterns. *Neuroscience.* (2006) 142:1263–71. doi: 10.1016/j.neuroscience.2006.07.009
40. Tamura S, Morikawa Y, Miyajima A, Senba E. Expression of oncostatin M receptor beta in a specific subset of nociceptive sensory neurons. *Eur J Neurosci.* (2003) 17:2287–98. doi: 10.1046/j.1460-9568.2003.02681.x
41. Arai I, Tsuji M, Miyagawa K, Takeda H, Akiyama N, Saito S. Repeated administration of IL-31 upregulates IL-31 receptor A (IL-31RA) in dorsal root ganglia and causes severe itch-associated scratching behaviour in mice. *Exp Dermatol.* (2015) 24:75–8. doi: 10.1111/exd.12587
42. Mishra SK, Hoon MA The cells and circuitry for itch responses in mice. *Science.* (2013) 340:968–71. doi: 10.1126/science.1233765
43. Sun YG, Zhao ZQ, Meng XL, Yin J, Liu XY, Chen ZF. Cellular basis of itch sensation. *Science.* (2009) 325:1531–4. doi: 10.1126/science.1174868
44. Aresh B, Freitag FB, Perry S, Blümel E, Lau J, Franck MCM, et al. Spinal cord interneurons expressing the gastrin-releasing peptide receptor convey itch through VGLUT2-mediated signaling. *Pain.* (2017) 158:945–61. doi: 10.1097/j.pain.0000000000000861
45. Mu D, Deng J, Liu KF, Wu ZY, Shi YF, Guo WM, et al. A central neural circuit for itch sensation. *Science.* (2017) 357:695–9. doi: 10.1126/science.aaf4918
46. Meng J, Moriyama M, Feld M, Buddenkotte J, Buhl T, Szöllösi A, et al. New mechanism underlying IL-31-induced atopic dermatitis. *J Allergy Clin Immunol.* (2018) 141:1677–89.e8. doi: 10.1016/j.jaci.2017.12.1002
47. Ma H, Gao T, Jakobsson JET, Weman HM, Xu B, Larhammar D, et al. The neuropeptide Y Y(2) receptor is coexpressed with Nppb in primary afferent neurons and Y(2) activation reduces histaminergic and IL-31-induced itch. *J Pharmacol Exp Ther.* (2020) 372:73–82. doi: 10.1124/jpet.119.262584
48. Feld M, Garcia R, Buddenkotte J, Katayama S, Lewis K, Muirhead G, et al. The pruritus- and TH2-associated cytokine IL-31 promotes growth of sensory nerves. *J Allergy Clin Immunol.* (2016) 138:500–8.e24. doi: 10.1016/j.jaci.2016.02.020
49. Yoshimoto T. The hunt for the source of primary interleukin-4: how we discovered that natural killer T cells and basophils determine T helper type 2 cell differentiation *in vivo*. *Front Immunol.* (2018) 9:716. doi: 10.3389/fimmu.2018.00716
50. Sokol CL, Medzhitov R. Role of basophils in the initiation of Th2 responses. *Curr Opin Immunol.* (2010) 22:73–7. doi: 10.1016/j.coi.2010.01.012
51. Kunsleben N, Rüdrich U, Gehring M, Novak N, Kapp A, Raap U. IL-31 induces chemotaxis, calcium mobilization, release of reactive oxygen species, and CCL26 in eosinophils, which are capable to release IL-31. *J Invest Dermatol.* (2015) 135:1908–11. doi: 10.1038/jid.2015.106
52. Zlotnik A, Burkhardt AM, Homey B. Homeostatic chemokine receptors and organ-specific metastasis. *Nat Rev Immunol.* (2011) 11:597–606. doi: 10.1038/nri3049
53. Griffith JW, Sokol CL, Luster AD. Chemokines and chemokine receptors: positioning cells for host defense and immunity. *Annu Rev*

Immunol. (2014) 32:659–702. doi: 10.1146/annurev-immunol-032713-120145
54. Jones SA, Jenkins BJ. Recent insights into targeting the IL-6 cytokine family in inflammatory diseases and cancer. *Nat Rev Immunol.* (2018) 18:773–89. doi: 10.1038/s41577-018-0066-7
55. Cornelissen C, Lüscher-Firzlaff J, Baron JM, Lüscher B. Signaling by IL-31 and functional consequences. *Eur J Cell Biol.* (2012) 91:552–66. doi: 10.1016/j.ejcb.2011.07.006
56. Singh B, Jegga AG, Shanmukhappa KS, Edukulla R, Khurana Hershey GH, Medvedovic M, et al. IL-31-driven skin remodeling involves epidermal cell proliferation and thickening that lead to impaired skin-barrier function. *PLoS ONE.* (2016) 11:e0161877. doi: 10.1371/journal.pone.0161877
57. Hänel KH, Pfaff CM, Cornelissen C, Amann PM, Marquardt Y, Czaja K, et al. Control of the physical and antimicrobial skin barrier by an IL-31-IL-1 signaling network. *J Immunol.* (2016) 196:3233–44. doi: 10.4049/jimmunol.1402943
58. Andoh T, Li S, Uta D. Involvement of thromboxane A(2) in interleukin-31-induced itch-associated response in mice. *Pharmacol Rep.* (2018) 70:251–7. doi: 10.1016/j.pharep.2017.10.001
59. Andoh T, Harada A, Kuraishi Y. Involvement of leukotriene B4 released from keratinocytes in itch-associated response to intradermal interleukin-31 in mice. *Acta Derm Venereol.* (2017) 97:922–7. doi: 10.2340/00015555-2697
60. Kahremany S, Hofmann L, Gruzman A, Cohen G. Advances in understanding the initial steps of pruritoceptive itch: how the itch hits the switch. *Int J Mol Sci.* (2020) 21:4883. doi: 10.3390/ijms21144883
61. Ip WK, Wong CK, Li ML, Li PW, Cheung PF, Lam CW. Interleukin-31 induces cytokine and chemokine production from human bronchial epithelial cells through activation of mitogen-activated protein kinase signalling pathways: implications for the allergic response. *Immunology.* (2007) 122:532–41. doi: 10.1111/j.1365-2567.2007.02668.x
62. Perrigoue JG, Zaph C, Guild K, Du Y, Artis D. IL-31-IL-31R interactions limit the magnitude of Th2 cytokine-dependent immunity and inflammation following intestinal helminth infection. *J Immunol.* (2009) 182:6088–94. doi: 10.4049/jimmunol.0802459
63. Yagi Y, Andoh A, Nishida A, Shioya M, Nishimura T, Hashimoto T, et al. Interleukin-31 stimulates production of inflammatory mediators from human colonic subepithelial myofibroblasts. *Int J Mol Med.* (2007) 19:941–6. doi: 10.3892/ijmm.19.6.941
64. Chakraborty D, Šumová B, Mallano T, Chen CW, Distler A, Bergmann C, et al. Activation of STAT3 integrates common profibrotic pathways to promote fibroblast activation and tissue fibrosis. *Nat Commun.* (2017) 8:1130. doi: 10.1038/s41467-017-01236-6
65. Kulczycka-Siennicka L, Cynkier A, Waszczykowska E, Wozniacka A, Zebrowska A. The role of intereukin-31 in pathogenesis of itch and its intensity in a course of bullous pemphigoid and dermatitis herpetiformis. *Biomed Res Int.* (2017) 2017:5965492. doi: 10.1155/2017/5965492
66. Salz M, Haeberle S, Hoffmann J, Enk AH, Hadaschik EN. Elevated IL-31 serum levels in bullous pemphigoid patients correlate with eosinophil numbers and are associated with BP180-IgE. *J Dermatol Sci.* (2017) 87:309–11. doi: 10.1016/j.jdermsci.2017.07.019
67. Rüdrich U, Gehring M, Papakonstantinou E, Illerhaus A, Engmann J, Kapp A, et al. Eosinophils are a major source of interleukin-31 in bullous pemphigoid. *Acta Derm Venereol.* (2018) 98:766–71. doi: 10.2340/00015555-2951
68. Hashimoto T, Kursewicz CD, Fayne RA, Nanda S, Shah SM, Nattkemper L, et al. Pathophysiologic mechanisms of itch in bullous pemphigoid. *J Am Acad Dermatol.* (2020) 83:53–62. doi: 10.1016/j.jaad.2019.07.060
69. Ohmatsu H, Sugaya M, Suga H, Morimura S, Miyagaki T, Kai H, et al. Serum IL-31 levels are increased in patients with cutaneous T-cell lymphoma. *Acta Derm Venereol.* (2012) 92:282–3. doi: 10.2340/00015555-1345
70. Nattkemper LA, Martinez-Escala ME, Gelman AB, Singer EM, Rook AH, Guitart J, et al. Cutaneous T-cell lymphoma and pruritus: the expression of IL-31 and its receptors in the skin. *Acta Derm Venereol.* (2016) 96:894–8. doi: 10.2340/00015555-2417
71. Singer EM, Shin DB, Nattkemper LA, Benoit BM, Klein RS, Didigu CA, et al. IL-31 is produced by the malignant T-cell population in cutaneous T-Cell lymphoma and correlates with CTCL pruritus. *J Invest Dermatol.* (2013) 133:2783–5. doi: 10.1038/jid.2013.227
72. Zeng X, Zhang Z, Gao QQ, Wang YY, Yu XZ, Zhou B, et al. Clinical significance of serum interleukin-31 and interleukin-33 levels in patients of endometrial cancer: a case control study. *Dis Markers.* (2016) 2016:9262919. doi: 10.1155/2016/9262919
73. Naumnik W, Naumnik B, Niewiarowska K, Ossolinska M, Chyczewska E. Novel cytokines: IL-27, IL-29, IL-31 and IL-33. Can they be useful in clinical practice at the time diagnosis of lung cancer? *Exp Oncol.* (2012) 34:348–53.
74. Lange M, Gleń J, Zabłotna M, Nedoszytko B, Sokołowska-Wojdyło M, Rebała K, et al. Interleukin-31 polymorphisms and serum IL-31 level in patients with mastocytosis: correlation with clinical presen-tation and pruritus. *Acta Derm Venereol.* (2017) 97:47–53. doi: 10.2340/00015555-2474
75. Ferretti E, Tripodo C, Pagnan G, Guarnotta C, Marimpietri D, Corrias MV, et al. The interleukin (IL)-31/IL-31R axis contributes to tumor growth in human follicular lymphoma. *Leukemia.* (2015) 29:958–67. doi: 10.1038/leu.2014.291
76. Ferretti E, Corcione A, Pistoia V. The IL-31/IL-31 receptor axis: general features and role in tumor microenvironment. *J Leukoc Biol.* (2017) 102:711–7. doi: 10.1189/jlb.3MR0117-033R

19

Electrically Evoked Itch in Human Subjects

Hans Jürgen Solinski and Roman Rukwied*

Department of Experimental Pain Research, Medical Faculty Mannheim, University of Heidelberg, Mannheim, Germany

***Correspondence:**
Roman Rukwied
roman.rukwied@medma.uni-heidelberg.de

Administration of chemicals (pruritogens) into the skin evokes itch based on signal transduction mechanisms that generate action potentials mainly in mechanically sensitive and *in*sensitive primary afferent C-fibers (pruriceptors). These signals from peripheral neurons are processed in spinal and supra-spinal centers of the central nervous system and finally generate the sensation of itch. Compared to chemical stimulation, electrical activation of pruriceptors would allow for better temporal control and thereby a more direct functional assessment of their activation. Here, we review the electrical stimulation paradigms which were used to evoke itch in humans in the past. We further evaluate recent attempts to explore electrically induced itch in atopic dermatitis patients. Possible mechanisms underlying successful pruritus generation in chronic itch patients by transdermal slowly depolarizing electrical stimulation are discussed.

Keywords: atopic dermatitis, rectangular pulses, sinusoidal stimulation, polymodal nociceptors, silent C-fibers, voltage-gated sodium channels, slow depolarization, peripheral (axonal) and central sensitization

TEXT

Traditionally, basic researchers administered histamine into the skin of human subjects to experimentally evoke an itch response (pruritus). An alternative approach to induce itch is a depletion of histamine from skin mast cells by e.g., administration of codeine (1) or compound 48/80 (2). In chronic itch conditions, however, histamine is apparently not the major contributor driving chronic itch (3) and over the past decades a plethora of compounds ("pruritogens") have been identified to cause histamine-independent itch. For example, the bovine adrenal medulla peptide 8–22 (BAM8-22), the anti-malarial drug chloroquine (CQ), the hexapeptide SLIGRL, but also endogenous substances such as cytokines (e.g., interleukine-31), proteases (e.g., trypsin), amino-acids (e.g., beta-alanine), peptide hormones (e.g., endothelin-1), and many others [for review see (4)]. These compounds act on their cognate receptors expressed on primary afferent neurons, for example Mas-related G protein-coupled receptors (Mrgprs) or protease-activated receptors (PARs) [e.g., see (5–7)]. Itch induced by these mediators involves signal transduction mechanisms that, in turn, induce the generation of action potentials (APs) in primary afferent neurons. Of these, unmyelinated nerve fibers—mechanically sensitive as well as mechanically *in*sensitive C-fibers—are instrumental for chemically evoked APs and their transmission to the central nervous system (CNS). This peripheral pruriceptive signal is processed in spinal and supra-spinal centers in the CNS to finally generate the sensation of pruritus (8, 9).

Electrically Evoked Itch in Healthy Human Subjects

In order to improve temporal control and assess the function of peripheral itch-inducing nerve fibers more directly and thereby circumvent above mentioned chemical signal transduction mechanisms, their electrical activation was pursued for decades. In 1943, Bishop developed a constant voltage stimulator for repetitive electrical skin stimulation through a fine wire being in skin contact, and when combining weak electrical shocks with high stimulation frequency of about 10 Hz a pure sensation of itch could be evoked (10). He noted that the higher the frequency the lower the strength must be for the purest sensation of itch. Instead of a transcutaneous electrical stimulation, Shelley and Arthur inserted an electrode just beneath the epidermis and delivered biphasic square-waves of variable frequency, duration and intensity (11). The most robust pruritogenic effects were observed at a stimulation frequency of 20 Hz, a 5 ms pulse duration and a voltage ranging from 0.5 to 1.5 V. However, the current level could not be controlled sufficiently to avoid that cells and nerve fibers surrounding the electrode were immediately cauterized. Therefore, Edwards and co-workers used a solid state constant current generator placed between the square-wave generator and the subject, thus enabling the control of the current amplitude, and attached a transcutaneous electrode of 5 cm^2 to the wrist of the subjects (12). The volar aspect of the wrist was chosen because at this site the greatest concentration of "itch points" was identified, i.e., areas at which an itch developed when stimulated electrically (11). Delivering monophasic repetitive current pulses of 50 Hz and 10 ms pulse duration induced reliable itch at threshold current levels of 15 μA and up to a maximum of 150 μA (12). On some occasions, subjects reported in addition to an itch a sensation of warmth or prickling, and the authors suggested a variation of the experimental procedure, for instance using bi-phasic rather than mono-phasic currents or other pulse forms than the delivered square-waves. Tuckett followed this suggestion, exploring the responses of feline "polymodal" nociceptors (mechanically- and heat-sensitive C-fibers) to different frequencies of electrical square-wave stimulation and correlating the results to the psychophysical assessment of electrical stimulation and application of cowhage spicules (*Mucuna pruriens*) in human subjects (13). One of his findings was that 10 Hz square-wave pulses of 7 ms duration and gradually increasing currents, delivered through 6 cm^2 gauze pads placed to the wrist, induced pure itch in 50% of the subjects (in addition, about 40% of the subjects reported a mixture of itch and pain), which was very similar to the sensation from cowhage stimulation. While polymodal nociceptors tended to fatigue and their average response rate remained constant between 10 and 40 Hz, human subjects reported increased sensations with increasing frequency of stimulation, and the author suggested that increased pruritus at higher stimulation frequencies is signaled by few neurons that can follow higher frequencies of stimulation (13). About 15 years ago, Ikoma and colleagues modified aforementioned electrical stimulation protocols by delivering trains of 50 rectangular pulses (2 ms pulse duration) every 3 s for a period of 90 s across a 0.1 × 7 mm stainless steel wire attached to the wrist skin. Varying pulse frequency and current intensity revealed a maximum itch response at frequencies exceeding 50 Hz and current intensities lower than 0.12 mA (14). Higher current intensities frequently induced a tapping and pain sensation accompanied by a reduction of itch. The phenomenon of itch reduction by painful stimuli is most likely attributed to central inhibitory mechanisms (15, 16). A comparable method of itch induction comprised the use of a pair of disk electrodes with a diameter of 1 cm attached to the wrist (17) or the volar forearm skin (18) of human subjects. At both skin sites, itch was induced by delivering rectangular electrical pulses of 0.1 ms duration with 50 Hz and a current intensity that continuously increased over 2 min at 0.05 mA/s up to a maximum of 5 mA (wrist) or 6.4 mA (forearm).

All aforementioned studies suggest that itch can be induced by electrical stimulation in human skin. Of note, the parameters for electrical stimulation (current intensity, pulse frequency, stimulus duration and electrode configuration) need to be considered carefully as these determine which primary sensory afferent nerve fibers will be preferentially activated. As already mentioned, primarily unmyelinated C-nociceptors (named "pruriceptors") are involved in itch signaling from the periphery to the CNS. Early recordings from the saphenous nerve of the cat provided evidence that the itching after-sensation to light touch results most probably from C-fiber activation (19). Isolation of small nerve fascicles and their separation into fine strands allowing for single-unit recordings of slowly conducting myelinated (20) and unmyelinated (21) neurons revealed that polymodal C-fibers most likely contribute to cowhage-induced itch. Single nerve fiber recordings in awake human subjects (microneurography), initially developed by Hagbarth and Vallbo (22) and adapted by Torebjörk and Hallin for C-fiber recordings (23), eventually demonstrated that a subgroup of mechanically insensitive ("silent") C-nociceptors were particularly responsive to histamine and thus most likely convey histamine-mediated itch (24), whereas mechanically sensitive ("polymodal") C-nociceptors were reliably activated by cowhage spicules (25) and thus, apparently mediate this form of histamine-independent itch (26). Notably, in addition to C-fibers also thinly myelinated A-delta nociceptors can be activated by cowhage spicules in monkeys (27). However, considering electrically induced itch (see **Table 1**) and the hitherto established profiles of transcutaneous high frequency (>50 Hz) stimulation with pulses of short duration (<2 ms), and bearing in mind the remarkably high electrical activation threshold of C-nociceptors compared to myelinated fibers (30), it remains open which primary sensory afferent nerve fibers explicitly had been activated in the investigations mentioned above (10–14, 17, 18). Both myelinated and unmyelinated fiber types are activated by high frequency electrical stimulation with rectangular pulses. The uncertainty of matching stimulus configuration to the activated nerve fiber class, however, is rather unsatisfying. This issue can be addressed by employing slowly depolarizing electrical stimuli of half-sine and sine wave shape delivered transcutaneously via small punctate electrodes that selectively activate C-fibers (33–36). Thereby, "polymodal" C-nociceptors are activated by a single 500 ms half-sine wave pulse responding with a current intensity dependent burst of action potential discharges (34). Notably, low-threshold unmyelinated tactile afferents also respond to that type of stimulus (34) but this fiber class is associated primarily with social touch rather than pain or itch processing (37, 38). In contrast, "silent" and "polymodal" C-nociceptors are activated by 4 Hz sine wave pulses (33, 36) of which "silent" nociceptors respond with one action potential per sinusoidal cycle compared

TABLE 1 | Parameters of electrical stimulation for experimental itch induction in humans.

Wave form	Electrode configuration and dimension	Pulse duration	Stimulation frequency	Stimulation intensity	Stimulation period	Optimal paramaters to elicit itch	Skin type and location	Fiber-class preferentially activated	Discharge pattern	References
rectangular 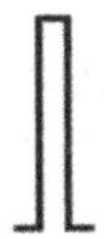	transdermal; 40G wire, 5 cm; 3,14 cm^2 disc	n.d.	10 Hz	n.d.	several seconds	n.d.	healthy; dorsum hand and forearm	A-fibers	1 AP/ pulse	(10)
	intra-cutaneous; pinpoint copper wire	5 ms	20 Hz	0.5–1.5 V	0.2 s	20 Hz; 5 ms	healthy	A- + C-fibers	1 AP/ pulse	(11)
	transdermal; 5 cm^2 gauze pad	10 ms	50 Hz	15–150 µA	>15 s	50–150 µA	healthy + AD non-lesional skin; volar wrist	A- + C-fibers	1 AP/ pulse	(12)
	transdermal; 6 cm^2 gauze pad	7 ms	10–40 Hz	supra-threshold	5 s	10 Hz; 7 ms	healthy	A- + C-fibers	1 AP/ pulse	(13)
	transdermal; stainless steel wire 0.1 x 7 mm	0.08–8 ms	2–200 Hz	<0.12 mA	90 s	50 Hz; 2 ms; 0.05–0.1 mA	healthy + AD non-lesional skin; volar wrist	A- + C-fibers	1 AP/ pulse	(14)
	transdermal; 3,14 cm^2 disc	0.1 ms	50 Hz	1.6–6.4 mA	2 min	50 Hz; 0.1 ms; 6.4 mA	healthy; volar forearm	A- > C-fibers	1 AP/ pulse	(17, 18)
half-sine 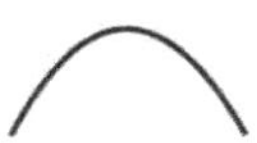	transdermal; pinpoint platinum wire 0.4 mm	500 ms	1 Hz	0.2–1 mA	500 ms	single pulse; 0.6–1 mA	AD lesional + non-lesional (volar forearm) skin	low-threshold and polymodal C-fibers	burst of APs/ pulse	(28)
sine 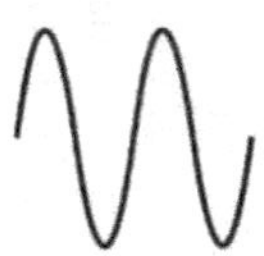	transdermal; 3,14 cm^2 disc	200 ms and 0.0005 ms per cycle	5–2000 Hz	2–140 µA	several seconds until itch threshold	5 Hz; 8–25 µA	healthy + AD/prurigo nodularis lesional + non-lesional	A- > C-fibers	1 AP/ cycle	(29)
	transdermal; pinpoint platinum wire 0.4 mm	250 ms per cycle	4 Hz	0.025–0.2 mA	1 min	4 Hz; 0.1–0.2 mA; continuous 30–60 s	AD lesional + non-lesional (volar forearm) skin	polymodal and silent C-nociceptors	1 AP/ cycle	(28)

Summary and references of the electrical stimulation protocols. Note that with a rectangular stimulation paradigm of 0.25 Hz and 0.5 ms pulse duration the transcutaneous electrical thresholds were >9 mA for C-nociceptor stimulation (electrode covering 30 mm^2) (30). If higher current densities are provided at the stimulation sites by using pointed (1 mm diameter) or bipolar (2 mm length, 3 mm distance) pin electrodes (stimulation frequency 1–10 Hz) current intensities exceeding 5 mA are required for C-fiber activation (31, 32). Given the low intensities and high frequencies used in the protocols summarized, most likely myelinated A-fibers had been stimulated.

n.d. not determined.

to the discharge burst recorded from "polymodal" units (34, 36). Hence, the selection of a slowly depolarizing stimulation profile applied through pinpointed electrodes can be used to differentially activate nociceptor sub-types, which of course provoke in healthy human skin rather pain than itch but may change under pathologic conditions (see below).

Limitations

The stimulation paradigms of electrical rectangular pulses delivered to human skin (10–14, 17, 18) do not differentiate nerve fibers that contribute to histaminergic vs. non-histaminergic itch. This can be seen as a limitation of electrically evoked itch in experimental human studies when compared with chemical stimulation (e.g., histamine vs. cowhage spicules). The use of antihistamines during the electrical stimulation protocol might be suggested to overcome a possible lack of specificity and to rule out an unintentional activation of skin mast cells, but electrical activation of C-fibers should not require G protein-coupled receptors (e.g., histamine receptors). In contrast, itch caused by chemical stimulation involves signal transduction processes at the sensory endings and knowledge of these itch mediating pathways, indeed, may lead to the development of biologics [e.g., interleukin-receptor antibodies (39, 40)] and eventually successful anti-pruritic therapies. However, the number of chemical substances causing an itch indicate a plethora of key mediators and pathways being involved [see (41) for review]. Direct depolarization of primary afferent axons by electrical stimulation and subsequent induction of APs would skip these transduction processes, thereby bypassing any (perhaps disease-induced) changes in cutaneous pruriceptive nerve endings but of course also losing the opportunity to investigate them further. On the other hand, bypassing these potential changes at terminal nerve fiber endings through direct electrical axonal induction of APs might enable the unconfounded investigation of spinal itch circuits that might have been sensitized e.g., under pathologic conditions. Furthermore, the advantage of a precise timing of electrically evoked "itch onset" and "itch offset" can be used in combination with CNS imaging techniques (e.g., fMRI) providing a promising tool to amend human itch research.

Electrically Evoked Itch in Atopic Dermatitis (AD) Patients

Based on the hypothesis that chronic inflammation might differentially modify neuronal excitability of skin afferents in pruritic skin, it is intriguing to investigate electrically induced itch in patients suffering from chronic itch. Until recently, only few studies explored this issue in atopic dermatitis (AD) patients (12, 14, 29). Edwards and colleagues demonstrated a faster response time of itch to different intensity levels of electrical stimulation. This was interpreted as a reduction of itch thresholds in AD, but unfortunately the authors did not record a dose-response for itch magnitude (12). The study by Ikoma and colleagues compared both histamine and electrically induced itch between healthy controls and AD patients (14). Read out parameters were electrically evoked itch, pain, tapping sensations, skin erythema and secondary areas of alloknesis, hyperknesis or punctuate hyperalgesia, but none of these measures were significantly different between healthy control subjects and AD patients (14). An explanation for these rather disappointing results might be that the peripheral primary afferent nerve fiber classes contributing to chronic itch in AD were not sufficiently activated by the electrical stimulation. Additionally, differences of sensation between healthy control subjects and patients might have been missed since AD patients were not stimulated in their itchy and/or eczematous skin. In another study, Pereira and colleagues stimulated peripheral nerve fibers of patients with chronic pruritus (AD and prurigo nodularis) by 5 Hz and 2 kHz transcutaneous electrical stimuli generated by a Neurometer® and delivered via a pair of gold electrodes (each 1 cm in diameter) attached the volar forearm skin (29). The Neurometer® is a device that produces a pure sine wave of up to 10 mA (42). It is commonly used to assess peripheral nerve fiber function and sensory symptoms in polyneuropathy patients (43). In six of the 78 investigated patients a sensation of itch was recorded upon 5 Hz stimulation and in two of 73 patients during 2 kHz stimuli (29). The relative small number of patients reporting electrically evoked itch might be due to the electrode configuration (diameter 1 cm) used for transcutaneous stimulation. High current densities facilitate the excitation of unmyelinated pruriceptors and therefore small pinpointed electrodes would be recommended for their recruitment (31). Also, the authors assessed the sensation of the patients at current perception thresholds, which may have hampered itch induction when compared with supra-threshold electrical stimulation.

Recent investigations demonstrated the differential activation of C-nociceptor subclasses by transcutaneous administration of a single electrical 1 Hz half-sine wave pulse (500 ms duration, current <1 mA) as well as a series of 4 Hz sine wave pulses (<0.4 mA), delivered through pinpointed electrodes (34, 36). Human psychophysics, skin erythema and sweat response measurements as well as compound action potential recordings *in vitro*, single nerve fiber discharge patterns monitored *in vivo* from pig saphenous nerve, and microneurography in humans thereby provided evidence that half-sine wave pulses activate primarily polymodal C-nociceptors. In particular, the C-fibers respond with a burst of APs in which the number of APs and their discharge frequency varies intensity-dependently to the single half-sine wave stimulus (34). In contrast, delivering 4 Hz sine wave pulses activates both, polymodal and "silent" C-nociceptors (36). Thereby, particularly "silent" C-fibers respond with a single AP per sine wave cycle revealing an activation pattern that is characterized by synchronized discharge at 4 Hz (34).

If slowly depolarizing sinusoidal stimuli of 4 Hz are applied continuously for a longer period (1 min), healthy human subjects report a gradual decline of the perceived burning pain sensation indicating a profound C-nociceptor accommodation to the electrical pulses. In contrast, neuropathic pain patients reported—particularly at their painful skin sites—an increased nociception without adaptation upon (supra-threshold) ongoing sine wave stimulation (36).

In a recent study, we used this electrical stimulation protocol of differential ("polymodal" and "silent") C-nociceptor activation to investigate electrically evoked sensations in AD patients (28). Half-sine wave and sine wave stimuli were delivered to eczematous skin areas that had been particularly itchy before the investigation, and the corresponding sensation was compared to the electrically induced responses obtained from the patients' non-affected (if possible site matched) skin sites. Single half-sine wave pulses (500 ms, 0.2–1 mA) induced itch in about 30% of the patients. Delivering sinusoidal pulses for a duration of 2.5 s (4 Hz, 0.025–0.4 mA) caused itch in only three of 25 patients, all others mentioned discomfort or pain upon stimulation. Importantly, when the sine wave pulses were delivered continuously for 1 min (4 Hz, max. 0.2 mA) to eczematous skin sites, the number of patients reporting itch increased progressively the longer the stimulation lasted, resulting in about 50% of AD patients perceiving an itch at 1 min (all of them also perceived half-sine wave itch) (28). When stimulating non-affected skin sites only three patients reported itch. These results indicate that activation of both, "polymodal" and "silent" nociceptors, can evoke pruritus in AD and the duration of stimulation might be essential to induce it. Notably, an inter-individual variability in the sensation of itch upon electrical stimulation has to be considered as pruritus could be evoked in only a part of the AD patients. Possible reasons for variable responses might be individual differences in skin pathophysiology [for instance hypo- vs. hyper-innervation (44, 45)] or psychological stress status (46), which both might be a target for future experimental studies.

Neuronal Pathways Mediating Itch

Currently, three models explain in general, why we feel an itch [reviewed in (47–49)]. In the mouse, dedicated pruriceptive sensory neurons exist and their activity is sufficient to produce pruritus (50, 51) along a so-called "labeled-line," leading to the *specificity theory of itch*. This specificity theory was based on the use of itch-specific neuropeptides by pruriceptive sensory neurons or the involvement of spinal itch-specific transmission pathways (52, 53). In humans, sensory neurons that constitute a labeled-line for itch have not yet been described, as neurons activated by pruritogens also respond to algogenic stimuli. However, it was postulated that pruritogens induce lower AP frequencies or different AP patterns as compared to algogenic stimuli in these neurons, leading to the *intensity/pattern theory of itch* (54). Finally, focal application of pruciceptive or algogenic stimuli can lead to itch (55), potentially because the CNS interprets a heightened spatial contrast of peripheral input as itch, leading to the *spatial contrast theory of itch* (56, 57).

Independent of the exact coding mechanism of pruritus, it is a striking observation that AD patients often feel itch during stimulation of their eczematous skin upon a stimulus that is normally perceived as painful (28, 58). One likely mechanism of such a shift from pain to itch can be a changed central processing of the pruriceptive and/or nociceptive input in AD. Altered central processing on spinal and supra-spinal levels could facilitate transmission of pruriceptive information in ascending sensory circuits. A switch from an intense nociceptive stimulus (e.g., the injection of protons) in healthy human skin to an itch in AD patients has already suggested such a central sensitization process (58). In addition, a reduced descending inhibition of itch may be suggested in chronic pruritus, given that the effect of conditioned pain modulation was decreased (59) and transcutaneous electrical nerve stimulation (TENS, 100 Hz up to 26 mA) did not reduce acute itch sensation in AD (60). Intriguingly, cutaneous field stimulation applied to itchy skin areas of AD patients via 16 needle electrodes fixed at 2 cm intervals on a 4 × 4 cm flexible rubber plate by delivering 1 ms rectangular pulses at 4 Hz and up to 0.8 mA per electrode for 25 min (61) initially enhanced the intensity of itch in AD but significantly reduced it by about 25% after cessation for 1–5 h post-treatment (60). Changes in spinal circuits that determine the link between peripheral sensory input and the output of the different classes of spinal projection neurons ascending into the brain could also explain the switch from pain to itch observed in AD patients when delivering sine wave pulses to the eczema sites for longer duration. However, slowly depolarizing electrical stimuli activate specific peripheral afferent nerve fiber classes and can evoke itch only inside the eczematous skin in some (but not all) AD patients. This indicates that the stimulation of "polymodal" and "silent" nerve fibers—alone or in combination—contributes to a peripheral mechanism for the induction of itch that takes place in AD patients in addition to potential central mechanisms.

Parameters Influencing Electrical Nerve Fiber Activation in the Skin

Excitability of sensory nerves to transdermal electrical stimulation depends—in principle—on three major cellular characteristics of a given nerve fiber: (a) the exact geometry of the nerve ending in the skin; (b) the membrane characteristics determining the extent of local depolarization upon electrical stimulation; (c) the encoding of the depolarization into discharges of single APs or bursts. All of these characteristics may be modified particularly by local inflammatory processes in eczematous skin and therefore could contribute to the observed itch upon normally painful electrical stimulation (28).

a) In various skin diseases, including AD, epidermal innervation patterns change. However, the direction of this change is under debate, potentially due to different quantification methods of epidermal nerve fiber density. Initially, hyper-innervation of eczematous skin was proposed as a structural rearrangement causing chronic pruritus in AD (45, 62, 63). However, more recently, investigations in bigger patient cohorts as well as the use of various microscopic methods that allow imaging of large dermal volumes point to an epidermal hypo-innervation of eczematous AD skin (59, 64, 65). In line with this finding, we did not find decreased sensory thresholds to sine wave stimulation between eczematous/itchy and un-affected skin of AD patients as well as between AD and control subjects (28), as would be predicted from hyper-innervated skin. However, due to the lack of established markers for human pruriceptive nerve fibers—the mentioned studies used the pan-fiber marker protein gene product 9.5 (PGP9.5)—the significance of such epidermal innervation changes for electrical induction of pruritus in AD patients remains unclear and needs further investigation. Epidermal thickening, especially prevalent in eczematous AD skin, adds an additional layer of complexity as it might increase the distance between the most superficial nerve fibers and the transdermal stimulation electrodes as well as the length and axonal branching pattern of the nerve terminals, both of which might influence their excitability (65, 66).

b) Most ion channels with established roles in the transduction of natural nociceptive stimuli, including the polymodal transient receptor potential (TRP) superfamily members TRP vanilloid 1 (TRPV1) and ankyrin 1 (TRPA1), are only weakly voltage dependent, limiting their contribution to electrically induced depolarization (67, 68). However, TRPV1 has been found to interact with voltage sensitive potassium channels (69) and might therefore also modulate neuronal excitability. Moreover, the voltage dependence of TRP channels is highly plastic in disease, thereby contributing to inflammatory pain states (70, 71). Interestingly, TRPV1- and TRPA1-expression was elevated in eczematous AD skin, an effect attributable to an increased expression per cell, as the number of TRPV1/TRPA1-immunopositive nerve fibers was unchanged (72). Thus, under inflamed conditions, in addition to a potential sensitization of their voltage dependence, the overexpression of TRPA1 and TRPV1 might increase the depolarizing effects of sinusoidal stimulation and thereby facilitate neuronal discharge. A potentially increased recruitment of TRPV1/TRPA1$^+$ fibers upon sinusoidal stimulation in AD and the accompanied perception of itch would be in line with a previous observation, in which the administration of protons (known to activate TRPV1) evoked itch in lesional and healthy appearing skin of AD patients, but burning pain in control subjects (58).

c) Receptor potentials are encoded into trains of APs at the so-called spike initiation zone. The position of this zone can be dynamically moved closer to the receptive endings under inflammatory conditions, thereby facilitating encoding of the receptor potential in APs as shown in corneal nociceptors in mouse (73). Such modulation of axonal excitability might also occur in inflamed human skin but has not yet been studied. With the advent of next-generation sequencing techniques, expression changes of ion channels in eczematous skin of AD patients have been investigated, using a dermal punch biopsy as input material (72, 74, 75). This bulk analysis, though powerful, also has some caveats. For instance, differences in the cellular constituents of the biopsy involuntarily lead to differences in gene expression. In line with this notion, genes selectively expressed by invading leukocytes show high overexpression in eczematous skin (72, 74, 75). Expression changes in nerve fibers are particularly hard to detect in punch biopsies, as they make up only a minute amount of the tissue's total RNA, are not specifically targetable by current single cell transcriptomic approaches (76) and only refer to axonally transported RNA. These problems also preclude to link global transcriptomic changes to specific nerve fiber classes, which is particularly warranted, given that sinusoidal transcutaneous electrical stimuli preferentially activate C-fibers (35, 36). However, despite these technical difficulties, one study found the voltage-gated sodium channels Nav1.3, Nav1.7, and Nav1.9 to be overexpressed in eczematous skin of AD patients and, importantly, this overexpression correlated with pruritus severity (72). Assuming that neurons were the only cell type expressing voltage-gated sodium channels in the skin, the authors concluded that their overexpression in the eczematous lesions might indicate a sensitized state, which could potentially explain increased responsiveness to slowly depolarizing sine wave stimulation. Particularly Nav1.7 might be a target of axonal hyper-excitability, as this channel can amplify slow depolarizations (77) by producing so called ramp currents that are based on the channels slow closed-state inactivation kinetics. As the time course of depolarization during the 4 Hz sinusoidal stimulation fits to such ramp currents, Nav1.7 might facilitate the electrically induced activation of axons (78, 79) and possibly contributes to the itch in AD patients.

In addition to voltage-gated sodium channels, potassium channels are major determinants of nociceptive discharge patterns. Indeed, Esaki and colleagues found a member of the Kv1 family of voltage-gated potassium channels (Kv1.3, encoded by KCNA3) to be upregulated in eczematous skin of AD patients (74). Specifically, this upregulation was only detectable in the dermis (72, 74). As Kv1 channels are involved in limiting the maximal AP frequency in nociceptors (80), it is possible that the observed upregulation of Kv1.3 limits electrically induced nociceptive input to the spinal cord that would have inhibited the spinal transmission of pruriceptive information to the brain under normal conditions (81).

Temporal Electrical Stimulation Patterns and Their Role in Itch Induction in AD Patients

The duration of electrically evoked ongoing primary afferent nerve fiber stimulation seems to play a pivotal role for itch induction in AD patients. Our recent studies demonstrated that eliciting pain or itch in patients does not only depend on the stimulation of the specific nerve fiber classes, but is also dependent on the actual duration of the stimulation (28, 36). In healthy human subjects, sinusoidal electrical stimulation evokes pain that adapts substantially upon ongoing electrical stimulation with 4 Hz sine waves (36). By contrast, the same stimulation protocol induced increasing pain in chronic pain patients, particularly at neuropathic painful skin sites (36). Similarly, we observed progressively increasing pruritus in AD patients when stimulating with ongoing sinusoidal stimulation, indicating that in both groups of patients the nerve fiber classes activated by the electrical stimulation appear resistant to adaptation. This kind of activity-dependent change of pruriceptor or C-nociceptor excitability upon ongoing stimulation is important to differentiate from acute activation thresholds of these nerve fibers to a single stimulus, in particular when trying to link it to a potential mechanism contributing to chronic itch (or chronic pain) that is based on spontaneous discharge of C-fibers lasting for prolonged periods. However, prolonged neuronal input has also implications for the spinal itch processing as sustained peripheral neuronal input may be required to facilitate spinal itch transmission. Such spinal circuit changes involve, for instance, the activation of gastrin-releasing peptide (GRP) receptor neurons (82). Zeilhofer and colleagues showed that the release of GRP from spinal interneurons is a prerequisite for the transmission of pruriceptive information to higher itch centers in the brain, which, importantly, requires ongoing peripheral input to induce several periods of burst-like activity in spinal GRP^{+} neurons (82). A sufficient interaction of GRP^{+} and GRP-sensing neurons, possibly triggered during our ongoing sinusoidal stimulation of primary afferent neurons, may have initiated itch in AD patients. On the other hand, our electrically induced neuronal input could also inhibit spinal itch processing via GABAergic (83) or glycinergic (84) signaling. Thus, long-lasting slowly depolarizing electrical stimulation protocols that cause itch in a sub-group of AD patients probably indicate facilitated spinal processing and/or weaker inhibition of itch and might therefore help to identify those patients that benefit from spinally acting antipruritic therapy.

Perspectives

Slowly depolarizing transcutaneous electrical stimulation provides functional assessment of both, pruriceptors (e.g., in AD patients) and nociceptors (e.g., in neuropathic pain patients). The precise electrical protocols, including the temporal profile of stimulation, are of particular importance to generate peripheral input from different classes of C-nociceptors and pruriceptors. Furthermore, the advantage of a controlled pruriceptive/nociceptive stimulus onset and offset can be exploited in various explorative directions, for instance when combining the stimulation profile with other techniques (like EEG or fMRI) to investigate the human brain. Future research may help to link specific functional attributes of electrically evoked responses and structural changes to the patient's symptoms. This would facilitate a better understanding of the peripheral and also central processing of pruriceptive and nociceptive inputs in general.

AUTHOR CONTRIBUTIONS

All authors contributed to the article and approved the submitted version.

REFERENCES

1. Perzanowska M, Malhotra D, Skinner SP, Rihoux JP, Bewley AP, Petersen LJ, et al. The effect of cetirizine and loratadine on codeine-induced histamine release in human skin in vivo assessed by cutaneous microdialysis. *InflammRes.* (1996) 45:486–90. doi: 10.1007/BF02252321
2. Church MK, Okayama Y, el Lati S. Mediator secretion from human skin mast cells provoked by immunological and non-immunological stimulation. *SkinPharmacol.* (1991) 4(Suppl. 1):15–24. doi: 10.1159/000210980
3. Hanifin JM. The role of antihistamines in atopic dermatitis. *J Allergy Clin Immunol.* (1990) 86:666–9. doi: 10.1016/S0091-6749(05)80237-4
4. Cevikbas F, Lerner EA. Physiology and pathophysiology of itch. *Physiol Rev.* (2020) 100:945–82. doi: 10.1152/physrev.00017.2019
5. Steinhoff M, Buddenkotte J, Shpacovitch V, Rattenholl A, Moormann C, Vergnolle N, et al. Proteinase-activated receptors: transducers of proteinase-mediated signaling in inflammation and immune response. *EndocrRev.* (2005) 26:1–43. doi: 10.1210/er.2003-0025
6. Liu Q, Weng HJ, Patel KN, Tang Z, Bai H, Steinhoff M, et al. The distinct roles of two GPCRs, MrgprC11 and PAR2, in itch and hyperalgesia. *Sci Signal.* (2011) 4:ra45. doi: 10.1126/scisignal.2001925
7. Bautista DM, Wilson SR, Hoon MA. Why we scratch an itch: the molecules, cells and circuits of itch. *Nat Neurosci.* (2014) 17:175–82. doi: 10.1038/nn.3619
8. Chen XJ, Sun YG. Central circuit mechanisms of itch. *Nat Commun.* (2020) 11:3052. doi: 10.1038/s41467-020-16859-5
9. Lay M, Dong X. Neural mechanisms of itch. *Annu Rev Neurosci.* (2020) 43:187–205. doi: 10.1146/annurev-neuro-083019-024537
10. Bishop GH. Responses to electrical stimulation of single sensory units of skin. *J Neurophysiol.* (1943) 6:361–82. doi: 10.1152/jn.1943.6.5.361
11. Shelley WB, Arthur RP. The neurohistology and neurophysiology of the itch sensation in man. *AMA Arch Derm.* (1957) 76:296–323. doi: 10.1001/archderm.1957.01550210020004
12. Edwards AE, Shellow WV, Wright ET, Dignam TF. Pruritic skin diseases, psychological stress, and the itch sensation. A reliable method for the induction of experimental pruritus. *Arch Dermatol.* (1976) 112:339–43. doi: 10.1001/archderm.112.3.339
13. Tuckett RP. Itch evoked by electrical stimulation of the skin. *J Invest Dermatol.* (1982) 79:368–73. doi: 10.1111/1523-1747.ep12529734
14. Ikoma A, Handwerker H, Miyachi Y, Schmelz M. Electrically evoked itch in humans. *Pain.* (2005) 113:148–54. doi: 10.1016/j.pain.2004.10.003
15. Murray FS, Weaver MM. Effects of ipsilateral and contralateral counterirritation on experimentally produced itch in human beings. *J Comp Physiol Psychol.* (1975) 89:819–26. doi: 10.1037/h0077028
16. Ward L, Wright E, McMahon SB. A comparison of the effects of noxious and innocuous counterstimuli on experimentally induced itch and pain. *Pain.* (1996) 64:129–38. doi: 10.1016/0304-3959(95)00080-1
17. van Laarhoven AI, Ulrich DJ, Wilder-Smith OH, van Loey NE, Nieuwenhuis M, van der Wee NJ, et al. Psychophysiological processing of itch in patients with chronic post-burn itch: an exploratory study. *Acta Derm Venereol.* (2016) 96:613–8. doi: 10.2340/00015555-2323
18. Andersen HH, van Laarhoven AIM, Elberling J, Arendt-Nielsen L. Modulation of itch by conditioning itch and pain stimulation in healthy humans. *J Pain.* (2017) 18:1437–50. doi: 10.1016/j.jpain.2017.07.002
19. Zotterman Y. Touch, pain and tickling: an electro-physiological investigation on cutaneous sensory nerves. *J Physiol.* (1939) 95:1–28. doi: 10.1113/jphysiol.1939.sp003707
20. Tuckett RP, Wei JY. Response to an itch-producing substance in cat. I. Cutaneous receptor populations with myelinated axons. *Brain Res.* (1987) 413:87–94. doi: 10.1016/0006-8993(87)90156-9
21. Tuckett RP, Wei JY. Response to an itch-producing substance in cat. II. Cutaneous receptor populations with unmyelinated axons. *Brain Res.* (1987) 413:95–103. doi: 10.1016/0006-8993(87)90157-0
22. Vallbo AB, Hagbarth KE. Acvtivity from skin mechanoreceptors recorded percutaneously in awake human subjects. *Exp Neurol.* (1968) 21:270–89. doi: 10.1016/0014-4886(68)90041-1
23. Torebjörk HE, Hallin RG. C-fibre units recorded from human sensory nerve fascicles in situ. A preliminary report. *Acta Soc Med Ups.* (1970) 75:81–4.
24. Schmelz M, Schmidt R, Bickel A, Handwerker HO, Torebjörk HE. Specific C-receptors for itch in human skin. *J Neurosci.* (1997) 17:8003–8. doi: 10.1523/JNEUROSCI.17-20-08003.1997

25. Namer B, Carr R, Johanek LM, Schmelz M, Handwerker HO, Ringkamp M. Separate peripheral pathways for pruritus in man. *JNeurophysiol.* (2008) 100:2062–9. doi: 10.1152/jn.90482.2008
26. Johanek LM, Meyer RA, Friedman RM, Greenquist KW, Shim B, Borzan J, et al. A role for polymodal C-fiber afferents in nonhistaminergic itch. *JNeurosci.* (2008) 28:7659–69. doi: 10.1523/JNEUROSCI.1760-08.2008
27. Ringkamp M, Schepers RJ, Shimada SG, Johanek LM, Hartke TV, Borzan J, et al. A role for nociceptive, myelinated nerve fibers in itch sensation. *JNeurosci.* (2011) 31:14841–9. doi: 10.1523/JNEUROSCI.3005-11.2011
28. Rukwied R, Schnakenberg M, Solinkski HJ, Schmelz M, Weisshaar E. Transcutaneous slowly depolarizing currents elicit pruritus in patients with atopic dermatitis. *Acta Derm Venereol.* (2020) 100:adv00302. doi: 10.2340/00015555-3658
29. Pereira MP, Agelopoulos K, Kollner J, Neufang G, Schmelz M, Stander S. Selective nerve fibre activation in patients with generalized chronic pruritus: hint for central sensitization? *Acta Derm Venereol.* (2019) 99:1009–15. doi: 10.2340/00015555-3261
30. Weidner C, Schmelz M, Schmidt R, Hansson B, Handwerker HO, Torebjork HE. Functional attributes discriminating mechano-insensitive and mechano-responsive C nociceptors in human skin. *JNeurosci.* (1999) 19:10184–90. doi: 10.1523/JNEUROSCI.19-22-10184.1999
31. Landmann G, Stockinger L, Lustenberger C, Schmelz M, Rukwied R. Effects of current density on nociceptor activation upon electrical stimulation in humans. *Pain Pract.* (2016) 16:273–81. doi: 10.1111/papr.12339
32. Schmelz M, Michael K, Weidner C, Schmidt R, Torebjörk HE, Handwerker HO. Which nerve fibers mediate the axon reflex flare in human skin? *Neuroreport.* (2000) 11:645–8. doi: 10.1097/00001756-200002280-00041
33. Jonas R, Namer B, Schnakenberg M, Soares S, Pakalniskis J, Carr R, et al. Sympathetic efferent neurons are less sensitive than nociceptors to 4 Hz sinusoidal stimulation. *Eur J Pain.* (2020) 24:122–33. doi: 10.1002/ejp.1467
34. Rukwied R, Thomas C, Obreja O, Werland F, Kleggetveit IP, Jorum E, et al. Slow depolarizing stimuli differentially activate mechanosensitive and silent C-nociceptors in human and pig skin. *Pain.* (2020) 161:2119–28. doi: 10.1097/j.pain.0000000000001912
35. Schnakenberg M, Thomas C, Schmelz M, Rukwied R. Nerve growth factor sensitizes nociceptors to C-fiber selective supra-threshold electrical stimuli in human skin. *Eur J Pain.* (2020) 1–13. doi: 10.1002/ejp.1678
36. Jonas R, Namer B, Stockinger L, Chisholm K, Schnakenberg M, Landmann G, et al. Tuning in C-nociceptors to reveal mechanisms in chronic neuropathic pain. *Ann Neurol.* (2018) 83:945–57. doi: 10.1002/ana.25231
37. Marshall AG, McGlone FP. Affective touch: the enigmatic spinal pathway of the C-tactile afferent. *Neurosci Insights.* (2020) 15:2633105520925072. doi: 10.1177/2633105520925072
38. McGlone F, Wessberg J, Olausson H. Discriminative and affective touch: sensing and feeling. *Neuron.* (2014) 82:737–55. doi: 10.1016/j.neuron.2014.05.001
39. Guttman-Yassky E, Blauvelt A, Eichenfield LF, Paller AS, Armstrong AW, Drew J, et al. Efficacy and safety of lebrikizumab, a high-affinity interleukin 13 inhibitor, in adults with moderate to severe atopic dermatitis: a phase 2b randomized clinical trial. *JAMA Dermatol.* (2020) 156:411–20. doi: 10.1001/jamadermatol.2020.0079
40. Kabashima K, Matsumura T, Komazaki H, Kawashima M. Trial of nemolizumab and topical agents for atopic dermatitis with pruritus. *N Engl J Med.* (2020) 383:141–50. doi: 10.1056/NEJMoa1917006
41. Pereira MP, Ständer S. Novel drugs for the treatment of chronic pruritus. *Exp Opin Investig Drugs.* (2018) 27:981–8. doi: 10.1080/13543784.2018.1548606
42. Masson EA, Veves A, Fernando D, Boulton AJ. Current perception thresholds: a new, quick, and reproducible method for the assessment of peripheral neuropathy in diabetes mellitus. *Diabetologia.* (1989) 32:724–8. doi: 10.1007/BF00274531
43. Lv SL, Fang C, Hu J, Huang Y, Yang B, Zou R, et al. Assessment of peripheral neuropathy using measurement of the current perception threshold with the neurometer® in patients with type 1 diabetes mellitus. *Diabetes Res Clin Pract.* (2015) 109:130–4. doi: 10.1016/j.diabres.2015.04.018
44. Tobin D, Nabarro G, Baart dlF, van Vloten WA, van der Putte SC, Schuurman HJ. Increased number of immunoreactive nerve fibers in atopic dermatitis. *J Allergy Clin Immunol.* (1992) 90:613–22. doi: 10.1016/0091-6749(92)90134-N
45. Emtestam L, Hagströmer L, Dou YC, Sartorius K, Johansson O. PGP 9.5 distribution patterns in biopsies from early lesions of atopic dermatitis. *Arch Dermatol Res.* (2012) 304:781–5. doi: 10.1007/s00403-012-1246-0
46. Mochizuki H, Lavery MJ, Nattkemper LA, Albornoz C, Valdes Rodriguez R, Stull C, et al. Impact of acute stress on itch sensation and scratching behaviour in patients with atopic dermatitis and healthy controls. *Br J Dermatol.* (2019) 180:821–7. doi: 10.1111/bjd.16921
47. LaMotte RH, Dong X, Ringkamp M. Sensory neurons and circuits mediating itch. *Nat Rev Neurosci.* (2014) 15:19–31. doi: 10.1038/nrn3641
48. Steinhoff M, Oaklander AL, Szabó IL, Ständer S, Schmelz M. Neuropathic itch. *Pain.* (2019) 160(Suppl. 1):S11–6. doi: 10.1097/j.pain.0000000000001551
49. Schmelz M. Itch and pain differences and commonalities. *Handb Exp Pharmacol.* (2015) 227:285–301. doi: 10.1007/978-3-662-46450-2_14
50. Han L, Ma C, Liu Q, Weng HJ, Cui Y, Tang Z, et al. A subpopulation of nociceptors specifically linked to itch. *Nat Neurosci.* (2013) 16:174–82. doi: 10.1038/nn.3289
51. Huang J, Polgar E, Solinski HJ, Mishra SK, Tseng PY, Iwagaki N, et al. Circuit dissection of the role of somatostatin in itch and pain. *Nat Neurosci.* (2018) 21:707–16. doi: 10.1038/s41593-018-0119-z
52. Mishra SK, Hoon MA. The cells and circuitry for itch responses in mice. *Science.* (2013) 340:968–71. doi: 10.1126/science.1233765
53. Sun YG, Zhao ZQ, Meng XL, Yin J, Liu XY, Chen ZF. Cellular basis of itch sensation. *Science.* (2009) 325:1531–4. doi: 10.1126/science.1174868
54. Davidson S, Zhang X, Khasabov SG, Moser HR, Honda CN, Simone DA, et al. Pruriceptive spinothalamic tract neurons: physiological properties and projection targets in the primate. *J Neurophysiol.* (2012) 108:1711–23. doi: 10.1152/jn.00206.2012
55. Sikand P, Shimada SG, Green BG, LaMotte RH. Similar itch and nociceptive sensations evoked by punctate cutaneous application of capsaicin, histamine and cowhage. *Pain.* (2009) 144:66–75. doi: 10.1016/j.pain.2009.03.001
56. Namer B, Reeh P. Scratching an itch. *Nat Neurosci.* (2013) 16:117–8. doi: 10.1038/nn.3316
57. Schmelz M. Itch and pain. *NeurosciBiobehavRev.* (2010) 34:171–6. doi: 10.1016/j.neubiorev.2008.12.004
58. Ikoma A, Fartasch M, Heyer G, Miyachi Y, Handwerker H, Schmelz M. Painful stimuli evoke itch in patients with chronic pruritus: central sensitization for itch. *Neurology.* (2004) 62:212–7. doi: 10.1212/WNL.62.2.212
59. Pogatzki-Zahn EM, Pereira MP, Cremer A, Zeidler C, Dreyer T, Riepe C, et al. Peripheral sensitization and loss of descending inhibition is a hallmark of chronic pruritus. *J Invest Dermatol.* (2020) 140:203–11.e4. doi: 10.1016/j.jid.2019.05.029
60. Nilsson HJ, Psouni E, Carstam R, Schouenborg J. Profound inhibition of chronic itch induced by stimulation of thin cutaneous nerve fibres. *J Eur Acad Dermatol Venereol.* (2004) 18:37–43. doi: 10.1111/j.1468-3083.2004.00724.x
61. Nilsson HJ, Schouenborg J. Differential inhibitory effect on human nociceptive skin senses induced by local stimulation of thin cutaneous fibers. *Pain.* (1999) 80:103–12. doi: 10.1016/S0304-3959(98)00205-X
62. Tominaga M, Takamori K. Itch and nerve fibers with special reference to atopic dermatitis: therapeutic implications. *J Dermatol.* (2014) 41:205–12. doi: 10.1111/1346-8138.12317
63. Tominaga M, Tengara S, Kamo A, Ogawa H, Takamori K. Psoralen-ultraviolet A therapy alters epidermal Sema3A and NGF levels and modulates epidermal innervation in atopic dermatitis. *J Dermatol Sci.* (2009) 55:40–6. doi: 10.1016/j.jdermsci.2009.03.007
64. Tan Y, Ng WJ, Lee SZX, Lee BTK, Nattkemper LA, Yosipovitch G, et al. 3-dimensional optical clearing and imaging of pruritic atopic dermatitis and psoriasis skin reveals downregulation of epidermal innervation. *J Invest Dermatol.* (2019) 139:1201–4. doi: 10.1016/j.jid.2018.11.006
65. Tsutsumi M, Kitahata H, Fukuda M, Kumamoto J, Goto M, Denda S, et al. Numerical and comparative three-dimensional structural analysis of peripheral nerve fibres in epidermis of patients with atopic dermatitis. *Br J Dermatol.* (2016) 174:191–4. doi: 10.1111/bjd.13974
66. Barkai O, Butterman R, Katz B, Lev S, Binshtok AM. The input-output relation of primary nociceptive neurons is determined by the morphology of the peripheral nociceptive terminals. *bioRxiv.* (2020) 40:9346–63. doi: 10.1101/2020.07.30.228015
67. Meents JE, Ciotu CI, Fischer MJM. TRPA1: a molecular view. *J Neurophysiol.* (2019) 121:427–43. doi: 10.1152/jn.00524.2018

68. Yang F, Xu L, Lee BH, Xiao X, Yarov-Yarovoy V, Zheng J. An unorthodox mechanism underlying voltage sensitivity of TRPV1 ion channel. *Adv Sci (Weinh).* (2020) 7:2000575. doi: 10.1002/advs.202000575
69. Wang Y, Mo X, Ping C, Huang Q, Zhang H, Xie C, et al. Site-specific contacts enable distinct modes of TRPV1 regulation by the potassium channel Kvbeta1 subunit. *J Biol Chem.* (2020) 295:17337–48. doi: 10.1074/jbc.RA120.015605
70. Meents JE, Fischer MJ, McNaughton PA. Agonist-induced sensitisation of the irritant receptor ion channel TRPA1. *J Physiol.* (2016) 594:6643–60. doi: 10.1113/JP272237
71. Voets T, Droogmans G, Wissenbach U, Janssens A, Flockerzi V, Nilius B. The principle of temperature-dependent gating in cold- and heat-sensitive TRP channels. *Nature.* (2004) 430:748–54. doi: 10.1038/nature02732
72. Nattkemper LA, Tey HL, Valdes-Rodriguez R, Lee H, Mollanazar NK, Albornoz C, et al. The genetics of chronic itch: gene expression in the skin of patients with atopic dermatitis and psoriasis with severe itch. *J Invest Dermatol.* (2018) 138:1311–7. doi: 10.1016/j.jid.2017.12.029
73. Goldstein RH, Barkai O, Inigo-Portugues A, Katz B, Lev S, Binshtok AM. Location and plasticity of the sodium spike initiation zone in nociceptive terminals *in vivo*. *Neuron.* (2019) 102:801–12.e5. doi: 10.1016/j.neuron.2019.03.005
74. Esaki H, Ewald DA, Ungar B, Rozenblit M, Zheng X, Xu H, et al. Identification of novel immune and barrier genes in atopic dermatitis by means of laser capture microdissection. *J Allergy Clin Immunol.* (2015) 135:153–63. doi: 10.1016/j.jaci.2014.10.037
75. Suarez-Farinas M, Ungar B, Correa da Rosa J, Ewald DA, Rozenblit M, Gonzalez J, et al. RNA sequencing atopic dermatitis transcriptome profiling provides insights into novel disease mechanisms with potential therapeutic implications. *J Allergy Clin Immunol.* (2015) 135:1218–27. doi: 10.1016/j.jaci.2015.03.003
76. He H, Suryawanshi H, Morozov P, Gay-Mimbrera J, Del Duca E, Kim HJ, et al. Single-cell transcriptome analysis of human skin identifies novel fibroblast subpopulation and enrichment of immune subsets in atopic dermatitis. *J Allergy Clin Immunol.* (2020) 145:1615–28. doi: 10.1016/j.jaci.2020.01.042
77. Cummins TR, Howe JR, Waxman SG. Slow closed-state inactivation: a novel mechanism underlying ramp currents in cells expressing the hNE/PN1 sodium channel. *J Neurosci.* (1998) 18:9607–19. doi: 10.1523/JNEUROSCI.18-23-09607.1998
78. Dib-Hajj SD, Yang Y, Black JA, Waxman SG. The Na(V)1.7 sodium channel: from molecule to man. *NatRevNeurosci.* (2013) 14:49–62. doi: 10.1038/nrn3404
79. Herzog RI, Cummins TR, Ghassemi F, Dib-Hajj SD, Waxman SG. Distinct repriming and closed-state inactivation kinetics of Nav1.6 and Nav1.7 sodium channels in mouse spinal sensory neurons. *J Physiol.* (2003) 551:741–50. doi: 10.1113/jphysiol.2003.047357
80. Zheng Y, Liu P, Bai L, Trimmer JS, Bean BP, Ginty DD. Deep sequencing of somatosensory neurons reveals molecular determinants of intrinsic physiological properties. *Neuron.* (2019) 103:598–616.e7. doi: 10.1016/j.neuron.2019.05.039
81. Kardon AP, Polgar E, Hachisuka J, Snyder LM, Cameron D, Savage S, et al. Dynorphin acts as a neuromodulator to inhibit itch in the dorsal horn of the spinal cord. *Neuron.* (2014) 82:573–86. doi: 10.1016/j.neuron.2014.02.046
82. Pagani M, Albisetti GW, Sivakumar N, Wildner H, Santello M, Johannssen HC, et al. How gastrin-releasing peptide opens the spinal gate for itch. *Neuron.* (2019) 103:102–17.e5. doi: 10.1016/j.neuron.2019.04.022
83. Bardoni R, Shen KF, Li H, Jeffry J, Barry DM, Comitato A, et al. Pain inhibits GRPR neurons via GABAergic signaling in the spinal cord. *Sci Rep.* (2019) 9:15804. doi: 10.1038/s41598-019-52316-0
84. Foster E, Wildner H, Tudeau L, Haueter S, Ralvenius WT, Jegen M, et al. Targeted ablation, silencing, and activation establish glycinergic dorsal horn neurons as key components of a spinal gate for pain and itch. *Neuron.* (2015) 85:1289–304. doi: 10.1016/j.neuron.2015.02.028

20

Itch in Scabies—What Do We Know?

Sascha Ständer[1] and Sonja Ständer[2]*

[1] Department of Dermatology, University of Lübeck, Lübeck, Germany, [2] Department of Dermatology, Center for Chronic Pruritus, University Hospital Münster, Münster, Germany

***Correspondence:**
Sascha Ständer
sascha.staender@uksh.de

Scabies is a common parasitic skin infestation characterized by severe itch and a heterogenous clinical presentation. Itch, as the cardinal symptom of scabies, is imposing a high burden on affected patients and is often difficult to manage. Decreased life quality and secondary complications, caused by an itch-related disruption of the epidermal barrier and subsequent superinfections, illustrate the need to treat scabies and to understand the underlying mechanisms of itch in respective patients. This review summarizes available data on itch in scabies with a special focus on the clinical aspects and its underlying pathomechanisms.

Keywords: scabies, itch, pruritus, itch mediators, itch and its pathways

SCABIES—AN OVERVIEW

Scabies is a highly contagious ectoparasitic skin infestation caused by Sarcoptes scabiei var. hominis. With a global prevalence of 204 million, scabies poses a remarkable burden on both infected individuals and on the healthcare system regardless of the socioeconomic standard of the respective country (1, 2). More specifically, in high income countries, delayed diagnosis of this neglected disease can lead to waves of institutional outbreaks. In middle-to-low income countries a lack of therapeutic resources often results in secondary scabies-related complications, such as chronic kidney disease since excoriations and the disruption of the epidermal barrier caused by itch may lead to impetigo and to a subsequent dissemination of streptococci to the glomeruli (1, 3). The increased disease-related morbidity and mortality further adds to the patients' burden. Depending on different populations, the prevalence of scabies is ranging from 0.2 to 71.4% (4), with a predominant affection of people living in tropical regions (5). While scabies can occur in every individual, current data reveal a greater susceptibility for the young, old, and, generally, immunocompromised patients (6). Accordingly, Mason et al. reported the highest prevalence of scabies in infants <1 year of age [34.1%, adjusted odds ratio (AOR) compared with adults: 3.6, 95%CI 2.2–6.0] and children aged 1–4 years (25.7%, AOR 2.6, 95%CI 1.7–3.9) in the Solomon Islands (7). Furthermore, the disability-adjusted life-years (DALY) burden was found to be the highest in children 1–4 years-old, eventually decreasing from age 5–24 years and recurrently rising after the age of 70 years in the Global Burden of Disease Study 2015 (5). Furthermore, in low-income countries, disadvantaged populations and children under the age of two bare a greater risk to get infected with scabies (4).

The mite Sarcoptes scabiei is an obligate human parasite that burrows into the epidermis mostly after intense skin to skin contact but also after contact to mites from textiles (i.e., sleeping in a bed with mites). The female mite lays eggs and after approximately 14 days the hatched larvae, and later the nymph, reach adulthood (8), provoking symptoms mostly after 2-5 weeks of latency after the first infestation. After a second infestation, the aforementioned symptoms can occur earlier (~ after 1–2 weeks) due to the immune memory. As scabies mites prefer areas with a higher body temperature and a rather thin stratum corneum, predilection sites are the interdigital spaces of hands and feet, the axillary and periumbilical region, the penis and the perianal skin, while the

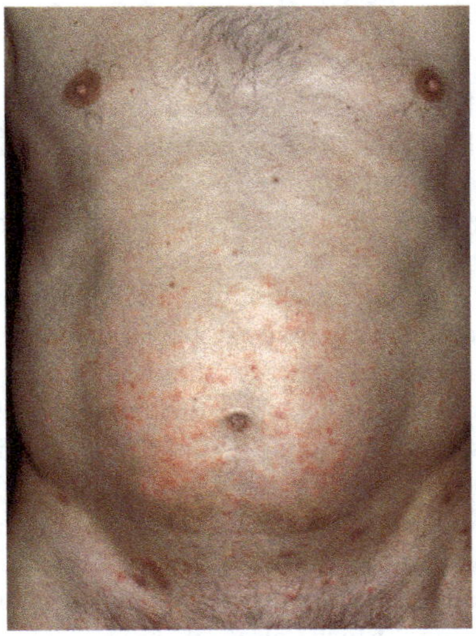

FIGURE 1 | Clinical presentation of a male patient infected with scabies: Multiple erythematous papules in the periumbilical region with several scratch lesions and excoriations.

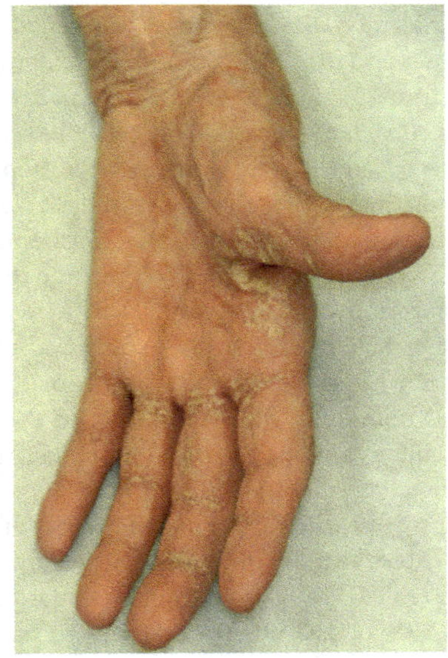

FIGURE 2 | Crusted scabies: Interdigitally located squamous plaques and disseminated erythematous papules.

head and neck are usually spared (exception in infants and old people) (9).

The clinical picture of the disease is caused by the infestation of the mites *per se* and by an immunologic reaction elicited by the contact toward the by-products of the mites (i.e., saliva, excrements). This delayed type reaction of cellular immunity is clinically apparent as an eczematous morphology with multiple disseminated erythematous papules and vesicles on red skin (**Figure 1**). Due to an intense pruritus, especially at night, secondary skin lesions, that is, excoriations and scratch marks occur frequently. Secondary superinfections in terms of impetigo can frequently be observed in children.

Scabies crustosa (norvegica), a comparably rare and severe form of scabies with a prevalence of <0.1%, is especially apparent in individuals with an underlying immunosuppression, that is, HIV (10). The localized or generalized hyperkeratotic clinical picture results from a massive mite proliferation and is associated with an increased mortality and a lower grade of itch (10, 11) (**Figure 2**).

Diagnosis of scabies is based on a characteristic history (intense pruritus with a nightly deterioration, frequent relapses and refractory to treatment with topical corticosteroids) and the clinical presentation with skin lesions along the predilection sites and typical findings in dermatoscopy and positive microscopy, that is, mites, feces, eggs or mite passages.

Currently, topical treatment with permethrin cream (5%) is considered as the gold standard, leading to a cure in most of the cases (12). Yet, increasing numbers of failures in treatment by permethrin have been recently reported also hinting toward the possibility of increased tolerance of permethrin (when applied under controlled conditions) or possible application errors (13, 14). Successful treatment, however, highly depends on the appropriate application of the cream (whole body from the neck) and concomitant treatment of persons with close contact and basic hygiene measures. Relapses, however, occur frequently; particularly in larger families and groups. Treatment with oral ivermectin has proven to remarkably decrease the prevalence of scabies in larger communities with a good tolerability and efficacy. Recent data is additionally hinting toward the safe and effective use of ivermectin in infants weighing <15 kg (6, 15). Besides these two most commonly used treatments in Europe and the US, various other options are available (16). Sulfur compounds are widely used in Afrika and South America due to good efficacy, however, skin irritations are frequent. Benzyl benzoate is highly antiscabietic but also bares high rates of skin irritation. Both treatment options are commonly used in poorer regions due to their efficacy and low cost. Crotamiton is a topical treatment that shows a good tolerability and is therefore used in children with unsatisfactory success (16).

CLINICAL CHARACTERISTICS OF ITCH IN PATIENTS INFECTED WITH SCABIES

The infestation with scabies poses a high burden on respective patients, often due to an intense unbearable itch. The symptom lasts as long as scabies lasts, however, it might become chronic due to persistence after therapy of the infestation. Thus, scabies should be excluded in cases of persisting pruritus especially with a history of itch in persons with close skin contact (17). In severe cases, the patients even develop papules due to scratching (prurigo), or eczema. Management of chronic itch is often challenging (18) and especially scabies-specific itch is poorly characterized and understood. Itch can deteriorate over the night (nocturnal crescendo). This, however, is not specifically applicable to scabies, as other common skin diseases also display a nighty worsening of itch, that is, atopic dermatitis and psoriasis (19–22). Concerning other clinical symptoms,

Brenaut et al. found that heat sensations accompanying the itch were significantly less frequent as compared to the other pruritic skin diseases (19). Sweating and hot water increased the intensity of itch in 73 and 67% of scabies patients, respectively. Scratching was considered pleasurable in 47% of scabies patients as compared to 69 and 65% of patients with atopic dermatitis and psoriasis, respectively. Interestingly, while scratching lesions in patients infected with scabies (63% of patients, $p < 0.01$) were significantly more frequent as compared to non-atopic eczema, psoriasis and urticaria, patients with scabies revealed the lowest rate of lichenification (8%) compared to 80, 61, and 33% of patients with atopic dermatitis, eczema and psoriasis, respectively. Of note, one major limitation of the study is the depiction of qualitative but not quantitative itch features between the aforementioned dermatosis (19).

The presence of pruritus is reported in most of the patients infected with scabies and the prevalence ranges from 90–99% in current literature (23). Nair et al. found a reported prevalence of pruritus in 99% of 102 adults and a nocturnal aggravation in nearly 80% of the patients leading to sleep disturbances in a prospective, observational cross-sectional study conducted at a tertiary center (24). Similar data regarding the manifestation of itch was reported from a cohort of 323 pediatric patients (25). Here, the overall itch prevalence accounted for 94.5% with a range from 90.3–96.9%. Interestingly, the authors showed that the sensation of itch increases with the age of the pediatric patients characterized in the cohort (25). Itch, however, is more difficult to assess in infant patients and is often displayed as discomfort, crying and an increased irritability what might explain the aforementioned observation.

Comparing classical scabies with scabies crustosa/norvegica, differences in pruritus have been reported, indicating that the itch intensity is lower in patients with crusted scabies. However, still most of the patients with crusted scabies had pruritus to some extend (10, 11). Interestingly, in the crusted scabies cohort characterized by Roberts et al. more than half of the patients bared an identifiable immunosuppressive risk. The authors stated that in patients without respective risks, the development of the crusted clinical appearance might result from an increased tendency to mount a Th2 immune response (10). Furthermore, crusted scabies is reported to affect predominantly individuals with malnutrition, Down's syndrome, the elderly and patients with deficient cognitive abilities or physical debilities who are unable to appropriately depict and to react to itch by scratching (10, 26, 27).

PATHOPHYSIOLOGY OF ITCH IN SCABIES

Yet, insights into the exact underlying pathomechanisms of itch in scabies remain scant while remarkable progress in understanding itch in principal had been made in the past 20 years (23). The pathophysiology of itch in general includes the direct stimulation of itch-sensory neurons in the skin by epithelial-cell-derived cytokines, that is, IL-33 and thymic stromal lymphopoietin (TSLP) and an indirect stimulation of itch by keratinocyte-derived kalikreins (KLK) like KLK7. Furthermore, the effector cytokines IL-4, IL-9, IL-13, and IL-31 and CXCL10 directly promote itch (28). Regarding the pruritogens IL-4, IL-13, and downstream JAK activation, no studies investigated this in scabies in detail.

However, hypothesis can be derived from the immunologic reaction ongoing in a patient infected with scabies and by using a novel porcine animal model for scabies, thus, deeper insights into the scabies-specific itch can be generated.

The major immune response to the mite infestation includes the innate immune system and the activation of the complement system that, so some extent, can be inhibited by components produced by the mites. Effectors of the immune response include activated mast cells, immunoglobulin E (IgE), eosinophils, and non-histaminergic effectors like PAR2 and IL-31. While in the classical non-crusted scabies, a Th1 mediated immune response plays a predominant role, a Th2 immune response seems to be more important in the pathogenesis of crusted scabies (29).

Albeit immunohistochemical analysis, using a basophil-specific BB1 antibody, revealed numerous basophils infiltrating lesional scabies-infested skin, the pathogenetic significance of this observation remains unclear and requires further investigations (30, 31).

Current hypothesis regarding the pathophysiology of itch in scabies can be subdivided into the direct action of the scabies mite and the immune response toward the mite itself (23).

Mite components can directly lead to an activation of the Toll-like receptor (TLR) pathway with a subsequent activation of TLR 3, 4, and 7 that are expressed on primary sensory neurons (32, 33). Mite feces contain proteases that can lead to an activation of protease-activated receptor 2 (34). The close interaction between the mites and the keratinocytes can lead to the release of protease activating protease-activated prurireceptors (23, 35). Furthermore, mite components that can be recognized as antigens and show a similar structure to antigens of the house dust mite, can induce an IgE-mediated mast cell activation with an aggravation of itch mediated by the degranulation of histamine, tumor necrosis factor (TNF) alpha and tryptase with a subsequent activation of histaminergic H1 and H4 prurireceptors and protease-activated prurireceptors by tryptase (36, 37). The itch sensation can further be enhanced by a release of leukotriens and prostaglandins implicated my macrophages (23).

In the Th1-mediated immune response that is primarily present in classical non-crusted scabies, a release of INF-gamma and interleukin(IL)-2 lead to an activation of cytokine prurireceptors, whereas an up-regulation of the Th2-mediated immune response in crusted scabies elevates eosinophils, IgE-activated mast cells and enhances the activation of cytokine prurireceptors by IL-31 (23, 37). Recently, it was shown that increased IL-31 levels from murine peritoneal macrophages were induced by an overexpression of thymic stromal lymphopoietin and periostin in an experimental mouse model (38). However, the relevance of this non-histaminergic pathway in the scabies itch is yet to be further investigated as compared to the histaminergic pathway.

In the recent years, a porcine model for scabies was established facilitating the investigation of specific scabies-related questions

(39–41). Recently, Sanders et al. investigated the potential mechanisms of scabies itch and found that non-histaminergic mediators of pruritus were significantly elevated in the skin of pigs experimentally infested with scabies as well as in human skin as compared to non-infected healthy controls (42). Accordingly, a significant upregulation of TRPV1, TRPA1, and PAR-2 expression in the epidermis and an increase of tryptase+ cells around the dermal-epidermal junction was found in both porcine and human scabies-infected skin. These data suggest that the non-histaminergic mediators might play an important role in scabies itch and might potentially serve as therapeutic targets. Furthermore, the similar results from human and pig skin biopsies indicate that the porcine model might serve as suitable animal model to investigate the scabies-specific itch in future experiments. Slight variances in the data might result from different biopsy sites, different durations of the disease, scratching and general differences between the species (42).

COMPLICATIONS LINKED TO ITCH IN SCABIES

Usually, secondary complications and morbidity of individuals infected with scabies are discussed as a direct consequence of the infestation with scabies. However, it is more accurate to refer to subsequent complications due to massive itch caused by an immune response toward the mites and the direct interaction of complement inhibitors produced by the mites and complement pathways in the skin enabling bacteria to grow more easily. Furthermore, severe itch and subsequent scratching leads to a disruption of the epidermal skin barrier (43) and thus to a skin more susceptible for bacterial skin infections. Due to the ability of the scabies mite to interfere with the human complement system by blocking all three complement initiation pathways and leading to decreased neutrophil functions, staphylococcal and streptococcal growth is promoted (44–50). A study performed using the porcine animal model provided evidence that the skin microbiome is changed due to the scabies infestation enabling the growth of opportunistic pathogens (51). In literature, impetigo is described as the most frequent complication of scabies-related itch. It commonly affects children and individuals living under crowded conditions in tropical regions (4, 52, 53). Excoriated deep skin lesions harboring bacteria, most frequently Staphylococcus aureus and group A Strepococcus (AGU), can further lead to a hematogenic dissemination with subsequent complications involving other organs. Interestingly, scratching lesions appear more frequently in patients infested with scabies as compared to other itching dermatosis i.e. eczema, psoriasis and uritcaria (19). The bacterial superinfection can lead to local infections (i.e., erysipelas, cellulitis, abscesses, staphyloderma) with/or without systemic affection and in the worst case to a sepsis. Post-streptococcal complications can affect the kidneys (glomerulonephritis), the heart (rheumatic heart disease) and the joints (acute rheumatic fever) and pose a high burden on respective patients and the healthcare system (54–57). Patients infected with scabies, thus, suffer from an impaired life quality that is directly linked to the severity of itch.

CONCLUSION

Scabies is a common and neglected skin infestation characterized by severe itch and a heterogenous clinical picture. Itch in scabies can be caused by direct mite actions and by a resulting immune response toward the mites. Recent data from the porcine animal model hint toward an important role of non-histaminergic itch mediators, that is, TRPV1, TRPA1, PAR-2, and tryptase+ cells. The exact pathomechanism of scabies-specific itch remains yet to be further investigated.

AUTHOR CONTRIBUTIONS

All authors contributed to the article and approved the submitted version.

REFERENCES

1. Thomas C, Coates SJ, Engelman D, Chosidow O, Chang AY. Ectoparasites: scabies. *J Am Acad Dermatol.* (2020) 82:533–48. doi: 10.1016/j.jaad.2019.05.109
2. GBD 2015 Disease and Injury Incidence and Prevalence Collaborators. Global, regional, and national incidence, prevalence, and years lived with disability for 310 diseases and injuries, 1990–2015: a systematic analysis for the Global Burden of Disease Study 2015. *Lancet.* (2016) 388:1545–602. doi: 10.1016/S0140-6736(16)31678-6
3. Chung S-D, Wang K-H, Huang C-C, Lin H-C. Scabies increased the risk of chronic kidney disease: a 5-year follow-up study. *J Eur Acad Dermatol Venereol.* (2014) 28:286–92. doi: 10.1111/jdv.12099
4. Romani L, Steer AC, Whitfeld MJ, Kaldor JM. Prevalence of scabies and impetigo worldwide: a systematic review. *Lancet Infect Dis.* (2015) 15:960–7. doi: 10.1016/S1473-3099(15)00132-2
5. Karimkhani C, Colombara DV, Drucker AM, Norton S, Hay R, Engelmann D, et al. The global burden of scabies: a cross-sectional analysis from the Global Burden of Disease Study 2015. *Lancet Infect Dis.* (2017) 17:1247–54. doi: 10.1016/S1473-3099(17)30483-8
6. Ständer S, Kirschstein DJ, Kohl-Sobania M, Zillikens D, Ludwig RJ, Anemüller W. Effectiveness and adverse events of ivermectin treatment for scabies in 30 infant patients: report from a German single centre. *J Eur Acad Dermatol Venereol.* (2020) 34:e736–7. doi: 10.1111/jdv.16554
7. Mason DS, Marks M, Sokana O, Solomon A, Mabey DC, Romani L, et al. The prevalence of scabies and impetigo in the Solomon Islands: a population-based survey. *PLoS Negl Trop Dis.* (2016) 10:e0004803. doi: 10.1371/journal.pntd.0004803
8. Arlian LG, Morgan MS. A review of Sarcoptes scabiei: past, present and future. *Parasit Vectors.* (2017) 10:297. doi: 10.1186/s13071-017-2234-1
9. Sunderkötter C, Mayser P, Fölster-Holst R, Maier WA, Kampen H, Hamm H. Scabies. *J Dtsch Dermatol Ges.* (2007) 5:424–30. doi: 10.1111/j.1610-0387.2007.06298.x
10. Roberts LJ, Huffam SE, Walton SF, Currie BJ. Crusted scabies: clinical and immunological findings in seventy-eight patients and a review of the literature. *J Infect.* (2005) 50:375–81. doi: 10.1016/j.jinf.2004.08.033
11. Karthikeyan K. Crusted scabies. *Indian J Dermatol Venereol Leprol.* (2009) 75:340–7. doi: 10.4103/0378-6323.53128
12. Salavastru CM, Chosidow O, Boffa MJ, Janier M, Tiplica GS. European guideline for the management of scabies. *J Eur Acad Dermatol Venereol.* (2017) 31:1248–53. doi: 10.1111/jdv.14351

13. Søreide EH, Ravn J. Scabies. *Tidsskr Nor Laegeforen.* (2020) 140. doi: 10.4045/tidsskr.20.0095
14. Hackenberg B, Horváth ON, Petachti M, Schult R, Yenigün N, Bannenberg P. Scabies therapy in Germany : Results of a nationwide survey with a special focus on the efficacy of first-line therapy with permethrin. *Hautarzt.* (2020) 71:374–9. doi: 10.1007/s00105-020-04561-y
15. Levy M, Martin L, Bursztejn A-C, Chiaverini C, Miquel J, Mahé E, et al. Ivermectin safety in infants and children under 15 kg treated for scabies: a multicentric observational study. *Br J Dermatol.* (2019) 182:1003–6. doi: 10.1111/bjd.18369
16. Chandler DJ, Fuller LC. A Review of scabies: an infestation more than skin deep. *DRM.* (2019) 235:79–90. doi: 10.1159/000495290
17. Hengge UR, Currie BJ, Jäger G, Lupi O, Schwartz RA. Scabies: a ubiquitous neglected skin disease. *Lancet Infect Dis.* (2006) 6:769–79. doi: 10.1016/S1473-3099(06)70654-5
18. Pereira MP, Zeidler C, Storck M, Agelopoulos K, Philipp-Dormston W, Ständer S, et al. Challenges in clinical research and care in pruritus. *Acta Derm Venereol.* (2020) 100:adv00028. doi: 10.2340/00015555-3348
19. Brenaut E, Garlantezec R, Talour K, Misery L. Itch characteristics in five dermatoses: non-atopic eczema, atopic dermatitis, urticaria, psoriasis and scabies. *Acta Derm Venereol.* (2013) 93:573–4. doi: 10.2340/00015555-1599
20. Li JC, Fishbein A, Singam V, Patel KR, Zee PC, Attarian H, et al. Sleep disturbance and sleep-related impairment in adults with atopic dermatitis: a cross-sectional study. *Dermatitis.* (2018) 29:270–7. doi: 10.1097/DER.0000000000000401
21. Kimball AB, Edson-Heredia E, Zhu B, Guo J, Maeda-Chubachi T, Shen W, et al. Understanding the relationship between pruritus severity and work productivity in patients with moderate-to-severe psoriasis: sleep problems are a mediating factor. *J Drugs Dermatol.* (2016) 15:183–8.
22. Lavery MJ, Stull C, Nattkemper LA, Sanders KM, Lee H, Valdes-Rodriguez R, et al. Nocturnal pruritus: prevalence, characteristics, and impact on ItchyQoL in a chronic itch population. *Acta Derm Venereol.* (2017) 97:513–5. doi: 10.2340/00015555-2560
23. Jannic A, Bernigaud C, Brenaut E, Chosidow O. Scabies itch. *Dermatol Clin.* (2018) 36:301–8. doi: 10.1016/j.det.2018.02.009
24. Nair PA, Vora RV, Jivani NB, Gandhi SS. A study of clinical profile and quality of life in patients with scabies at a rural tertiary care centre. *J Clin Diagn Res.* (2016) 10:WC01–5. doi: 10.7860/JCDR/2016/20938.8703
25. Boralevi F, Diallo A, Miquel J, Guerin-Moreau M, Bessis D, Chiavérini C, et al. Clinical phenotype of scabies by age. *Pediatrics.* (2014) 133:e910–6. doi: 10.1542/peds.2013-2880
26. Chosidow O. Scabies and pediculosis: neglected diseases to highlight. *Clin Microbiol Infect.* (2012) 18:311–2. doi: 10.1111/j.1469-0691.2012.03791.x
27. Sullivan JR, Watt G, Barker B. Successful use of ivermectin in the treatment of endemic scabies in a nursing home. *Australas J Dermatol.* (1997) 38:137–40. doi: 10.1111/j.1440-0960.1997.tb01130.x
28. Wang F, Kim BS. Itch: a paradigm of neuroimmune crosstalk. *Immunity.* (2020) 52:753–66. doi: 10.1016/j.immuni.2020.04.008
29. Bhat SA, Mounsey KE, Liu X, Walton SF. Host immune responses to the itch mite, Sarcoptes scabiei, in humans. *Parasit Vectors.* (2017) 10:385. doi: 10.1186/s13071-017-2320-4
30. Ito Y, Satoh T, Takayama K, Miyagishi C, Walls AF, Yokozeki H. Basophil recruitment and activation in inflammatory skin diseases. *Allergy.* (2011) 66:1107–13. doi: 10.1111/j.1398-9995.2011.02570.x
31. Hashimoto T, Rosen JD, Sanders KM, Yosipovitch G. Possible roles of basophils in chronic itch. *Exp Dermatol.* (2019) 28:1373–9. doi: 10.1111/exd.13705
32. He R, Gu X, Lai W, Peng X, Yang G. Transcriptome-microRNA analysis of Sarcoptes scabiei and host immune response. *PLoS ONE.* (2017) 12:e0177733. doi: 10.1371/journal.pone.0177733
33. Taves S, Ji R-R. Itch control by toll-like receptors. *Handb Exp Pharmacol.* (2015) 226:135–50. doi: 10.1007/978-3-662-44605-8_7
34. Lavery MJ, Stull C, Kinney MO, Yosipovitch G. Nocturnal pruritus: the battle for a peaceful night's sleep. *Int J Mol Sci.* (2016) 17:425. doi: 10.3390/ijms17030425
35. Raap U, Ständer S, Metz M. Pathophysiology of itch and new treatments. *Curr Opin Allergy Clin Immunol.* (2011) 11:420–7. doi: 10.1097/ACI.0b013e32834a41c2
36. Morgan MS, Rider SD, Arlian LG. Identification of antigenic Sarcoptes scabiei proteins for use in a diagnostic test and of non-antigenic proteins that may be immunomodulatory. *PLoS Negl Trop Dis.* (2017) 11:e0005669. doi: 10.1371/journal.pntd.0005669
37. Azimi E, Xia J, Lerner EA. Peripheral mechanisms of itch. *Curr Probl Dermatol.* (2016) 50:18–23. doi: 10.1159/000446012
38. Hashimoto T, Satoh T, Yokozeki H. Pruritus in ordinary scabies: IL-31 from macrophages induced by overexpression of thymic stromal lymphopoietin and periostin. *Allergy.* (2019) 74:1727–37. doi: 10.1111/all.13870
39. Bernigaud C, Fang F, Fischer K, Lespine A, Aho LS, Dreau D, et al. Preclinical study of single-dose moxidectin, a new oral treatment for scabies: efficacy, safety, and pharmacokinetics compared to two-dose ivermectin in a porcine model. *PLoS Negl Trop Dis.* (2016) 10:e0005030. doi: 10.1371/journal.pntd.0005030
40. Bernigaud C, Fang F, Fischer K, Lespine A, Aho LS, Mullins AJ, et al. Efficacy and pharmacokinetics evaluation of a single oral dose of afoxolaner against sarcoptes scabiei in the porcine scabies model for human infestation. *Antimicrob Agents Chemother.* (2018) 62:e02334–17. doi: 10.1128/AAC.02334-17
41. Mounsey K, Ho M-F, Kelly A, Willis C, Pasay C, Kemp DJ, et al. A tractable experimental model for study of human and animal scabies. *PLoS Negl Trop Dis.* (2010) 4:e756. doi: 10.1371/journal.pntd.0000756
42. Sanders KM, Nattkemper LA, Rosen JD, Andersen HH, Hsiang J, Romanelli P, et al. Non-Histaminergic itch mediators elevated in the skin of a porcine model of scabies and of human scabies patients. *J Invest Dermatol.* (2019) 139:971–3. doi: 10.1016/j.jid.2018.09.032
43. Yosipovitch G, Misery L, Proksch E, Metz M, Ständer S, Schmelz M. Skin barrier damage and itch: review of mechanisms, topical management and future directions. *Acta Derm Venereol.* (2019) 99:1201–9. doi: 10.2340/00015555-3296
44. Swe PM, Christian LD, Lu HC, Sriprakash KS, Fischer K. Complement inhibition by Sarcoptes scabiei protects Streptococcus pyogenes—an in vitro study to unravel the molecular mechanisms behind the poorly understood predilection of S. pyogenes to infect mite-induced skin lesions. *PLoS Negl Trop Dis.* (2017) 11:e0005437. doi: 10.1371/journal.pntd.0005437
45. Swe PM, Reynolds SL, Fischer K. Parasitic scabies mites and associated bacteria joining forces against host complement defence. *Parasite Immunol.* (2014) 36:585–93. doi: 10.1111/pim.12133
46. Swe PM, Fischer K. A scabies mite serpin interferes with complement-mediated neutrophil functions and promotes staphylococcal growth. *PLoS Negl Trop Dis.* (2014) 8:e2928. doi: 10.1371/journal.pntd.0002928
47. Mika A, Reynolds SL, Mohlin FC, Willis C, Swe PM, Pickering DA, et al. Novel scabies mite serpins inhibit the three pathways of the human complement system. *PLoS ONE.* (2012) 7:e40489. doi: 10.1371/journal.pone.0040489
48. Mika A, Reynolds SL, Pickering D, McMillan D, Sriprakash K, Kemp DJ, et al. Complement inhibitors from scabies mites promote streptococcal growth–a novel mechanism in infected epidermis? *PLoS Negl Trop Dis.* (2012) 6:e1563. doi: 10.1371/journal.pntd.0001563
49. Bergström FC, Reynolds S, Johnstone M, Pike RN, Buckle AM, Kemp DJ, et al. Scabies mite inactivated serine protease paralogs inhibit the human complement system. *J Immunol.* (2009) 182:7809–17. doi: 10.4049/jimmunol.0804205
50. Reynolds SL, Pike RN, Mika A, Blom AM, Hofmann A, Wijeyewickrema L, et al. Scabies mite inactive serine proteases are potent inhibitors of the human complement lectin pathway. *PLoS Negl Trop Dis.* (2014) 8:e2872. doi: 10.1371/journal.pntd.0002872
51. Swe PM, Zakrzewski M, Kelly A, Krause L, Fischer K. Scabies mites alter the skin microbiome and promote growth of opportunistic pathogens in a porcine model. *PLoS Negl Trop Dis.* (2014) 8:e2897. doi: 10.1371/journal.pntd.0002897
52. Romani L, Marks M, Sokana O, Nasi T, Kamoriki B, Cordell B, et al. Efficacy of mass drug administration with ivermectin for control of scabies and impetigo, with coadministration of azithromycin: a single-arm community intervention trial. *Lancet Infect Dis.* (2019) 19:510–8. doi: 10.1016/S1473-3099(18)30790-4
53. Reid HF, Birju B, Holder Y, Hospedales J, Poon-King T. Epidemic scabies in four Caribbean islands, 1981-1988. *Trans R Soc Trop Med Hyg.* (1990) 84:298–300. doi: 10.1016/0035-9203(90)90296-Q

54. Streeton CL, Hanna JN, Messer RD, Merianos A. An epidemic of acute post-streptococcal glomerulonephritis among aboriginal children. *J Paediatr Child Health.* (1995) 31:245–8. doi: 10.1111/j.1440-1754.1995.tb00795.x
55. Lawrence G, Leafasia J, Sheridan J, Hills S, Wate J, Wate C, et al. Control of scabies, skin sores and haematuria in children in the Solomon Islands: another role for ivermectin. *Bull World Health Organ.* (2005) 83:34–42.
56. Steer AC, Jenney AWJ, Kado J, Batzloff MR, La Vincente S, Waqatakirewa L, et al. High burden of impetigo and scabies in a tropical country. *PLoS Negl Trop Dis.* (2009) 3:e467. doi: 10.1371/journal.pntd.0000467
57. Carapetis JR, Steer AC, Mulholland EK, Weber M. The global burden of group A streptococcal diseases. *Lancet Infect Dis.* (2005) 5:685–94. doi: 10.1016/S1473-3099(05)70267-X

21

Itch: A Global Problem?

*Elke Weisshaar**

Occupational Dermatology, Department of Dermatology, Ruprecht-Karls University Heidelberg, Heidelberg, Germany

Keywords: itch, global itch, pruritus, prevalence, prurigo, epidemiology

***Correspondence:**
Elke Weisshaar
elke.weisshaar@med.uni-heidelberg.de

INTRODUCTION: THE GLOBAL BURDEN OF ITCH

Chronic itch (CI) is defined as itch occurring for 6 weeks and longer (1). Both the frequency and the causes of CI depend on age, predisposition like atopy, underlying diseases, ethnicity, climate/humidity, and especially access to the regional healthcare system (2–5). Different living conditions and rituals in human beings as well as migration also contribute to acute and chronic itch (5, 6). The prevalence of itch appears to differ worldwide (2, 3, 5). Direct comparisons between continents or countries are unusual and rare. There are only a few epidemiological studies on itch outside Europe and North America (2, 3, 5). This may be mainly caused by the facts that there is a lack of dermatological care in many countries, no direct access to a dermatologist in most countries, and several countries do not allow access to health care without any insurance certificate or cash payment. Comparing studies from different countries all over the world is difficult because of different and/or unclear, especially non-standardized definitions of itch, lacking to differentiate acute and chronic itch and especially of a lack of defining prevalence estimates. A very recent meta-analysis in atopic dermatitis (AD) and its clinical characteristics stated itch to be almost universally reported and the most common feature in AD (7). Chronic urticaria affects about 1% of the world population, presents with severe itch, and constitutes a global burden (8). Dermatological diseases (frequently accompanied by itch) have a worldwide distribution, but their prevalence is related to the geographical location. For example, otomycoses is much more frequent in subtropical and tropical climate (9) and does hardly contribute to the differential diagnoses of CI in countries with Western lifestyle. Scabies is considered to be the most frequent cause of acute itch but rather rare in CI. Scabies was recently added to the World Health Organization's list of neglected tropical diseases (NTDs), and its occurrence has been increasing in poor countries, countries with low standard of living, and especially in times of wars, migration, and in reception centers for asylum seekers (10). As infections and infestations are more prevalent in subtropical and tropical countries, scabies is a major cause of acute itch in these countries but is considered to be a less frequent cause in Western countries that are more affected by CI. All this may explain why itch is mentioned as a global burden of skin diseases, also in the elderly (11, 12). A large-scale implementation of a mass drug administration campaign of scabies in Ethiopia was called "stop the itch" (13).

Itch, especially CI, strongly reduces health-related quality of life (HRQOL) (2, 3, 5, 14–16). CI can be an additional burden in chronically ill patients leading to an additional reduction in QOL and affecting mortality in patients (14–16). CI can be a symptom or precursor of another (frequently) severe disease (17), but diagnostics are limited and not accessible in most countries; for example, radiological diagnostics and allergy testing are not reimbursed in many countries or excluded in insurance policy (18, 19). Common treatments like antihistamines do not relive itch, even in combination (19, 20). All this makes the topic of itch so important.

ETIOLOGIES OF ITCH WORLDWIDE: EXAMPLES

Itch is highly prevalent in European dermatological outpatient clinics. The prevalence of itch among adult dermatological patients was 54.4 and 8% among the controls (21). The intensity was highest among patients with prurigo. It is also prevalent in dermatological practices. In a German

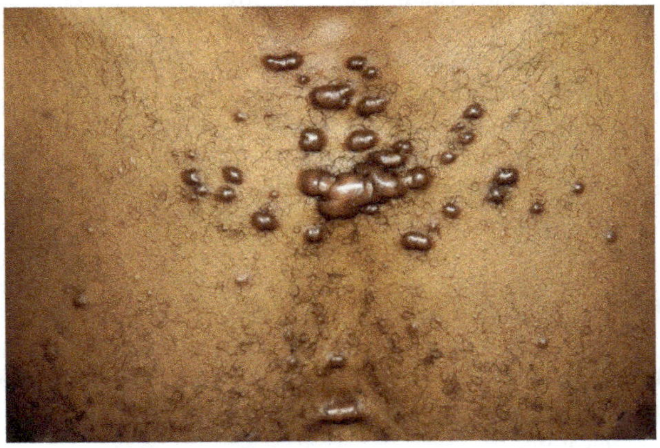

FIGURE 1 | Ritual behavior like cutting the skin in many African and Asian countries contribute to chronic itch caused by keloid manifestation in variable shape and extent.

private practice, the prevalence of itch in a 1-week period was 36.2% (87.6% of whom had chronic itch) (22).

Itch may reflect a malignant disease. A Danish cohort study investigated the association between hospital inpatient and outpatient diagnosis of itch and cancer incidence (23). The 1-year absolute cancer risk was 1.63%. Among patients with itch, a 13% higher than expected number of cases with hematological and various solid cancers were found (23). However, the study was unable to differentiate between acute and chronic itch. In a Danish acute outpatient dermatological clinic, "pruritus and prurigo" were among the most prevalent diagnoses, accounting for 2.5% of all referred patients, but when considering all diagnoses, one may assume that itch was an accompanying symptom in more than 50% of referred cases (24).

Xerosis cutis, systemic diseases, and drug intake are frequent in elderly patients and may all contribute to the occurrence of CI (2, 3, 25). Dry skin, itchy dermatoses, and diabetes all contribute to chronic itch in the elderly.

Itch is also prevalent in the general population and is not always addressed by a medical doctor (MD). The Heidelberg Pruritus Prevalence Study showed a point prevalence of 13.5%, a 12-month prevalence of 16.4%, and a lifetime prevalence of 22% of CI in the general population (26). In the follow-up study, the 12-month cumulative incidence of chronic itch was 7%, and the lifetime prevalence was 25.5% (27). Women were more affected than men, and female sex was associated with an increased but non-significant risk for incident CI during the past 12-months (27).

Itch is prevalent in chronic diseases, especially in Western societies. CI in patients with end-stage renal disease (ESRD) is a considerable problem, and regional differences need to be taken into account because in (developing) countries, patients have limited access to hemodialysis (HD) with differing dialysis quality standards. There are no epidemiological studies on itch HD in developing countries because this treatment is hardly available. A representative cross-sectional prospective prevalence study on chronic itch (CI) in HD patients [German Epidemiological Hemodialysis Itch Study (GEHIS)] showed CI to affect 25.2% (point prevalence) of HD patients (28). No significant differences in prevalence estimates were shown concerning ethnic origin, schooling, or patients' marital status (28).

HIV infection and AIDS contribute to acute and CI worldwide (2, 3, 5, 29). Some diseases vary according to country and its most frequent diseases. Pruritic papular eruption (PPE) is a substantial cause of HIV-related morbidity in Sub-Saharan Africa. Its prevalence varies from 12 to 46% depending on the geographical region. More than half of HIV-infected patients report the eruption of PPE as their initial disease manifestation. We could show that none of the Ugandan itch patients had an underlying systemic disease, and in all HIV patients, itching was caused by dermatoses (5). It is likely that Ugandan patients with severe systemic diseases do not have a survival period that allows the initiation of itch, such as uremic itch, or access to certain therapies such as hemodialysis. Various etiologies from skin disease and keloids to drugs and burns contribute to a high prevalence of itch in African countries (30–34) (**Figure 1**).

DISCUSSION AND FUTURE THOUGHTS

Itch is a big challenge for clinicians and researchers all over the world, especially in regard to the structure of the regional healthcare system and the accessibility to medical care and specialists particularly in Non-Western countries. True epidemiological studies are lacking, especially in Asian and African countries as well as in South America. There is a lack of awareness, depending on, for example, the MD's speciality; other symptoms may be rated higher and/or itch is ignored. This is also caused by a lack of knowledge on itch. However, the rise in clinical and experimental research and findings resulting in an increased number of publications and networks like International Forum for the Study of Itch (IFSI) (1, 35, 36), the EDAV Task Force Pruritus (37, 38), and scientific meetings like The World Congress of Itch (WCI) have helped to increase itch being regarded as a global problem. Social networking platforms like, e.g., Instagram, connect patients looking for the support regarding itch (39). All this has increased the awareness of itch beyond dermatology. It has also improved the capacity to diagnose itch. More and specific clinical studies have enhanced the spectrum of treatments; local and systemic treatments were developed, which are also reflected in an updated S2k guideline on chronic pruritus (19). However, there is still a need for new and more specific treatments of itch including combination of treatments. The demographic situation in Western countries with an increasing number of aged patients, most of them chronically ill, will additionally increase the need for dermatological care including the treatment of itch. This also includes improving patients' motivation and the assistance to seek the specialist's help. Even if there is access, chronically ill patients tend to limit their visits to MDs especially when they already have chronic procedures/treatments like HD. This results in limited itch treatment, even in a Western country (40). In recent years, utilizing technology like telehealth services and teledermatology are useful to provide diagnoses like prurigo by consulting physicians (41). A global look makes one realize that all this is not accessible for most of the countries out of Europe and North America. The inequalities in health are also present in itch and its handling. There is a gross mismatch between the burden of itch and the skills and medications to treat them. To change this is basically not only a medical challenge but an economic and political one of all societies including the global economy. In the end, it is the task of any society to decide how to disseminate medical care and how to provide resources.

SOME OPEN QUESTIONS

How does the perception and the impact of itch differ according to continent and climate?

Will the climate change affect the frequency and etiologies of itch?

Does the awareness of itch and its health care depend on life expectancy and standard of living?

How can we improve education of MDs and healthcare providers to enhance the awareness for especially chronic itch?

Could we initiate a global network to better provide the care of chronic itch?

AUTHOR CONTRIBUTIONS

The author confirms being the sole contributor of this work and has approved it for publication.

REFERENCES

1. Ständer S, Weisshaar E, Mettang T, Szepietowski JC, Carstens E, Ikoma A, et al. Clinical classification of itch: a position paper of the International Forum for the Study of Itch. *Acta Derm Venereol.* (2007) 87:291–4. doi: 10.2340/00015555-0305
2. Weisshaar E, Dalgard F. Epidemiology of Itch: adding to the Burden of Skin Morbidity. *Acta Derm Venereol.* (2009) 89:339–50. doi: 10.2340/00015555-0662
3. Weisshaar E. Epidemiology of itch. *Curr Probl Dermatol.* (2016) 50:5–10. doi: 10.1159/000446010
4. Dalgard F, Holm JØ, Svensson A, Kumar B, Sundby J. Self-reported skin morbidity and ethnicity: a population-based study in a Western community. *BMC Dermatol.* (2007) 7:4. doi: 10.1186/1471-5945-7-4
5. Weisshaar E, Apfelbacher C, Jager G, Zimmermann E, Bruckner T, Diepgen TL, et al. Pruritus as a leading symptom: clinical characteristics and quality of life in German and Ugandan patients. *Br J Dermatol.* (2006) 155:957–64. doi: 10.1111/j.1365-2133.2006.07430.x
6. Padovese V, Knapp A. Challenges of managing skin diseases in refugees and migrants. *Dermatol Clin.* (2021) 39:101–15. doi: 10.1016/j.det.2020.08.010
7. Yew YW, Thyssen JP, Silverberg JI. A systematic review and meta-analysis of the regional and age-related differences in atopic dermatitis clinical characteristics. *J Am Acad Dermatol.* (2019) 80:390–401. doi: 10.1016/j.jaad.2018.09.035
8. Gonçalo M, Gimenéz-Arnau A, Al-Ahmad M, Ben-Shoshan M, Bernstein JA, Ensina LF, et al. The global burden of chronic urticaria for the patient and society. *Br J Dermatol.* (2021) 184:226–36. doi: 10.1111/bjd.19561
9. Gharaghani M, Seifi Z, Zarei Mahmoudabadi A. Otomycosis in Iran: a review. *Mycopathologia.* (2015) 179:415–24. doi: 10.1007/s11046-015-9864-7
10. Stamm LV, Strowd LC. Ignoring the "Itch": the global health problem of scabies. *Am J Trop Med Hyg.* (2017) 97:1647–9. doi: 10.4269/ajtmh.17-0242
11. Hay RJ, Johns NE, Williams HC, Bolliger IW, Dellavalle RP, Margolis DJ, et al. The global burden of skin disease in 2010: an analysis of the prevalence and impact of skin conditions. *J Invest Dermatol.* (2014) 134:1527–34. doi: 10.1038/jid.2013.446
12. Hay RJ, Fuller LC. Global burden of skin disease in the elderly: a grand challenge to skin health. *G Ital Dermatol Venereol.* (2015) 150:693–8.
13. Enbiale W, Baynie TB, Ayalew A, Gebrehiwot T, Getanew T, Ayal A, et al. "Stopping the itch": mass drug administration for scabies outbreak control covered for over nine million people in Ethiopia. *J Infect Dev Ctries.* (2020) 14:28–35S. doi: 10.3855/jidc.11701
14. Weiss M, Mettang T, Tschulena U, Weisshaar E. Health-related quality of life in haemodialysis patients suffering from chronic itch: results from GEHIS (German Epidemiology Haemodialysis Itch Study). *Qual Life Res.* (2016) 25:3097–106. doi: 10.1007/s11136-016-1340-4
15. Grochulska K, Ofenloch RF, Mettang T, Weisshaar E. Mortality of haemodialysis patients with and without chronic itch: a follow-up study of the German Epidemiological Hemodialysis Itch Study (GEHIS). *Acta Derm Venereol.* (2019) 99:423–8. doi: 10.2340/00015555-3125
16. Plewig N, Ofenloch R, Mettang T, Weisshaar E. The course of chronic itch in hemodialysis patients: results of a 4-year follow-up study of GEHIS (German Epidemiological Hemodialysis Itch Study). *J Eur Acad Dermatol Venereol.* (2019) 33:1429–35. doi: 10.1111/jdv.15483
17. Beigi M, Häberle M, Gschwendtner A, Baum U, Weisshaar E. Generalized chronic itch as a first sign of malignancy resembling paraneoplastic sensomotoric neuropathy. *Acta Derm Venereol.* (2018) 98:526–27. doi: 10.2340/00015555-2910
18. Weisshaar E, Molin S, Darsow U, Geier J. Contact sensitization in prurigo patients. *Contact Dermatitis.* (2016) 75:173–9. doi: 10.1111/cod.12564
19. Weisshaar E, Szepietowski JC, Dalgard F, Garcovich S, Gieler U, Gimenez-Arnau A, et al. S2k European guideline on chronic pruritus. *Acta Derm Venereol.* (2019) 99:469–506. doi: 10.2340/00015555-3164
20. Matterne U, Böhmer MM, Weisshaar E, Jupiter A, Carter B, Apfelbacher CJ. Oral H1 antihistamines as 'add-on' therapy to topical treatment for eczema. *Cochrane Database Syst Rev.* (2019) 1:CD012167. doi: 10.1002/14651858.CD012167.pub2
21. Halvorsen JA, Kupfer J, Dalgard F. The prevalence and intensity of itch among dermatological patients in 13 European countries. *Acta Derm Venereol.* (2013) 91:620.
22. Kopyciok ME, Ständer HF, Osada N, Steinke S, Ständer S. Prevalence and characteristics of pruritus: a one-week cross-sectional study in a German dermatology practice. *Acta Derm Venereol.* (2016) 96:50–5. doi: 10.2340/00015555-2166
23. Johannesdottir SA, Farkas DK, Vinding GR, Pedersen L, Lamberg A, Lamberg A, et al. Cancer incidence among patients with a hospital diagnosis of pruritus: a nationwide Danish cohort study. *Br J Dermatol.* (2014) 171:839–46. doi: 10.1111/bjd.13157
24. Fett N, Haynes K, Propert KJ, Margolis DJ. Five-year malignancy incidence in patients with chronic pruritus: a population-based cohort study aimed at limiting unnecessary screening practices. *J Am Acad Dermatol.* (2014) 70:651–8. doi: 10.1016/j.jaad.2013.11.045
25. Valdes-Rodriguez R, Mollanazar NK, González-Muro J, Nattkemper L, Torres-Alvarez B, López-Esqueda FJ, et al. Itch prevalence and characteristics in a Hispanic geriatric population: a comprehensive study using a standardized itch questionnaire. *Acta Derm Venereol.* (2015) 95:417–21. doi: 10.2340/00015555-1968
26. Matterne U, Apfelbacher CJ, Loerbroks A, Schwarzer T, Büttner M, Ofenloch R, et al. Prevalence, correlates and characteristics of chronic pruritus: a population-based cross-sectional study. *Acta Derm Venereol.* (2011) 91:674–9. doi: 10.2340/00015555-1159
27. Matterne U, Apfelbacher CJ, Vogelgsang L, Loerbroks A, Weisshaar E. Incidence and determinants of chronic pruritus: a population-based cohort study. *Acta Derm Venereol.* (2013) 93:532–7. doi: 10.2340/00015555-1572
28. Weiss M, Mettang T, Tschulena U, Passlick-Deetjen J, Weisshaar E. Prevalence of chronic itch and associated factors in hemodialysis patients: a representative cross-sectional study. *Acta Derm Venereol.* (2015) 98:816–21. doi: 10.2340/00015555-2087

29. Xu T, Shetty AK, Badiger S, Chan YH, Yosipovitch G. Prevalence and characteristics of pruritus and association with quality of life in people living with HIV: a cross-sectional study. *J Pain Symp Manag.* (2018) 55:e4–7. doi: 10.1016/j.jpainsymman.2018.01.014
30. Mirembe SK, Mulyowa GK, Jaeger G, Ofenloch R, Diepgen TL, Weisshaar E. Hand eczema in Africa: clinical findings and experiences from South-West Uganda. *Acta Derm Venereol.* (2016) 96:388–9. doi: 10.2340/00015555-2246
31. Mahboob F. Frequency and aetiology of pruritis in admitted patients in a medical ward of Mayo Hospital, Lahore. *J Ayub Med Coll Abbottabad.* (2004) 16:42–3.
32. Nyembue TD, Jorissen M, Hellings PW, Muyunga C, Kayembe JM. Prevalence and determinants of allergic diseases in a Congolese population. *Int Forum Allergy Rhinol.* (2012) 2:285–93. doi: 10.1002/alr.21017
33. Obebi Cliff-Eribo K, Sammons H, Star K, Ralph Edwards I, Osakwe A, Choonara I. Adverse drug reactions in Nigerian children: a retrospective review of reports submitted to the Nigerian Pharmacovigilance Centre from 2005 to 2012. *Paediatr Int Child Health.* (2016) 36:300–4. doi: 10.1179/2046905515Y.0000000059
34. Otene CI, Onumaegbu OO. Post-burn pruritus: need for standardization of care in Nigeria. *Ann Burns Fire Disasters.* (2013) 26:63–7.
35. Ständer S, Augustin M, Reich A, Blome C, Ebata T, Phan NQ, et al. Pruritus assessment in clinical trials: consensus recommendations from the International Forum for the Study of Itch (IFSI) Special Interest Group Scoring Itch in Clinical Trials. *Acta Derm Venereol.* (2013) 93:509–14. doi: 10.2340/00015555-1620
36. Weisshaar E, Weiss M, Mettang T, Yosipovitch G, Zylicz Z, Special Interest Group of the International Forum on the Study of Itch. Paraneoplastic itch: an expert position statement from the Special Interest Group (SIG) of the International Forum on the Study of Itch (IFSI). *Acta Derm Venereol.* (2015) 95:261–5. doi: 10.2340/00015555-1959
37. Ständer S, Zeidler C, Riepe C, Steinke S, Fritz F, Bruland P, et al. European EADV network on assessment of severity and burden of Pruritus (PruNet): first meeting on outcome tools. *J Eur Acad Dermatol Venereol.* (2016) 30:1144–7. doi: 10.1111/jdv.13296
38. Pereira MP, Steinke S, Zeidler C, Forner C, Riepe C, Augustin M, et al. European Academy of Dermatology and Venereology European Prurigo Project: expert consensus on the definition, classification and terminology of chronic prurigo. *J Eur Acad Dermatol Venereol.* (2018) 32:1059–65. doi: 10.1111/jdv.14570
39. Braunberger T, Mounessa J, Rudningen K, Dunnick CA, Dellavalle RP. Global skin diseases on Instagram hashtags. *Dermatol Online J.* (2017) 23:13030/qt7sk410j3.
40. Hayani K, Weiss M, Weisshaar E. Clinical findings and provision of care in haemodialysis patients with chronic itch: new results from the German Epidemiological Haemodialysis Itch Study. *Acta Derm Venereol.* (2016) 96:361–6. doi: 10.2340/00015555-2280
41. Lotfizadeh A, Sultonov RA, Morim A, Tavakol S, Daneshvar M, Qosimov A, et al. Utilizing technology for dermatology care in Tajikistan. A health systems perspective. *Dermatol Clin.* (2021) 39:33–41. doi: 10.1016/j.det.2020.08.004

22

Formalin Itch Test: Low-Dose Formalin Induces Histamine-Independent, TRPA1-Mediated Itch in Mice

Xu Liu[1,2†], Jiang-Tao Zhang[2†], Yue Hu[2†], Wen-Qi Shan[2], Zhi-Hong Wang[2], Qing-Yue Fu[2], Dan-Ni Fu[2], Jiang Ji[1] and Tong Liu[3,4*]*

[1] Department of Dermatology, The Second Affiliated Hospital of Soochow University, Suzhou, China, [2] Jiangsu Key Laboratory of Neuropsychiatric Diseases and Institute of Neuroscience, Soochow University, Suzhou, China, [3] Institute of Pain Medicine and Special Environmental Medicine, Nantong University, Nantong, China, [4] College of Life Sciences, Yanan University, Yanan, China

***Correspondence:**
Tong Liu
tongliu@ntu.edu.cn
Jiang Ji
jijiang2222@126.com

† These authors have contributed equally to this work

Chronic itch is a common distressing symptom of many diseases, which reduced patient's quality of life. The mechanistic study on itch and screening for new anti-itch drugs require the development of new pre-clinical itch animal models. Herein, we established an acute itch model by intradermal (i.d.) injection of low-dose formalin into the neck or cheek in mice. In mice, i.d. injection of formalin (0.1–5%) in the nape of the neck evoked robust scratching behavior in a dose-dependent manner and the dose–response curves showed an inverted "U" shape. I.d. injection of formalin (0.3–0.6%) into the cheek evoked scratching in mice but wiping in rats, while formalin (1.25–5%) induced mixed wiping and scratching behavior in both mice and rats. Further, we found that 0.3% formalin-induced scratching was histamine-independent and significantly attenuated by transient receptor potential ion channel A1 (TRPA1) inhibitor (HC030031) or in TRPA1 knockout (KO) mice, but not affected by transient receptor potential ion channel V1 (TRPV1) inhibitor (capsazepine) or in TRPV1 KO mice. Additionally, 0.3% formalin-induced up-regulation of phosphorylation of extracellular regulated protein kinases (p-ERK) in the dorsal root ganglion (DRG) and scratching were suppressed by intrathecal injection of MEK inhibitor U0126 in mice. Incubation of 0.03% formalin induced the accumulation of intracellular reactive oxygen species (ROS) in the cultured DRG-derived cell line ND7-23, and formalin-induced itch was suppressed by antioxidants in mice. Finally, perfusion of 0.03% formalin induced elevation of intracellular calcium in a subset of primary cultured DRG neurons of mice. Thus, these results indicate that low-dose formalin induced non-histaminergic itch by activation of TRPA1 in mice, which may be employed as a useful acute itch model for screening potential anti-itch drugs.

Keywords: itch, pain, formalin, TRPA1, dorsal root ganglion

INTRODUCTION

Itch (pruritus) is defined as a common unpleasant sensation that causes desire or reflex to scratch (1, 2). Itch can be divided into acute itch and chronic itch (3). Acute itch may have a protective function for the body in order to remove potential harmful substances by scratching behavior (4). However, chronic itch is a common symptom in the complications of skin diseases (e.g., atopic dermatitis and psoriasis) (5, 6), metabolic diseases (e.g., diabetes) (7), liver diseases (e.g., cholestasis) (8), kidney diseases (e.g., uremic pruritus) (9), and seriously affecting patient's quality of life. Based on mechanisms, itch can be further divided into histamine-dependent itch and histamine-independent itch (10). Generally, histamine-dependent itch (such as allergy itch) is mediated by the histamine receptor H1 and H4, which is clinically treated with antihistamine drugs (11). However, chronic itch is often resistant for the treatment of antihistamines (3), which suggests histamine-independent mechanisms involved. Thus, to elucidate the mechanisms of histamine-independent itch and to screen new anti-itch compounds, it is urgently needed to develop new pre-clinical itch animal models (12).

Traditionally, formalin test has been long-term used for studying the underlying mechanism of acute inflammatory pain and screening potential analgesics in rodents (13, 14). In the past decades, it was found that formalin is able to directly activate several ion channels that are involved in the generation of pain, including transient receptor potential ion channel A1 (TRPA1) (15), transient receptor potential ion channel V1 (TRPV1) (16), or transient receptor potential ion channel V4 (TRPV4) (17). Recently, it was demonstrated that several TRP channels, including TRPV1, TRPA1, and TRPV4, are important mediators for both acute and chronic itch (18, 19). For example, TRPV1 was demonstrated to mediate histamine-dependent itch (20). TRPA1 plays a critical role in the genesis of histamine-independent itch, such as Mas-related G protein-coupled receptors (Mrgprs)-mediated itch (21, 22), oxidative stress-induced itch (23, 24), endothelin-induced itch (25), and 5-HT_7 receptor-mediated itch (26). In addition, it was demonstrated that TRPA1 also contributed to the pathogenesis of chronic itch, including dry skin-induced itch (27), bile acids TGR5-mediated cholestatic itch (28), tacrolimus-induced contact dermatitis pruritus (29), and imiquimod-induced psoriatic itch (30, 31). In addition, TRPV4 has also been shown to contribute to serotonin-induced itch and chronic allergic itch in mice (32, 33). Interestingly, several studies have provided several important clues that show that formalin-induced behavioral responses may have some itch component (34, 35). However, whether and how formalin induces itch is still unclear.

In the present study, we found that intradermal (i.d.) injection of low-dose formalin (0.3%) was able to evoke obvious scratching behavior in both neck and cheek models of mice, in a histamine-independent manner. Furthermore, the activation of TRPA1, oxidative stress, and extracellular regulated protein kinase (ERK) signaling were involved in low-dose formalin-induced itch in mice. Together, our results indicated low-dose formalin-induced histamine-independent itch in mice, and this new "formalin itch test" may be used for screening potential novel anti-itch compounds, especially for histamine-independent itch.

MATERIALS AND METHODS

Animals

Male ICR mice, C57BL/6J mice, and Sprague–Dawley (SD) rats (6–8 weeks old) were obtained from the Shanghai SLAC Laboratory Animal CO., LTD. (Shanghai, China). Male *Trpa1*$^{-/-}$and *Trpv1*$^{-/-}$ mice were purchased from Jackson Laboratories (Bar Harbor, ME, USA). *Trpv4*$^{-/-}$ mice were produced by Cam-Su Genomic Resource Center, Soochow University. All animals were kept on a 12-h light/dark cycle with free access to food and water, and the rooms were maintained at 22 ± 2°C and 40–60% humidity. All animal experiments were conducted in accordance with the National Institutes of Health Guide for the Care and Use of Laboratory Animals and the guidelines of the International Association for the Study of Pain.

Neck Model of Acute Itch

As previously reported (36, 37), mice or rats were shaved at the nape of the neck more than 2 days before experiments. On the day of behavioral testing, mice or rats were placed in separate small plastic chambers (for mice: 10 × 10 × 12.5 cm^3; for rats: 20 × 20 × 25 cm^3) on an elevated metal mesh floor at least 30 min for habituation. Under brief anesthesia with isoflurane, 50 μl of compound 48/80 (100 μg), chloroquine (CQ, 200 μg), formalin (0.03–5%), and allyl isothiocyanate (AITC, 10–400 μg) were injected i.d. into the neck of mice through a 26G needle. Rats were injected with 100 μl of formalin (0.03–5%) into the nape of the neck. Immediately after the injection, mice were returned to the chambers and video-recorded for 30 min (Sony HDRCX610, Shanghai, China). The video was then played back offline and scratching behavior was quantified in a blinded manner. Scratching behavior occurred when mice lifted their hindpaws to scratch shaved skin and returned the paws to the floor or to their mouths. The drugs are different doses of formalin (0.03, 0.3, 0.6, 1.25, 2.5, and 5%) and different doses of AITC (10, 50, 100, 200, and 400).

Cheek Model

As previously reported (38), mice or rats were shaved at the cheek more than 2 days prior to experiments. One day after shaving, the animals were moved to small plastic chambers (for mice: 10 × 10 × 12.5 cm^3; for rats: 20 × 20 × 25 cm^3) on an elevated metal mesh floor and allowed to acclimate for at least 30 min. Under brief anesthesia with isoflurane, mice or rats were given an i.d. injection of drugs into the cheek (for mice: 20 μl; for rats: 25 μl). After injection, the mice were immediately returned to the chambers and recorded for 30 min (Sony HDRCX610, Shanghai, China). The video was subsequently played back offline; scratching behavior and wiping behaviors were quantified in a blinded manner. Count scratch bouts and wiping behaviors, respectively. The wiping behavior means that mice or rats raise a forelimb toward the cheek times over 1 s or a few seconds, then put their forelimb down. This series of actions were counted as one wiping. Formalin (0.03, 0.3, 0.6, 1.25, 2.5, and 5%) and AITC (10, 50, 100, 200, and 400 μg) were used.

Formalin Test

As previously reported (13), mice were acclimated to the environment (small plastic chambers 10 × 10 × 12.5 cm^3) 1 h before the behavioral testing. Mice were given an intraperitoneal (i.p.) injection of morphine (3 mg/kg in saline) or saline. After 30 min, mice were given an intraplantar injection of 20 μl of 5 or 0.3% formalin in the right hindpaw. The behaviors of the animals were observed for 45 min to evaluate the total time each animal spent in lifting, licking, shaking, or biting their injected hindlimb. Nociceptive behavior was video-recorded (Sony HDRCX610, Shanghai, China) at 45° below the observation chamber. Analysis of the acute phase (0–10 min; phase 1) and the inflammatory phase (10–45 min; phase 2) was performed by experimenters that were blinded to the treatments.

Western Blotting

Mice were deeply anesthetized with isoflurane and underwent cardiac perfusion with normal saline, after i.d. injection of 0.3 and 5% formalin in the neck of mice for 10 and 30 min. The dorsal root ganglion (DRG) of the C1–C8 segments were obtained and homogenized in a RIPA buffer containing a mixture of phosphatase inhibitors and protease inhibitors. The protein concentration in the RIPA buffer was measured by Pierce bicinchoninic acid (BCA) protein assay (Thermo), and sodium dodecyl-sulfate polyacrylamide gel electrophoresis (SDS-PAGE) sample loading buffer was added into the RIPA buffer, and the proteins were separated by SDS-PAGE. After transfer, the blots were blocked with 5% non-fat milk in Tris–HCl Buffer Saline (TBS) for 1 h at room temperature and the PVDF membranes were incubated overnight at 4°C with primary monoclonal anti-p-ERK (mouse, 1:1000; Santa Cruz Biotechnology, CA) or primary monoclonal anti-ERK (mouse, 1:1000, Vazyme, Nanjing, China). The blots were washed and incubated with horseradish peroxidase-conjugated goat anti-mouse IgG secondary antibody (1:2000, Vazyme). Protein bands were visualized using an enhanced chemiluminescence detection kit (Pierce), and the band densities were assessed and analyzed with NIH ImageJ software (NIH, Bethesda, MD).

Measurement of Intracellular Reactive Oxygen Species in ND7-23 Cells

ROS level was detected by the DCFDA/H2DCFDA–cellular ROS assay kit (ab113852). The ND7-23 cells were cultured in the six-well plate up to 60–70%, and 0.03% formalin was added in the plate after pre-treatment with NAC (100 μmol/L) for 15 min and then incubating at 37°C for 30 min. The medium was removed and cells were stained with DCFH-DA (25 μmol/L) and incubated at 37°C for 30 min. The cells were washed times later and transferred to 1.5-ml tubes for flow cytometry (FC500; Beckman Coulter, Brea, CA). Similarly, DRG neurons were stained with DCFH-DA, and the AXIO SCOPE A1 was used to take images. Finally, fluorescence intensity was analyzed by ImageJ.

Dorsal Root Ganglion Neuron Culture, Calcium Imaging, and Analysis

Extirpated cervical DRGs of neonatal mouse were dissociated by incubation for 30 min at 37°C in a culture medium (Neurobasal with 10% fetal bovine serum and 1% penicillin–streptomycin) containing 0.2% Collagenase D (Roche) followed by a 9-min incubation in 4 ml of culture media with 0.125% Trypsin–EDTA (NCM). Cells were fully dissociated with a pipette and filtered with a 70-μm cell strainer (NEST). Dissociated neurons were seeded on poly-L-lysine/laminin (Sigma) microscope cover glass (NEST). The neurons were incubated in an incubator (Thermo Fisher Scientific) humidified at 37°C, with 5% CO_2. Culture media were supplemented with 2% B-27. For Ca^{2+} imaging experiments, primary cultured DRG neurons were loaded with 1 μg/ml Fura-2 AM (1:1000, Thermo Fisher) and 0.01% F-127 (w/v; Invitrogen) for 30 min in the dark at 37°C and perfusion DRG neurons with calcium imaging buffer (CIB) (130 mM NaCl, 5.6 mM KCl, 2.6 mM $CaCl_2$, 1.2 mM $MgCl_2$, 10 mM Hepes, and 5.6 mM D-glucose at pH 7.4). In chambers equipped with a custom four-channel perfusion valve control system, neurons were incubated with 0.03% formalin for 1 min and then infused with CIB to baseline, then with 0.06% formalin again for 1 min and infused with CIB to baseline, and finally with 56 mM KCl for 1 min and infused with CIB to baseline. To monitor changes in intracellular $[Ca^{2+}]$ with fluorescence images that were acquired using a Nikon Eclipse Ti microscope, emission at 510 nm was monitored from excitation at both 340 nm and 380 nm.

Drugs and Administration

Formalin, compound 48/80 (Cat#C2313), CQ (Cat#C6628), Loratadine, N-acetyl-L-cysteine (NAC, Cat#A7250), N-tert-butyl-a-phenylnitrone (PBN, Cat#B7263), and AITC (Cat#377430) were obtained from Sigma-Aldrich (St. Louis, MO). Nalfurafine was purchased from MCE. HC-030031 (Cat#2896), Capsazepine (CPZ, Cat#0464), HC067047 (Cat#4100), and U0126 (Cat#U120) were obtained from Tocris (Bristol, UK). Morphine hydrochloride was obtained from China Northeast Pharmaceutical Group Shenyang No.1 Pharmaceutical CO., Ltd (Shenyang City, Liaoning Province, China). Naloxone hydrochloride was obtained from China Sinopharm Group Guorui Pharmaceutical CO., Ltd. (Huainan City, Anhui Province, China). PBN, capsazepine, and HC030031 were dissolved in 10% DMSO. Other reagents were dissolved in sterile saline unless specified otherwise. Formalin was dissolved in CIB for Ca^{2+} imaging analysis.

Statistical Analysis

Data were analyzed using GraphPad Prism 6.1 (GraphPad, La Jolla, CA). All data were expressed as the mean ± standard error of the mean (SEM). Two-tailed Student's *t*-test was used for two-group comparisons. One-way ANOVA followed by *post-hoc* Bonferroni test was used for multiple comparisons. Two-way ANOVA followed by *post-hoc* Bonferroni test was used to analyze the data with repeated measures over a time course. Difference with $P < 0.05$ was considered to be statistically significant.

RESULTS

Low-Dose Formalin Induces Itch Behavior in Mice, but Not in Rats

First, we investigated whether administration of formalin is able to induce itch in rodent or not. We found that i.d. injection of the different doses of formalin (0.03–5% in 50 μl) in the nape of the neck of mice were able to evoke scratching behavior in a dose-dependent manner [$F_{(6, 48)} = 25.76$, $P < 0.0001$; **Figures 1A,B**]. Formalin began to evoke scratching at 0.3% and research a peak at the dosage of 1.25%. However, the highest dose of formalin (5%) induced significantly less scratches than that of 1.25% formalin ($t_{13} = 4.601$, $P = 0.0005$; **Figure 1A**), which suggested an inverted "U" shape for the dose–response curve. The cheek model showed that the low-dose formalin (0.3%) only induces itch-indicative scratching but not pain-indicative wiping. However, the higher doses of formalin (1.25–5%) induced both wiping [$F_{(6, 51)} = 19.81$, $P < 0.0001$; **Figure 1C**] and scratching behaviors in mice [$F_{(6, 51)} = 9.737$, $P < 0.0001$; **Figure 1D**]. In addition, i.d. injection of a TRPA1 selective agonist AITC (10–400 μg) into the nape of the neck also evoked scratching behavior in a dose-dependent manner in mice [$F_{(5, 29)} = 4.529$, $P = 0.0036$; **Figures 1E,F**]. For the cheek model, it was demonstrated that low-dose AITC (50 μg) only induces itch-indicative scratching but not pain-indicative wiping, while the higher doses of AITC (100–400 μg) induce both wiping [$F_{(5, 30)} = 8.286$, $P < 0.0001$; **Figure 1G**] and scratching [$F_{(5, 31)} = 4.335$, $P = 0.0042$; **Figure 1H**]. Thus, the results indicated that the low-dose formalin is able to induce acute itch behavior in mice.

We further compared the differences of formalin-induced scratching behavior between mice and rats, in order to see whether there are species differences or not. In rats, we found that i.d. injection of formalin (0.03–5%) in the nape of the neck also similarly induced scratching behavior in a dose-dependent manner [$F_{(6, 48)} = 46.91$, $P < 0.0001$; **Figures 2A,B**]. However, in sharp contrast, the dose–response curve of formalin-induced scratching in rats did not show an inverted "U" shape. In contrast, in the cheek model, we found that low-dose formalin (0.03–0.6%) only induced pain-indicative wiping behavior, but not itch-indicative scratching behavior in rats (**Figures 2C,D**). Furthermore, higher doses of formalin (1.25–5%) induce mixed wiping [$F_{(6, 49)} = 12.64$, $P < 0.0001$; **Figure 2C**] and scratching [$F_{(6, 46)} = 29.34$, $P < 0.0001$; **Figure 2D**] in rats. Together, these data indicated that low-dose formalin induced itch in mice. In contrast, low-dose formalin induced pain in rats, but not in mice. Thus, it indicated that there are significant species differences for low-dose formalin-induced itch behavior.

Involvement of Opioid Receptors in Low-Dose Formalin-Induced Itch in Mice

We subsequently explored that possible role of opioid receptors in low-dose formalin-induced itch in mice. Opioid receptors can be divided into three classes: μ-, κ-, and δ-opioid receptors, which are distributed in the central nervous system (CNS) and peripheral nervous system (PNS) (39). It has been reported that μ-opioid receptor agonists evoke itch, while κ-opioid receptor agonists inhibit itch in both animal models and human (40). Consistently, μ-opioid receptor antagonists inhibit itch, while κ-opioid receptor antagonists evoke itch (41). In the present study, μ-opioid receptors agonist morphine (1 mg/kg) and the μ-opioid receptors antagonist naloxone (1 mg/kg) were administered intraperitoneally (i.p.) 30 min before i.d. injection of 0.3% formalin in mice. The results showed that pre-treatment of morphine was not able to affect 0.3% formalin-induced itch ($t_{10} = 1.610$, $P = 0.1385$), while pre-treatment of naloxone was able to significantly reduce 0.3% formalin-induced itch in the neck model of mice ($t_{10} = 3.417$, $P = 0.0066$; **Figure 3A**). In addition, pre-treatment of morphine also failed to reduce 5% formalin-induced scratching in mice ($t_{14} = 0.8992$, $P = 0.3837$; **Figure 3B**). Moreover, nalfurafine, a κ-opioid receptor agonist, significantly reduced 0.3% formalin-induced itch in a dose-dependent manner in mice [$F_{(3, 28)} = 7.962$, $P = 0.0005$; **Figure 3C**].

To further investigate the effects of morphine on behavioral responses induced by intraplantar (i.pl.) injection of 5 or 0.3% formalin into hindpaw in mice, we recorded the total time of licking, shaking, and biting of the injected hindpaw induced by i.pl. injection of formalin. We found that 5% formalin induced licking, shaking, and biting behaviors in phase 1 (1–10 min; $t_{10} = 11.45$, $P < 0.0001$) and phase 2 (10–45 min; $t_{10} = 6.718$, $P < 0.0001$). In addition, pre-treatment of morphine (3 mg/kg; i.p.) significantly reduced 5% formalin-induced phase 1 ($t_9 = 3.612$, $P = 0.0056$) and phase 2 ($t_9 = 2.433$, $P = 0.0378$) nociceptive behaviors in mice (**Figures 3D,E**). In contrast, pre-treatment of morphine (3 mg/kg; i.p.) did not affect 0.3% formalin-induced licking, shaking, and biting behaviors in mice (**Figures 3F,G**). Thus, these data indicated i.pl. injection of low-dose formalin-induced responses were insensitive to morphine treatment, suggesting these responses may also be itch-related behaviors.

Low-Dose Formalin-Induced Itch Is Histamine-Independent in Mice

Traditionally, itch is divided into histamine-dependent and histamine-independent itch (42). For example, i.d. injection of compound 48/80 evokes histamine-dependent itch through mast cell degranulation and histamine release (1). CQ, an anti-malarial drug, has been demonstrated to induce histamine-independent itch via activation of Mas-related G protein-coupled receptor A3 (MrgprA3) and TRPA1 in primary sensory neurons in mice (21, 22). Then, we asked whether low-dose formalin-induced itch was histamine-dependent or -independent. Antihistamine loratadine was used as a blocker for histamine H1 receptor (H1R). I.p. injection of loratadine (10 mg/kg) was applied 30 min before i.d. injection of compound 48/80 (100 μg) and 0.3% formalin into the nape of the neck, we found that loratadine failed to inhibit 0.3% formalin-induced itch ($t_{12} = 0.5733$, $P = 0.5770$; **Figure 4A**). In sharp contrast, loratadine significantly attenuated compound 48/80-induced histamine-dependent itch in mice ($t_{12} = 4.384$, $P = 0.0009$; **Figure 4B**). In addition, co-administration of 0.3% formalin and CQ (50 μg) significantly increased CQ-induced itch (Saline vs. 50 μg CQ, $t_{10} = 5.611$, $P = 0.0002$; Saline vs. 0.3% Formalin, $t_{10} = 6.555$, $P < 0.0001$; Saline vs. 50 μg CQ + 0.3% Formalin, $t_{10} = 15.78$, $P < 0.0001$; 50 μg

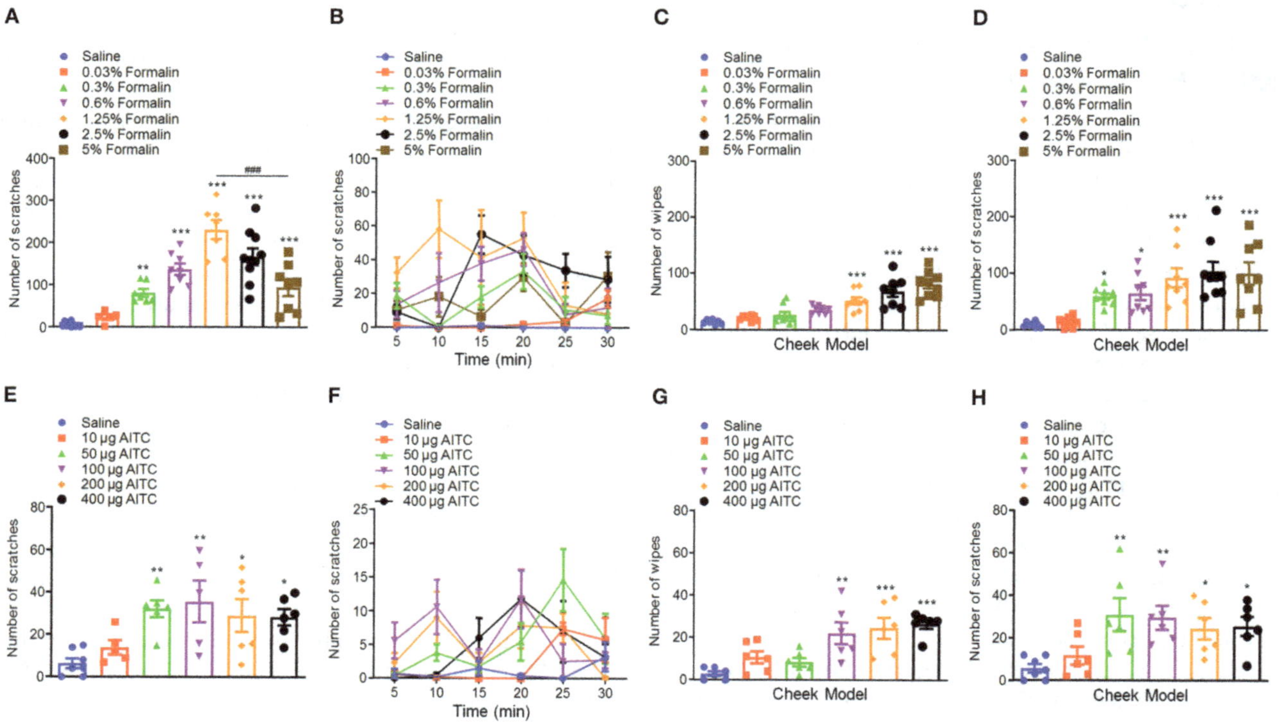

FIGURE 1 | Low-dose formalin evoked scratching behavior in the neck and cheek models of mice. **(A,B)** The total number **(A)** and time course **(B)** of scratching behavior induced by intradermal (i.d.) injection of the different doses of formalin (0.03–5%) in the nape of the neck in mice. **(C,D)** The total number of wiping **(C)** and scratching behavior **(D)** induced by i.d. injection of the different doses of formalin (0.03–5%) in the cheek in mice. **(E,F)** The total number **(E)** and time course **(F)** of scratching behavior induced by i.d. injection of the different doses of AITC (10–400 µg) in the nape of the neck in mice. **(G,H)** The total number of wiping **(G)** and scratching behavior **(H)** induced by i.d. injection of the different doses of AITC (10–400 µg) in the cheek in mice (*$P < 0.05$, **$P < 0.01$, ***$P < 0.001$ vs. Saline, ###$P < 0.001$ vs. 1.25% Formalin, one-way AVOVA following *post-hoc* Bonferroni's test and unpaired Student's *t*-test; $n = 5$–10). All data are expressed by means ± SEM.

CQ vs. 50 µg CQ + 0.3% Formalin, $t_{10} = 7.458$, $P < 0.0001$; 0.3% Formalin vs. 50 µg CQ + 0.3% Formalin, $t_{10} = 4.999$, $P = 0.0005$; **Figure 4C**). Co-administration of 0.3% formalin and compound 48/80 (25 µg) also significantly increased compound 48/80-induced itch in mice (Saline vs. 25 µg compound 48/80, $t_{10} = 9.946$, $P < 0.0001$; Saline vs. 0.3% Formalin, $t_{10} = 8.544$, $P < 0.0001$; Saline vs. 25 µg compound 48/80 + 0.3% Formalin, $t_{10} = 7.720$, $P < 0.0001$; 25 µg compound 48/80 vs. 25 µg compound 48/80 + 0.3% Formalin, $t_{10} = 2.490$, $P = 0.0320$; 0.3% Formalin vs. 25 µg compound 48/80 + 0.3% Formalin, $t_{10} = 2.835$, $P = 0.0177$; **Figure 4D**). Therefore, low-dose formalin is able to induce histamine-independent itch in mice.

TRPA1, but Not TRPV1 or TRPV4, Contributes to Low-Dose Formalin-Induced Itch in Mice

Previous extensive studies have provided evidence showing TRP ion channels as molecular sensors for chemical, thermal, mechanical, painful, and/or itchy stimuli (43). Previous reports demonstrated that formalin is able to directly activate several TRP channels, including TRPA1 (15), TRPV1 (16), and TRPV4 (17). Then, we explored whether and which TRP ion channels participate in 0.3% formalin-induced itch in mice. We found that co-administration of TRPA1 blockers HC030031 (50 µg) significantly reduced 0.3% formalin-evoked acute itch in mice [$F_{(2, 17)} = 7.565$, $P = 0.0045$; **Figure 5A**]. However, co-administration of TRPV1 blockers capsazepine (50 µg; $t_{10} = 1.787$, $P = 0.1043$; **Figure 5B**) or TRPV4 blockers HC067047 (50 µg; $t_{12} = 1.824$, $P = 0.0932$; **Figure 5C**) failed to affect 0.3% formalin-evoked itch in mice. Consistently, 0.3% formalin-induced acute itch in mice was abolished in *Trpa1*$^{-/-}$ mice compared with WT mice ($t_{12} = 6.630$, $P < 0.0001$; **Figure 5D**). In sharp contrast, 0.3% formalin-evoked acute itch was affected in neither *Trpv1*$^{-/-}$ mice ($t_{10} = 1.087$, $P = 0.3026$; **Figure 5E**) nor *Trpv4*$^{-/-}$ mice ($t_{10} = 1.819$, $P = 0.0989$; **Figure 5F**). Therefore, activation of TRPA1 (but not TRPV1 or TRPV4) is required for low-dose formalin-induced acute itch.

Oxidative Stress Contributes to Low-Dose Formalin-Induced Itch in Mice

Our previous studies have demonstrated that oxidative stress plays a critical role in the genesis of histamine-independent itch (23, 24). In the present study, we investigated whether 0.3% formalin directly increases the level of intracellular ROS in the ND7-23 cells, a DRG-derived cell line (23). The intracellular ROS generation and scavenging were measured using DCFH-DA, a fluorescent probe for the highly-selective detection of superoxide in live cells (23). We found that incubation with 0.03% formalin

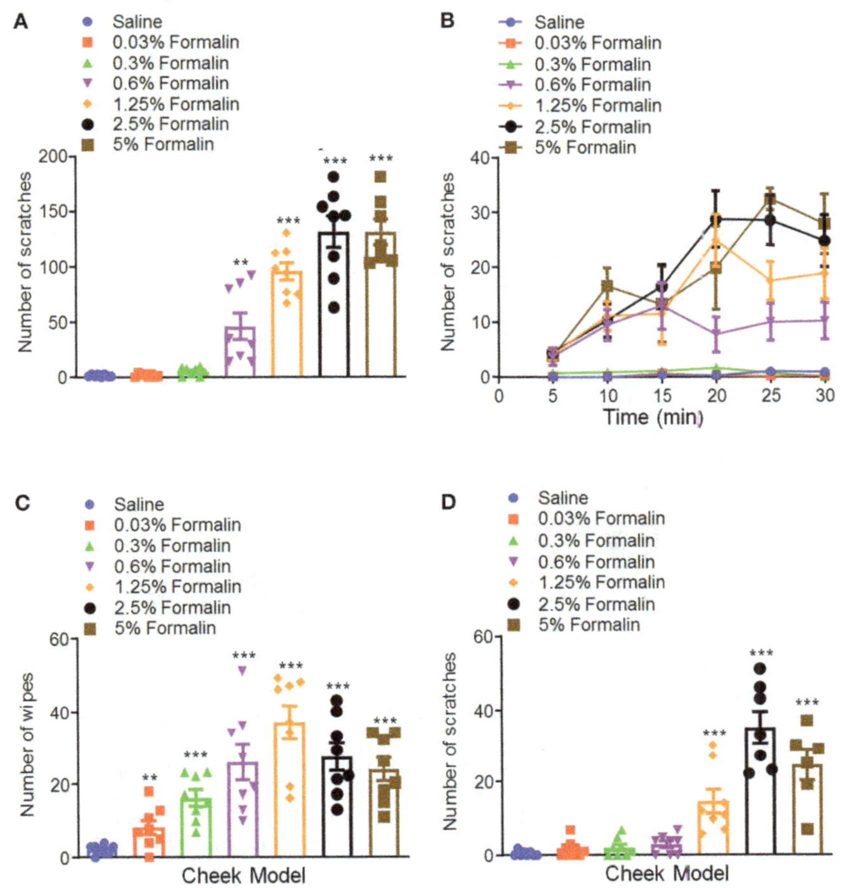

FIGURE 2 | Low-dose formalin evoked wiping behavior in cheek model of rats. **(A,B)** The total number **(A)** and time course **(B)** of scratching behavior induced by i.d. injection of the different doses of formalin (0.03–5%) in the nape of the neck in rats. **(C,D)** The total number of wiping **(C)** and scratching behavior **(D)** induced by i.d. injection of the different doses of formalin (0.03–5%) in the cheek in rats (**$P < 0.01$, ***$P < 0.001$ vs. Saline, one-way AVOVA following Bonferroni's test; $n = 6$–8). All data are expressed by means ± SEM.

significantly increased intracellular ROS in the ND7-23 cells, as reflected by enhanced DCFH-DA fluorescence intensity compared with control, while antioxidant NAC remarkably decreased it (**Figure 6A**). Moreover, we used flow cytometry to quantify intracellular ROS generation (**Figures 6B,C**). When ND7-23 cells were exposed to 0.03% formalin, the mean fluorescence intensity (MFI) was higher than with vehicle treatment, and this was attenuated by pre-treatment with NAC (PBS vs. PBS + Formalin, $t_4 = 9.709$, $P = 0.0006$, PBS + Formalin vs. NAC + Formalin, $t_4 = 9.373$, $P = 0.0007$; **Figure 6C**). Thus, our results demonstrated that 0.03% formalin directly caused the accumulation of intracellular ROS in ND7-23 cells and antioxidants attenuated it. Furthermore, two commonly used antioxidants, NAC and PBN, were i.p. administered 30 min before i.d. injection of 0.3% formalin into the nape of the neck in mice. The results showed that low-dose formalin-induced scratching was significantly reduced by pre-treatment with NAC ($t_{12} = 7.817$, $P < 0.0001$; **Figure 6D**) or PBN ($t_{11} = 3.938$, $P = 0.0023$; **Figure 6E**) in mice.

Activation of p-ERK Signaling in the Dorsal Root Ganglion Contributes to Low-Dose Formalin-Induced Itch in Mice

Previous reports demonstrated that phosphorylation of extracellular signal-regulated kinase (ERK) in the DRG and spinal cord contributes to the genesis of both pain (44) and itch (45). In our study, we confirmed that i.d. injection of 0.3% formalin (Saline vs. 0.3% Formalin 10 min, $t_3 = 3.898$, $P = 0.0107$) and 5% formalin (Saline vs. 5% Formalin 10 min, $t_4 = 5.722$, $P = 0.0046$; Saline vs. 5% Formalin 30 min, $t_4 = 4.074$, $P = 0.0152$) up-regulated p-ERK in the DRG in 10 and 30 min, respectively (**Figures 7A,B**). Moreover, intrathecal (i.t.) injection of the mitogen-activated protein kinase (MEK) inhibitor U0126 (1 nmol) inhibited both low-dose ($t_{13} = 2.808$, $P = 0.0148$; **Figure 7C**) and high-dose ($t_{12} = 2.922$, $P = 0.0128$; **Figure 7D**) formalin-induced acute itch in mice. Thus, our results demonstrated that p-ERK activation in the DRG was involved in formalin-induced acute itch in mice.

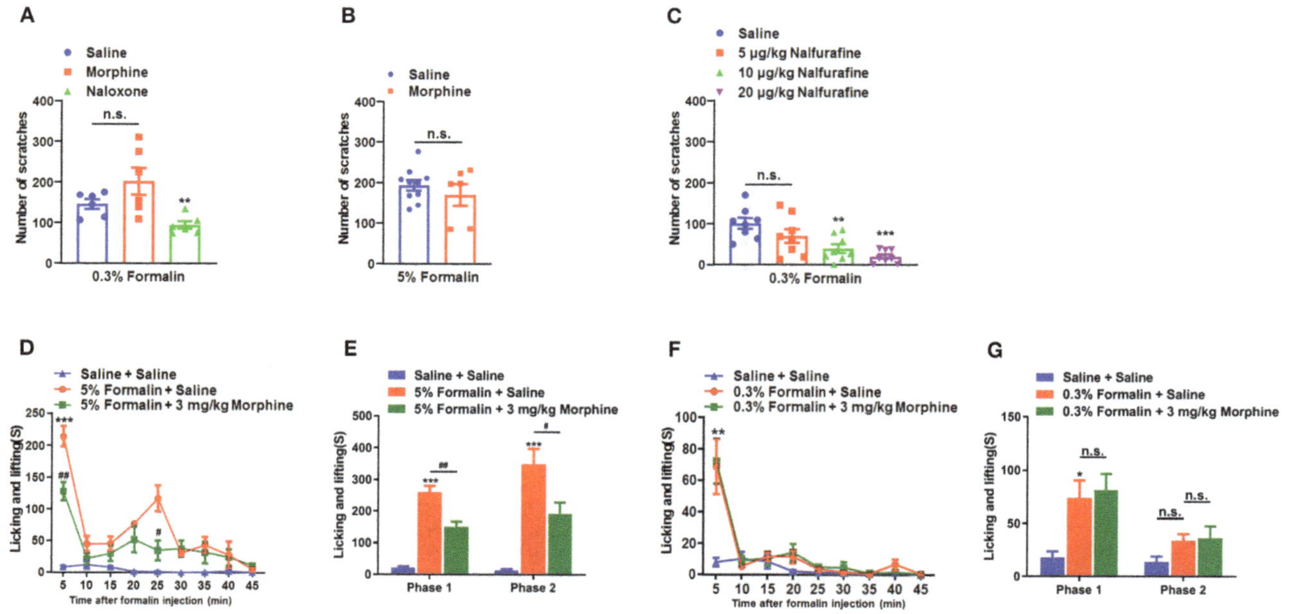

FIGURE 3 | Opioid receptors were involved in the low-dose formalin-induced itch in mice. **(A)** The effects of systemic administration of morphine (1 mg/kg) and naloxone (1 mg/kg), on scratching behavior induced by 0.3% formalin in mice. **(B)** The effects of morphine (1 mg/kg) on 5% formalin-induced itch in mice ($^{*}P < 0.05$, $^{**}P < 0.01$, $^{***}P < 0.001$ vs. Saline, unpaired Student's *t*-test; $n = 6$–10). **(C)** The effects of systemic administration of nalfurafine on scratching behavior induced by 0.3% formalin in mice ($^{*}P < 0.05$, $^{**}P < 0.01$,$^{***}P < 0.001$ vs. Saline, one-way AVOVA following Bonferroni's test; $n = 8$). **(D,E)** The time course **(D)** and total time **(E)** in nociceptive responses induced by i.pl. 5% formalin and the effects of intraperitoneal (i.p.) injection of morphine (3 mg/kg) on it ($^{*}P < 0.05$, $^{**}P < 0.01$,$^{***}P < 0.001$ vs. Saline + Saline, $^{\#}P < 0.05$, $^{\#\#}P < 0.01$, $^{\#\#\#}P < 0.001$ vs. 5% Formalin + Saline, two-way ANOVA following *post hoc* Bonferroni test; $n = 6$–9). **(F,G)** The time course **(F)** and total time **(G)** in nociceptive responses induced by i.pl. 0.3% formalin and the effects of i.p. injection of morphine (3 mg/kg) on it ($^{*}P < 0.05$, $^{**}P < 0.01$,$^{***}P < 0.001$ vs. Saline + Saline, $^{\#}P < 0.05$, $^{\#\#}P < 0.01$ vs. 5% Formalin + Saline, unpaired Student's *t*-test; $n = 6$–9). All data are expressed by means ± SEM. n.s., not significant.

Incubation of Low-Dose Formalin Increases Intracellular Calcium in Primary Cultured Dorsal Root Ganglion Neurons From Mice

We further explored the direct activation of the primary cultured DRG neurons with different doses of formalin by calcium imaging experiments. We found that a subset of DRG neurons (about 13.17 ± 3.61%) could be activated by low-dose formalin (0.03%), while significantly more neurons (32.52 ± 1.91%) could be activated by high-dose formalin (0.06%) ($P < 0.01$; **Figures 8A–C**). Thus, these results indicate that low-dose formalin activates a small subset of neurons, while higher-dose formalin activates a larger population of DRG neurons.

DISCUSSION

Itch is a distinct sensory modality of the somatosensory system of mammals. Acute itch is considered as a protective mechanism to remove potentially harmful stimuli. However, chronic itch is a clinical challenging problem in many dermatological or systemic diseases. To elucidate the mechanisms of itch and to screen new anti-itch compounds, reliable pre-clinical itch animal models are urgently needed to be developed. In the present study, we established an acute histamine-independent itch mouse model by i.d. injection of low-dose formalin in the neck or the cheek. It was found that 0.3% formalin induced histamine-independent itch by activation of TRPA1 in mice, but not in rats. Furthermore, 0.3% formalin-induced itch was inhibited by κ-receptor agonist, antioxidants, and MEK inhibitor. Thus, these data supported the idea that this new "formalin itch test" may be useful for the screening of novel anti-itch drugs.

Low-Dose Formalin Induces Itch in Mice: A New Acute Itch Model?

To date, there are several acute itch models that were developed for studying underlying mechanisms or screening anti-itch drugs, including acute itch induced by histamine (46), compound 48/80 (47), CQ (21), endothelin-1 (48), 5-HT (49), H_2O_2 (23), and imiquimod (31). Given different pruritogens may induce itch through a distinct mechanism, different acute itch models are still needed to be developed. Since first reported over 40 years ago, the formalin test has been widely used in pain research and evaluation of analgesic drugs in laboratory animals (50), and formalin test is known to capture some mechanisms that are likely to be relevant to many pain patients in clinic (51). The nociceptive responses induced by formalin are marked by licking, biting, lifting, and shaking the injected hindpaw in rodents (52). The formalin test is well-known with a biphasic (early and late) nociceptive response in rodent (53). The early

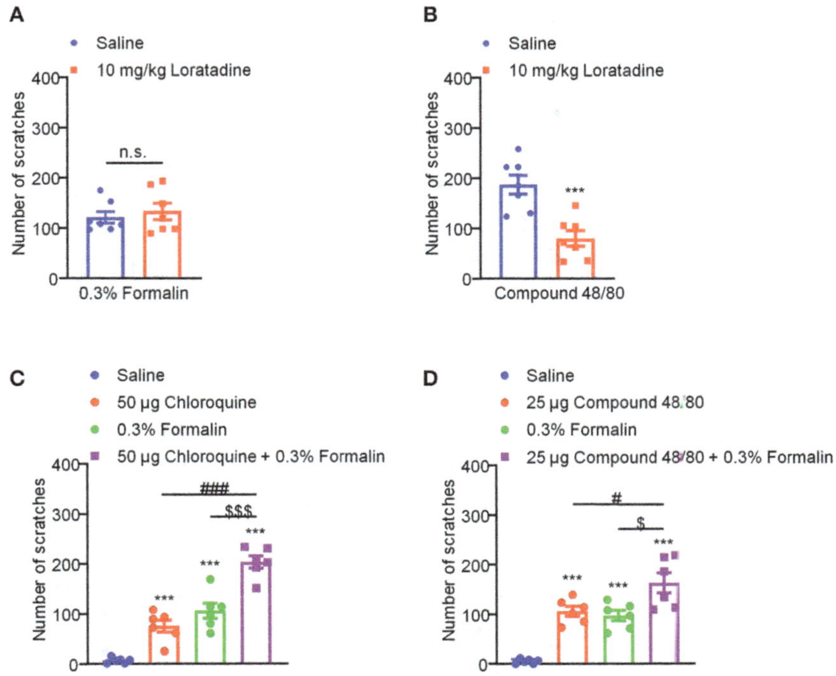

FIGURE 4 | Low-dose formalin-induced itch in a histamine-independent manner in mice. **(A)** The effects of systemic administration of loratadine (10 mg/kg) on 0.3% formalin-induced itch. **(B)** The effects of systemic administration of loratadine (10 mg/kg) on compound 48/80-induced itch ($^{***}P < 0.001$ vs. Saline, unpaired Student's *t*-test; $n = 7$). **(C)** 0.3% formalin significantly increased chloroquine-induced itch in mice. **(D)** 0.3% formalin significantly increased compound 48/80-induced itch in mice [$^{***}P < 0.001$ vs. Saline, $^{\#\#\#}P < 0.001$ vs. 50 µg Chloroquine, $^{\$\$\$}P < 0.001$ vs. 0.3% Formalin, unpaired Student's *t*-test; $n = 6$, **(C)**; $^{***}P < 0.001$ vs. Saline, $^{\#}P < 0.001$ vs. 25 µg Compound 48/80, $^{\$}P < 0.001$ vs. 0.3% Formalin, unpaired Student's *t*-test; $n = 6$ **(D)**]. All data are expressed by means ± SEM. n.s., not significant.

phase (phase 1) is characterized by acute peripheral activation of C and Aδ fibers, while the late phase (phase 2) involves persistent inflammatory nociceptive inputs and the development of central sensitization (54). However, whether and how formalin induces itch are unclear. In a previous report, subcutaneous (s.c.) injections of pruritogenic agents, such as compound 48/80 and substance P, in the rostral back induced scratching in mice (50). In contrast, s.c. injection of algesiogenic agents, such as capsaicin (30 and 100 µg) and dilute formalin (5 mg formaldehyde), into the rostral back was without significant effects in mice (55). Thus, they concluded that pruritogenic (but not algesiogenic) agents are able to induce scratching behavior in mice, and scratching behavior was considered to be a reliable measurement for itch testing (55). Interestingly, there were several studies that suggested that i.d. injection of formalin may be able to evoke itch-associated scratching in mice (34, 35). In the present study, we demonstrated that i.d. injection of the different doses of formalin (0.3–5%) in mice can evoke scratching behavior in a dose-dependent manner. The dose–response curve of formalin-induced scratching showed an inverted "U" shape, which was consistent with our previous reports (7, 23). Further, the cheek model showed that the low-dose formalin (0.3–0.6%) only induced itch-indicative scratching; however, the higher doses of formalin (1.25–5%) induce mixed itch and pain in mice. Low-dose formalin-induced itch was significantly inhibited by κ-receptor agonist nalfurafine, but not µ-opioid receptor agonist morphine. After i.pl. injection of formalin, we found that both 0.3% formalin and 5% formalin induced acute pain in phase 1, and 5% formalin evoked inflammatory pain in phase 2. In addition, systemic application of morphine reduced i.pl. injection of 5% formalin-induced acute pain and inflammatory pain, while it failed to reduce 0.3% formalin-evoked responses in mice. Thus, we provided strong behavioral and pharmacological evidence to support that low-dose formalin induced itch behaviors in mice.

Furthermore, we also found that i.d. injection of the different doses of formalin into the nape of the neck induced scratching behavior in a dose-dependent manner in rats without an inverted "U" shape for the dose–response curve. In sharp contrast, the cheek model indicated that low-dose formalin only induced pain-indicative wiping, but the higher doses of formalin (1.25–5%) induced mixed itch and pain in rats. Thus, although higher-dose formalin induced mixed itch and pain in both mice and rats, low-dose formalin induced only itch in mice, but not in rats. Although formalin test in both mice and rats was widely used for pain research, these results indicated that there are significant species differences for low-dose formalin-induced itch between mice and rats.

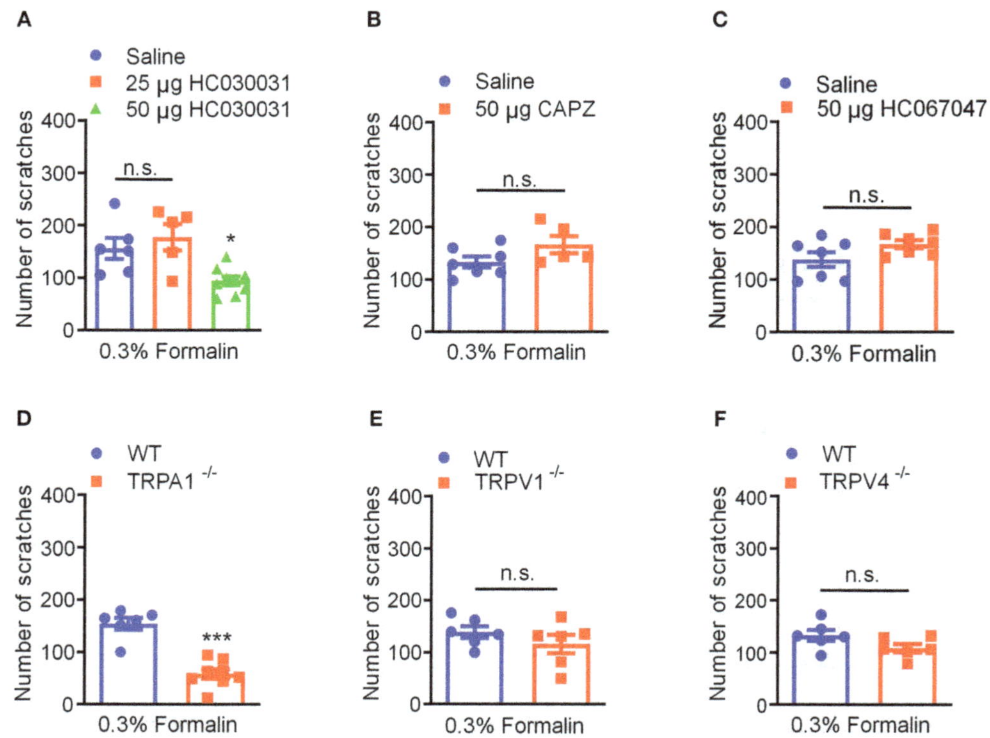

FIGURE 5 | Activation of TRPA1 was required for 0.3% formalin-induced itch in mice. **(A)** The effects of co-administration TRPA1 blocker HC030031 on 0.3% formalin-induced itch in mice. **(B)** The effects of co-administration TRPV1 blocker capsazepine on 0.3% formalin-induced itch in mice. **(C)** The effects of co-administration TRPV4 blocker HC067047 on 0.3% formalin-induced itch in mice. **(D–F)** 0.3% formalin-induced acute itch in mice was abolished in *Trpa1*$^{-/-}$ mice (D), but neither in *Trpv1*$^{-/-}$ mice **(E)** nor in *Trpv4*$^{-/-}$ mice **(F)** [$^{*}P < 0.05$, $^{***}P < 0.001$ vs. 0.3% Formalin, one-way AVOVA following Bonferroni's test; $n = 5$–9, A; $^{*}P < 0.05$, $^{**}P < 0.01$, $^{***}P < 0.001$ vs. 0.3% Formalin, WT, unpaired Student's *t*-test; $n = 5$–9, **(B–F)**]. All data are expressed by means ± SEM. n.s., not significant.

TRPA1 Mediates Low-Dose Formalin-Induced Itch in Mice

We asked which TRP channels are involved in low-dose formalin-induced itch in mice. First, we found that systemic administration of the histamine H1R blocker loratadine fails to inhibit 0.3% formalin-induced itch, indicating 0.3% formalin-induced itch in a histamine-independent manner. Co-administration of TRPA1 blockers HC030031 significantly reduced 0.3% formalin-evoked acute itch in mice, but not for TRPV1 and TRPV4 inhibitors. In addition, 0.3% formalin-induced acute itch was abolished in *Trpa1*$^{-/-}$ mice, but not affected in *Trpv1*$^{-/-}$ and *Trpv4*$^{-/-}$ mice. Thus, these data indicated that activation of TRPA1 is required for low-dose formalin-induced itch in mice. Although previous studies demonstrated that formalin is able to activate several TRP channels, including TRPV1 (16), TRPA1 (15), and TRPV4 (17), our results indicated that only TRPA1 activation contributes to low-dose formalin-induced itch in mice, indicating that different TRP channels mediate different behaviors induced by formalin. Our results also emphasized that TRPA1 acts as receptor for many pruritogens, including H_2O_2 (23), methylglyoxal (7), imiquimod (30), and low-dose formalin in this study. Recently, it was reported that a non-covalent agonist (GNE551) had distinct binding pocket and ligand-interaction mechanism for TRPA1 (56). Unlike the covalent agonist AITC, GNE551 activated TRPA1 without desensitization and induced persistent pain (51). Thus, targeting TRPA1 may be a novel strategy for developing new anti-nociception or anti-itch compounds, which is consistent with previous reports (7, 22, 23).

The Roles of Oxidative Stress and p-ERK Signaling in Low-Dose Formalin-Induced Itch

Previous reports have shown that oxidative stress plays a key role in the pathogenesis of acute and chronic itch (23, 24). In the present study, we found that accumulation of intracellular ROS induced by 0.03% formalin in cultured DRG-derived cell line ND7-23, which was suppressed by perfusion of antioxidant NAC. In line with this observation, incubation of compound 48/80 or CQ also significantly increased the level of intracellular ROS in ND7-23 cells (24). Thus, these data indicated that intracellular ROS may act as second messengers for itch signaling transduction. In addition, systemic administration of the antioxidants NAC and PBN markedly reduced low-dose formalin-induced itch in mice. Thus, it indicated that oxidative stress in the DRGs is involved in low-dose

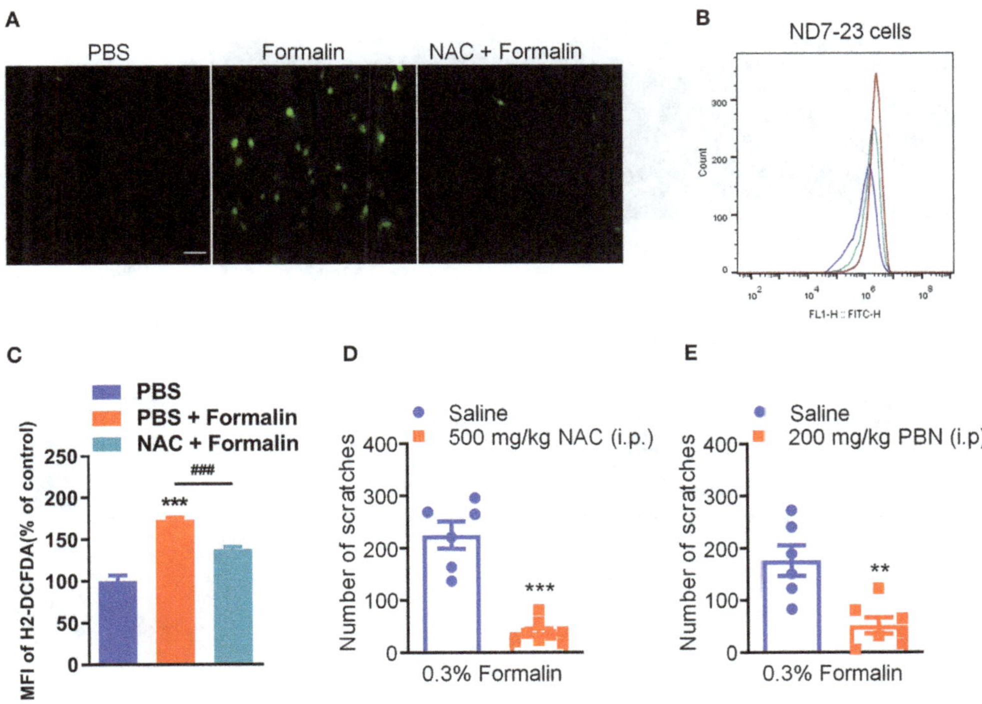

FIGURE 6 | The effects of antioxidants on low-dose formalin-induced itch. **(A)** Representative fluorescence images of intracellular ROS stained with DCFH-DA probe showing that 0.03% formalin-induced significant accumulation of intracellular ROS, which was suppressed by the antioxidants NAC. **(B,C)** Flow cytometry **(B)** and quantification **(C)** confirmed that incubation with 0.03% formalin increased intracellular ROS, which was inhibited by the antioxidants NAC (**$P < 0.01$; ***$P < 0.001$ vs. PBS, ###$P < 0.001$ vs. PBS + Formalin, unpaired Student's *t*-test; $n = 3$). **(D,E)** The effects of systemic administration of NAC (500 mg/kg) and PBN (200 mg/kg) on 0.3% formalin-induced itch in mice [**$P < 0.01$, ***$P < 0.001$ vs. Saline, unpaired Student's *t*-test; $n = 6–8$, **(D,E)**]. All data are expressed by means ± SEM. n.s., not significant.

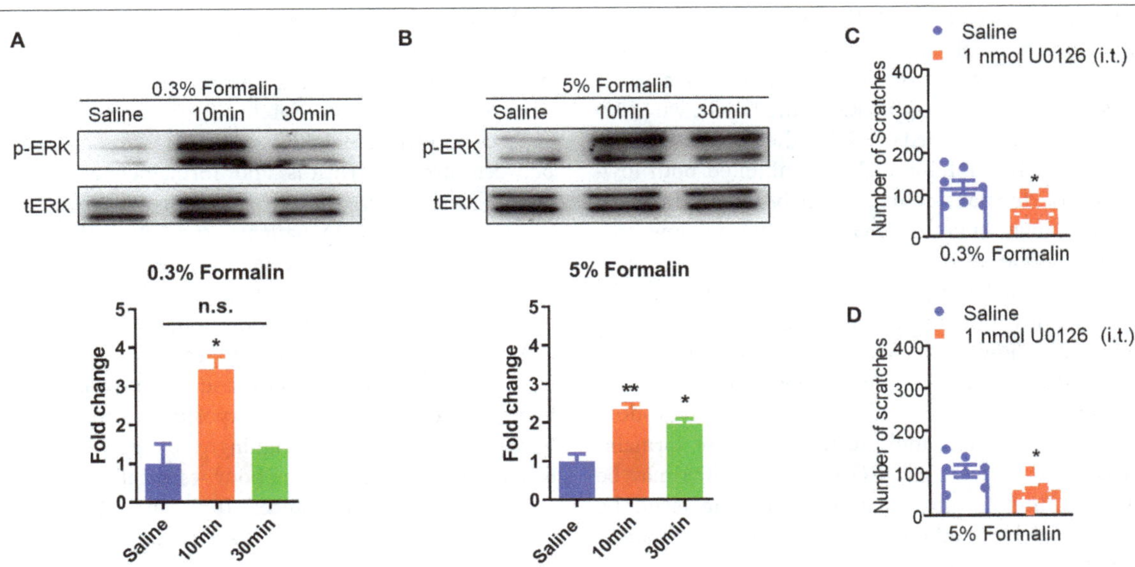

FIGURE 7 | Activation of p-ERK in the DRGs was involved in low-dose formalin-induced itch in mice. **(A,B)** Western blots (upper panel) and quantification (lower panel) showing that p-ERK expression was significantly increased in 10 min and 30 min in the DRG after i.d. injection of 0.3% **(A)** and 5% formalin **(B)** (*$P < 0.05$, **$P < 0.01$ vs. Saline, unpaired Student's *t*-test; $n = 3$). **(C,D)** Intrathecal (i.t.) injection of U0126 (1 nmol) decreased both 0.3% **(C)** and 5% formalin **(D)**-induced scratching behavior in mice (*$P < 0.05$, **$P < 0.01$ vs. Saline, unpaired Student's *t*-test; $n = 7–8$). All data are expressed by means ± SEM. n.s., not significant.

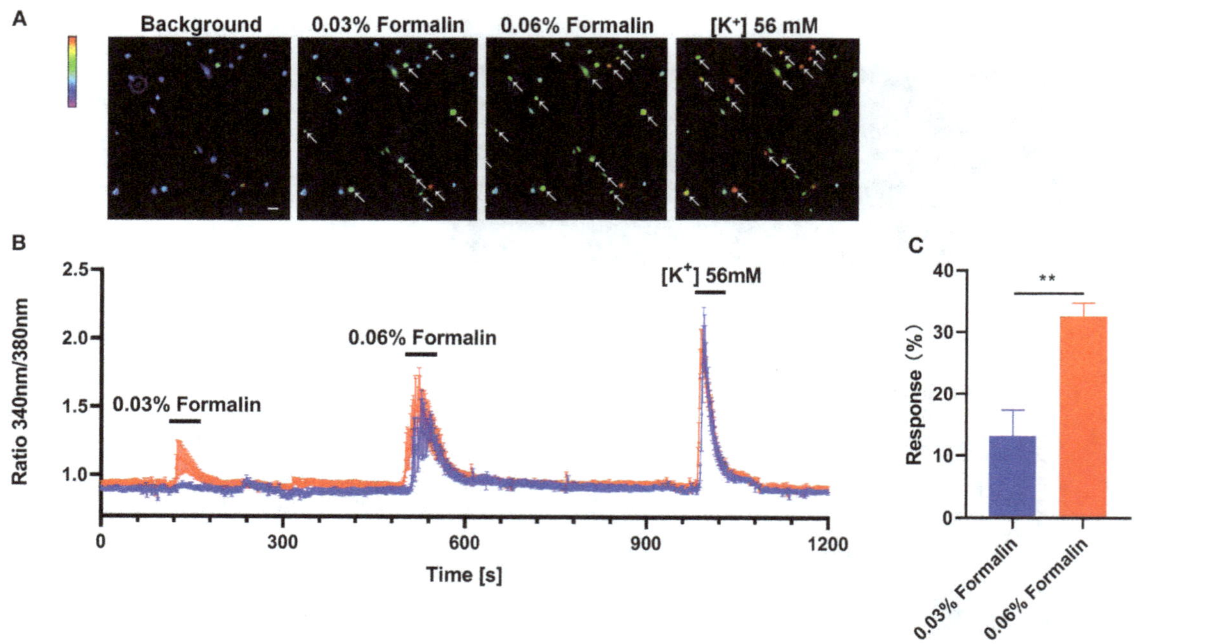

FIGURE 8 | Direct activation of DRG neurons by low-dose formalin. Ca^{2+} imaging of primary cultured DRG neurons with the indicator Fluo-2 AM **(A)** Representative Fura-2 fluorescence heat map images of DRG neurons before and after application of 0.03% formalin, 0.06% formalin, and 56 mM KCl (scale bar, 100 μm). **(B)**. Representative traces of intracellular Ca^{2+} responses induced by application of 0.03% formalin, 0.06% formalin, and 56 mM KCl (blue traces, $n = 5$; red traces, $n = 7$). **(C)** The response (%) of primary DRG neurons with 0.03% and 0.06% formalin and 56 mM KCl treatment. All data are expressed by means ± SEM. n.s., not significant (**$P < 0.01$ vs. 0.03% formalin, unpaired Student's t-test; $n = 4$).

formalin-induced itch and antioxidants may act as promising anti-itch compounds.

Previous work suggested that p-ERK activation in the DRGs and the spinal cord is involved in the genesis of itch (24, 45). In the present work, it was found that i.d. injection of 0.3% formalin transiently up-regulated p-ERK in the DRGs, while 5% formalin persistently up-regulated p-ERK in the DRG. Moreover, i.t. injection of the MEK inhibitor U0126 inhibited both low-dose and high-dose formalin-induced itch behaviors in mice. Thus, p-ERK up-regulation in the DRG was involved in low-dose formalin-induced itch in mice.

Finally, we found that the primary DRG neurons could be directly activated by low-dose formalin by using calcium imaging analysis. The results showed that a subset of DRG neurons are sensitive to low-dose formalin, while a subpopulation of DRG neurons are responsive to both low-dose (0.03%) and high-dose (0.06%) formalin. The results indicate that low-dose formalin may directly activate a subset of DRG neurons, which may be selectively involved in itch signaling transduction. However, the identity, function, and sex difference of this subpopulation of DRG neurons that are sensitive to low-dose formalin remain to be investigated.

Is Formaldehyde a Novel Pruritogen?

Our study has developed a novel acute histamine-independent itch model, which may be useful for itch mechanistic studies and screening for anti-itch drugs. Furthermore, I wondered whether there is clinical relevance for low-dose formalin-induced itch or not. A previous study showed that exposure to formaldehyde aggravated pruritus and skin inflammation in a rat model of atopic dermatitis (57). In addition, many patients undergoing chronic hemodialysis are suffering from chronic itch (9). Interestingly, these patients are often exposed to formaldehyde (58), although the causal relationship between uremic pruritus and formaldehyde is unclear. For atopic dermatitis, exposure to formaldehyde causes skin barrier dysfunction in patients, suggesting that formaldehyde may exacerbate atopic dermatitis (59). Repeated exposure of formaldehyde can cause allergic contact dermatitis in both human (60) and animal models (61). Given many cytokines (especially IL-31) contribute to the pathogenesis of chronic itch, the roles of cytokines and/or chemokines in chronic itch induced by repeated exposure formaldehyde warrant further investigation. Intriguingly, endogenous formaldehyde can also be produced in the body, especially under pathological conditions, such as cancer (62) and Alzheimer's disease (63). The roles of endogenous formaldehyde in chronic itch remain unclear.

In summary, we have provided strong evidence that the low-dose formalin is able to induce histamine-independent itch in mice (but not in rats), which is mediated by the activation of the TRPA1 channel. Thus, we have developed a new pre-clinical itch animal model, which may be helpful to pruritus research.

ETHICS STATEMENT

The animal study was reviewed and approved by the Ethics Committee for the Use of Experimental Animals in Soochow University Animal Committee.

AUTHOR CONTRIBUTIONS

XL, J-TZ, YH, W-QS, Z-HW, Q-YF, D-NF, JJ, and TL contributed to the work design, performed experiments, and analyzed and interpreted data from all the experiments. XL, J-TZ, YH, W-QS, Z-HW, Q-YF, and D-NF carried out *in vivo* animal experiments. J-TZ, YH, W-QS, and Q-YF performed *in vitro* experiments. J-TZ, YH, JJ, and TL prepared and finalized the manuscript. All authors have critically revised and approved the final manuscript and agreed to be accountable for all aspects of the work.

REFERENCES

1. Lay M, Dong X. Neural Mechanisms of Itch. *Annu Rev Neurosci.* (2020) 43:187–205. doi: 10.1146/annurev-neuro-083019-024537
2. Yosipovitch G, Greaves MW, Schmelz M. Itch. *Lancet.* (2003) 361:690–4. doi: 10.1016/S0140-6736(03)12570-6
3. Yosipovitch G, Bernhard JD. Clinical practice. Chronic pruritus. *N Engl J Med.* (2013) 368:1625–34. doi: 10.1056/NEJMcp1208814
4. Ikoma A, Steinhoff M, Stander S, Yosipovitch G, Schmelz M. The neurobiology of itch. *Nat Rev Neurosci.* (2006) 7:535–47. doi: 10.1038/nrn1950
5. Andersen HH, Elberling J, Solvsten H, Yosipovitch G, Arendt-Nielsen L. Non-histaminergic and mechanical itch sensitization in atopic dermatitis. *Pain.* (2017) 158:1780–91. doi: 10.1097/j.pain.0000000000000980
6. Sakai K, Sanders KM, Youssef MR, Yanushefski KM, Jensen L, Yosipovitch G, et al. Mouse model of imiquimod-induced psoriatic itch. *Pain.* (2016) 157:2536–43. doi: 10.1097/j.pain.0000000000000674
7. Cheng RX, Feng Y, Liu D, Wang ZH, Zhang JT, Chen LH, et al. The role of Nav1.7 and methylglyoxal-mediated activation of TRPA1 in itch and hypoalgesia in a murine model of type 1 diabetes. *Theranostics.* (2019) 9:4287–307. doi: 10.7150/thno.36077
8. Patel SP, Vasavda C, Ho B, Meixiong J, Dong X, Kwatra SG. Cholestatic pruritus: emerging mechanisms and therapeutics. *J Am Acad Dermatol.* (2019) 81:1371–8. doi: 10.1016/j.jaad.2019.04.035
9. Mettang T, Kremer AE. Uremic pruritus. *Kidney Int.* (2014) 87:685–91. doi: 10.1038/ki.2013.454
10. Patel KN, Dong X. Itch: cells, molecules, and circuits. *ACS Chem Neurosci.* (2011) 2:17–25. doi: 10.1021/cn100085g
11. Bell JK, McQueen DS, Rees JL. Involvement of histamine H4 and H1 receptors in scratching induced by histamine receptor agonists in Balb C mice. *Br J Pharmacol.* (2004) 142:374–80. doi: 10.1038/sj.bjp.0705754
12. Mogil JS, Davis KD, Derbyshire SW. The necessity of animal models in pain research. *Pain.* (2010) 151:12–7. doi: 10.1016/j.pain.2010.07.015
13. Saddi G, Abbott FV. The formalin test in the mouse: a parametric analysis of scoring properties. *Pain.* (2000) 89:53–63. doi: 10.1016/S0304-3959(00)00348-1
14. Abbott FV, Franklin KB, Westbrook RF. The formalin test: scoring properties of the first and second phases of the pain response in rats. *Pain.* (1995) 60:91–102. doi: 10.1016/0304-3959(94)00095-V
15. McNamara CR, Mandel-Brehm J, Bautista DM, Siemens J, Deranian KL, Zhao M, et al. TRPA1 mediates formalin-induced pain. *Proc Natl Acad Sci USA.* (2007) 104:13525–30. doi: 10.1073/pnas.0705924104
16. Tong Z, Luo W, Wang Y, Yang F, Han Y, Li H, et al. Tumor tissue-derived formaldehyde and acidic microenvironment synergistically induce bone cancer pain. *PLoS ONE.* (2010) 5:e10234. doi: 10.1371/journal.pone.0010234
17. Chen Y, Kanju P, Fang Q, Lee SH, Parekh PK, Lee W, et al. TRPV4 is necessary for trigeminal irritant pain and functions as a cellular formalin receptor. *Pain.* (2014) 155:2662–72. doi: 10.1016/j.pain.2014.09.033
18. Moore C, Gupta R, Jordt SE, Chen Y, Liedtke WB. Regulation of pain and itch by TRP channels. *Neurosci Bull.* (2018) 34:120–42. doi: 10.1007/s12264-017-0200-8
19. Xie Z, Hu H. TRP Channels as drug targets to relieve itch. *Pharmaceuticals.* (2018) 11:100. doi: 10.3390/ph11040100
20. Shim WS, Tak MH, Lee MH, Kim M, Kim M, Koo JY, et al. TRPV1 mediates histamine-induced itching via the activation of phospholipase A2 and 12-lipoxygenase. *J Neurosci.* (2007) 27:2331–7. doi: 10.1523/JNEUROSCI.4643-06.2007
21. Liu Q, Tang Z, Surdenikova L, Kim S, Patel KN, Kim A, et al. Sensory neuron-specific GPCR Mrgprs are itch receptors mediating chloroquine-induced pruritus. *Cell.* (2009) 139:1353–65. doi: 10.1016/j.cell.2009.11.034
22. Wilson SR, Gerhold KA, Bifolck-Fisher A, Liu Q, Patel KN, Dong X, et al. TRPA1 is required for histamine-independent, mas-related G protein-coupled receptor-mediated itch. *Nat Neurosci.* (2011) 14:595–602. doi: 10.1038/nn.2789
23. Liu T, Ji RR. Oxidative stress induces itch via activation of transient receptor potential subtype ankyrin 1 in mice. *Neurosci Bull.* (2012) 28:145–54. doi: 10.1007/s12264-012-1207-9
24. Zhou FM, Cheng RX, Wang S, Huang Y, Gao YJ, Zhou Y, et al. Antioxidants attenuate acute and chronic itch: peripheral and central mechanisms of oxidative stress in pruritus. *Neurosci Bull.* (2017) 33:423–35. doi: 10.1007/s12264-016-0076-z
25. Kido-Nakahara M, Buddenkotte J, Kempkes C, Ikoma A, Cevikbas F, Akiyama T, et al. Neural peptidase endothelin-converting enzyme 1 regulates endothelin 1-induced pruritus. *J Clin Invest.* (2014) 124:2683–95. doi: 10.1172/JCI67323
26. Morita T, McClain SP, Batia LM, Pellegrino M, Wilson SR, Kienzler MA, et al. HTR7 mediates serotonergic acute and chronic itch. *Neuron.* (2015) 87:124–38. doi: 10.1016/j.neuron.2015.05.044
27. Wilson SR, Nelson AM, Batia L, Morita T, Estandian D, Owens DM, et al. The ion channel TRPA1 is required for chronic itch. *J Neurosci.* (2013) 33:9283–94. doi: 10.1523/JNEUROSCI.5318-12.2013
28. Lieu T, Jayaweera G, Zhao P, Poole DP, Jensen D, Grace M, et al. The bile acid receptor TGR5 activates the TRPA1 channel to induce itch in mice. *Gastroenterology.* (2014) 147:1417–28. doi: 10.1053/j.gastro.2014.08.042
29. Wong LS, Otsuka A, Yamamoto Y, Nonomura Y, Nakashima C, Kitayama N, et al. TRPA1 channel participates in tacrolimus-induced pruritus in a chronic contact hypersensitivity murine model. *J Dermatol Sci.* (2017) 89:207–9. doi: 10.1016/j.jdermsci.2017.10.012
30. Esancy K, Condon L, Feng J, Kimball C, Curtright A, Dhaka A. A zebrafish and mouse model for selective pruritus via direct activation of TRPA1. *Elife.* (2018) 7:e32036. doi: 10.7554/eLife.32036
31. Liu T, Xu ZZ, Park CK, Berta T, Ji RR. Toll-like receptor 7 mediates pruritus. *Nat Neurosci.* (2010) 13:1460–2. doi: 10.1038/nn.2683

32. Snyder LM, Kuzirian MS, Ross SE. An unexpected role for TRPV4 in serotonin-mediated itch. *J Invest Dermatol.* (2016) 136:7–9. doi: 10.1016/j.jid.2015.11.010
33. Luo J, Feng J, Yu G, Yang P, Mack MR, Du J, et al. Transient receptor potential vanilloid 4-expressing macrophages and keratinocytes contribute differentially to allergic and non-allergic chronic itch. *J Allergy Clin Immunol.* (2017) 141:608–19.e7. doi: 10.1016/j.jaci.2017.05.051
34. Imamachi N, Park GH, Lee H, Anderson DJ, Simon MI, Basbaum AI, et al. TRPV1-expressing primary afferents generate behavioral responses to pruritogens via multiple mechanisms. *Proc Natl Acad Sci USA.* (2009) 106:11330–5. doi: 10.1073/pnas.0905605106
35. Ross SE, Mardinly AR, McCord AE, Zurawski J, Cohen S, Jung C, et al. Loss of inhibitory interneurons in the dorsal spinal cord and elevated itch in Bhlhb5 mutant mice. *Neuron.* (2010) 65:886–98. doi: 10.1016/j.neuron.2010.02.025
36. Miao X, Huang Y, Liu TT, Guo R, Wang B, Wang XL, et al. TNF-α/TNFR1 signaling is required for the full expression of acute and chronic itch in mice via peripheral and central mechanisms. *Neurosci Bull.* (2018) 34:42–53. doi: 10.1007/s12264-017-0124-3
37. Liu T, Berta T, Xu ZZ, Park CK, Zhang L, Lu N, et al. TLR3 deficiency impairs spinal cord synaptic transmission, central sensitization, and pruritus in mice. *J Clin Invest.* (2012) 122:2195–207. doi: 10.1172/JCI45414
38. Shimada SG, LaMotte RH. Behavioral differentiation between itch and pain in mouse. *Pain.* (2008) 139:681–7. doi: 10.1016/j.pain.2008.08.002
39. Zhang L, Zhang JT, Hang L, Liu T. Mu opioid receptor heterodimers emerge as novel therapeutic targets: recent progress and future perspective. *Front Pharmacol.* (2020) 11:1078. doi: 10.3389/fphar.2020.01078
40. Nojima H, Simons CT, Cuellar JM, Carstens MI, Moore JA, Carstens E. Opioid modulation of scratching and spinal c-fos expression evoked by intradermal serotonin. *J Neurosci.* (2003) 23:10784–90. doi: 10.1523/JNEUROSCI.23-34-10784.2003
41. Kardon AP, Polgar E, Hachisuka J, Snyder LM, Cameron D, Savage S, et al. Dynorphin acts as a neuromodulator to inhibit itch in the dorsal horn of the spinal cord. *Neuron.* (2014) 82:573–86. doi: 10.1016/j.neuron.2014.02.046
42. Dong X, Dong X. Peripheral and central mechanisms of itch. *Neuron.* (2018) 98:482–94. doi: 10.1016/j.neuron.2018.03.023
43. Clapham DE. TRP channels as cellular sensors. *Nature.* (2003) 426:517–24. doi: 10.1038/nature02196
44. Cheng JK, Ji RR. Intracellular signaling in primary sensory neurons and persistent pain. *Neurochem Res.* (2008) 33:1970–8. doi: 10.1007/s11064-008-9711-z
45. Zhang L, Jiang GY, Song NJ, Huang Y, Chen JY, Wang QX, et al. Extracellular signal-regulated kinase (ERK) activation is required for itch sensation in the spinal cord. *Mol Brain.* (2014) 7:25. doi: 10.1186/1756-6606-7-25
46. Shim WS, Oh U. Histamine-induced itch and its relationship with pain. *Mol Pain.* (2008) 4:29. doi: 10.1186/1744-8069-4-29
47. Sun YG, Chen ZF. A gastrin-releasing peptide receptor mediates the itch sensation in the spinal cord. *Nature.* (2007) 448:700–3. doi: 10.1038/nature06029
48. McQueen DS, Noble MA, Bond SM. Endothelin-1 activates ETA receptors to cause reflex scratching in BALB/c mice. *Br J Pharmacol.* (2007) 151:278–84. doi: 10.1038/sj.bjp.0707216
49. Akiyama T, Ivanov M, Nagamine M, Davoodi A, Carstens MI, Ikoma A, et al. Involvement of TRPV4 in serotonin-evoked scratching. *J Invest Dermatol.* (2016) 136:154–60. doi: 10.1038/JID.2015.388
50. Dubuisson D, Dennis SG. The formalin test: a quantitative study of the analgesic effects of morphine, meperidine, and brain stem stimulation in rats and cats. *Pain.* (1977) 4:161–74. doi: 10.1016/0304-3959(77)90130-0
51. Lopes DM, Cater HL, Thakur M, Wells S, McMahon SB. A refinement to the formalin test in mice. *F1000Res.* (2019) 8:891. doi: 10.12688/f1000research.18338.1
52. Tjølsen A, Berge OG, Hunskaar S, Rosland JH, Hole K. The formalin test: an evaluation of the method. *Pain.* (1992) 51:5–17. doi: 10.1016/0304-3959(92)90003-T
53. Fischer M, Carli G, Raboisson P, Reeh P. The interphase of the formalin test. *Pain.* (2014) 155:511–21. doi: 10.1016/j.pain.2013.11.015
54. Woolf CJ. Central sensitization: implications for the diagnosis and treatment of pain. *Pain.* (2011) 152(Suppl. 3):S2–15. doi: 10.1016/j.pain.2010.09.030
55. Kuraishi Y, Nagasawa T, Hayashi K, Satoh M. Scratching behavior induced by pruritogenic but not algesiogenic agents in mice. *Eur J Pharmacol.* (1995) 275:229–33. doi: 10.1016/0014-2999(94)00780-B
56. Liu C, Reese R, Vu S, Rougé L, Shields SD, Kakiuchi-Kiyota S, et al. A Non-covalent ligand reveals biased agonism of the TRPA1 Ion channel. *Neuron.* (2020) 109:273-84.e4. doi: 10.1016/j.neuron.2020.10.014
57. Han RT, Back SK, Lee H, Lee J, Kim HY, Kim HJ, et al. Formaldehyde-induced aggravation of pruritus and dermatitis is associated with the elevated expression of Th1 cytokines in a rat model of atopic dermatitis. *PLoS ONE.* (2016) 11:e0168466. doi: 10.1371/journal.pone.0168466
58. Bousquet J, Rivory JP, Maurice F, Skassa-Brociek W, Larrson P, Johansson SG, et al. Allergy in chronic haemodialysis. 1. Double-blind intravenous challenge with formaldehyde. *Clin Allergy.* (1987) 17:499–506. doi: 10.1111/j.1365-2222.1987.tb02045.x
59. Kim J, Han Y, Ahn JH, Kim SW, Lee SI, Lee KH, et al. Airborne formaldehyde causes skin barrier dysfunction in atopic dermatitis. *Br J Dermatol.* (2016) 175:357–63. doi: 10.1111/bjd.14357
60. Kuritzky LA, Pratt M. Systemic allergic contact dermatitis after formaldehyde-containing influenza vaccination. *J Cutan Med Surg.* (2015) 19:504–6. doi: 10.1177/1203475415582306
61. Saito A, Tanaka H, Usuda H, Shibata T, Higashi S, Yamashita H, et al. Characterization of skin inflammation induced by repeated exposure of toluene, xylene, and formaldehyde in mice. *Environ Toxicol.* (2011) 26:224–32. doi: 10.1002/tox.20547
62. Dorokhov YL, Sheshukova EV, Bialik TE, Komarova TV. Human endogenous formaldehyde as an anticancer metabolite: its oxidation downregulation may be a means of improving therapy. *Bioessays.* (2018) 40:e1800136. doi: 10.1002/bies.201800136
63. Tulpule K, Dringen R. Formaldehyde in brain: an overlooked player in neurodegeneration? *J Neurochem.* (2013) 127:7–21. doi: 10.1111/jnc.12356

23

Pruriplastic Itch—A Novel Pathogenic Concept in Chronic Pruritus

Laurent Misery*

Univ Brest, LIEN, Brest, France

***Correspondence:**
Laurent Misery
laurent.misery@chu-brest.fr

The International Association for the Study of Pain (IASP) defined three descriptors for pain: nociceptive pain is "pain that arises from actual or threatened damage to non neural tissue and is due to the activation of nociceptors"; neuropathic pain is "pain caused by a lesion or disease of the somatosensory nervous system"; and nociplastic pain is "pain that arises from altered nociception despite no clear evidence of actual or threatened tissue damage causing the activation of peripheral nociceptors or evidence for disease or lesion of the somatosensory system causing the pain." Based on clinical and pathophysiological arguments, a similar definition of "pruriplastic pruritus" should be made. Pruriplastic pruritus would include psychogenic pruritus, as well as some cases of pruritus ani, vulvar pruritus, sensitive skin or other poorly understood cases of pruritus. This new descriptor of itch could serve as systematic screening for altered pruriceptive function in patients who suffer from chronic itch and it may also help in defining better tailored treatment by identifying patients who are likely to respond better to centrally rather than to peripherally targeted therapies.

Keywords: pruritus, psychogenic, sensitization, itch, neuropathic

INTRODUCTION

In 2007, the International Forum for the Study of Itch (IFSI) proposed a classification of chronic itch based on clinical signs and distinguished between diseases with and without primary or secondary skin lesions (1). Three groups of conditions were proposed: pruritus on diseased (inflamed) skin (group I), pruritus on non-diseased (non-inflamed) skin (group II), and pruritus presenting with severe chronic secondary scratch lesions, such as prurigo nodularis (group III). The next part classified the underlying diseases according to different categories: dermatological diseases, systemic diseases including diseases of pregnancy and drug-induced pruritus; and neurological and psychiatric diseases. In some patients, more than one cause may account for pruritus (category "mixed"), while in others, no underlying disease can be identified (category "others"). Thus, it was concluded that our knowledge regarding neurophysiological and pathophysiological aspects of chronic pruritus has developed and that this initial classification will undoubtedly require future revisions.

Patients with pruritic diseases of systemic, neurological or psychosomatic/psychiatric origin should be included in group II or group III. It was recommended that the term pruritus sine materia should no longer be used because this term has multiple interpretations, such as idiopathic pruritus, pruritus without any skin changes, pruritus in systemic diseases without any initially visible skin changes, pruritus characterized by the absence of specific cutaneous lesions of an itching dermatosis, pruritus in the elderly or psychosomatic pruritus (1).

Indeed, there is a psychosomatic definition of pruritus sine materia in the ICD-10 classification of F45.8 as somatoform pruritus, which was considered the more acceptable term by the

IFSI (1). Neuropathic itch should refer to pruritus caused by neuronal or glial damage (2), whereas psychogenic itch is related to psychological disorders (3). Nonetheless, the concept of somatoform or psychogenic itch remains controversial.

CONTROVERSIES RELATED TO PSYCHOGENIC ITCH

Psychogenic itch is known as psychogenic pruritus, somatoform pruritus (4), functional itch disorder (5), non-organic pruritus, psychosomatic pruritus, or functional pruritus, but "psychogenic itch" is the most commonly used denomination (6).

The 11th revision of the International Classification of Diseases (ICD-11) clearly separates psychogenic pruritus (EC90.4, using this term), from pruritus of unknown origin (EC90.6) among other causes of pruritus (EC90).

European guideline on chronic pruritus proposes that somatoform pruritus is defined as pruritus where psychic, psychiatric and psychosomatic factors play a critical role in the onset, intensity, aggravation or persistence of the pruritus (7).

The French Psycho-Dermatology Group (FPDG) is an expert group from the French Society of Dermatology that includes dermatologists, psychologists and psychiatrists. This group has proposed a definition of psychogenic pruritus as "an itch disorder where itch is at the center of the symptomatology and where psychological factors play an evident role in the triggering, intensity, aggravation or persistence of the pruritus" and has suggested calling it "functional itch disorder" (FID) (5). The FPDG also proposed 10 diagnostic criteria (3 compulsory and 7 optional) to assess the diagnosis, with both negative (no somatic cause) and positive criteria (clinical characteristics, association with psychological disorders or stressful life events).

Previous psycho-dermatological classifications (associated skin and psychological disorders) had included psychogenic pruritus among the "psychological disorders responsible for skin sensations" (8), "functional cutaneous and mucous disorders" (9) or "conditions in which strong psychogenic factors are imputed" (10). It is of particular interest to separate psychogenic excoriations (11), dermatitis artefacta and all other self-inflicted skin lesions (SISLs) (12) from psychogenic pruritus. SISLs are related to impulsive, compulsive or other psychopathological mechanisms. In contrast, psychogenic pruritus is related to an illusion of pruritus, but this pruritus is felt by the patient and is the main complaint.

Psychogenic pruritus was not precisely cited in the 4th edition of the Diagnostic and Statistical Manual of Mental Disorders (DSM-IV) (13), but it could be recognized among the following 4 diagnoses (6) listed in the DSM-IV:

- Conversion disorder (300.11): Unexplained symptoms or deficits affecting voluntary motor or sensory function that suggest a neurological or other general medical condition. Psychological factors are judged to be associated with the symptoms or deficits.
- Undifferentiated somatoform disorders (300.81): One or several somatic complaints lasting 6 months or more with no medical or mental disease available to explain the presence or intensity of these symptoms. This symptom is not intentionally self-induced or simulated.
- Unspecified somatoform disorder (300.82): All disorders with somatoform symptoms that do not fit the criteria of any specific somatoform disorder.
- Pain disorder associated with psychological factors (307.80): Psychological factors play a critical role in the triggering, intensity, aggravation or persistence of the pain.

The 5th edition of the Diagnostic and Statistical Manual of Mental Disorders (DSM-5) (14) defined a new diagnosis of "somatic symptom disorder" (SSD), which is characterized by "somatic symptoms that are either very distressing or result in significant disruption of functioning, as well as excessive and disproportionate thoughts, feelings and behaviors regarding those symptoms. To be diagnosed with SSD, the individual must be persistently symptomatic (typically for at least 6 months)."

The DSM-IV disorders of somatization disorder, hypochondriasis, pain disorder, and undifferentiated somatoform disorder were removed. The DSM-IV diagnosis of somatization disorder required a specific number of complaints from among four symptom groups while the SSD criteria must only be significantly distressing or disruptive to daily life and must be accompanied by excessive thoughts, feelings, or behaviors. While medically unexplained symptoms were a key feature for many of the disorders in the DSM-IV, a diagnosis of SSD does not require that the somatic symptoms are medically unexplained. Consequantly, symptoms may or may not be associated with another medical diagnosis. Furthermore, it is not appropriate to diagnose individuals with a mental disorder solely because a medical cause cannot be demonstrated. Regardless of whether the somatic symptoms can be medically explained, the individual would still have to meet the remaining criteria to receive a diagnosis of SSD.

As in the case of psychogenic pain (15), the concept of SSD overpsychologizes people with chronic pain and may contribute to misdiagnosis and unnecessary stigma (16). In contrast, the DSM-5 SSD criteria may be more restrictive than the DSM-IV criteria for somatoform disorders for a population of patients with medically unexplained physical symptoms (MUPS) (17).

Because SSD include both psychogenic pruritus and pruritus of a somatic origin, this disproportionate resounding is very confusing (6). Nonetheless, we have to admit that it is very difficult to separate in clinical practice patients with a pure psychogenic pruritus from those with a large but not exclusive contribution of psychological factors in the pathogenesis of their pruritus. Numerous psychological factors could influence the perception and modulation of pruritus (18–24).

UNIFIED PATHOPHYSIOLOGY

In case of pruritus or even if we think about pruritus or scratching sensory, motor and affective areas of the brain are activated (25–28). Consequently, a new definition of pruritus could be "a sensation accompanied by the contralateral activation of the anterior cortex and the predominantly ipsilateral activation of the supplementary motor areas and the inferior parietal lobule;

scratching may follow" (29), reflecting the fact that "it is the brain that itches, not the skin" (30). Hence, a psychological component may occur in all cases of pruritus (31) and that a specific psychogenic pruritus can exist (30).

Convergent visceral-somatic processing and neuroimaging studies in somatoform disorders have demonstrated that somatosensory amplification may, in part, develop through stress-mediated neuroplastic changes and the neuromodulatory effects of inflammation (32). Neural correlates of cognitive-affective amplifiers are integrated into a network for somatosensory amplification, including anterior cingulate cortex, insula, amygdala, hippocampal formation, and striatum.

Transient scratching inhibits the itch sensation, but repeted and increasing scratching is involved in peripheral and central sensitizations to itch (30, 33–35). Similarly to pain sensitizations, inflammatory mediators are released by pruriceptors (peripheral sensitization), whereas chronic skin inflammation facilitates spinal and cerebral itch processing, resulting in touch-evoked pruritus (central sensitization). Clinical consequences are alloknesis and hyperknesis (36), which could be confused with psychological involvement in itch, extending up to itch catastrophizing.

All humans can suffer from itch in the course of their life (37, 38). Witnessing your neighbor scratching, discussing or reading about itch, watching movies showing people scratching and viewing pictures of affected skin or insects can induce itch in healthy persons and to a greater degree in chronic itch patients and subjects with neurotic personalities (39). The underlying course of contagious itch seems to be related to human mirror neurons that are active when we imitate actions and/or negative affects (38). Brain imaging evidenced an important functional coupling of the insula and basal ganglia in initiating the urge to scratch when provided with itch-evoking visual stimuli (40).

Several studies suggest that mechanisms of central modulation play an important role in the development and maintenance of chronic itch (41). The management of the neurosensory aspects of itch is an important part of the management of chronic itch. The reason for our underlying desire to itch may be an overactive limbic system, particularly the anterior cingulate cortex, which is essential in modulating emotional and cognitive activities (39). The co-activation of the prefrontal cortex in conjunction with the limbic system upon application of itch stimuli suggests interplay of this network on motivation and emotion (42). The role of the prefrontal cortex has been highlighted in reward processing for addictive behaviors (39). The reward circuit, particularly in the midbrain, may be part of the neural basis of the vicious itch-scratch-itch circle and appears to be linked to the development of an urge to scratch to achieve the "pleasure" derived from scratching (40). The involvement of the midbrain strongly suggests a role for the dopaminergic system in the addictive nature such a circle (43). Central mechanisms of itch have been previously reviewed (41, 44–46). More recently, the growing number of brain imaging studies has allowed meta-analyses (47, 48).

In addition to clinical considerations, pathophysiological data on the brain processing of itch support that it not possible to separate psychogenic from non psychogenic itch.

LESSONS FROM PAIN RESEARCH

Because mechanisms of chronic itch are close to those of chronic pain (36, 44, 49–52) or chronic cough (50, 53), it is very interesting to observe the evolution of thoughts in these fields.

The first definition for neuropathic pain was given in 1994 by the International Association for the Study of Pain (IASP) as "pain initiated or caused by a primary lesion or dysfunction in the nervous system." This definition was changed to a new one in 2005 when the nociceptive terminology appeared. Nociceptive pain was defined as "pain due to stimulation of primary nociceptive nerve endings," and neuropathic pain was defined as "pain due to lesion or dysfunction of the nervous system" (54). Consequently, we could modify the definition of neuropathic pruritus (2). Both definitions are periodically reviewed, and currently, nociceptive pain is "pain that arises from actual or threatened damage to nonneural tissue and is due to the activation of nociceptors," and neuropathic pain is "pain caused by a lesion or disease of the somatosensory nervous system" (54).

Because this dichotomy between pain mechanistic definitions created a gap for numerous patients without activation of neither nociceptors nor lesion or disease of the nervous system, a third descriptor was proposed in 2016 (55) then adopted by the IASP council in 2017, although it is not yet universally agreed: nociplastic pain. This choice was supported by abundant literature confirming changes in cerebral activation in once-called "dysfunctional diseases" (56, 57) and changes in cerebral connectivity across multiple chronic pain conditions (58). More recent studies have shown that central pain processing is augmented after psychological trauma (alterations in painful and non-painful areas), whereas there are only alterations in the painful area without such a trauma (59). The relationship between anxiety or depression symptoms, and pain intensity is completely mediated by central sensitization while the relationship between catastrophic thinking and pain intensity is partially mediated by central sensitization (60).

The chosen definition of nociplastic pain is "pain that arises from altered nociception despite no clear evidence of actual or threatened tissue damage causing the activation of peripheral nociceptors or evidence for disease or lesion of the somatosensory system causing the pain" (55).

Patients can have a combination of nociceptive and nociplastic pain (55). The concept of mixed pain, which is defined as "a complex overlap of the different known pain types (nociceptive, neuropathic, and nociplastic) in any combination, acting simultaneously and/or concurrently to cause pain in the same body area. Either mechanism may be more clinically predominant at any point in time. That mixed pain can be acute or chronic" has also been proposed (61).

CONCLUSIONS

Hence, it should be proposed to use three descriptors for itch (**Table 1**):

TABLE 1 | Comparisons between pruriceptive, neuropathic and pruriplastic itch.

	Pruriceptive	Neuropathic	Pruriplastic
Origin	Pruriceptor	Lesions of peripheral or central nervous system	Dysfunctions of itch processing (central sensitization, loss of downstream controls)
Characteristics	Variables	Associated with other unpleasant sensations (paresthesia, dysesthesia)	Atypical*
Localization	Locoregional or diffuse	According to involved nervous system	Local or diffuse
Neurological examination	Normal	Abnormal	Normal
Evolution	Acute or chronic	Chronic	Chronic
Treatment	Etiological Symptomatic	Gabapentinoids Antidepressants**	Antidepressants**

***There is a need for confirmation by clinical trials.*
**Examples: association with extra-cutaneous sensory or other disorders.*

- Pruriceptive itch: itch that arises from actual or threatened damage to non-neural tissue and is due to the activation of pruriceptors
- Neuropathic itch: itch caused by a lesion or disease of the somatosensory nervous system
- Pruriplastic itch: itch that arises from altered pruriception despite no clear evidence of actual or threatened tissue damage causing the activation of peripheral pruriceptors or evidence of disease or lesions of the somatosensory system causing the itch
- Mixed itch: overlap of the different known itch types (nociceptive, neuropathic, and nociplastic) in any combination, acting simultaneously and/or concurrently to cause itch in the same body area.

Pruriceptive and neuropathic pruritus are not new concepts but pruriplastic pruritus is a new one. Pruriplastic pruritus would include psychogenic pruritus, as well as some cases of pruritus ani, vulvar pruritus, sensitive skin or other poorly understood cases of pruritus. It would be the pruritic equivalent of nociplastic pain, including vulvodynia, burning mouth syndrome, fibromyalgia and all SSDs.

In clinical practice, the diagnosis of pruriplastic pruritus could be a neutral, more acceptable and understandable diagnosis for patients with these disorders, avoiding oppositions between neurogenic and psychogenic hypotheses. Indeed, many patients are afraid by psychogenic hypotheses or refuse diagnoses of psychogenic diseases because that challenges them personally. In the absence of direct evidence of skin or somatosensory disorders, it would be useful to have a category of "pruriplastic itch" to reassure the patient that their itch is real.

Finally, it could be used for further clinical research and diagnostic criteria might be defined. Like nociplastic pain (54), this new descriptor of itch could serve as systematic screening for altered pruriceptive function in patients who have chronic itch and it may also help in defining better tailored treatment by identifying those who are likely to respond better to centrally rather than to peripherally targeted therapies.

Like nociplastic pain, there is likely an organic basis for pruriplastic itch such as central sensitization of itch pathways, although central sensitization may also occur in all causes of chronic itch, in the absence of overt evidence of disease or lesions of the somatosensory system. The loss of descending pathways has been recently evidenced as a hallmark of chronic itch patients, who have reduced conditioned pain modulation (CPM) which might contribute to enhanced itch (62). Otherwise there is little clinical evidence based on quantitative sensory testing (QST) to suggest that chronic itch patients exhibit altered pruriception (e.g., alloknesis or hyperknesis). This proposal would be strengthened by including any studies that have investigated pruriception in patients suffering from chronic itch of different origins including psychogenic/pruriplastic itch.

Hence, I propose this new concept of pruriplastic itch, which needs discussion by colleagues and a final validation by the IFSI.

AUTHOR CONTRIBUTIONS

The author confirms being the sole contributor of this work and has approved it for publication.

REFERENCES

1. Stander S, Weisshaar E, Mettang T, Szepietowski JC, Carstens E, Ikoma A, et al. Clinical classification of itch: a position paper of the International Forum for the Study of Itch. *Acta Derm Venereol.* (2007) 87:291–4. doi: 10.2340/00015555-0305
2. Misery L, Brenaut E, Le Garrec R, Abasq C, Genestet S, Marcorelles P, et al. Neuropathic pruritus. *Nat Rev Neurol.* (2014) 10:408–16. doi: 10.1038/nrneurol.2014.99
3. Yosipovitch G, Samuel LS. Neuropathic and psychogenic itch. *Dermatol Ther.* (2008) 21:32–41. doi: 10.1111/j.1529-8019.2008.00167.x
4. Harth W, Hermes B, Niemeier V, Gieler U. Clinical pictures and classification of somatoform disorders in dermatology. *Eur J Dermatol.* (2006) 16:607–14.
5. Misery L, Alexandre S, Dutray S, Chastaing M, Consoli SG, Audra H, et al. Functional itch disorder or psychogenic pruritus: suggested diagnosis criteria from the French psychodermatology group. *Acta Derm Venereol.* (2007) 87:341–4. doi: 10.2340/00015555-0266
6. Misery L, Dutray S, Chastaing M, Schollhammer M, Consoli SG, Consoli SM. Psychogenic itch. *Transl Psychiatry.* (2018) 8:52. doi: 10.1038/s41398-018-0097-7
7. Weisshaar E, Szepietowski JC, Dalgard FJ, Garcovich S, Gieler U, Giménez-Arnau AM, et al. European S2k guideline on chronic pruritus. *Acta Derm Venereol.* (2019) 99:469–506. doi: 10.2340/00015555-3164
8. Misery L, Chastaing M. Joint consultation by a psychiatrist and a dermatologist. *Dermatol Psychosom.* (2003) 4:160–4. doi: 10.1159/000073994
9. Consoli SG. *Psychiatrie et dermatologie.* Paris: Elsevier (2001).
10. Koblenzer CS. Psychosomatic concepts in dermatology. *Arch Dermatol.* (1983) 119:501–12. doi: 10.1001/archderm.1983.01650300055017
11. Misery L, Chastaing M, Touboul S, Callot V, Schollhammer M, Young P, et al. Psychogenic skin excoriations: diagnostic criteria, semiological

analysis and psychiatric profiles. *Acta Derm Venereol.* (2012) 92:416–8. doi: 10.2340/00015555-1320

12. Gieler U, Consoli SG, Tomás-Aragones L, Linder DM, Jemec GB, Poot F, et al. Self-inflicted lesions in dermatology: terminology and classification–a position paper from the European Society for Dermatology and Psychiatry (ESDaP). *Acta Derm Venereol.* (2013) 93:4–12. doi: 10.2340/00015555-1506
13. Association AP. *Diagnostic and Statistical Manual of Mental Disorders.* 4th ed. Arlington: American Psychiatric Publishing (1994).
14. Association AP. *DSM-5: Diagnostic and Statistical Manual of Mental Disorders.* 5th ed. Washington: American Psychiatric Association(2013).
15. Katz J, Rosenbloom BN, Fashler S. Chronic pain, psychopathology, and DSM-5 somatic symptom disorder. *Can J Psychiatry.* (2015) 60:160–7. doi: 10.1177/070674371506000402
16. Levenson JL, Sharma AA, Ortega-Loyza AG. Somatic symptom disorder in dermatology. *Clin Dermatol.* (2017) 35:246–51. doi: 10.1016/j.clindermatol.2017.01.010
17. Van Dessel NC, Van Der Wouden JC, Dekker J, Van Der Horst HE. Clinical value of DSM IV and DSM 5 criteria for diagnosing the most prevalent somatoform disorders in patients with medically unexplained physical symptoms (MUPS). *J Psychosom Res.* (2016) 82:4–10. doi: 10.1016/j.jpsychores.2016.01.004
18. Schneider G, Driesch G, Heuft G, Evers S, Luger TA, Stander S. Psychosomatic cofactors and psychiatric comorbidity in patients with chronic itch. *Clin Exp Dermatol.* (2006) 31:762–7. doi: 10.1111/j.1365-2230.2006.02211.x
19. Halvorsen JA, Dalgard F, Thoresen M, Bjertness E, Lien L. Itch and mental distress: a cross-sectional study among late adolescents. *Acta Derm Venereol.* (2009) 89:39–44. doi: 10.2340/00015555-0554
20. Dalgard FJ, Gieler U, Tomas-Aragones L, Lien L, Poot F, Jemec GB, et al. The psychological burden of skin diseases: a cross-sectional multicenter study among dermatological out-patients in 13 European countries. *J Invest Dermatol.* (2015) 135:984–91. doi: 10.1038/jid.2014.530
21. Misery L, Ständer S. *Pruritus.* London: Springer (2017).
22. Stumpf A, Schneider G, Ständer S. Psychosomatic and psychiatric disorders and psychologic factors in pruritus. *Clin Dermatol.* (2018) 36:704–8. doi: 10.1016/j.clindermatol.2018.08.015
23. Schut C, Dalgard FJ, Halvorsen JA, Gieler U, Lien L, Tomas Aragones L, et al. Occurrence, chronicity and intensity of itch in a clinical consecutive sample of patients with skin diseases: a multi-centre study in 13 European Countries. *Acta Derm Venereol.* (2019) 99:146–51. doi: 10.2340/00015555-3040
24. Golpanian RS, Lipman Z, Fourzali K, Fowler E, Nattkemper L, Chan YH, et al. Psychiatric comorbidities in non-psychogenic chronic itch, a US based study. *Acta Derm Venereol.* (2020) 100:adv00169. doi: 10.2340/00015555-3487
25. Darsow U, Drzezga A, Frisch M, Munz F, Weilke F, Bartenstein P, et al. Processing of histamine-induced itch in the human cerebral cortex: a correlation analysis with dermal reactions. *J Invest Dermatol.* (2000) 115:1029–33. doi: 10.1046/j.1523-1747.2000.00193.x
26. Drzezga A, Darsow U, Treede RD, Siebner H, Frisch M, Munz F, et al. Central activation by histamine-induced itch: analogies to pain processing: a correlational analysis of O-15 H2O positron emission tomography studies. *Pain.* (2001) 92:295–305. doi: 10.1016/S0304-3959(01)00271-8
27. Mochizuki H, Tashiro M, Kano M, Sakurada Y, Itoh M, Yanai K. Imaging of central itch modulation in the human brain using positron emission tomography. *Pain.* (2003) 105:339–46. doi: 10.1016/S0304-3959(03)00249-5
28. Walter B, Sadlo MN, Kupfer J, Niemeier V, Brosig B, Stark R, et al. Brain activation by histamine prick test-induced itch. *J Invest Dermatol.* (2005) 125:380–2. doi: 10.1111/j.0022-202X.2005.23817.x
29. Savin JA. How should we define itching? *J Am Acad Dermatol.* (1998) 39:268–9. doi: 10.1016/S0190-9622(98)70087-8
30. Paus R, Schmelz M, Biro T, Steinhoff M. Frontiers in pruritus research: scratching the brain for more effective itch therapy. *J Clin Invest.* (2006) 116:1174–85. doi: 10.1172/JCI28553
31. Van Os-Medendorp H, Eland- De Kok PCM, Grypdonck M, Bruijnzeel-Koomen CA, Ros WJG. Prevalence and predictors of psychosocial morbidity in patients with chronic pruritic skin. *J Eur Acad Dermatol Venereol.* (2006) 20:810–7. doi: 10.1111/j.1468-3083.2006.01647.x
32. Perez DL, Barsky AJ, Vago DR, Baslet G, Silbersweig DA. A neural circuit framework for somatosensory amplification in somatoform disorders. *J Neuropsychiatry Clin Neurosci.* (2015) 27:e40–50. doi: 10.1176/appi.neuropsych.13070170
33. Yosipovitch G, Greaves MW, Schmelz M. Itch. *Lancet.* (2003) 361:690–4. doi: 10.1016/S0140-6736(03)12570-6
34. Ikoma A, Steinhoff M, Stander S, Yosipovitch G, Schmelz M. The neurobiology of itch. *Nat Rev Neurosci.* (2006) 7:535–47. doi: 10.1038/nrn1950
35. Stander S, Schmelz M. Chronic itch and pain–similarities and differences. *Eur J Pain.* (2006) 10:473–8. doi: 10.1016/j.ejpain.2006.03.005
36. Andersen HH, Akiyama T, Nattkemper LA, Van Laarhoven A, Elberling J, Yosipovitch G, et al. Alloknesis and hyperknesis-mechanisms, assessment methodology, and clinical implications of itch sensitization. *Pain.* (2018) 159:1185–97. doi: 10.1097/j.pain.0000000000001220
37. Niemeier V, Kupfer J, Gieler U. Observations during an itch-inducing lecture. *Dermatol Psychosom.* (1999) 1:15–9. doi: 10.1159/000057993
38. Schut C, Grossman S, Gieler U, Kupfer J, Yosipovitch G. Contagious itch: what we know and what we would like to know. *Front Hum Neurosci.* (2015) 9:57. doi: 10.3389/fnhum.2015.00057
39. Lee HG, Stull C, Yosipovitch G. Psychiatric disorders and pruritus. *Clin Dermatol.* (2017) 35:273–80. doi: 10.1016/j.clindermatol.2017.01.008
40. Mochizuki H, Baumgartner U, Kamping S, Ruttorf M, Schad LR, Flor H, et al. Cortico-subcortical activation patterns for itch and pain imagery. *Pain.* (2013) 154:1989–98. doi: 10.1016/j.pain.2013.06.007
41. Mochizuki H, Schut C, Nattkemper LA, Yosipovitch G. Brain mechanism of itch in atopic dermatitis and its possible alteration through non-invasive treatments. *Allergol Int.* (2017) 66:14–21. doi: 10.1016/j.alit.2016.08.013
42. Mochizuki H, Yosipovitch G. Neuroimaging of itch as a tool of assessment of chronic itch and its management. *Handb Exp Pharmacol.* (2015) 226:57–70. doi: 10.1007/978-3-662-44605-8_4
43. Papoiu AD, Nattkemper LA, Sanders KM, Kraft RA, Chan YH, Coghill RC, et al. Brain's reward circuits mediate itch relief. A functional MRI study of active scratching *PLoS ONE.* (2013) 8:e82389. doi: 10.1371/journal.pone.0082389
44. Akiyama T, Carstens E. Neural processing of itch. *Neuroscience.* (2013) 250:697–714. doi: 10.1016/j.neuroscience.2013.07.035
45. Mochizuki H, Kakigi R. Central mechanisms of itch. *Clin Neurophysiol.* (2015) 126:1650–60. doi: 10.1016/j.clinph.2014.11.019
46. Dong X, Dong X. Peripheral and central mechanisms of itch. *Neuron.* (2018) 98:482–94. doi: 10.1016/j.neuron.2018.03.023
47. Roberts CA, Stancak A, Fallon N, Thomas A, Kirkham TC. Where is itch represented in the brain, and how does it differ from pain? an activation likelihood estimation meta-analysis of experimentally-induced itch. *J Invest Dermatol.* (2019) 139:2245–8. doi: 10.1016/j.jid.2019.04.007
48. Najafi P, Carré JL, Ben Salem D, Brenaut E, Misery L, Dufor O. Central mechanisms of itch: a systematic literature review and meta-analysis. *J Neuroradiol.* (2020) 47:450–7. doi: 10.1016/j.neurad.2019.11.005
49. Van Laarhoven AIM, Vogelaar ML, Wilder-Smith OH, Van Riel PLCM, Van De Kerkhof PCM, Kraaimaat FW, et al. Induction of nocebo and placebo effects on itch and pain by verbal suggestions. *Pain.* (2011) 152:1486–94. doi: 10.1016/j.pain.2011.01.043
50. Ji RR. Neuroimmune interactions in itch: do chronic itch, chronic pain, and chronic cough share similar mechanisms? *Pulm Pharmacol Ther.* (2015) 35:81–6. doi: 10.1016/j.pupt.2015.09.001
51. Schmelz M. Neurophysiology and itch pathways. *Handb Exp Pharmacol.* (2015) 226:39–55. doi: 10.1007/978-3-662-44605-8_3
52. Evers AWM, Colloca L, Blease C, Atlas LY, Benedetti F, Bingel U, et al. Implications of placebo and nocebo effects for clinical practice: expert consensus. *Psychother Psychosom.* (2018) 87:204–10. doi: 10.1159/000490354
53. Misery L. Are pruritus and scratching the cough of the skin? *Dermatology.* (2008) 216:3–5. doi: 10.1159/000109351
54. Trouvin AP, Perrot S. New concepts of pain. *Best Pract Res Clin Rheumatol.* (2019) 33:101415. doi: 10.1016/j.berh.2019.04.007
55. Kosek E, Cohen M, Baron R, Gebhart GF, Mico JA, Rice ASC, et al. Do we need a third mechanistic descriptor for chronic pain states? *Pain.* (2016) 157:1382–6. doi: 10.1097/j.pain.0000000000000507
56. Giesecke T, Gracely RH, Grant MA, Nachemson A, Petzke F, Williams DA, et al. Evidence of augmented central pain processing in idiopathic chronic low back pain. *Arthritis Rheum.* (2004) 50:613. doi: 10.1002/art.20063

57. Burgmer M, Pfleiderer B, Maihöfner C, Gaubitz M, Wessolleck E, Heuft G, et al. Cerebral mechanisms of experimental hyperalgesia in fibromyalgia. *Eur J Pain.* (2012) 16:636. doi: 10.1002/j.1532-2149.2011.00058.x
58. Baliki MN, Mansour AR, Baria AT, Apkarian AV. Functional reorganization of the default mode network across chronic pain conditions. *PLoS ONE.* (2014) 9:e106133. doi: 10.1371/journal.pone.0106133
59. Tesarz J, Gerhardt A, Leisner S, Janke S, Treede RD, Eich W. Distinct quantitative sensory testing profiles in nonspecific chronic back pain subjects with and without psychological trauma. *Pain.* (2016) 156:577–86. doi: 10.1097/01.j.pain.0000460350.30707.8d
60. Shigetoh H, Tanaka Y, Koga M, Osumi M, Morioka S. The mediating effect of central sensitization on the relation between pain intensity and psychological factors: a cross-sectional study with mediation analysis. *Pain Res Manag.* (2019) 2019:3916135. doi: 10.1155/2019/3916135
61. Freynhagen R, Arevalo Parada H, Calderon-Ospina CA, Chen J, Emril DR, Fernández-Villacorta FJ, et al. Current understanding of the mixed pain concept: a brief narrative review. *Curr Med Res Opin.* (2018) 27:e16. doi: 10.1080/03007995.2018.1552042
62. Pogatzki-Zahn EM, Pereira MP, Cremer A, Zeidler C, Dreyer T, Riepe C, et al. Peripheral sensitization and loss of descending inhibition is a hallmark of chronic pruritus. *J Invest Dermatol.* (2020) 140:203–11. doi: 10.1016/j.jid.2019.05.029

24

Mindfulness as Predictor of Itch Catastrophizing in Patients with Atopic Dermatitis: Results of a Cross-Sectional Questionnaire Study

Kjell Lüßmann[1], *Kerry Montgomery*[2], *Andrew Thompson*[3†], *Uwe Gieler*[4], *Christoph Zick*[5], *Joerg Kupfer*[1] *and Christina Schut*[1*]

[1] Institute of Medical Psychology, Justus-Liebig-University, Giessen, Germany, [2] Department of Psychology, University of Sheffield, Sheffield, United Kingdom, [3] South Wales Doctorate in Clinical Psychology, Cardiff University, Wales, United Kingdom, [4] Uwe Gieler, Department of Dermatology, Justus-Liebig-University, Giessen, Germany, Clinic of Psychosomatics, Vitos Clinic, Giessen, Germany, [5] Department of Dermatology, Rehabilitation Center Borkum Riff, Borkum, Germany

***Correspondence:**
Christina Schut
Christina.Schut@mp.jlug.de

†ORCID:
Andrew Thompson
orcid.org/0000-0001-6788-7222

Itch and worry about itch are predominant symptoms in atopic dermatitis (AD). Mindfulness refers to paying attention in a certain way, non-judgementally and on purpose. In patients with chronic pain, which shares several similarities with chronic itch, a significant relationship between pain intensity, mindfulness and pain catastrophizing has been found. The aim of this study was to investigate whether itch intensity and mindfulness are related to itch catastrophizing in AD patients. Participants receiving treatment for AD ($n = 155$; 58 male; mean age: 46.5 ± 12 years) completed measures of itch-related catastrophizing (Itch Cognitions Questionnaire; ICQ) and mindfulness (Comprehensive Inventory of Mindfulness; CHIME) during their stay at a rehabilitation center in Borkum, Germany. In addition to other variables, their average itch intensity during the last 2 weeks was assessed by means of a visual analog scale. A positive relationship between itch intensity and itch catastrophizing was found ($r = 0.409$; $p < 0.01$). Moreover, the mindfulness scales "acting with awareness," "accepting and non-judgemental orientation," and "non-reactive orientation" were negatively related to itch catastrophizing. A linear regression analysis revealed that itch intensity in combination with "acting with awareness" was able to explain more than 27 % (corrected $R^2 = 0.274$; $p < 0.001$) of the variance of itch catastrophizing. Thus, itch intensity and certain facets of mindfulness were associated with itch catastrophizing in AD patients. Psychological interventions aiming to increase acting with awareness might have a buffering effect on itch catastrophizing, which in turn could lead to lower itch intensity in patients with AD. Future RCTs should test this hypothesis.

Keywords: itch, atopic dermatitis, mindfulness, rehabilitation, itch catastrophizing

INTRODUCTION

Itch or pruritus is an unpleasant bodily sensation usually accompanied by scratching behavior (1). When itch lasts longer than 6 weeks, it is regarded as chronic (2). Chronic itch is a common symptom in patients with skin diseases like atopic dermatitis (AD) (3). It has been shown that itch and scratching behavior play a role in the maintenance and exacerbation of AD as the mechanic stimulation of the skin through scratching can provoke increased inflammation whilst also removing any topical treatments that have been applied (4). Further inflammation then subsequently triggers an additional itch sensation.

In addition to the direct behavior of scratching, psychological, and social factors play an important role in the maintenance and worsening of the itch-scratch cycle in AD. The biopsychosocial model of chronic itch (5) proposes that internal (e.g., personality) and external factors (e.g., stress) can lead to illness cognitions, social reactions, and behaviors, which can increase physiological responses (e.g., activation of certain brain areas) leading to itch (5). Studies have reported that excessive worrying about the skin condition is associated with the severity of physical symptoms in AD and psoriasis (6). Schut et al. (7) found a significant correlation between perceived stress, cognitive coping, and itch intensity in patients with AD. In this study, the relationship between stress and itch was mediated by itch-related cognitions and patients, who reacted to stress with negative itch-related cognitions reported higher itch intensities than patients with the opposite cognitive reaction (7).

Mindfulness has been defined as "paying attention to the present moment, non-judgmentally and on purpose" [(8), p4]. Sometimes, the term mindfulness is understood as synonym of meditation. However, psychological models of "mindfulness" posit that the construct is made up of a number of different facets (9). Further, these facets are believed to be present to varying degrees in all individuals and as such are thought to some extent to represent "personality" variables. Thus, mindfulness comprises more than just emotional awareness, but also e.g., awareness of surrounding others, things, acting consciously (9). These facets of mindfulness have been found to be significantly associated with wellbeing (10). As postulated by Shenefelt (11) mindfulness could help via psychoneuroimmunological pathways to reduce itch. In a dermatology sample mindfulness explained a significant proportion of the variance in social anxiety, anxiety, depression, and health-related quality of life after controlling for subjective severity of the skin condition (12). Moreover, there is some evidence that mindfulness based interventions can have a positive effect on the skin status and wellbeing of patients with psoriasis that can also be accompanied by itch [e.g., (13–15)]. Whether also participation in a *short* 2-week-mindfulness-based intervention delivered at a German rehabilitation clinic is beneficial in patients with the chronic, in many cases itchy skin disease psoriasis is investigated at the moment (16).

Itch shares some similarity with pain (17) as both are unpleasant sensations with common pathophysiological features (18). In patients with chronic pain, mindfulness predicted pain catastrophizing and moderated the relationship between pain intensity and pain catastrophizing (19). Increasing levels of mindfulness can be effective in reducing the experience of pain (20), which may have important implications for people living with AD given the significant association between itch and chronic pain (21). Therefore, the current study aims to investigate the relationship between itch intensity, mindfulness and itch catastrophizing in patients with chronic itch. It is hypothesized that in addition to itch intensity, levels of mindfulness will be significant predictors of itch catastrophizing. In this context, catastrophizing refers to a negative way of thinking about the bodily symptom itch, e.g., the course or consequences of it. Such negative thoughts measured in this study are "The itching will never stop," "I will scratch myself again until I look horrible" (22).

MATERIALS AND METHODS

Inclusion and Exclusion Criteria and Procedure

Participants were receiving treatment at the rehabilitation clinic on Borkum, Germany and were assessed for eligibility and recruited to the study by KL (medical student) and CZ (Consultant and Lead Dermatologist). Inclusion criteria included being between the ages of 18–70 and having a verified diagnosis of atopic dermatitis of at least 1 year duration. In order to ensure that participants could complete the survey, proficiency in the German language was also required. Exclusion criteria included having a comorbid severe psychological or psychiatric condition or another skin disease associated with itch, or having another long-term disease which was in the focus at the time of investigation. Participants were asked to complete the questionnaires and return them during their 1st week at the clinic.

Ethics

Ethical approval was gained at the University of Gießen (AZ: 210/15). Information on the study was provided to all participants who signed the consent form before filling in the questionnaires.

Measures

Mindfulness

The Comprehensive inventory of mindfulness experiences (CHIME) (9) was used to measure different facets of mindfulness. It provides a multi-dimensional assessment of mindfulness and consists of 37 items measured on a six-point scale (1-6). Participants were asked to rate levels of mindfulness over the last 2 weeks. Eight subscales of mindfulness were measured; (1) awareness toward internal experiences, (2) awareness toward external experiences, (3) acting with awareness, (4) accepting and non-judgemental orientation, (5) non-reactivity, (6) openness to experiences, (7) relativity of thoughts, and (8) insightful understanding.

Itch Catastrophizing

The Itch Cognitions Questionnaire (22, 23) was used to measure itch catastrophizing. Participants were asked to rate the frequency of thoughts they had regarding itch over the past 2 weeks, for

TABLE 1 | Description of the sample ($n = 155$ patients with atopic dermatitis).

Gender	Female 97 (62.6%)	Male 58 (37.4%)	Missing data /
Age (x ± SD)	46.8 ± 11.5	46 ± 13.0	/
Education	No formal qualification: $n = 1$ Secondary school qualification: $n = 70$ College or university degree: $n = 26$	No formal qualification: $n = 2$ Secondary school qualification: $n = 41$ College or university degree: $n = 15$	/
Self-reported physical comorbidities	Yes: $n = 48$	Yes: $n = 38$	/
CHIME 1 (x ± SD)	4.49 ± 0.89	4.39 ± 0.86	/
CHIME 2 (x ± SD)	4.84 ± 0.96	4.57 ± 0.81	/
CHIME 3 (x ± SD)	3.97 ± 1.00	3.95 ± 0.89	/
CHIME 4 (x ± SD)	3.25 ± 1.07	3.34 ± 0.99	/
CHIME 5 (x ± SD)	3.48 ± 0.98	3.47 ± 0.89	1
CHIME 6 (x ± SD)	3.75 ± 1.00	3.74 ± 0.68	1
CHIME 7 (x ± SD)	3.84 ± 1.01	3.73 ± 0.72	1
CHIME 8 (x ± SD)	3.91 ± 0.89	3.75 ± 0.81	/
Itch Inten (x ± SD)	5.32 ± 2.68	5.89 ± 2.27	2
Itch Cat (x ± SD)	2.34 ± 0.87	2.33 ± 0.95	5
PO-SCORAD (x ± SD)	46.69 ± 20.55	49.74 ± 18.96	20

Itch Cat, Itch Catastrophizing; Itch Inten, Itch Intensity; values for the CHIME-scales can range from 1 to 6 and values for Itch Cat can range from 0 to 4. x, mean; SD, standard deviation.
CHIME 1: awareness toward internal experiences.
CHIME 2: awareness toward external experiences.
CHIME 3: acting with awareness.
CHIME 4: accepting and non-judgemental orientation.
CHIME 5: non-reactivity.
CHIME 6: openness to experiences.
CHIME 7: relativity of thoughts.
CHIME 8: insightful understanding.

example "*The itching will get worse and worse.*" The questionnaire consists of 20 statements measured on a five-point Likert scale ranging from 0 (thought never occurs) to 4 (the thought usually occurs) which can be combined to the two scales "itch catastrophizing" and "itch coping." In the current study we were only interested in the scale "itch catastrophizing."

Itch Intensity

Itch intensity during the last 2 weeks was measured by a visual analog scale ranging from 0 to 10. The item to measure itch was "Please evaluate on this scale how intense your itch was on average during the last 2 weeks."

Atopic Dermatitis Severity—Self Report

The Patient Orientated SCORing Dermatitis Index (PO-SCORAD) (24) was used to measure the self-rated severity of AD. Participants indicate the area of the body affected (POSCORAD-A), the severity of the condition including redness, scratch lesions, skin dryness, edema, and skin thickening (POSCORAD-B). In addition, using visual analog scales participants indicated the severity of itching and insomnia (POSCORAD-C). As for the SCORAD, also POSCORAD scores can range from 0 to 103 with higher scores indicating a more severe AD. SCORAD-scores below 25 indicate a mild AD, scores between 25 and 50 indicate a moderate AD and scores > 50 indicate a severe AD (25). In former studies, it was shown that SCORAD scores rated by clinicians and PO-SCORAD scores rated by patients highly correlate (24, 26).

Other Variables

Besides the before mentioned variables, further data on alexithymia, self-rated causes of itch, sociodemographic variables and comorbidities were gathered which are included in the doctoral thesis of the first author of this article.

Statistical Analysis

Statistical analyses were conducted using SPSS 24. Due to the fact that variables were not normally distributed in all cases, Spearman-Rank-correlations were conducted in addition to Pearson correlations to investigate the associations between mindfulness, itch catastrophizing, and itch intensity. These analyses did not reveal substantially different results (differences in r's < 0.045). After testing whether the assumptions for a linear regression analysis (27) were fulfilled this method was used to investigate how much variance in itch catastrophizing could be predicted by itch intensity and the mindfulness subscales related to itch catastrophizing in the correlation analyses ("method of best predictors"). In the regression model, the control variables age and sex were entered in the first step of the analysis, itch intensity during the last 2 weeks was entered in the second step and the mindfulness subscales were entered in step three of the analysis.

TABLE 2 | Results of the *correlation* analyses.

		0: Itch Cat	1	2	3	4	5	6	7	8	9	10
1	Itch Inten	**0.409****	1									
2	CHIME 1	0.039	−0.071	1								
3	CHIME 2	−0.088	−0.044	**0.635*****	1							
4	CHIME 3	**−0.373*****	−0.130	**0.190***	**0.250****	1						
5	CHIME 4	**−0.198***	−0.129	**0.243****	**0.333*****	**0.352*****	1					
6	CHIME 5	**−0.260****	−0.053	**0.383*****	**0.503*****	**0.375*****	**0.577*****	1				
7	CHIME 6	0.084	−0.085	−0.003	0.054	**−0.264*****	**−0.214****	−0.029	1			
8	CHIME 7	0.006	−0.087	**0.425*****	**0.359*****	0.000	0.138	**−258****	**0.189***	1		
9	CHIME 8	−0.028	−0.074	**0.401*****	**0.445*****	0.014	**0.261*****	**0.441*****	**0.163***	**0.608*****	1	
10	Age	−0.157	**−0.166***	−0.034	0.119	**0.189***	0.041	0.154	−0.109	−0.063	−0.006	1
11	Sex	0.004	−0.109	0.059	0.089	0.012	−0.040	0.005	0.006	0.062	0.089	0.031

Shown are correlations between itch catastrophizing, average itch intensity during the last 2 weeks, the eight mindfulness scales measured by CHIME and sex and age. Bold numbers indicate significant correlations.
****Indicate that the correlation is significant on the 0.001 niveau,*
***indicate that the correlation is significant on the 0.01 niveau, *indicates that the correlation is significant on the 0.05 niveau.*
The number of patients included in the analyses varies between n = 149 and 155.
Itch Cat, Itch Catastrophizing; Itch Inten, Itch Intensity.
CHIME 1: awareness toward internal experiences.
CHIME 2: awareness toward external experiences.
CHIME 3: acting with awareness.
CHIME 4: accepting and non-judgmental orientation.
CHIME 5: non-reactivity.
CHIME 6: openness to experiences.
CHIME 7: relativity of thoughts.
CHIME 8: insightful understanding.

RESULTS

Sample Characteristics

One hundred and sixty three AD patients took part in the study, 8 had to be excluded from the analyses, because they did not fulfill the inclusion criteria. Thus, the final sample size consisted of 155 AD patients (58 men and 97 women). Their mean age (data available from all $n = 155$) was 46.5 ± 12 years. Their mean AD severity (data available from $n = 135$ patients) measured by the PO-SCORAD was 47.9 ± 19.9, which indicates that on average patients suffered from a moderate AD. Twenty-one patients had mild AD, 72 moderate and 42 severe AD. Patients who reported to have a physical comorbidity did not differ from patients without self-reported physical comorbidity regarding itch-catastrophizing ($p = 0.763$) or itch-intensity ($p = 0.337$). For more information regarding the sample characteristics, please see **Table 1**.

Results of the Correlation Analyses

The Pearson correlation analyses revealed that itch catastrophizing and itch intensity during the last 2 weeks were significantly positively related ($r = 0.409$). Moreover, itch catastrophizing was significantly negatively related to the mindfulness subscales acting with awareness ($r = -0.373$), accepting and non-judgemental orientation ($r = -0.198$) and non-reactivity ($r = -0.260$). For the full correlation matrix, please see **Table 2**. Spearman-Rank-correlations also revealed significant correlations between itch-catastrophizing and the mindfulness subscales "acting with awareness," "accepting and non-judgemental orientation," and "non-reactivity" ($p < 0.05$).

Results of the Regression Analyses

The regression analysis showed that 27.4 % of the variance of itch catastrophizing could be predicted by itch intensity and the mindfulness-scale "acting with awareness" ($R^2 = 0.284$; corrected $R^2 = 0.274$; $F = 28.728$; $p < 0.001$). Hereby, 17.1% of the variance were explained by itch-intensity and 10.3% by the mindfulness-scale "acting with awareness" (also see **Figure 1**).

DISCUSSION

The current study is the first to examine the relationship between mindfulness and itch and mindfulness and itch-catastrophizing in patients with AD. There was no significant relationship between itch intensity and mindfulness; however, there was a significant negative relationship between the mindfulness scale "acting with awareness" and itch catastrophizing.

This finding is in line with the results of previous studies in which mindfulness and especially the mindfulness facets "acting with awareness" and non-reactivity were related to pain catastrophizing and other types of psychological distress (12, 19). This is an important finding as catastrophic thoughts and physiological reactivity are important maintaining factors to itch (6). Furthermore, studies using itch induction suggest that a focus on bodily sensations and catastrophizing of upcoming itch stimuli

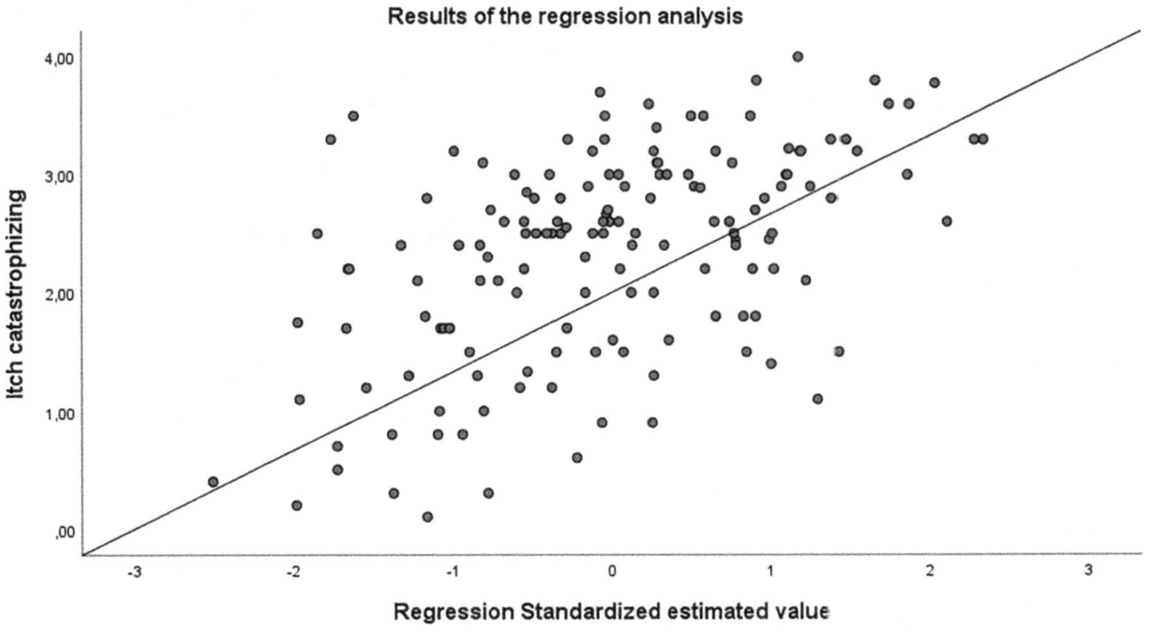

FIGURE 1 | Results of the regression analysis. 27.4% of itch catastrophizing could be explained by itch intensity during the last 2 weeks and the mindfulness scale "acting with awareness".

lead to greater itch intensity or more profound scratching behavior (28, 29).

Our findings suggest that acting with awareness, essentially being more aware of bodily sensations and not reacting to them automatically, may reduce the likelihood of automatic scratching in response to itch. This in turn could then lead to less negative thinking about the skin as skin lesions would not occur that often anymore. In this context, it has already been shown that higher levels of present moment awareness can reduce negative thinking, a characteristic of depression and anxiety (30).

Intervention studies have shown promising results for mindfulness interventions in patients living with long term health conditions and chronic pain (31, 32). In dermatology, mindfulness interventions have been used in patients living with psoriasis with promising results (13, 14, 33). Audio-guided meditations used as an adjunct to light treatment increased the rates of skin clearing (13), and a structured 8-week mindfulness intervention, Mindfulness-based cognitive group therapy, was found to improve dermatology quality of life and self-reported psoriasis severity (14). In atopic dermatitis first results of positive effects in a small patient therapy group were demonstrated (34). However, D'Alton et al. (33) conducted a randomized controlled trial of mindfulness-based interventions in psoriasis and found that whilst participants reported perceiving the interventions as beneficial, there was no significant difference found on distress, symptom burden, or quality of life at completion, or at 6 or 12-month follow-up. Clearly, whilst mindfulness interventions show promise, and our study further supports the theoretical rationale for using it as an intervention where itch is a factor, further examination of mindfulness interventions in a range of skin conditions is required.

Limitations

There are limitations to the current study. First, this study is a cross-sectional study and therefore conclusions on causation cannot be drawn. Randomized, controlled trials in which "acting with awareness" as one important facet of mindfulness is manipulated by participation in a mindfulness based intervention could provide answers on causal relationships between mindfulness and itch/itch catastrophizing. Further, as participants were recruited at a rehabilitation clinic and were experiencing moderate or severe AD in most cases, the generalisability of our findings to community samples needs to be acknowledged, and be investigated in future studies. In addition, given that AD is known to be associated with anxiety and depression future studies might investigate the role that both "acting with awareness" and catastrophizing play in significant psychological distress associated with AD.

CONCLUSION

The current study findings indicate that higher levels of a specific facet of mindfulness termed "acting with awareness" are related to lower levels of itch catastrophizing. This finding is important as it suggests that psychological interventions should seek to increase acting with awareness in patients with AD as a way of improving patient outcomes associated with problematic itch.

ETHICS STATEMENT

The studies involving human participants were reviewed and approved by Ethics Committee of the Department of Medicine at Justus-Liebig-University. The patients/participants provided their written informed consent to participate in this study.

AUTHOR CONTRIBUTIONS

KL collected the data in this project, contributed to the statistical analyses, and presentation of the results. KM contributed to the first draft of the paper and analyses of the data. AT contributed to study design, writing the theoretical background, and discussion section of the article. UG contributed to the study design. CZ contributed to data collection. JK contributed to the study design and the analyses of the data. CS contributed to the study design, statistical analyses, presentation of the study results and writing the manuscript. All authors critically reviewed the manuscript.

ACKNOWLEDGMENTS

Part of these data have been presented by Dr. CS at the World Congress of Itch in Wroclaw in 2017 as well as at the Conference on Health Psychology in Siegen, Germany, in 2017. These data are part of the doctoral thesis of KL, who presented some of the data also during the second Science Day at the Justus-Liebig-University in Gießen in November 2018.

REFERENCES

1. Hafenreffer S. *Nosodochium, in quo cutis, eique adaerentium partium, affectus omnes, singulari methodo, et cognoscendiet curandi fidelissime traduntur.* Ulm: Kühn (1660).
2. Ständer S, Weisshaar E, Mettang T, Szepietowski JC, Carstens E, Ikoma A, et al. Clinical classification of itch: a position paper of the International Forum for the Study of Itch. *Acta Derm Venereol.* (2007) 87:291–4. doi: 10.2340/00015555-0305
3. Hanifin JM, Rajka G. Diagnostic features of atopic dermatitis. *Acta Derm Venereol.* (1980) 1980:44–7.
4. Leung DY, Boguniewicz M, Howell MD, Nomura I, Hamid QA. New insights into atopic dermatitis. *J Clin Invest.* (2004) 113:651–7. doi: 10.1172/JCI21060
5. Verhoeven EW, de Klerk S, Kraaimaat FW, van de Kerkhof PC, de Jong EM, Evers A, et al. Biopsychosocial mechanisms of chronic itch in patients with skin diseases: a review. *Acta Derm Venereol.* (2008) 88:211–8. doi: 10.2340/00015555-0452
6. Verhoeven L, Kraaimaat F, Duller P, van de Kerkhof P, Evers, A. Cognitive, behavioral, and physiological reactivity to chronic itching: analogies to chronic pain. *Int J Behav Med.* (2006) 13:237–43. doi: 10.1207/s15327558ijbm1303_7
7. Schut C, Weik U, Tews N, Gieler U, Deinzer R, Kupfer J. Coping as mediator of the relationship between stress and itch in patients with atopic dermatitis: a regression and mediation analysis. *Exp Dermatol.* (2015) 24:148–50. doi: 10.1111/exd.12578
8. Kabat-Zinn J. *Wherever You Go, There You Are: Mindfulness Meditation in Everyday Life.* New York, NY: Hyperion (1994).
9. Bergomi C, Tschacher W, Kupper Z. Construction and first validation of the comprehensive inventory of mindfulness experiences. *Diagnostica.* (2014) 60:111–25. doi: 10.1026/0012-1924/a000109
10. Baer RA, Smith GT, Hopkins J, Krietemeyer J, Toney L. Using self-report assessment methods to explore facets of mindfulness. *Assessment.* (2006) 13:27–45. doi: 10.1177/1073191105283504
11. Shenefelt PD. Mindfulness-based cognitive hypnotherapy and skin disorders. *Am J Clin Hypn.* (2018) 61:34–44. doi: 10.1080/00029157.2017.1419457
12. Montgomery K, Norman P, Messenger AG, Thompson AR. The importance of mindfulness in psychosocial distress and quality of life in dermatology patients. *Br J Dermatol.* (2016) 175:930–6. doi: 10.1111/bjd.14719
13. Kabat-Zinn J, Wheeler E, Light T, Skillings A, Scharf MJ, Cropley TG, et al. Influence of a mindfulness meditation-based stress reduction intervention on rates of skin clearing in patients with moderate to severe psoriasis undergoing phototherapy (UVB) and photochemotherapy (PUVA). *Psychosom Med.* (1998) 60:625–32. doi: 10.1097/00006842-199809000-00020
14. Fordham B, Griffiths CE, Bundy C. A pilot study examining mindfulness-based cognitive therapy in psoriasis. *Psychol Health Med.* (2015) 20:121–27. doi: 10.1080/13548506.2014.902483
15. Montgomery K, Thompson AR. The potential role of mindfulness in psychosocial support for dermatology patients. *Clinics Dermatol.* (2018) 36:743–7. doi: 10.1016/j.clindermatol.2018.08.010
16. Stadtmüller L, Eckardt M, Zick C, Kupfer J, Schut C. Investigation of predictors of interest in a brief mindfulness-based intervention and its effects in patients with psoriasis at a rehabilitation clinic (SkinMind): an observational study and randomised controlled trial. *BMJ Open.* (2020) 10:e033952. doi: 10.1136/bmjopen-2019-033952
17. Andrew D, Craig AD. Spinothalamic lamina I neurons selectively sensitive to histamine: a central neural pathway for itch. *Nat Neurosci.* (2001) 4:72–7. doi: 10.1038/82924
18. Yosipovitch G, Greaves MW, Schmelz M. Itch. *Lancet.* (2003) 361:690–4. doi: 10.1016/S0140-6736(03)12570-6
19. Schütze R, Rees C, Preece M, Schütze M. Low mindfulness predicts pain catastrophizing in a fear-avoidance model of chronic pain. *Pain.* (2010) 148:120–7. doi: 10.1016/j.pain.2009.10.030
20. Chiesa A, Serretti A. Mindfulness-based interventions for chronic pain: a systematic review of the evidence. *J Altern Complement Med.* (2011) 17:83–93. doi: 10.1089/acm.2009.0546
21. Dalgard F, Dawn AG, Yosipovitch G. Are itch and chronic pain associated in adults? Results of a large population survey in Norway. *Dermatology.* (2007) 214:305–9. doi: 10.1159/000100881
22. Heckman CJ, Schut C, Riley M, Ehlers A, Valdes-Rodriguez R, Kupfer J. Development and psychometrics of the English version of the Itch Cognitions Questionnaire. *PLoS One.* (2020) 15:e0230585. doi: 10.1371/journal.pone.0230585
23. Ehlers A, Stangier U, Dohn D, Gieler U. Kognitive Faktoren beim juckreiz: entwicklung und validierung eines fragebogens. *Verhaltenstherapie.* (1993) 3:112–9. doi: 10.1159/000258752
24. Stalder JF, Barbarot S, Wollenberg A, Holm EA, De Raeve L, Seidenari S, et al. Patient-Oriented SCORAD (PO-SCORAD): a new self-assessment scale in atopic dermatitis validated in Europe. *Allergy.* (2011) 66:1114–21. doi: 10.1111/j.1398-9995.2011.02577.x
25. Oranje AP. Practical issues on interpretation of scoring atopic dermatitis: SCORAD index, objective SCORAD, patient-oriented SCORAD and three- item severity score. *Curr Probl Dermatol.* (2011) 41:149–55. doi: 10.1159/000323308
26. Coutanceau C, Stalder F. Analysis of correlations between patient-oriented SCORAD (PO-SCORAD) and other assessment scores of atopic dermatitis severity and quality of life. *Dermatology.* (2014) 229:248–255. doi: 10.1159/000365075
27. Field A. *Discovering Statistics Using IBM SPSS Statistics: And Sex and Drugs and Rock "N" Roll,* 4th edn. *Sage* (2013).

28. Van Laarhoven AI, Kraaimaat FW, Wilder-Smith OH, Evers AW. Role of attentional focus on bodily sensations in sensitivity to itch and pain. *Acta Derm Venereol.* (2010) 90:46–51. doi: 10.2340/00015555-0743
29. Schut C, Rädel A, Frey L, Gieler U, Kupfer J. Role of personality and expectations for itch and scratching induced by audiovisual itch stimuli. *Eur J Pain.* (2016) 20:14–8. doi: 10.1002/ejp.751
30. Teasdale JD, Segal Z, Williams JMG. How does cognitive therapy prevent depressive relapse and why should attentional control (mindfulness) training help? *Behav Res Ther.* (1995) 33:25–39.
31. Baer RA. Mindfulness training as a clinical intervention: A conceptual and empirical review. *Clin Psychol Sci Pract.* (2003) 10:125–43. doi: 10.1093/clipsy.bpg015
32. Creswell JD, Lindsay EK, Villalba DK, Chin B. Mindfulness training and physical health. *Psychosom Med.* (2019) 81:224–32. doi: 10.1097/PSY.0000000000000675
33. D'Alton P, Kinsella L, Walsh O, Timoney I, Lynch M, O'Connor M, et al. Mindfulness-based interventions for psoriasis: a randomized controlled trial. *Mindfulness* (2019) 10:288–300. doi: 10.1007/s12671-018-0973-5
34. Hedman-Lagerlöf E, Bergman A, Lindefors N, Bradley M. Exposure-based cognitive therapy for atopic dermatitis: an open trial. *Cogn Behav Ther.* (2019) 48:300–10. doi: 10.1080/16506073.2018.1504320

25

Affective Touch Reduces Electrically Induced Itch Experience

Larissa L. Meijer, Zoë A. Schielen, Kim Y. van Ree and H. Chris Dijkerman*

Experimental Psychology/Helmholtz Institute, Utrecht University, Utrecht, Netherlands

***Correspondence:**
Larissa L. Meijer
l.l.meijer@uu.nl

Introduction: Itch is a common symptom in dermatologic and other diseases and can have a severe impact on quality of life and mental health. As a proportion of patients with itch-symptoms is resistant to commonly used anti-histamine treatments, development of new treatments is desirable. Past research on pain, itch and affective touch (i.e. slow, gentle stroking of the skin activating C-tactile fibers) revealed an inhibitory relationship between affective touch and pain and between pain and itch. Given the overlap in neural processing between these three sensory submodalities, a possible interaction between affective touch and itch might be expected. This study investigated whether there is a relationship between itch and affective touch, and if so, whether affective touch inhibits itch.

Methodology: Itch was electrically induced with the use of electrodes that were placed at the ventral side of the wrist of 61 participants. A within-subject design was conducted with two conditions. An experimental -affective touch- condition (stroking the forearm with a soft brush at 3 cm/s) and a control -non-affective touch- condition (stroking the forearm with a soft brush at 18 cm/s). Touch was applied on the dorsal side of the forearm, the same arm as were the electrodes were placed. For each condition itch was induced for 20 min, with every 2 min a VAS-scale measurement of the level of experienced itch.

Results: Both types of touch reduced the experienced itch compared to baseline ($p < 0.01$, partial $\eta^2 = 0.67$). However, affective touch had an additional significant relieving effect compared to non-affective touch ($p = 0.03$, partial $\eta^2 = 0.08$). The alleviation of itch started after 2 min of stroking and continued to increase up till 6 min, where after the relieving effect stabilized but still persisted.

Conclusion: This finding suggest that affective touch, as with acute pain, has a relieving effect on electrically induced itch.

Keywords: itch, affective touch, C-fibers, somatosensory, relief

INTRODUCTION

Itch is a common symptom in dermatological diseases and is defined as "an unpleasant sensation causing the urge to scratch" (1). Itch is a commonly experienced problem, with a prevalence of 8.4% in the general population. In addition, the lifetime prevalence of chronic itch is even higher with 22%, meaning that one out of five people will experience chronic itch (2). Furthermore, the burden of itch is comparable to the burden that is experienced during chronic pain and itch symptoms can significantly impact quality of life and mental health as well (3–7). Studies indicated that higher scores on an itch intensity scale in patients with dermatological diseases causing itch were related to a higher score on depression scales (7, 8). In addition, a study by Schneider et al. (9) showed that 70% of the patients in a sample of 109 participants with dermatological diseases causing itch had one to six psychiatric disorders. Given the high prevalence and impact of itch, it seems a worldwide problem (3).

One aspect of itch that has been researched considerably is the neurophysiological basis of itch. In 1997, itch-selective neurons were discovered in humans (10). Research indicated that these neurons were part of a broader category of neurons called C-afferents. These C-afferents are characterized by their lack of myelination and therefore have a slow conducting speed (1, 10, 11). After activation of the C-fibers, the signal is transported to the dorsal horn of the spinal cord from which signals are projected to the thalamus, somatosensory cortex, sensorimotor cortex, posterior cingulate cortex (PCC), anterior cingulate cortex (ACC), insular cortex, and the basal ganglia with the putamen (12, 13). The involvement of the ACC contributes to the affective component of itch (13).

Furthermore, subsequent research implied that the itch-selective neurons were sensitive to histamine, mostly associated with acute itch experience (14, 15). However, recent research revealed that some of these neurons do not respond to histamine, but are activated by other substances and stimuli (16). Consequently, a proportion of patients with itch symptoms is resistant to commonly used anti-histamine treatments (16, 17). It seems that especially chronic itch conditions are associated with non-histamine sensitive neurons and therefore respond better to treatments targeting the nerves than the immune system (14). Given the impact of (chronic) itch, development of new suitable treatments is needed.

The development of new treatments could be inspired by research on another sensory modality that affects itch, namely pain. During the processing of pain, brain areas such as the insular cortex, cingulate cortex and premotor areas are activated (18). As mentioned, these brain areas are also highly involved in the processing of itch (13). This shows the close relationship between these senses at supraspinal level (11, 15, 18). In addition, itch and pain also seem to affect each other at a behavioral level: research confirmed that painful sensations can reduce itch sensations, which explains why we scratch our skin during itch (11, 15, 19). Scratching activates interneurons in the dorsal horn of the spinal cord. These interneurons subsequently inhibit the transduction of C-afferent signals involved in itch (20–22). Because the itch-signal is inhibited by pain, the transduction of the signal from the dorsal horn of the spinal cord toward the thalamus is reduced which results in a reduction of itch sensations.

Reducing itch by evoking pain (e.g., scratching) can only be a temporary solution as it is unpleasant and can cause serious skin inflammation when used on a permanent basis. However, the interaction between pain and other systems might provide useful information on which new interventions to reduce itch can be based. An example is the interaction between pain and affective touch. Affective touch activates another subgroup of C-afferents, known as C-tactile or CT-afferents (23–25). CT-afferents are located mainly in the hairy skin and respond to slow and gentle stroking of the skin, consisting of velocities between 1 and 10 centimeters per second, with an optimal response at 3 centimeter per second, which provides a pleasant sensation (23, 26, 27). The CT-afferents transmit signals through the dorsal horn of the spinal cord to the thalamus, insula, anterior cingulate cortex (ACC), prefrontal cortex and amygdala (28). Recent research shows that affective touch and pain influence each other as well: affective touch has an inhibitory effect on acute pain (29, 30). It seems that affective touch can inhibit pain at the level of the dorsal horn of the spinal cord by a specific inhibitory pathway related to CT-fiber input (31). In addition, Gursul et al. (32) and von Mohr et al. (33) showed that at a supraspinal level, affective touch reduces activation of areas related to pain processing, namely the insula and anterior cingulate cortex. In sum, affective touch and pain share neural characteristics that are comparable to the similarities between pain and itch. Furthermore, affective touch seems to inhibit pain, as is the case for the effect of pain on itch.

The evident similarities between brain areas involved in itch, pain and affective touch, and the inhibitory behavioral effects of pain on itch and affective touch on pain, suggest that affective touch might have a relieving effect on itch (20) and the current study will research this. Itch will be induced by an electrical current stimulator, as recent research shows that this is a reliable way of inducing itch (17, 34). The relieving effect of affective touch on itch will be evaluated by testing the decrease in perceived itch in two conditions. Affective touch will be used in the experimental condition, and non-affective touch (stroking with a velocity of 18 cm/s) will be used in the control condition. Itch induction and touch stimulation will be provided simultaneously for 20 min. This time-frame is based on recent research of Sailer et al. (35) showing that the activation of brain areas related to affective touch and the perceived pleasantness of affective touch stabilizes after 20 min. Therefore, we expect that, if there is a relieving effect of affective touch, it will persist for ~20 min. In addition, perceived pleasantness of affective touch will be monitored, and the relationship between pleasantness of affective touch and its relieving effect on itch will be researched. It is expected that experiencing affective touch as more pleasant is associated with experiencing more itch relief from affective touch (36, 37). A factor that modulates how intensely itch is experienced is the amount of attentional focus. Research suggests that a high attentional focus to bodily sensations such as itch, increases the amount of experienced itch (38). Therefore, we will additionally investigate whether there is a relation between high awareness to bodily sensations and the alleviation of itch by affective touch. We expect that people who have a high attentional focus to bodily sensations, experience less relief from affective touch (39).

METHODS AND MATERIALS

Participants

An a priori calculation for the repeated measures ANOVA ($f = 0.2$, α err prob. $= 0.05$, power $= 0.95$, number of groups $= 2$, number of measurements $= 11$) recommend a sample size of 30. Eventually, 69 participants signed up for participation out of which 61 participants were eligible for participation. The study group consisted of 12 men (Mage = 27.50, range age = 18–28) and 49 women (Mage = 21.61, range age= 18–53). Of the participants, 54.1% were following or had finished tertiary education, 45.9% had finished secondary education. The participants were recruited through the Social and Behavioral Sciences research participation system (SONA) of Utrecht University. Participants from the age of 18 and older, and fluent in the Dutch language were eligible to participate in this experiment. People suffering from a skin condition where itch is a present symptom, like chronic itch or psoriasis, or people using a pacemaker, were excluded from this experiment. People using a pacemaker were not allowed to participate because of the electrical stimulation that could interfere with the functioning of the pacemaker. The faculty ethical review board of the University of Utrecht approved the study's protocol and all participants gave permission for participating in this experiment by means of a written informed consent.

Materials

Demographical Information

To verify the inclusion and exclusion criteria the participants were asked to state their age, gender, highest completed education, whether they were suffering from skin conditions, and whether they were using a pacemaker.

Pain and Vigilance Attention Questionnaire (PVAQ)

To examine the awareness to bodily sensations, an adjusted version of the Pain Vigilance and Awareness Questionnaire (PVAQ) was used (40). Originally, this questionnaire was focused on pain. As claimed by van Laarhoven et al. (34), the questionnaire is suitable to investigate itch, when changing the word "pain" to "physical sensations." This alteration had no consequences for the reliability or validity of the PVAQ. The questions of the PVAQ focus on sensing, ignoring and monitoring bodily sensations. The PVAQ consists of 16 items, which are scored on a 6-point Likert scale. Zero represents "never," 5 represents "always." Items 8 and 16 should be reverse-scored before the total score of the PVAQ can be calculated. A relatively low score on the PVAQ indicated low attention to bodily sensations. A relatively high score represented high attentional focus on bodily sensations.

Itch Induction

An electrical stimulus was used to induce itch. According to Ikoma et al. (17) and van Laarhoven et al. (34), using a constant current stimulator (Isolated Bipolar Constant Current Stimulator DS7, Digitimer, United Kingdom) is a reliable way to induce itch. Nerve stimulation electrodes were attached to the ventral side of the wrist, alternately to the right or left wrist equally divided among the participants. The DS7 had a default setting where the pulse duration was set at 100 milliseconds and the compliance voltage was set at 200 volts. E-prime 2.0 (Psychology Software Tools, 2015) was used to alter the pulse duration of the DS7. A transmission of a constant stimulation of 50 Hz by having a pulse duration of 20 milliseconds was programmed. These pulses were active for 0.2 milliseconds and inactive for 19.8 milliseconds. The level of amperage (in milliampere) was individually adjusted prior to the experiment and was determined based on the participants' experienced level of itch. A stimulation period of 4 s was used to test the itch stimulation, the experienced itch was rated on the VAS. After each VAS rating, the amperage was increased, by steps of 0.1–0.2 mA, until the participants considered the experienced itch a 7 or higher on the VAS. If participants did experience itch but did not report higher than a 7 on the VAS, the highest rating of the experienced itch was registered. The corresponding amperage was used in the experiment. The level of amperage ranged from 1.80 to 4.90 ($M_{amperage} = 3.02$, $SD_{amperage} = 0.76$). When participants did not experience any itch or the experienced itch intensity was not rated with a three or higher, the experiment was discontinued.

Affective and Non-Affective Touch

The (non-)affective touch stimulation was executed by stroking with a soft foundation brush. The velocity of stroking in the experimental affective touch condition was 3 centimeters per second. The velocity of stroking in the control non-affective touch condition was 18 centimeters per second. The researcher marked the length of 6 centimeters on the dorsal side of the arm to which the electrode was attached. This enabled the researcher to stroke with the correct velocity during the affective touch and non-affective touch condition (thus in the affective touch condition, the 6 cm length was stroked over 2 s, while in the non-affective touch condition the 6 cm length was stroked 3 times per second).

Monitoring Sensations

Visual Analog Scale (VAS) for Itch

To measure itch, participants were asked to indicate the degree of itch they experienced on a scale of 0 to 10. Zero represented "no itch" and 10 represented "unbearable itch."

VAS for Pleasantness

To measure the experienced pleasantness of stroking, participants were asked to rate the experienced pleasantness on a scale that ranged from 0 to 10, where 0 represented "very unpleasant" and 10 represented "very pleasant." The VAS is evaluated as a reliable and valid assessment to measure itch and pleasantness (35, 41).

Procedure

Prior to the experiment participants filled in the demographical details and the PVAQ. The baseline itch intensity was registered before each condition. Hereafter, the baseline pleasantness of touch was determined and registered by stroking the arm for 10 s over the 6 cm outline at either affective or non-affective touch velocities. The participant underwent an experimental and control condition which both had a duration of 20 min, the order was randomized between subjects. Between the conditions there was a 10 min break. Each condition had 10 blocks of 2 min simultaneous stimulation from the DS7 and stroking. Immediately following every 2 min of itch stimulation and stroking, the participants were asked to rate the experienced itch

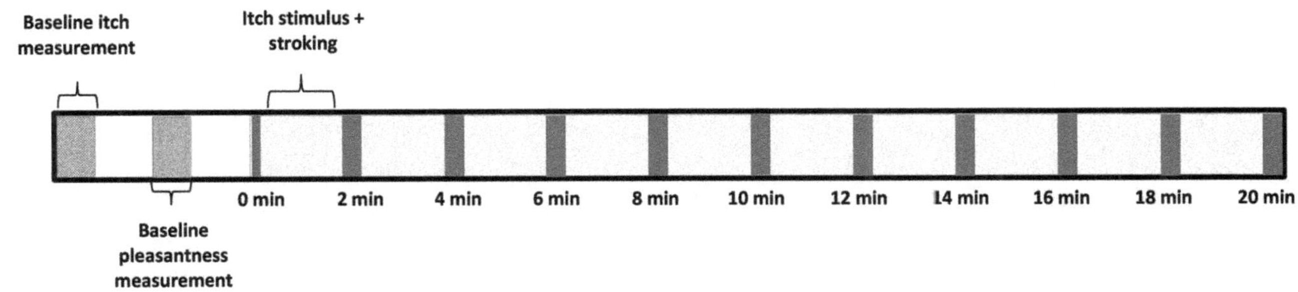

FIGURE 1 | Outline in time of a single condition.

TABLE 1 | The mean scores, SE and range of VAS scores of the affective and non-affective touch condition, the PVAQ score and the difference scores of itch and pleasantness ($N = 61$).

	Mean ± SE	Range
Affective touch		
Baseline itch VAS score	6.80 ± 0.16	3.00–9.00
2-min measurement itch VAS score	3.83 ± 0.29	0.00–8.50
4-min measurement itch VAS score	3.57 ± 0.29	0.00–8.00
6-min measurement itch VAS score	3.39 ± 0.32	0.00–9.00
8-min measurement itch VAS score	3.60 ± 0.32	0.00–9.00
10-min measurement itch VAS score	3.80 ± 0.34	0.00–9.00
12-min measurement itch VAS score	3.82 ± 0.35	0.00–9.00
14-min measurement itch VAS score	4.06 ± 0.33	0.00–9.00
16-min measurement itch VAS score	4.17 ± 0.35	0.00–9.00
18-min measurement itch VAS score	4.16 ± 0.35	0.00–9.00
20-min measurement itch VAS score	4.24 ± 0.38	0.00–9.00
Baseline pleasantness VAS score	6.82 ± 0.22	0.00–10.00
Non-Affective touch		
Baseline itch VAS score	6.75 ± 0.21	2.00–10.00
2-min measurement itch VAS score	4.00 ± 0.34	0.00–9.00
4-min measurement itch VAS score	4.24 ± 0.34	0.00–9.00
6-min measurement itch VAS score	4.37 ± 0.34	0.00–9.00
8-min measurement itch VAS score	4.22 ± 0.35	0.00–9.00
10-min measurement itch VAS score	4.40 ± 0.33	0.00–9.00
12-min measurement itch VAS score	4.41 ± 0.36	0.00–9.00
14-min measurement itch VAS score	4.34 ± 0.35	0.00–9.00
16-min measurement itch VAS score	4.56 ± 0.36	0.00–9.00
18-min measurement itch VAS score	4.77 ± 0.37	0.00–9.50
20-min measurement itch VAS score	4.77 ± 0.38	0.00–9.50
Baseline pleasantness VAS score	5.24 ± 0.23	1.00–9.00
PVAQ Score	37.25 ± 1.35	13–62
Difference score of VAS scores for itch	0.55 ± 0.24	−3.20–5.00
Difference score of VAS scores for pleasantness	−1.58 ± 0.31	−6.00–8.50

*Data of **Table 1** are partly visualized in **Figures 2, 3**.*

on the VAS. This took ~10 s. Hereafter the next 2 min of itch stimulation and stroking started (**Figure 1**).

Statistical Analysis

Data was analyzed using SPSS Statistics (version 26). Eight participants were excluded and the experiment was discontinued because they did not experience itch. Data was checked for normal distribution. For the VAS itch intensity scores, which were analyzed with a repeated measures ANOVA, the residuals were used. According to the Shapiro–Wilk test most variables were not normally distributed, but the Shapiro–Wilk test is shown to be too sensitive in a large sample size (>50). Therefore, data was also visually inspected using the Q-Q plots and histograms, these showed that the data was approximately normally distributed. Based on these factors, together with the large sample size (>60), we decided that parametric testing was permitted (42, 43). The sphericity was mildly violated, therefore the Greenhouse-Geisser Epsilon output was used.

The VAS pleasantness scores were also checked for normality. The VAS scores for pleasantness in the affective touch condition violated the assumption of normality. The VAS scores for pleasantness in the non-affective condition did not violate the assumption of normality. The differences between the pleasantness of touch in the affective and non-affective condition were checked with a paired t-test.

In order to analyze the difference between the effect of affective touch and non-affective touch on itch, a repeated measures ANOVA was conducted, with touch (affective and non-affective touch) and time (baseline and the 10 timepoints within a 20-min period on which itch was measured) as independent variables and the experienced itch measured with VAS scores as dependent variable.

To analyze the changes in the relieving effect of affective touch on itch over time, a repeated measures ANOVA with contrasts (follow-up analysis) was conducted with the itch ratings from the experimental and control conditions excluding the baseline itch measurements. Every 2-min itch measurement was compared to the first 2-min itch measurement. This resulted in nine contrast analyses.

To assess the effect that attention to bodily sensations has on the effect of affective touch on itch, a Spearman correlation with the difference scores between itch ratings in the non-affective and affective touch conditions and the PVAQ scores was conducted. The mean of the 10 measurements in the non-affective condition was subtracted from that of the affective condition. Two assumptions for the Pearson correlation were violated, therefore a non-parametric Spearman correlation was conducted.

To analyze the influence of individual differences in experienced pleasantness on the relieving effect of affective touch,

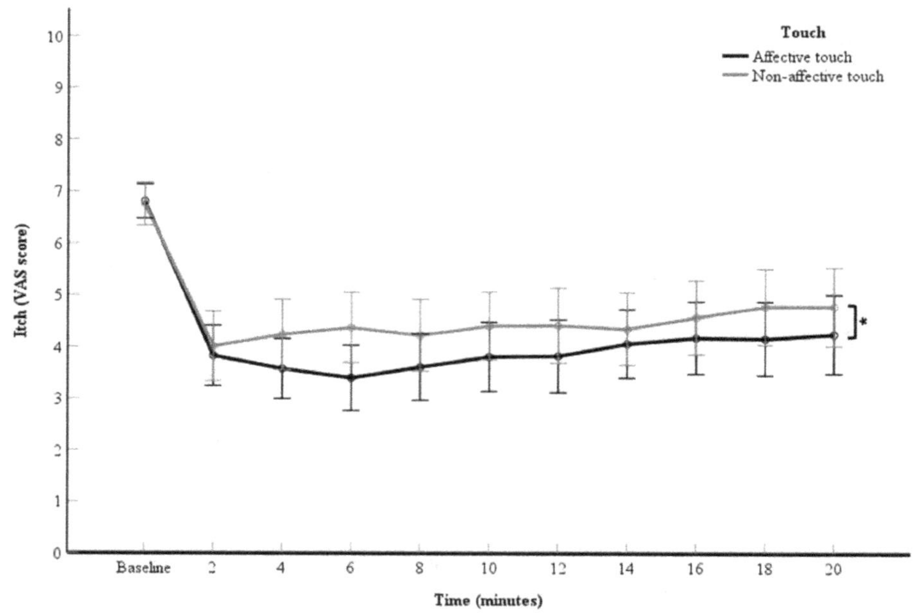

FIGURE 2 | Mean of VAS scores for itch per 2-min itch measurement including the baseline measurement. The data points represent the means of the VAS scores for itch (with error bars depicting standard error). The black line represents affective touch and the gray line represents non-affective touch ($N = 61$). $^{*}p < 0.05$; Displaying significant difference between type of touch.

the difference scores of pleasantness were correlated with the difference scores of itch. The difference scores of pleasantness were calculated by subtracting the VAS pleasantness score in the non-affective condition from those in the affective condition. The difference score of itch was calculated by subtracting the mean itch VAS scores in the non-affective touch conditions from those in the affective touch condition. The assumptions of normality and linearity were violated, a Spearman correlation was conducted. All results displayed are means ± SE, unless otherwise stated. A $p < 0.05$ is considered statistically significant.

RESULTS

The baseline data and experimental data of itch and pleasantness and the PVAQ scores are displayed in **Table 1**. The baseline itch measured in the affective and non-affective condition were comparable (6.80 ± 0.16 and 6.75 ± 0.21, respectively, $t_{(60)} = 0.23, p = 0.82$).

A two tailed, paired samples t-test was used to compare the VAS scores of pleasantness for the affective touch and non-affective touch condition (**Table 1**). The VAS scores for pleasantness in the affective touch condition were statistically significantly higher than the VAS scores for pleasantness in the non-affective touch condition, $t_{(60)} = 5.07, p < 0.01$. Cohen's d for this test was 0.89, which can be described as large.

Relieving Effect of Touch Relative to Baseline Itch Measurements

A 2 (touch: affective touch vs. non-affective touch) × 11 (time point: the VAS scores of the baseline itch measurement and the 10 itch measurements of after each 2-min itch stimulation) repeated measures ANOVA was used to investigate the relieving effect of touch on itch. A significant main effect for touch was obtained, $F_{(1, 60)} = 4.87$, $p = 0.03$, partial $\eta^2 = 0.08$ (**Figure 2**). The VAS scores for itch were significantly lower during the affective touch condition than during the non-affective touch condition (**Table 1, Figure 2**). A significant main effect was also reported for time point, $F_{(2.58,154.61)} = 28.72$, $p < 0.01$, partial $\eta^2 = 0.32$ (**Figure 2**). A contrast analysis was conducted to compare the baseline VAS scores with the other timepoints. There were significant differences between the baseline itch VAS score and the experimental itch VAS scores in both the affective and non-affective touch conditions $F_{(1, 60)} = 121.24$, $p < 0.01$, partial $\eta^2 = 0.67$). The interaction between touch and time point was not significant, $F_{(4.92,295.14)} = 1.75$, $p = 0.12$, partial $\eta^2 = 0.03$ (**Figure 2**).

Relieving Effect of Touch for Experimental Itch Ratings

A 2 (touch: affective touch vs. non-affective touch) × 10 (time point: the VAS scores the 10 itch measurements after each 2-min itch stimulation) repeated measures ANOVA was conducted to measure the effect of touch over time. The VAS scores for itch in the affective touch condition were significantly lower than the VAS scores for itch in the non-affective touch condition, which illustrates a main effect for touch, $F_{(1, 60)} = 5.01$, $p = 0.03$, partial $\eta^2 = 0.07$. The VAS scores for itch within each condition differed significantly over time, which illustrates a main effect for time point, $F_{(2.08,124.79)} = 3.33$, $p = 0.04$.

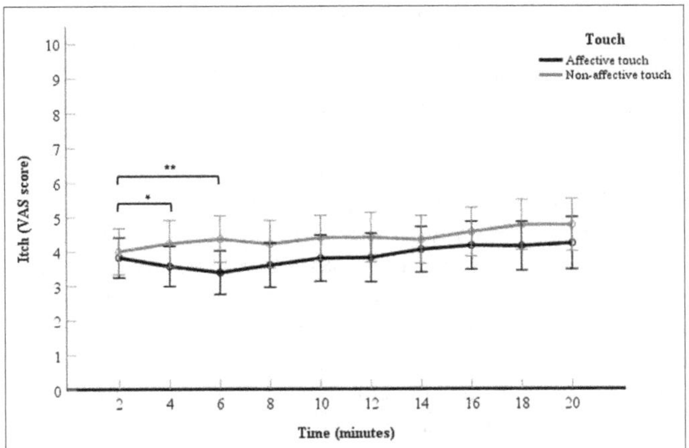

FIGURE 3 | Mean of VAS scores for itch per 2-min itch measurement including the baseline measurement. The data points represent the mean of the VAS scores for itch (with error bars depicting standard error). The black line represents affective touch and the gray line represents non-affective touch ($N = 61$).

TABLE 2 | Results of the interaction effect between touch and itch, derived from a 2 × 10 repeated measures ANOVA contrast analysis.

	Touch × Time point	
Contrasts	***F***	***p***
2 vs. 4 min	4.66	0.035*
2 vs. 6 min	9.19	0.004**
2 vs. 8 min	2.14	0.148
2 vs. 10 min	1.31	0.257
2 vs. 12 min	1.25	0.268
2 vs. 14 min	0.08	0.773
2 vs. 16 min	0.34	0.564
2 vs. 18 min	1.29	0.261
2 vs. 20 min	0.78	0.380

For every contrast analysis, the degrees of freedom are 1.60.
$^*p < 0.05$; $^{**}p < 0.01$.

There was no significant interaction effect found for touch × time point, $F_{(4.10,245.71)} = 1.30$, $p = 0.27$, in the ANOVA analysis. Although the interaction was not significant, as we did expect changes over time with respect to the difference in itch between conditions and after visual inspection of the data (**Figure 3**), it seemed of interest to conduct a follow up contrast analyses for the interaction. The 2- vs. 4-min itch measurements differed significantly, thus the difference in itch ratings between affective and non-affective touch were significantly larger at 4-min compared to 2 min, $F_{(1, 60)} = 4.66, p = 0.03$, partial $\eta^2 = 0.07$ (**Table 2, Figure 3**). A similar difference was found for the VAS scores for itch at 6-min compared to the 2-min measurement, $F_{(1, 60)} = 9.19, p = < 0.01$, partial $\eta^2 = 0.13$ (**Table 2, Figure 3**). Further details about the contrast analyses are stated in **Table 2.**

Relieving Effect of Touch and Pleasantness

Spearman's correlation indicated no correlation between the difference in experienced pleasantness for affective and non-affective touch and the difference in itch ratings for the affective and non-affective touch conditions, $\rho_s = -0.18$, $p = 0.17$, two-tailed, $N = 61$.

Relieving Effect of Touch and PVAQ

Spearman's rho indicated the presence of a negative correlation between the PVAQ score (**Table 1**) and the relieving effect of affective touch, ρ_s =-0.30, $p = 0.02$, two-tailed, $N = 61$ (**Figure 4**).

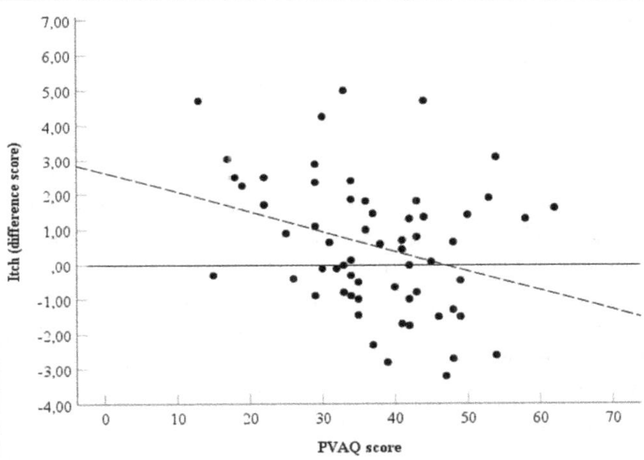

FIGURE 4 | Relationship between PVAQ scores and itch. Spearman's $\rho = -0.30$. Black line represents point zero reference line. Dotted line represents the line of best fit.

DISCUSSION

Past studies revealed an inhibitory relationship between affective touch and pain and between pain and itch (11, 15, 19, 30). However, as far as we know, no research has been reported on the relationship between itch and affective touch. Therefore, this study investigated whether there is a relationship between itch and affective touch and in particular, whether affective touch inhibits itch. The results showed that applying touch, either affective touch or non-affective touch, reduces itch experience. Several factors might account for this effect. First, it could be that the stroking of the arm is such a different sensation in comparison to electrically stimulated itch, that it is hard to feel both itch and stroking at the same time. Being touched might be a distraction on its own, independent of type of touch, which could explain why both types of touch reduced itch compared to baseline. On the other hand, there are studies showing that rubbing reliefs itch by activating low-threshold mechanosensitive A-fibers which inhibit itch signals in the spinal dorsal horn (44, 45). The velocity of rubbing could be compared to that of non-affective touch and might explain our findings. However, compared to rubbing, non-affective touch is applied with less force. This could influence the underlying mechanism regarding the inhibitory role on itch. Indeed, recent research in mice shows that a higher strength of stroking has a stronger inhibitory effect on itch. This implies that the strength of stroking plays an important role in itch inhibition (44). Therefore, it may be unlikely that the decline in itch experience by non-affective touch in our study is based on the underlying mechanisms of rubbing.

Interestingly, affective touch had an additional relieving effect on itch experience compared to non-affective touch. These findings suggest that affective touch alleviates itch experience more than non-affective touch. This implies that affective touch interferes with the processing of itch, resulting in a reduction of itch experience. How affective touch exactly interferes with itch is not known yet, but answers may be found in recent research into the pleasurability of scratching (46–49). As described, when we feel itchy we tend to scratch the itchy site. In addition, scratching provides a pleasant and rewarding feeling which explains its addictive property (49). Scratching activates brain regions involved in the processing of pleasantness, affection and reward e.g., insula, ACC and prefrontal regions (48–51). The involvement of this pleasant reward network in the brain could represent a top-down mechanism initiating a decrease in itch experience (49, 52). Furthermore, the pleasurability of scratching is associated with inhibition of the insula and ACC, regions which are associated with the emotional and affective evaluation of itch (49). Interestingly, these regions are also involved in the processing of affective touch (53). In addition, the pleasurability of scratching is mostly dependent on tactile sensations and it seems that on hairy parts of the body i.e., the arm or the back, CT-afferents are involved, which are also important for affective touch (47, 52). Taken together, the overlap in brain regions involved in scratching and affective touch, the involvement of CT-afferents in the pleasurability of scratching and our results show that affective touch possibly modulates itch through activation of regions involved in pleasantness and reward resulting in a decrease in itch experience. To confirm, further research should focus on the underlying process of this inhibitory relationship, for example by measuring brain activity through EEG or fMRI.

In addition, the optimal duration of applying affective touch to experience a relieving effect was investigated. Based on Sailer et al. (35), it was expected that the reduction in itch would persist for ~20 min. They stated that after 20 min, the brain areas activated by affective touch habituated to the stroking, which caused a decrease in brain activity and stabilized the experienced pleasantness of affective touch. Results of the current study showed that affective touch seems to reduce itch from 2 min after the start of appliance of affective touch and that this reduction in itch increased until 6 min after the start of stroking. After 6 min, this effect stabilized, but itch is still reduced compared to baseline. Importantly, even after 6 min, affective touch alleviated itch more than non-affective touch. The current study reported different temporal effects in comparison to the study of Sailer et al. (35), however they only researched the temporal effects of experienced pleasantness of affective touch and the accompanying brain activity. It could be that the temporal dynamics of the inhibitory effect of affective touch on itch do not depend on the perceived pleasantness of affective touch. Our results indeed show that the experienced pleasantness of affective touch does not correlate with the degree to which affective touch has a relieving effect on itch. This suggests that, even if affective touch is not experienced as pleasant, it still alleviates itch. This could be explained by CT-fiber activation and its possible independence of perceived pleasant, which is also hypothesized by Nagi et al. (54).

In addition, this research contributes to the evidence for an influence of attentional focus on the experience of bodily sensations. van Laarhoven et al. (38) stated that a high attentional focus on bodily sensations is associated with a more intense experience of itch, suggesting that attention to bodily sensation does play a role in how much affective touch will relief itch. The results of the current study showed that higher attention to bodily sensations indeed mediated the experienced itch. Being more susceptible to experiencing bodily sensations can intensify the feeling of itch or will diminish the relief from affective touch, which is in agreement with the hypothesis.

The current study was not without limitations. First, different durations of the baseline itch measurement (4 s) and the experimental itch measurements (2 min) were used, limiting the comparability of the results. We also did not assess the time course of electrical stimulated itch experience over the 20-min period without stroking. Any habituation to the electrical stimulus could therefore not be taken into account. In further research, it is recommended to add an extra control condition in which itch experience over time is measured without tactile input.

Secondly, electrical stimulation as a way to induce itch has its limitation. It has been reported that not everybody experienced the electrical stimulation as itch (55). An alternative way for future research to induce itch is using cowhage, a plant-based itch inducing substance evoking a mild itch (56).

Thirdly, 80% of the participants was female. This imbalance could have influenced the results. A recent meta-analysis into affective touch shows that females perceive affective touch as more pleasant than men (57). Furthermore, research into sex difference and itch experience shows that women report higher itch intensities compared to men. However, there was no difference in reduction of itch intensity between men and women when distracted (58). As our results show that pleasantness does not correlate with the degree of itch reduction and itch reduction itself is not influenced by gender, it may be unlikely that the skewed male/female ratio in our study influences the results. Nevertheless, the imbalance between male and female in our study should be taken into account when generalizing outcomes to the general population.

To expand fundamental knowledge on affective touch and its potential to contribute to clinical applications, future research should take individual differences into account. While some participants did not experience relief from affective touch, others reacted extremely well and experienced no itch at all after only 2 min of affective touch. These different responses could be caused by individual differences concerning tactile communication and touch perception (59). For example, Luong et al. (60) suggest that people have a stable preferred velocity of affective touch. These findings propose that individuals might respond differently to affective touch and that stroking should be adjusted to their preferred velocity.

To summarize, the current study showed that affective touch has a relieving effect on electrical stimulated itch. The relieving effect of affective touch is noticeable 2 min after the affective stroking has started, it stabilizes after 6 min, but persists up to 20 min. In addition, this effect is independent of the experienced pleasantness of affective touch. Lastly, a higher awareness of bodily sensations interferes with the relieving effect of affective touch on itch. The current study can serve as groundwork for future research in the application of affective touch as therapy for patient groups who experience itch as a significant burden. For this, it is necessary to determine how individuals with different kinds of non-histaminergic itch respond to affective touch and which characteristics result in maximal itch relief.

ETHICS STATEMENT

The studies involving human participants were reviewed and approved by Faculty Ethics Review Board, Faculty of Social Sciences, Utrecht University. The participants provided their written informed consent to participate in this study.

AUTHOR CONTRIBUTIONS

LM: concept, supervision, writing, and editing. ZS and KR: concept, data collection, and writing. HD: concept, supervision, and writing. All authors contributed to the article and approved the submitted version.

REFERENCES

1. Drzezga A, Darsow U, Treede RD, Siebner H, Frisch M, Munz F, et al. Central activation by histamine-induced itch: analogies to pain processing: a correlational analysis of O-15 H2O positron emission tomography studies. *Pain.* (2001) 92:295–305. doi: 10.1016/S0304-3959(01)00271-8
2. Weisshaar E. Epidemiology of itch. *Curr Probl Dermatol.* (2016) 50:5–10. doi: 10.1159/000446010
3. Bathe A, Matterne U, Dewald M, Grande T, Weisshaar E. Educational multidisciplinary training programme for patients with chronic pruritus. *Acta Derm Venereol.* (2009) 89:498–501. doi: 10.2340/00015555-0684
4. Desai NS, Poindexter GB, Monthrope YM, Bendeck SE, Swerlick RA, Chen SC. A pilot quality-of-life instrument for pruritus. *J Am Acad Dermatol.* (2008) 59:234–44. doi: 10.1016/j.jaad.2008.04.006
5. Jafferany M, Davari ME. Itch and psyche: psychiatric aspects of pruritus. *Int J Dermatol.* (2019) 58:3–23. doi: 10.1111/ijd.14081
6. Kini SP, DeLong LK, Veledar E, McKenzie-Brown AM, Schaufele M, Chen SC. The impact of pruritus on quality of life: the skin equivalent of pain. *Arch Dermatol.* (2011) 147:1153–6. doi: 10.1001/archdermatol.2011.178
7. Lee HG, Stull C, Yosipovitch G. Psychiatric disorders and pruritus. *Clin Dermatol.* (2017) 35:273–80. doi: 10.1016/j.clindermatol.2017.01.008
8. Misery L, Alexandre S, Dutray S, Chastaing M, Consoli SG, Audra H, et al. Functional itch disorder or psychogenic pruritus: suggested diagnosis criteria from the French psychodermatology group. *Acta Derm Venereol.* (2007) 87:341–4. doi: 10.2340/00015555-0266
9. Schneider G, Driesch G, Heuft G, Evers S, Luger TA, Ständer S. Psychosomatic cofactors and psychiatric comorbidity in patients with chronic itch. *Clin Exp Dermatol.* (2006) 31:762–7. doi: 10.1111/j.1365-2230.2006.02211.x
10. Schmelz M, Schmidt R, Bickel A, Handwerker HO, Torebjörk HE. Specific C-receptors for itch in human skin. *J Neurosci.* (1997) 17:8003–8. doi: 10.1523/JNEUROSCI.17-20-08003.1997
11. Ikoma A, Steinhoff M, Ständer S, Yosipovitch G, Schmelz M. The neurobiology of itch. *Nat Rev Neurosci.* (2006) 7:535–47. doi: 10.1038/nrn1950
12. Dhand A, Aminoff MJ. The neurology of itch. *Brain.* (2014) 137:313–22. doi: 10.1093/brain/awt158
13. Wallengren J. Neuroanatomy and neurophysiology of itch. *Dermatol Ther.* (2005) 18:292–303. doi: 10.1111/j.1529-8019.2005.00041.x
14. Fowler E, Yosipovitch G. Chronic itch management: therapies beyond those targeting the immune system. *Ann Allergy Asthma Immunol.* (2019) 123:158–65. doi: 10.1016/j.anai.2019.01.016
15. Ständer S, Schmelz M. Chronic itch and pain—Similarities and differences. *Eur J Pain.* (2006) 10:473. doi: 10.1016/j.ejpain.2006.03.005
16. Johanek LM, Meyer RA, Hartke T, Hobelmann JG, Maine DN, LaMotte RH, et al. Psychophysical and physiological evidence for parallel afferent pathways mediating the sensation of itch. *J Neurosci.* (2007) 27:7490–7. doi: 10.1523/JNEUROSCI.1249-07.2007
17. Ikoma A, Handwerker H, Miyachi Y, Schmelz M. Electrically evoked itch in humans. *Pain.* (2005) 113:148–54. doi: 10.1016/j.pain.2004.10.003
18. Bourne S, Machado AG, Nagel SJ. Basic anatomy and physiology of pain pathways. *Neurosurge Clinics.* (2014) 25:629–38. doi: 10.1016/j.nec.2014.06.001
19. Ikoma A, Rukwied R, Ständer S, Steinhoff M, Miyachi Y, Schmelz M. Neurophysiology of pruritus: interaction of itch and pain. *Arch Dermatol.* (2003) 139:1475–8. doi: 10.1001/archderm.139.1 1.1475
20. Chuquilin M, Alghalith Y, Fernandez KH. Neurocutaneous disease: cutaneous neuroanatomy and mechanisms of itch and pain. *J Am Acad Dermatol.* (2016) 74:197–212. doi: 10.1016/j.jaad.2015.04.060
21. Davidson S, Giesler GJ. The multiple pathways for itch and their interactions with pain. *Trends Neurosci.* (2010) 33:550–8. doi: 10.1016/j.tins.2010.09.002
22. Liu T, Ji R-R. New insights into the mechanisms of itch: are pain and itch controlled by distinct mechanisms? *Pflugers Arch.* (2013) 465:1671–85. doi: 10.1007/s00424-013-1284-2
23. Gordon I, Voos AC, Bennett RH, Bolling DZ, Pelphrey KA, Kaiser MD. Brain mechanisms for processing affective touch. *Hum Brain Mapp.* (2013) 34:914–22. doi: 10.1002/hbm.21480
24. Olausson H, Lamarre Y, Backlund H, Morin C, Wallin BG, Starck G, et al. Unmyelinated tactile afferents signal touch and project to insular cortex. *Nat Neurosci.* (2002) 5:900–4. doi: 10.1038/nn896
25. Triscoli C, Olausson H, Sailer U, Ignell H, Croy I. CT-optimized skin stroking delivered by hand or robot is comparable. *Front Behav Neurosci.* (2013) 7:208. doi: 10.3389/fnbeh.2013.00208
26. Löken LS, Wessberg J, Morrison I, McGlone F, Olausson H. Coding of pleasant touch by unmyelinated afferents in humans. *Nat Neurosci.* (2009) 12:547–8. doi: 10.1038/nn.2312
27. Morrison I, Löken LS, Minde J, Wessberg J, Perini I, Nennesmo I, et al. Reduced C-afferent fibre density affects perceived pleasantness and empathy for touch. *Brain.* (2011) 134:1116–26. doi: 10.1093/brain/awr011
28. Morrison I. ALE meta-analysis reveals dissociable networks for affective and discriminative aspects of touch. *Hum Brain Mapp.* (2016) 37:1308–20. doi: 10.1002/hbm.23103
29. Habig K, Schänzer A, Schirner W, Lautenschläger G, Dassinger B, Olausson H, et al. Low threshold unmyelinated mechanoafferents can modulate pain. *BMC Neurol.* (2017) 17:184. doi: 10.1186/s12883-017-0963-6

30. Liljencrantz J, Strigo I, Ellingsen DM, Krämer HH, Lundblad LC, Nagi SS, et al. Slow brushing reduces heat pain in humans. *Eur J Pain.* (2017) 21:1173–85. doi: 10.1002/ejp.1018
31. Lu Y, Perl E. A specific inhibitory pathway between substantia gelatinosa neurons receiving direct C-fiber input. *J Neurosci.* (2003) 23:8752–8. doi: 10.1523/JNEUROSCI.23-25-08752.2003
32. Gursul D, Goksan S, Hartley C, Mellado GS, Moultrie F, Hoskin A, et al. Stroking modulates noxious-evoked brain activity in human infants. *Current Biol.* (2018) 28:R1380–1. doi: 10.1016/j.cub.2018.11.014
33. von Mohr M, Krahé C, Beck B, Fotopoulou A. The social buffering of pain by affective touch: a laser-evoked potential study in romantic couples. *Soc Cogn Affect Neurosci.* (2018) 13:1121–30. doi: 10.1093/scan/nsy085
34. van Laarhoven AIM, van Damme S, Lavrijsen ASPM, van Ryckeghem DM, Crombez G, Evers AWM. Do tonic itch and pain stimuli draw attention towards their location? *Biomed Res Int.* (2017) 2017:2031627. doi: 10.1155/2017/2031627
35. Sailer U, Triscoli C, Häggblad G, Hamilton P, Olausson H, Croy I. Temporal dynamics of brain activation during 40 minutes of pleasant touch. *NeuroImage.* (2016) 139:360–7. doi: 10.1016/j.neuroimage.2016.06.031
36. Pawling R, Cannon PR, McGlone FP, Walker SC. C-tactile afferent stimulating touch carries a positive affective value. *PLoS ONE.* (2017) 12:e0173457. doi: 10.1371/journal.pone.0173457
37. Perini I, Olausson H, Morrison I. Seeking pleasant touch: neural correlates of behavioral preferences for skin stroking. *Front Behav Neurosci.* (2015) 9:1–9. doi: 10.3389/fnbeh.2015.00008
38. van Laarhoven AIM, Kraaimaat FW, Wilder-Smith OH, Evers AWM. Role of attentional focus on bodily sensations in sensitivity to itch and pain. *Acta Derm Venereol.* (2010) 90:46–51. doi: 10.2340/00015555-0743
39. Verhoeven L, Kraaimaat F, Duller P, van de Kerkhof P, Evers A. Cognitive, behavioral, and physiological reactivity to chronic itching: analogies to chronic pain. *Int J Behav Med.* (2006) 13:237–43. doi: 10.1207/s15327558ijbm1303_7
40. McCracken LM. "Attention" to pain in persons with chronic pain: a behavioral approach. *Behav Ther.* (1997) 28:271–84. doi: 10.1016/S0005-7894(97)80047-0
41. Phan NQ, Blome C, Fritz F, Gerss J, Reich A, Ebata T, et al. Assessment of pruritus intensity: prospective study on validity and reliability of the visual analogue scale, numerical rating scale and verbal rating scale in 471 patients with chronic pruritus. *Acta Derm Venereol.* (2012) 92:502–7. doi: 10.2340/00015555-1246
42. Field A. *Discovering Statistics Using IBM SPSS. (2013)* Statistics: Sage Publications Ltd.
43. Ghasemi A, Zahediasl S. Normality tests for statistical analysis: a guide for non-statisticians. *Int J Endocrinol Metab.* (2012) 10:486–9. doi: 10.5812/ijem.3505
44. Sakai K, Sanders KM, Lin S-H, Pavlenko D, Funahashi H, Lozada T, et al. Low-threshold mechanosensitive VGLUT3-lineage sensory neurons mediate spinal inhibition of itch by touch. *J Neurosci.* (2020) 40:7688–701. doi: 10.1523/JNEUROSCI.0091-20.2020
45. Yosipovitch G, Greaves MW, Schmelz M. Itch. *Lancet.* (2003) 361:690–4. doi: 10.1016/S0140-6736(03)12570-6
46. Bin Saif GA, Papoiu ADP, Banari L, McGlone F, Kwatra SG, Chan YH, et al. The pleasurability of scratching an itch: a psychophysical and topographical assessment. *Br J Dermatol.* (2012) 166:981–5. doi: 10.1111/j.1365-2133.2012.10826.x
47. Mochizuki H, Shevchenko A, Nattkemper LA, Valdes-Rodriguez R, Yosipovitch G. Suppression of scratching-induced pleasurable sensation by compression nerve blocking and its association with itch relief. *Itch.* (2017) 2:e7. doi: 10.1097/itx.0000000000000007
48. Mochizuki H, Tanaka S, Morita T, Wasaka T, Sadato N, Kakigi R. The cerebral representation of scratching-induced pleasantness. *J Neurophysiol.* (2014) 111:488–98. doi: 10.1152/jn.00374.2013
49. Papoiu AD, Nattkemper LA, Sanders KM, Kraft RA, Chan YH, Coghill RC, et al. Brain's reward circuits mediate itch relief. A functional MRI study of active scratching. *PLoS ONE.* (2013) 8:e82389. doi: 10.1371/journal.pone.0082389
50. Lloyd DM, McGlone FP, Yosipovitch G. Somatosensory pleasure circuit: from skin to brain and back. *Exp Dermatol.* (2015) 24:321–4. doi: 10.1111/exd.12639
51. Mochizuki H, Hernandez LE, Yosipovitch G, Sadato N, Kakigi R. The functional network processing acute electrical itch stimuli in humans. *Front Physiol.* (2019) 10:555. doi: 10.3389/fphys.2019.00555
52. Hashimoto T, Yosipovitch G. Itchy body: topographical difference of itch and scratching and C Nerve fibres. *Exp Dermatol.* (2019) 28:1385–9. doi: 10.1111/exd.14054
53. McGlone F, Wessberg J, Olausson H. Discriminative and affective touch: sensing and feeling. *Neuron.* (2014) 82:737–55. doi: 10.1016/j.neuron.2014.05.001
54. Nagi SS, Rubin TK, Chelvanayagam DK, Macefield VG, Mahns DA. Allodynia mediated by C-tactile afferents in human hairy skin. *J Physiol.* (2011) 589:4065–75. doi: 10.1113/jphysiol.2011.211326
55. Yuan T, Li J, Shen L, Zhang W, Wang T, Xu Y, et al. Assessment of Itch and Pain in Animal Models and Human Subjects. In C. Ma & Y. Huang (Eds.), *Translational Research in Pain and Itch.* Dordrecht: Springer Netherlands (2016). p. 1-22. doi: 10.1007/978-94-017-7537-3_1
56. Andersen HH, Sørensen AR, Nielsen GA, Mølgaard MS, Stilling P, Boudreau SA, et al. A test-retest reliability study of human experimental models of histaminergic and non-histaminergic itch. *Acta Derm Venereol.* (2017) 97:198–207. doi: 10.2340/00015555-2502
57. Russo V, Ottaviani C, Spitoni GF. Affective touch: a meta-analysis on sex differences. *Neurosci Biobehav Rev.* (2020) 108:445–52. doi: 10.1016/j.neubiorev.2019.09.037
58. Stumpf A, Burgmer M, Schneider G, Heuft G, Schmelz M, Phan NQ, et al. Sex differences in itch perception and modulation by distraction– an FMRI pilot study in healthy volunteers. *PLoS ONE.* (2013) 8:e79123. doi: 10.1371/journal.pone.0079123
59. Harjunen VJ, Spapé M, Ahmed I, Jacucci G, Ravaja N. Individual differences in affective touch: behavioral inhibition and gender define how an interpersonal touch is perceived. *Pers Individ Dif.* (2017) 107:88–95. doi: 10.1016/j.paid.2016.11.047
60. Luong A, Bendas J, Etzi R, Olausson H, Croy I. The individual preferred velocity of stroking touch as a stable measurement. *Physiol Behav.* (2017) 177:129–34. doi: 10.1016/j.physbeh.2017.04.022

26

Neuropathic Itch: Routes to Clinical Diagnosis

Manuel Pedro Pereira, Henning Wiegmann, Konstantin Agelopoulos and Sonja Ständer*

Department of Dermatology and Center for Chronic Pruritus, University Hospital Münster, Münster, Germany

***Correspondence:**
Manuel Pedro Pereira
manuelpedro.pereira@ukmuenster.de*

Neuropathic itch occurs due to damage of neurons of the peripheral or central nervous system. Several entities, including metabolic, neurodegenerative, orthopedic, infectious, autoimmune, malignant, and iatrogenic conditions, may affect the somatosensory system and induce neuropathic itch. Due to the complex nature of neuropathic itch, particularly concerning its clinical presentation and possible etiological factors, diagnostic work-up of this condition is challenging. A detailed medical history, especially in regard to the itch, and a comprehensive physical examination are relevant to detect characteristic signs and symptoms of neuropathic itch and to rule out other possible causes for chronic itch. Complementary diagnostic exams, especially laboratory tests, determination of the intraepidermal nerve fiber density via a skin biopsy and radiological examinations may be indicated to confirm the diagnosis of neuropathic itch and to identify underlying etiological factors. Functional assessments such as quantitative sensory testing, nerve conduction studies, evoked potentials, or microneurography may be considered in particular cases. This review article provides a comprehensive overview of the diagnostic work-up recommended for patients with neuropathic itch.

Keywords: neuropathic itch, chronic itch, dysesthesia, pain, small-fiber neuropathy, diagnostic work-up, intraepidermal nerve fiber density, magnet resonance imaging

INTRODUCTION

The International Forum for the Study of Itch (IFSI) defines neuropathic itch as itch occurring due to an injury of neurons of the peripheral or central nervous system (1). It is estimated that 8% of chronic itch cases have a neuropathic origin (2). However, epidemiological studies investigating the prevalence and incidence of neuropathic itch are still missing.

Damage at any site of the somatosensory system, including peripherally nerve fibers, nerve plexuses and ganglia, and centrally the spinal cord, brainstem, thalamus or cortex, may lead to neuropathic itch (3).

Several conditions affecting the peripheral nervous system are associated with neuropathic itch (**Table 1**). In small-fiber neuropathy (SFN), which results from injured C- and Aδ fibers (4), itch and pain may occur localized (mostly distally at the feet) or generalized. It may result from a myriad of conditions such as metabolic (e.g., diabetes), infectious, autoimmune and genetic diseases. Also drugs (e.g., chemotherapy) and alcohol may induce SFN (5, 6). Scars and burn-injuries are often associated with itch, likely due to damage of cutaneous nerves (7, 8). Postherpetic neuralgia is a frequent cause of neuropathic itch at the site of the affected peripheral nerve (9). Compression or irritation of different neural structures may induce localized neuropathic itch along the corresponding dermatome, as is the case in brachioradial pruritus (radiculopathy at C3–C6), notalgia paresthetica (dorsal rami of posterior nerves at T2–T6), cheiralgia paresthetica

TABLE 1 | Neuropathic pruritic conditions.

Disease	Etiology	Clinical features	Main work-up
Peripheral nervous system			
Small fiber neuropathy	Metabolic, drug-induced, infectious, or genetic origin	Itch starts usually distally and may generalize	IENFD, QST
Scars and burns	Iatrogenic or traumatic	Itch on lesional tissue	Clinical diagnosis
Radiculopathies	Compression of a peripheral nerve by degenerative alterations or space-occupying lesions	Itch and dysesthesias at the affected dermatome	MRI or CT scan, IENFD
Postherpetic neuralgia	Damage of peripheral nerve by the varicella zoster virus	Itch and dysesthesias at the affected dermatome	Clinical diagnosis
Trigeminal trophic syndrome	Injury of the sensory fibers of the trigeminal nerve	Unilateral dysesthesia and hypoesthesia of the central face. Self-induced ulceration of the nasal ala, cheek, and upper lip	Clinical diagnosis, MRI
Central nervous system			
Space occupying lesions	Tumors, abscesses, vascular lesions, syringomyelia	Clinical features according to affected neural structures	Neuroimaging (MRI/CT scan)
Stroke	Ischemic or hemorrhagic	Generalized or unilateral itch	Neuroimaging (CT scan)
Multiple sclerosis	Demyelinating disease	Generalized itch or localized at the head and upper back	MRI, analysis of cerebrospinal fluid (IgG oligoclonal bands), evoked potentials
Neuromyelitis optica	Demyelinating disease	Depending on injured spinal level	MRI, autoantibodies against aquaporin 4
Infectious diseases	Meningitis, encephalitis, prion disease	Depending on damaged neural structures	Neuroimaging (MRI/CT scan), analysis of cerebrospinal fluid, blood tests
Traumatic brain or spinal cord lesions	Accidents or iatrogenic lesions	Depending on damaged neural structures	Neuroimaging (MRI/CT scan)

Etiological factors, clinical features and diagnostic work-up of neuropathic pruritic conditions are shown. CT, computed tomography; IENFD, intraepidermal nerve fiber density; QST, quantitative sensory testing; MRI, magnet resonance imaging.

(radial nerve), meralgia paresthetica (lateral femoral cutaneous nerve), and gonyalgia paresthetica (infrapatellar branch of the saphenous nerve) (2, 10–13). Genitoanal itch, a common pruritic condition, can also have a neuropathic origin, due to a lumbosacral radiculopathy. Injury of the trigeminal nerve may cause facial itch leading often to manipulation of the skin with ulceration, a condition termed trigeminal trophic syndrome (14).

At central level, space-occupying lesions such as abscesses, cysts, tumors, vascular malformations or syringomyelia may originate neuropathic itch (15, 16). Also neural damage induced by trauma or meningitis has been associated with the occurrence of itch, while unilateral itch has been reported after a stroke (17, 18). Additionally, itch has been reported in neuroinflammatory conditions as for instance multiple sclerosis or neuromyelitis optica (19, 20).

Neuropathic itch should be differentiated from other etiologies possibly underlying itch. **Table 2** provides an overview of potential etiologies of chronic itch as defined by the IFSI, including clinical examples and distinctive clinical features.

Owing to the multidimensional nature of neuropathic itch, particularly regarding its clinical presentation and possible underlying causes, substantial diagnostic efforts are necessary in the management of these patients. This review article focuses on the diagnostic work-up of patients with neuropathic itch, including the medical history and physical examination (**Table 3**), use of standardized questionnaires, laboratory tests, skin biopsies for the assessment of neurocutaneous alterations, radiological examinations, and functional tests (**Table 4**).

Abbreviations: CT, computed tomography; DN4, *doleur neuropathique*; IENFD, intraepidermal nerve fiber density; IFSI, International Forum for the Study of Itch; QST, quantitative sensory testing; MRI, magnet resonance imaging; NP5, Neuropathic Pruritus 5; SFN, small-fiber neuropathy.

MEDICAL HISTORY

A detailed medical history is essential for the diagnosis of neuropathic itch and to exclude other possible etiologies for chronic pruritus. The itch characteristics should be asked in detail. The beginning of the pruritus and possible associated relevant events (e.g., herpes zoster prior to postherpetic neuralgia, or treatment with chemotherapy resulting in SFN) may give important clues of its etiology. Additionally, the appearance of the skin at the onset of the disease should be asked. Neuropathic itch starts on normal appearing skin, as no primary skin condition is present, but excoriations or chronic scratch lesions (e.g., chronic nodular prurigo or lichen simplex) may develop at a later stage due to ongoing scratching behavior (**Figure 1**) (21).

Also the localization of itch at the beginning and during the course of the disease should be addressed. The affected site of

TABLE 2 | Etiological classification of itch.

Etiology	Clinical examples	Clinical features
Dermatological	Atopic dermatitis, cutaneous T-cell lymphoma, psoriasis, urticaria	Primary skin alterations (e.g., eczema) can be found upon inspection
Systemic	Cholestasis, diabetes, drug-induced, myeloproliferative disorders, renal insufficiency, solid tumors	Temporal correlation between onset of systemic disease and begin of itch may hint toward a systemic origin of itch Onset of itch at the trunk is typical for diabetes, while begin of itch at the palms and soles suggests a liver disease as an underlying cause
Neuropathic	Brachioradial pruritus, notalgia paresthetica, postherpetic neuralgia, small-fiber neuropathy	Itch usually starts localized according to the affected nerves. Symptomatic alleviation with application of cold or ice
Psychosomatic/psychiatric	Delusional parasitosis, somatoform pruritus	Onset of itch may occur after a significant life event (e.g., death of the partner, job loss)
Mixed	If more than one etiology is found	Occurs more frequently in older or multimorbid patients
Unknown	If no underlying etiology is found after diagnostic work-up	Diagnostic work-up should be repeated yearly if the cause for chronic itch remains unknown

Adapted from Ständer et al. (1).

TABLE 3 | Medical history and physical examination: relevant aspects for neuropathic itch.

	Parameter	Comment
Medical history		
Itch specific history	Intensity	Itch intensity informs about the disease severity and should be monitored during the course of the disease
	Sensory symptoms	Dysesthesias such as stinging, tingling or sensation like electroshocks are typical for neuropathic itch
	Daily pattern	Itch usually occurs in attacks in neuropathic itch
	Localization at onset	Localization of the itch at onset gives important hints regarding the affected site of the somatosensory system
	Localization in the course of disease	Generalization of itch beyond the initial localization at onset may occur, suggesting neuronal sensitization
	Alleviating factors	Alleviation of sensory symptoms with application of cool-packs or cold water is characteristic for neuropathic itch (ice-pack sign)
	Performed therapies	Neuropathic itch is expected to improve with gabapentinoids or opioid modulators, while antihistamines are usually ineffective
General medical history	Comorbidities	Assessment of comorbidities including atopic conditions is important to rule out non-neuropathic conditions leading to chronic pruritus. Additionally, systemic conditions (e.g., renal insufficiency) may limit therapeutic options
	Co-medication	Co-medication should be assessed to exclude possible drug interactions when planning an antipruritic therapy
Physical examination		
Dermatological examination	Dermatoses	Primary skin conditions as a possible cause for chronic itch should be ruled out by clinical examination (and eventually with skin biopsies). Importantly, dermatoses should be differentiated from secondary scratch lesions
	Scratch lesions	The distribution of scratch lesions (along with the sensory symptoms) may inform on the affected site of the somatosensory system. Additionally the amount of scratch lesions may serve as an indirect indicator of disease severity
Neurological examination	Alloknesis, Hyperknesis	Pruritic response to a non-pruritic stimulus (e.g., cotton swab) and augmented pruritic response to a pruritic stimulus (e.g., skin challenge with cowhage) suggest neuronal sensitization
	Mapping of dysesthesias	Mapping areas of dysesthesia (and alloknesis/hyperknesis) is helpful in localized pruritic neuropathic syndromes, as it may give hints on the affected neural structure

the somatosensory system is of paramount importance for the localization of itch. However, generalization of itch may occur after initial localized begin (22).

Pruritus intensity, accompanying sensory symptoms, fluctuation of the itch during the day and alleviating factors should be assessed. Typical for neuropathic itch is the presence of additional dysesthesias such as stinging and tingling, occurrence of itch in attacks and alleviation of the symptoms after application of cool-packs or cold water (**Figure 1**) (5, 23).

Moreover, information on previous antipruritic therapies and their effect and tolerance may help guiding the decision on further therapeutic proceedings (24, 25).

In addition to the itch specific history, the general medical history, especially regarding comorbidities and co-medication are important to rule other possible factors contributing to the

TABLE 4 | Complementary diagnostic procedures in neuropathic itch.

Diagnostic procedure	Comment
Laboratory tests	• Exclusion of systemic disease as underlying cause for chronic pruritus • Exploratory work-up to investigate possible conditions inducing small-fiber neuropathy • Confirmatory tests of neurological disease (e.g., oligoclonal bands in multiple sclerosis) • Genetic work-up if hereditary conditions (e.g., genetic small-fiber neuropathy and channelopathy) is suspected
Skin biopsy	• Determination of the intraepidermal nerve fiber density to detect alterations of the cutaneous neuroanatomical architecture • Histology and/or direct immunofluorescence to rule out a primary skin condition
Radiological examinations	• Magnet resonance imaging (MRI)/computed tomography (CT) to identify space-occupying lesions affecting the central or peripheral nervous system • MRI (alternatively CT) to detect spinal disorders (e.g., degenerative alterations of the vertebral column, disc prolapse or herniation, compression of nerve roots or spinal nerves, neuroforaminal stenosis) in patients with pruritic compression syndromes • Diagnosis of neurological conditions potentially inducing itch (e.g., stroke, meningitis, multiple sclerosis)
Functional assessments	• Quantitative sensory testing to assess gain or loss of function of different populations of peripheral nerve fibers, including C and Aδ-fibers, and to detect possible signs of neuronal sensitization • Nerve conduction studies and electromyography to investigate impairment of large sensory (and motor) nerves • Microneurography and evoked potentials allow the assessment of selective nerve fibers, but are mostly used in research

development of pruritus and to inform on eventual limitations of therapeutic options due to drug interactions or systemic conditions as for instance impairment of renal or liver function (24, 25).

PHYSICAL EXAMINATION

A comprehensive dermatological examination of the entire skin including mucosae is advised (24, 25). In neuropathic itch, no primary skin diseases are expected to be found. These should be differentiated from secondary lesions resulting from scratching such as excoriations or lichenification (24, 25). The distribution pattern of possible scratch marks and/or of the reported symptoms in localized pruritic conditions is essential for the correct diagnosis of the neuropathy. For instance, SFN manifests initially distally at the feet and advance proximally with the course of the disease, whereas neuropathic itch due to postherpetic neuralgia occurs at the affected dermatome. Brachioradial pruritus affects the outer aspects of the arms, while in notalgia paresthetica a circumscribed hyperpigmented area due to rubbing, mostly between the scapulae at the back, is characteristic (26). Unilateral itch should raise suspicion of a past stroke (17).

Alloknesis, i.e., induction of itch after application of a non-pruritic stimulus, and hyperknesis, i.e., augmented itch response to a pruritic stimulus, may occur in neuropathic itch (27) and should be assessed in these patients. A typical example for alloknesis often reported by patients is an intense itch perception after light touch of the skin in an affected site. These phenomena argue for neuronal sensitization processes, which contribute to the chronicity of the itch (28).

STANDARDIZED QUESTIONNAIRES

Standardized questionnaires, as for instance the *doleur neuropathique* (DN4) (29), PainDetect (30), or the Brief Pain Inventory (31), have been successfully developed to screen for neuropathic pain (32). For neuropathic itch no such tools were available until recently, when a score to differentiate neuropathic from non-neuropathic itch based on patient reported outcomes was proposed. Independent factors for neuropathic itch were the presence of twinges, absence of burning, worsening of the itch with activity, no worsening with stress and relief of itch with cold temperature. As a result, the Neuropathic Pruritus 5 (NP5) score was suggested based on the 5 independent factors for neuropathic itch. The presence of two out of five criteria yield a sensitivity of 76% and a specificity of 77% in discriminating neuropathic from non-neuropathic itch (33). For SFN a patient oriented survey including a question on itchy skin is in development (34).

SKIN BIOPSY: INTRAEPIDERMAL NERVE FIBER DENSITY

Neurocutaneous morphological alterations are observed in neuropathic pruritic conditions. The determination of the intraepidermal nerve fiber density (IENFD) is the gold standard for the diagnosis of a SFN (5). Additionally, a reduction of the IENFD is also observed in neuropathic compression syndromes as for instance brachioradial pruritus (35). Thus, the examination of the epidermal neural architecture may provide important hints for the diagnosis of a neuropathic pruritic condition. Clinically, the magnitude of the decrease in IENFD seems to influence the perception of dysesthesias (5).

In order to determine the IENFD when neuropathic itch is suspected, a skin sample is obtained via a punch biopsy from non-lesional pruritic skin. Importantly, scratch lesions, scars or other skin conditions (e.g., eczema, skin infections) should be avoided when choosing the biopsy site, since such alterations may lead to false pathological findings. After staining of the skin sample with an axonal marker (e.g., protein gene

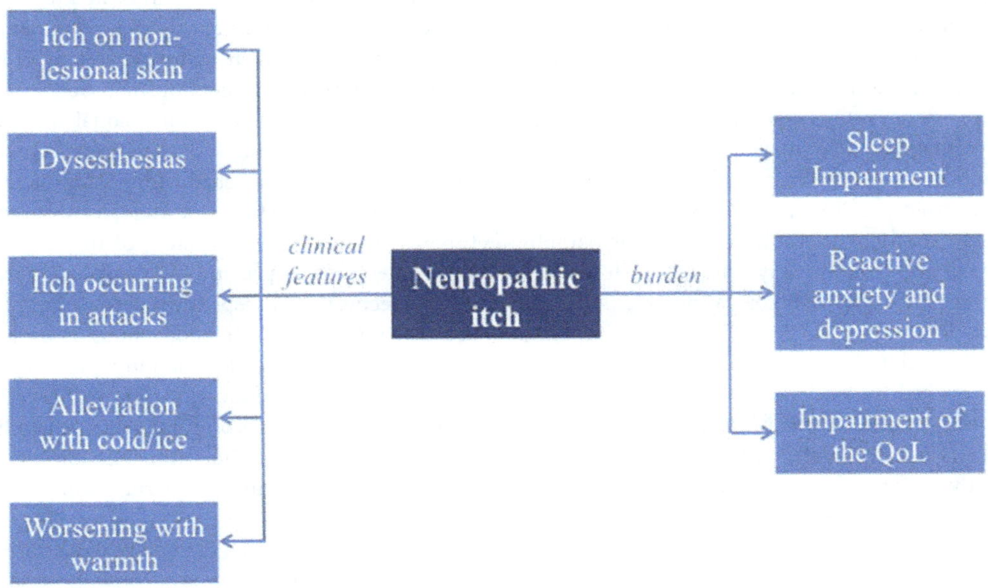

FIGURE 1 | Neuropathic itch: clinical features and burden.

product 9.5), nerve fibers crossing the basal membrane from the dermis into the epidermis are counted and divided by the length of the dermoepidermal junction. Fragments of nerve fibers in the epidermis and branching are not considered for the IENFD (36). Reference values are currently only available for the innervation site of the sural nerve (37). Therefore, this area (lateral lower leg) should be chosen for the biopsy, if patients report dysesthesias there. If another body site is affected, a skin sample from a non-affected symmetrical region should be obtained for comparison.

LABORATORY TESTS

Laboratory tests are indicated to rule out non-neuropathic conditions potentially inducing chronic itch, as for instance renal retention parameters to exclude renal insufficiency, cholestasis parameters or complete blood count to screen for hemato-oncological diseases (24, 25). Moreover, disease specific tests should be performed in selected patients with suspicion of a neurologic condition (e.g., analysis of cerebrospinal fluid including histology if a brain tumor is suspected, or oligoclonal bands for the diagnosis of multiple sclerosis) (24).

Additionally, after a SFN is diagnosed laboratory investigations should be performed in order to identify possible causes. The assessment of glycosylated hemoglobin to rule out diabetes, vitamin B12 and folate serum levels, HIV and hepatitis B and C serology, TSH, and antinuclear antibodies constitute the most relevant assessments. Additionally, genetic tests may be considered for young patients with SFN of unclear origin to exclude a hereditary condition. However, in spite of a comprehensive work-up, the etiology of SFN remains unknown in a substantial number of cases (38).

RADIOLOGICAL EXAMINATIONS

Diagnostic imaging, especially magnet resonance imaging (MRI) and computed tomography (CT), is helpful to detect space-occupying lesions such as tumors, abscesses, vascular or inflammatory lesions and their anatomical relationship to peripheral or central neural structures. Medical imaging plays also a relevant role in the diagnosis of neurological conditions as e.g., stroke, meningitis or degenerative neuroinflammatory diseases, which potentially induce neuropathic itch.

MRI [alternatively CT, high-resolution sonography or MR neurography (39)] is oftentimes used in the diagnostic work-up of pruritic neuropathic compression syndromes to identify underlying pathologies such as compression of nerve roots or of the spinal cord, disc prolapse or herniation, degenerative vertebral alterations, osteophytes or neuroforaminal stenosis (10, 11, 26). While in brachioradial pruritus there is a clear correlation between MRI findings and the localization of dysesthesias, such a relationship is not so clear for notalgia paresthetica (40).

FUNCTIONAL ASSESSMENTS

Morphological investigations of neuroanatomical alterations may be complemented with functional assessments in patients with neuropathic itch. The small unmyelinated C-fibers and thinly myelinated Aδ-fibers are of particular interest, as they transmit itch (41, 42). In quantitative sensory testing (QST), a validated test battery using thermal and mechanical standardized stimuli, detection and pain thresholds as well as response to suprathreshold stimuli are measured, allowing to infer a possible gain or loss of function of different nerve fiber populations (43–45). Additionally, QST informs about signs of neuronal sensitization, for instance by assessing mechanical allodynia and wind-up ratio (46). Although this non-invasive method provides a comprehensive neurophysiological profiling of sensory neuropathies, it is time-consuming, requires specialized personnel and the collaboration of the patient.

Large myelinated sensory fibers are not involved in itch transmission. Nevertheless, SFN may occur as part of a polyneuropathy with involvement of large fibers. Therefore, in patients with neuropathic pruritus due to a SFN, referral to a neurologist for nerve conduction studies or electromyography should be considered (3). Additionally patients with pruritic compression diseases may show pathological nerve conduction studies, as has been reported in brachioradial pruritus (47) and anogenital neuropathic itch (48).

Assessment of evoked potentials and microneurography constitute additional methods, in which functional impairment of selective nerve fibers are investigated (49, 50). These diagnostic procedures are mostly performed in research studies, but may be considered in selected clinical cases.

DISCUSSION

The diagnosis of neuropathic itch is challenging and may be overlooked in routine care. Neuropathic itch should be suspected in patients with chronic itch on normal appearing skin without a relevant systemic condition causing itch. A detailed medical history, especially in relation to the sensory symptoms, can further suggest the presence of a neuropathic origin. Typical is the presence of additional dysesthesias such as stinging and tingling, the occurrence of symptoms in attacks rather than continuously and alleviation with cool-packs or cold temperature. These clinical symptoms have been proposed as diagnostic criteria for pruritic SFN (5). However, these symptoms are not exclusive of neuropathic pruritic conditions. For instance, sensory symptoms other than itch such as crawling, tickling, and stinging have been reported in atopic dermatitis (51), while pain is perceived by the majority of patients with atopic dermatitis and psoriasis (52).

The localization of the dysesthesias, especially when distributed along a dermatome (e.g., in post-herpetic neuralgia or brachioradial pruritus) or in a *stocking-and-glove* distribution (e.g., in SFN), may yield further clues to the diagnosis of neuropathic itch and to the localization of the pathology within the somatosensory system (26).

Moreover, alloknesis, which can be easily tested by stimulating the affected skin area with a cotton wool or a brush, should be included in the evaluation of patients, as this phenomenon is characteristic of neuropathic itch, especially when neuronal sensitization has ensued (28).

Complementary exams are indicated to confirm a suspicious case of neuropathic itch. The determination of the IENFD, which is frequently reduced in neuropathic itch, is the gold-standard test to diagnose involvement of small-fibers. The biopsy needs to be performed at a pruritic non-lesional site, since the IENFD is also reduced in chronic scratch lesions (53) and in dermatoses (54–56), suggesting a neuropathic component of inflammatory pruritic conditions. However, while in chronic scratch lesions the IENFD normalizes with healing of the lesions, in neuropathic syndromes such as pruritic SFN and brachioradial pruritus the IENFD seems to be independent of the amount of scratch lesions present, arguing for an endogenous neuropathic mechanism leading to the rarefication of intraepidermal fibers (5, 35). A reduced IENFD is found not only in SFN, but also in extra-cutaneous neuropathic conditions such as brachioradial pruritus, likely due to anterograde transmission of neuromodulating factors leading to cutaneous neuroanatomical changes (57, 58).

Radiological exams, especially MRI, are useful when a neuropathic compression syndrome is suspected to identify orthopedic pathologies compromising neural structures. It should however be taken into account that in some cases anatomical abnormalities leading to neuropathic itch may be difficult to identify with medical imaging, as is the case in notalgia paresthetica (40).

In the management of patients with suspected neuropathic itch, diagnostic efforts focus on confirming the diagnosis and identifying the underlying pathological processes at the somatosensory system. With the advance of the understanding of the neurobiological mechanisms leading to neuropathic itch and their association with clinical signs and symptoms, a mechanism driven diagnostic work-up may be possible in the future, allowing the use of target specific drugs, which hopefully will result in a better care.

AUTHOR CONTRIBUTIONS

MP planned the manuscript, performed the literature search, wrote the manuscript, and approved the final version of the manuscript. HW performed the literature search, wrote the manuscript, and approved the final version of the manuscript. KA wrote the manuscript and approved the final version of the manuscript. SS planned the manuscript, wrote the manuscript, and approved the final version of the manuscript. All authors contributed to the article and approved the submitted version.

REFERENCES

1. Ständer S, Weisshaar E, Mettang T, Szepietowski JC, Carstens E, Ikoma A, et al. Clinical classification of itch: a position paper of the International Forum for the Study of Itch. *Acta Derm Venereol.* (2007) 87:291–4. doi: 10.2340/00015555-0305
2. Stumpf A, Ständer S. Neuropathic itch: diagnosis and management. *Dermatol Ther.* (2013) 26:104–9. doi: 10.1111/dth.12028
3. Misery L, Brenaut E, Le Garrec R, Abasq C, Genestet S, Marcorelles P, et al. Neuropathic pruritus. *Nat Rev Neurol.* (2014) 10:408–16. doi: 10.1038/nrneurol.2014.99

4. Oaklander AL. Neuropathic itch. In: Carstens E, Akiyama T, editors. *Itch: Mechanisms and Treatment.* Boca Raton, FL: CRC Press/Taylor and Francis Group, LLC (2014), 89–118.
5. Pereira MP, Derichs L, Meyer Zu Horste G, Agelopoulos K. Generalized chronic itch induced by small-fibre neuropathy: clinical profile and proposed diagnostic criteria. *J Eur Acad Dermatol Venereol.* (2019) 34:1795–802. doi: 10.1111/jdv.16151
6. Misery L, Bodere C, Genestet S, Zagnoli F, Marcorelles P. Small-fibre neuropathies and skin: news and perspectives for dermatologists. *Eur J Dermatol.* (2014) 24:147–53. doi: 10.1684/ejd.2013.2189
7. Lee SS, Yosipovitch G, Chan YH, Goh CL. Pruritus, pain, and small nerve fiber function in keloids: a controlled study. *J Am Acad Dermatol.* (2004) 51:1002–6. doi: 10.1016/j.jaad.2004.07.054
8. Chung BY, Kim HB, Jung MJ, Kang SY. Post-burn pruritus. *Int J Mol Sci.* (2020) 21:3880. doi: 10.3390/ijms21113880
9. Lee HJ, Kim GW, Kim WJ, Mun JH, Song M, Kim HS, et al. Clinical characteristics of postherpetic pruritus: assessment using a questionnaire, von Frey filaments and Neurometer. *Br J Dermatol.* (2015) 172:1672–3. doi: 10.1111/bjd.13569
10. Marziniak M, Phan NQ, Raap U, Siepmann D, Schurmeyer-Horst F, Pogatzki-Zahn E, et al. Brachioradial pruritus as a result of cervical spine pathology: the results of a magnetic resonance tomography study. *J Am Acad Dermatol.* (2011) 65:756–62. doi: 10.1016/j.jaad.2010.07.036
11. Huesmann T, Cunha PR, Osada N, Huesmann M, Zanelato TP, Phan NQ, et al. Notalgia paraesthetica: a descriptive two-cohort study of 65 patients from Brazil and Germany. *Acta Derm Venereol.* (2012) 92:535–40. doi: 10.2340/00015555-1344
12. Shumway NK, Cole E, Fernandez KH. Neurocutaneous disease: neurocutaneous dysesthesias. *J Am Acad Dermatol.* (2016) 74:215–28. doi: 10.1016/j.jaad.2015.04.059
13. Massey EW. Sensory mononeuropathies. *Semin Neurol.* (1998) 18:177–83. doi: 10.1055/s-2008-1040871
14. Sadeghi P, Papay FA, Vidimos AT. Trigeminal trophic syndrome–report of four cases and review of the literature. *Dermatol Surg.* (2004) 30:807–12. doi: 10.1111/j.1524-4725.2004.30220.x
15. Magilner D. Localized cervical pruritus as the presenting symptom of a spinal cord tumor. *Pediatr Emerg Care.* (2006) 22:746–7. doi: 10.1097/01.pec.0000238735.14532.2e
16. Waseem M, Raja A, Jeun E, Prokhorov S, Dobrenkov K. Paroxysmal neuropathic pain in an adolescent female with syringomyelia: a review of literature. *Pediatr Emerg Care.* (2012) 28:472–4. doi: 10.1097/PEC.0b013e318253907f
17. Ganguly S, Krishna CV, Parmar NV, Kuruvila S, Phansalkar DS. Unilateral pruritus following stroke. *Indian J Dermatol Venereol Leprol.* (2015) 81:186–8. doi: 10.4103/0378-6323.152294
18. Massey EW. Unilateral neurogenic pruritus following stroke. *Stroke.* (1984) 15:901–3. doi: 10.1161/01.STR.15.5.901
19. Yamamoto M, Yabuki S, Hayabara T, Otsuki S. Paroxysmal itching in multiple sclerosis: a report of three cases. *J Neurol Neurosurg Psychiatry.* (1981) 44:19–22. doi: 10.1136/jnnp.44.1.19
20. Xiao L, Qiu W, Lu Z, Li R, Hu X. Intractable pruritus in neuromyelitis optica. *Neurol Sci.* (2016) 37:949–54. doi: 10.1007/s10072-016-2523-z
21. Pereira MP, Kremer AE, Mettang T, Ständer S. Chronic pruritus in the absence of skin disease: pathophysiology, diagnosis and treatment. *Am J Clin Dermatol.* (2016) 17:337–48. doi: 10.1007/s40257-016-0198-0
22. Kwatra SG, Ständer S, Bernhard JD, Weisshaar E, Yosipovitch G. Brachioradial pruritus: a trigger for generalization of itch. *J Am Acad Dermatol.* (2013) 68:870–3. doi: 10.1016/j.jaad.2012.11.026
23. Misery L. Pruritus in cutaneous T-cell lymphomas. In: Carstens E, Akiyama T, editors. *Itch: Mechanisms and Treatment.* Boca Raton, FL: CRC Press/Taylor and Francis Group, LLC (2014), 119–28.
24. Weisshaar E, Szepietowski JC, Dalgard FJ, Garcovich S, Gieler U, Gimenez-Arnau AM, et al. European S2k guideline on chronic pruritus. *Acta Derm Venereol.* (2019) 99:469–506. doi: 10.2340/00015555-3164
25. Ständer S, Zeidler C, Augustin M, Bayer G, Kremer AE, Legat FJ, et al. S2k-Leitlinie zur diagnostik und therapie des chronischen pruritus - update - kurzversion. *J Dtsch Dermatol Ges.* (2017) 15:860–73. doi: 10.1111/ddg.13304_g
26. Steinhoff M, Schmelz M, Szabo IL, Oaklander AL. Clinical presentation, management, and pathophysiology of neuropathic itch. *Lancet Neurol.* (2018) 17:709–20. doi: 10.1016/S1474-4422(18)30217-5
27. Andersen HH, Akiyama T, Nattkemper LA, van Laarhoven A, Elberling J, Yosipovitch G, et al. Alloknesis and hyperknesis-mechanisms, assessment methodology, and clinical implications of itch sensitization. *Pain.* (2018) 159:1185–97. doi: 10.1097/j.pain.0000000000001220
28. Carstens E, Akiyama T. Central mechanisms of itch. *Curr Probl Dermatol.* (2016) 50:11–7. doi: 10.1159/000446011
29. VanDenKerkhof EG, Stitt L, Clark AJ, Gordon A, Lynch M, Morley-Forster PK, et al. Sensitivity of the DN4 in screening for neuropathic pain syndromes. *Clin J Pain.* (2018) 34:30–6. doi: 10.1097/AJP.0000000000000512
30. Freynhagen R, Tolle TR, Gockel U, Baron R. The painDETECT project - far more than a screening tool on neuropathic pain. *Curr Med Res Opin.* (2016) 32:1033–57. doi: 10.1185/03007995.2016.1157460
31. Poquet N, Lin C. The Brief Pain Inventory (BPI). *J Physiother.* (2016) 62:52. doi: 10.1016/j.jphys.2015.07.001
32. Bouhassira D, Attal N, Alchaar H, Boureau F, Brochet B, Bruxelle J, et al. Comparison of pain syndromes associated with nervous or somatic lesions and development of a new neuropathic pain diagnostic questionnaire (DN4). *Pain.* (2005) 114:29–36. doi: 10.1016/j.pain.2004.12.010
33. Huguen J, Brenaut E, Clerc CJ, Poizeau F, Marcorelles P, Quereux G, et al. Comparison of characteristics of neuropathic and non-neuropathic pruritus to develop a tool for the diagnosis of neuropathic pruritus: the NP5. *Front Med.* (2019) 6:79. doi: 10.3389/fmed.2019.00079
34. Treister R, Lodahl M, Lang M, Tworoger SS, Sawilowsky S, Oaklander AL. Initial development and validation of a patient-reported symptom survey for small-fiber polyneuropathy. *J Pain.* (2017) 18:556–63. doi: 10.1016/j.jpain.2016.12.014
35. Pereira MP, Luling H, Dieckhofer A, Steinke S, Zeidler C, Agelopoulos K, et al. Application of an 8% capsaicin patch normalizes epidermal TRPV1 expression but not the decreased intraepidermal nerve fibre density in patients with brachioradial pruritus. *J Eur Acad Dermatol Venereol.* (2018) 32:1535–41. doi: 10.1111/jdv.14857
36. Lauria G, Hsieh ST, Johansson O, Kennedy WR, Leger JM, Mellgren SI, et al. European Federation of Neurological Societies/Peripheral Nerve Society Guideline on the use of skin biopsy in the diagnosis of small fiber neuropathy. Report of a joint task force of the European Federation of Neurological Societies and the Peripheral Nerve Society. *Eur J Neurol.* (2010) 17, 903–12, e944-9. doi: 10.1111/j.1468-1331.2010.03023.x
37. Lauria G, Bakkers M, Schmitz C, Lombardi R, Penza P, Devigili G, et al. Intraepidermal nerve fiber density at the distal leg: a worldwide normative reference study. *J Peripher Nerv Syst.* (2010) 15:202–7. doi: 10.1111/j.1529-8027.2010.00271.x
38. Lauria G, Merkies IS, Faber CG. Small fibre neuropathy. *Curr Opin Neurol.* (2012) 25:542–9. doi: 10.1097/WCO.0b013e32835804c5
39. Pham M, Bäumer T, Bendszus M. Peripheral nerves and plexus: imaging by MR-neurography and high-resolution ultrasound. *Curr Opin Neurol.* (2014) 27:370–9. doi: 10.1097/WCO.0000000000000111
40. Pereira MP, Luling H, Dieckhofer A, Steinke S, Zeidler C, Ständer S. Brachioradial pruritus and notalgia paraesthetica: a comparative observational study of clinical presentation and morphological pathologies. *Acta Derm Venereol.* (2017) 98:82–8. doi: 10.2340/00015555-2789
41. Ringkamp M, Schepers RJ, Shimada SG, Johanek LM, Hartke TV, Borzan J, et al. A role for nociceptive, myelinated nerve fibers in itch sensation. *J Neurosci.* (2011) 31:14841–9. doi: 10.1523/JNEUROSCI.3005-11.2011
42. Schmelz M. Neuronal sensitivity of the skin. *Eur J Dermatol.* (2011) 21(Suppl. 2):43–7. doi: 10.1684/ejd.2011.1265
43. Rolke R, Baron R, Maier C, Tolle TR, Treede RD, Beyer A, et al. Quantitative sensory testing in the German Research Network on Neuropathic *Pain* (DFNS): standardized protocol and reference values. *Pain.* (2006) 123:231–43. doi: 10.1016/j.pain.2006.01.041
44. Maier C, Baron R, Tolle TR, Binder A, Birbaumer N, Birklein F, et al. Quantitative sensory testing in the German Research Network on Neuropathic *Pain* (DFNS): somatosensory abnormalities in 1236 patients

with different neuropathic pain syndromes. *Pain.* (2010) 150:439–50. doi: 10.1016/j.pain.2010.05.002

45. Magerl W, Krumova EK, Baron R, Tolle T, Treede RD, Maier C. Reference data for quantitative sensory testing (QST): refined stratification for age and a novel method for statistical comparison of group data. *Pain.* (2010) 151:598–605. doi: 10.1016/j.pain.2010.07.026
46. Walk D, Sehgal N, Moeller-Bertram T, Edwards RR, Wasan A, Wallace M, et al. Quantitative sensory testing and mapping: a review of nonautomated quantitative methods for examination of the patient with neuropathic pain. *Clin J Pain.* (2009) 25:632–40. doi: 10.1097/AJP.0b013e3181a68c64
47. Cohen AD, Masalha R, Medvedovsky E, Vardy DA. Brachioradial pruritus: a symptom of neuropathy. *J Am Acad Dermatol.* (2003) 48:825–8. doi: 10.1067/mjd.2003.494
48. Cohen AD, Vander T, Medvendovsky E, Biton A, Naimer S, Shalev R, et al. Neuropathic scrotal pruritus: anogenital pruritus is a symptom of lumbosacral radiculopathy. *J Am Acad Dermatol.* (2005) 52:61–6. doi: 10.1016/j.jaad.2004.04.039
49. Donadio V, Liguori R. Microneurographic recording from unmyelinated nerve fibers in neurological disorders: an update. *Clin Neurophysiol.* (2015) 126:437–45. doi: 10.1016/j.clinph.2014.10.009
50. Merkies IS, Faber CG, Lauria G. Advances in diagnostics and outcome measures in peripheral neuropathies. *Neurosci Lett.* (2015) 596:3–13. doi: 10.1016/j.neulet.2015.02.038
51. Yosipovitch G, Goon AT, Wee J, Chan YH, Zucker I, Goh CL. Itch characteristics in Chinese patients with atopic dermatitis using a new questionnaire for the assessment of pruritus. *Int J Dermatol.* (2002) 41:212–6. doi: 10.1046/j.1365-4362.2002.01460.x
52. O'Neill JL, Chan YH, Rapp SR, Yosipovitch G. Differences in itch characteristics between psoriasis and atopic dermatitis patients: results of a web-based questionnaire. *Acta Derm Venereol.* (2011) 91:537–40. doi: 10.2340/00015555-1126
53. Pogatzki-Zahn EM, Pereira MP, Cremer A, Zeidler C, Dreyer T, Riepe C, et al. Peripheral sensitization and loss of descending inhibition is a hallmark of chronic pruritus. *J Invest Dermatol.* (2020) 140:203–11.e204. doi: 10.1016/j.jid.2019.05.029
54. Maddison B, Parsons A, Sangueza O, Sheehan DJ, Yosipovitch G. Retrospective study of intraepidermal nerve fiber distribution in biopsies of patients with nummular eczema. *Am J Dermatopathol.* (2011) 33:621–3. doi: 10.1097/DAD.0b013e3181fe4c3c
55. Hashimoto T, Kursewicz CD, Fayne RA, Nanda S, Shah SM, Nattkemper L, et al. Pathophysiologic mechanisms of itch in bullous pemphigoid. *J Am Acad Dermatol.* (2019) 83:53–62. doi: 10.1016/j.jaad.2019.07.060
56. Milian-Ciesielska K, Chmura L, Dyduch G, Jagers C, Radwanska E, Adamek D. Intraepidermal nerve fiber density in vulvar lichen sclerosus and normal vulvar tissues. *J Physiol Pharmacol.* (2017) 68:453–8.
57. Brewer KL, Lee JW, Downs H, Oaklander AL, Yezierski RP. Dermatomal scratching after intramedullary quisqualate injection: correlation with cutaneous denervation. *J Pain.* (2008) 9:999–1005. doi: 10.1016/j.jpain.2008.05.010
58. Zhong W, Yang M, Zhang W, Visocchi M, Chen X, Liao C. Improved neural microcirculation and regeneration after peripheral nerve decompression in DPN rats. *Neurol Res.* (2017) 39:285–91. doi: 10.1080/01616412.2017.1297557

Permissions

All chapters in this book were first published by Frontiers; hereby published with permission under the Creative Commons Attribution License or equivalent. Every chapter published in this book has been scrutinized by our experts. Their significance has been extensively debated. The topics covered herein carry significant findings which will fuel the growth of the discipline. They may even be implemented as practical applications or may be referred to as a beginning point for another development.

The contributors of this book come from diverse backgrounds, making this book a truly international effort. This book will bring forth new frontiers with its revolutionizing research information and detailed analysis of the nascent developments around the world.

We would like to thank all the contributing authors for lending their expertise to make the book truly unique. They have played a crucial role in the development of this book. Without their invaluable contributions this book wouldn't have been possible. They have made vital efforts to compile up to date information on the varied aspects of this subject to make this book a valuable addition to the collection of many professionals and students.

This book was conceptualized with the vision of imparting up-to-date information and advanced data in this field. To ensure the same, a matchless editorial board was set up. Every individual on the board went through rigorous rounds of assessment to prove their worth. After which they invested a large part of their time researching and compiling the most relevant data for our readers.

The editorial board has been involved in producing this book since its inception. They have spent rigorous hours researching and exploring the diverse topics which have resulted in the successful publishing of this book. They have passed on their knowledge of decades through this book. To expedite this challenging task, the publisher supported the team at every step. A small team of assistant editors was also appointed to further simplify the editing procedure and attain best results for the readers.

Apart from the editorial board, the designing team has also invested a significant amount of their time in understanding the subject and creating the most relevant covers. They scrutinized every image to scout for the most suitable representation of the subject and create an appropriate cover for the book.

The publishing team has been an ardent support to the editorial, designing and production team. Their endless efforts to recruit the best for this project, has resulted in the accomplishment of this book. They are a veteran in the field of academics and their pool of knowledge is as vast as their experience in printing. Their expertise and guidance has proved useful at every step. Their uncompromising quality standards have made this book an exceptional effort. Their encouragement from time to time has been an inspiration for everyone.

The publisher and the editorial board hope that this book will prove to be a valuable piece of knowledge for researchers, students, practitioners and scholars across the globe.

List of Contributors

Antoinette I. M. van Laarhoven and Jennifer M. Becker
Health, Medical, and Neuropsychology Unit, Faculty of Social and Behavioural Sciences, Leiden University, Leiden, Netherlands
Leiden Institute for Brain and Cognition, Leiden University, Leiden, Netherlands

Dimitri M. L. van Ryckeghem
Department of Experimental-Clinical and Health Psychology, Ghent University, Ghent, Belgium
Research Unit Integrative Research Unit on Social and Individual Development (INSIDE), Institute of Health and Behaviour, Faculty of Humanities and Social Sciences, University of Luxembourg, Esch-sur-Alzette, Luxembourg
Section Experimental Health Psychology, Clinical Psychological Science Departments, Faculty of Psychology and Neuroscience, Maastricht University, Maastricht, Netherlands

Stefaan Van Damme
Department of Experimental-Clinical and Health Psychology, Ghent University, Ghent, Belgium

Geert Crombez
Department of Experimental-Clinical and Health Psychology, Ghent University, Ghent, Belgium
Centre for Pain Research, University of Bath, Bath, United Kingdom

Reinout W. H. J. Wiers
Addiction Development and Psychopathology Laboratory, Department of Psychology, University of Amsterdam, Amsterdam, Netherlands

Sarina B. Elmariah
Tufts University School of Medicine, Boston, MA, United States

Haya S. Raef
Tufts University School of Medicine, Boston, MA, United States
Massachusetts General Hospital, Boston, MA, United States

Katarzyna Stępień and Adam Reich
Department of Dermatology, Institute of Medical Sciences, Medical College of Rzeszow University, Rzeszów, Poland

Kenji Kabashima and Hiroyuki Irie
Department of Dermatology, Graduate School of Medicine, Kyoto University, Kyoto, Japan

Martin Schmelz
Department of Experimental Pain Research, Medical Faculty Mannheim, University

Yujuan Li, Wencui Zhang, Tainning Sun, Baowen Liu and Hong-Bing Xiang
Department of Anesthesiology, Tongji Hospital, Tongji Medical College, Huazhong University of Science and Technology, Wuhan, China

Anne Manyande
School of Human and Social Sciences, University of West London, London, United Kingdom

Weiguo Xu
Department of Orthopedics, Tongji Hospital of Tongji Medical College, Huazhong University of Science and Technology, Wuhan, China

Claudia Zeidler
Department of Dermatology and Center for Chronic Pruritus, University Hospital Münster, Münster, Germany

Manuel Pedro Pereira and Sonja Ständer
Department of Dermatology and Center for Chronic Pruritus, University Hospital Münster, Münster, Germany

Peyman Najafi
Univ Brest, LIEN, Brest, France Paris-Saclay Institute of Neuroscience, Centre National de la Recherche Scientifique/Université Paris-Saclay, Gif-sur-Yvette, France

Douraied Ben Salem
Univ Brest, LATIM, INSERM UMR, Brest, France
University Hospital of Brest, Department of Radiology, Brest, France

Olivier Dufor
Univ Brest, LIEN, Brest, France
L@bISEN Yncréa Ouest, ISEN, Brest, France

Laurent Misery
Department of Dermatology, CHU Brest, Brest, France
University of Brest, LIEN, Brest, France
Department of Dermatology, University Hospital of Brest, Brest, France

Jean-Luc Carré
Univ Brest, LIEN, Brest, France

Aylin Ruppenstein and Maren M. Limberg
Division of Experimental Allergy and Immunodermatology, Faculty of Medicine and Health Sciences, University of Oldenburg, Oldenburg, Germany

Karin Loser
Division of Immunology, Faculty of Medicine and Health Sciences, University of Oldenburg, Oldenburg, Germany

Andreas E. Kremer
Department of Medicine 1, University Hospital Erlangen and Friedrich-Alexander-University Erlangen-Nürnberg, Erlangen, Germany

Ulrike Raap
Division of Experimental Allergy and Immunodermatology, Faculty of Medicine and Health Sciences, University of Oldenburg, Oldenburg, Germany
University Clinic of Dermatology and Allergy, Oldenburg Clinic, Oldenburg, Germany

Bernhard Homey
Department of Dermatology, Medical Faculty, University Hospital Düsseldorf, Heinrich-Heine-University Düsseldorf, Düsseldorf, Germany

Peter Dietrich
Department of Medicine 1, University Hospital Erlangen and Translational Research Center, Friedrich-Alexander-University Erlangen-Nürnberg, Erlangen, Germany
Emil-Fischer-Zentrum, Institute of Biochemistry, Friedrich-Alexander-University Erlangen-Nürnberg, Erlangen, Germany

Miriam M. Düll, Katharina Wolf, Marcel Vetter and Andreas E. Kremer
Department of Medicine 1, University Hospital Erlangen and Translational Research Center, Friedrich-Alexander-University Erlangen-Nürnberg, Erlangen, Germany

Markus F. Neurath
Department of Medicine 1, University Hospital Erlangen and Translational Research Center, Friedrich-Alexander-University Erlangen-Nürnberg, Erlangen, Germany
Deutsches Zentrum Immuntherapie DZI, Erlangen, Germany

Nadia Salinas, Maxime Etienne, Delphine Legoupil and Maxime Fouchard
Department of Dermatology, University Hospital of Brest, Brest, France
Université de Brest, LIEN, Brest, France

Emilie Brenaut
Department of Dermatology, CHU Brest, Brest, France
University of Brest, LIEN, Brest, France
Department of Dermatology, University Hospital of Brest, Brest, France

Emmanuel Nowak
INSERM CIC 1412, University Hospital of Brest, Brest, France

Cécile Legeas
Department of Dermatology, CHU Brest, Brest, France

Alain-Claude Roudot and Anne-Sophie Ficheux
University of Brest, LIEN, Brest, France

Guan Donglang, Liu Tongtong, Chen Dan, Zhu Chan, Wang Changming, Yu Guang, Yang Yan and Tang Zongxiang
School of Medicine & Holistic Integrative Medicine, Nanjing University of Chinese Medicine, Nanjing, China

Jacqueline A. G. M. Langedijk, Ulrich H. Beuers and Ronald P. J. Oude Elferink
Amsterdam University Medical Centers, Tytgat Institute for Liver and Intestinal Research, Research Institute Amsterdam Gastroenterology, Endocrinologyand Metabolism (AGEM), University of Amsterdam, Amsterdam, Netherlands

Piotr K. Krajewski and Jacek C. Szepietowski
Department of Dermatology, Venereology and Allergology, Wroclaw Medical University, Wroclaw, Poland

Piotr Olczyk and Magdalena Krajewska
Department of Nephrology and Transplantation Medicine, Wroclaw Medical University, Wroclaw, Poland

Wojciech Krajewski
Department of Urology and Oncologic Urology, Wrocław Medical University, Wrocław, Poland

Franz J. Legat
Department of Dermatology, Medical University of Graz, Graz, Austria

Xin Jia and Ling Zhang
The First Rehabilitation Hospital of Shanghai, Tongji University School of Medicine, Shanghai, China
Key Laboratory of Spine and Spinal Cord Injury Repair and Regeneration of Ministry of Education, Orthopaedic Department of Tongji Hospital, School of Medicine, Tongji University, Shanghai, China

Meng-Han Dai
The First Rehabilitation Hospital of Shanghai, Tongji University School of Medicine, Shanghai, China
Department of Anesthesiology, Renmin Hospital, Hubei University of Medicine, Shiyan, China

An-Jing Ren
Department of Pathophysiology, Naval Medical University, Shanghai, China

Ting-Ting Wang
The First Rehabilitation Hospital of Shanghai, Tongji University School of Medicine, Shanghai, China
Department of Dermatology, Tongren Hospital Shanghai Jiao Tong University School of Medicine, Shanghai, China

Weiping J. Zhang
Department of Pathophysiology, Naval Medical University, Shanghai, China
NHC Key Laboratory of Hormones and Development, Tianjin Institute of Endocrinology, Tianjin Medical University Chu Hsien-I Memorial Hospital, Tianjin, China

Jana Maria Nemmer and Marcus Kuchner
Department of Dermatology, Medical Faculty, University Hospital Düsseldorf, Heinrich-Heine-University Düsseldorf, Düsseldorf, Germany

Angeliki Datsi
Department of Dermatology, Medical Faculty, University Hospital Düsseldorf, Heinrich-Heine-University Düsseldorf, Düsseldorf, Germany
Medical Faculty, Institute for Transplantation Diagnostics and Cell Therapy, University Hospital Düsseldorf, Heinrich-Heine-University Düsseldorf, Düsseldorf, Germany

Péter Oláh
Department of Dermatology, Medical Faculty, University Hospital Düsseldorf, Heinrich-Heine-University Düsseldorf, Düsseldorf, Germany
Department of Dermatology, Venereology and Oncodermatology, Medical Faculty, University of Pécs, Pécs, Hungary

Valérie Julia
Galderma Pharmaceuticals, Vevey, Switzerland

Hans Jürgen Solinski and Roman Rukwied
Department of Experimental Pain Research, Medical Faculty Mannheim, University of Heidelberg, Mannheim, Germany

Sascha Ständer
Department of Dermatology, University of Lübeck, Lübeck, Germany

Elke Weisshaar
Occupational Dermatology, Department of Dermatology, Ruprecht-Karls University Heidelberg, Heidelberg, Germany

Jiang Ji
Department of Dermatology, The Second Affiliated Hospital of Soochow University, Suzhou, China

Xu Liu
Department of Dermatology, The Second Affiliated Hospital of Soochow University, Suzhou, China
Jiangsu Key Laboratory of Neuropsychiatric Diseases and Institute of Neuroscience, Soochow University, Suzhou, China
Jiang-Tao Zhang, Yue Hu, Wen-Qi Shan, Zhi-Hong

Wang, Qing-Yue Fu and Dan-Ni Fu
Jiangsu Key Laboratory of Neuropsychiatric Diseases and Institute of Neuroscience, Soochow University, Suzhou, China

Tong Liu
Institute of Pain Medicine and Special Environmental Medicine, Nantong University, Nantong, China
College of Life Sciences, Yanan University, Yanan, China

Kjell Lüßmann, Joerg Kupfer and Christina Schut
Institute of Medical Psychology, Justus-Liebig-University, Giessen, Germany

Kerry Montgomery
Department of Psychology, University of Sheffield, Sheffield, United Kingdom

Andrew Thompson
South Wales Doctorate in Clinical Psychology, Cardiff University, Wales, United Kingdom

Uwe Gieler
Department of Dermatology, Justus-Liebig-University, Giessen, Germany, Clinic of Psychosomatics, Vitos Clinic, Giessen, Germany

Christoph Zick
Department of Dermatology, Rehabilitation Center Borkum Riff, Borkum, Germany

Larissa L. Meijer, Zoë A. Schielen, Kim Y. van Ree and H. Chris Dijkerman
Experimental Psychology/Helmholtz Institute, Utrecht University, Utrecht, Netherlands

Henning Wiegmann and Konstantin Agelopoulos
Department of Dermatology and Center for Chronic Pruritus, University Hospital Münster, Münster, Germany

Index

www.ingramcontent.com/pod-product-compliance
Lightning Source LLC
LaVergne TN
LVHW082137200926
848484LV00008B/2069